INTEGRATING BEHAVIORAL HEALTH AND PRIMARY CARE

INTEGRATING BEHAVIORAL HEALTH AND PRIMARY CARE

EDITED BY

ROBERT E. FEINSTEIN, MD
Professor of Psychiatry and Vice Chair
The University of Colorado School of Medicine
Aurora, CO

JOSEPH V. CONNELLY, MD
Assistant Clinical Professor of Medicine
Columbia University College of Physicians and Surgeons
New York, NY
Chairman, Department of Family Medicine
Stamford Hospital
Stamford, CT

MARILYN S. FEINSTEIN, ACC, LCSW, USPTA
Associated Certified Coach
International Coaching Federation
Licensed Clinical Social Worker LCSW
Elite Pro, United States Tennis Association
Centennial, CO

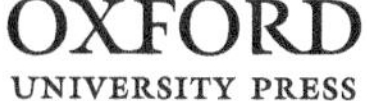

OXFORD
UNIVERSITY PRESS

OXFORD
UNIVERSITY PRESS

Oxford University Press is a department of the University of Oxford. It furthers the University's objective of excellence in research, scholarship, and education by publishing worldwide. Oxford is a registered trade mark of Oxford University Press in the UK and certain other countries.

Published in the United States of America by Oxford University Press
198 Madison Avenue, New York, NY 10016, United States of America.

CIP data is on file at the Library of Congress
ISBN 978–0–19–027620–1

3 5 7 9 8 6 4 2

Printed by Sheridan Books, Inc., United States of America

CONTENTS

Foreword *by Robert Freedman, MD* *vii*
Foreword *by Paul Summergrad, MD* *ix*
Preface *xi*
Acknowledgments *xv*
Personal Acknowledgments (*Robert E. Feinstein, MD*) *xvii*
Personal Acknowledgments (*Joseph V. Connelly, MD*) *xix*
Personal Acknowledgments (*Marilyn S. Feinstein, ACC, LCSW, USPTA*) *xxi*
Contributors *xxiii*

PART I: *Models of Integrated Care*

1. Conceptual Framework for Integrated Care: Multiple Models to Achieve Integrated Aims 3
   ALEXIS A. GIESE AND MARYANN WAUGH
2. Integrated Health Care at Cherokee Health Systems 17
   PARINDA KHATRI, GREGG PERRY, AND FRANK V. deGRUY III
3. Canadian Approach to Integrated Care 31
   NICK KATES AND ELLEN ANDERSON
4. Team-Based Integrated Primary Care 46
   TZIPORAH ROSENBERG, COLLEEN T. FOGARTY, MICHAEL R. PRIVITERA, AND SUSAN H. MCDANIEL
5. The Patient-Centered Medical Home 65
   COLLEEN CONRY, SHANDRA BROWN LEVEY, AND BONNIE T. JORTBERG
6. Financing Integrated Care Models 76
   BRUCE J. SCHWARTZ, GILLIAN STEIN, AND SCOTT WETZLER
7. Integrating Physical and Mental Health Care in the Veterans Health Administration: A Path to the Future 90
   LISA V. RUBENSTEIN
8. Aging Brain Care: A Model of Integrated Care for Dementia and Depression 107
   CATHERINE A. ALDER, MARY GUERRIERO AUSTROM, MICHAEL A. LAMANTIA, AND MALAZ A. BOUSTANI
9. Telehealth in an Integrated Care Environment 121
   MARYANN WAUGH, DEBBIE VOYLES, JAMES H. SHORE, L. CHAROLETTE LIPPOLIS, AND COREY LYON
10. Automated Mental Health Assessment for Integrated Care: The Quick PsychoDiagnostics Panel Meets Real-World Clinical Needs 134
    JONATHAN SHEDLER

PART II: *Integrative Care for Psychiatry and Primary Care*

11. Integrated Care for Anxiety Disorders 149
    ROBERT D. DAVIES, ISABELLE GUILLEMET, AND ADAM TROSTERMAN
12. Treating Depression and Bipolar Disorder in Integrated Care Settings 169
    CHRISTOPHER D. SCHNECK

13. The Treatment of Schizophrenia Spectrum and Other Psychotic Disorders in Integrated Primary Care *199*
ELIZABETH LOWDERMILK, NICOLE JOSEPH, AND ROBERT E. FEINSTEIN

14. Treating Substance Use Disorders in Integrated Care Settings *223*
PATRICIA PADE, LAURA MARTIN, AND SOPHIE COLLINS

15. Integrated Care for Binge Eating and Other Eating Disorders *256*
JOEL YAGER, PHILIP S. MEHLER, EILEEN D. YAGER, AND ALISON R. YAGER

16. Treating Somatic Symptom Disorder and Illness Anxiety in Integrated Care Settings *276*
ALLA LANDA, MARINA MAKOUS, AND BRIAN A. FALLON

17. Working with Personality Disorders in an Integrated Care Setting *303*
ROBERT E. FEINSTEIN AND JOSEPH V. CONNELLY

18. Violence and Suicide *326*
ROBERT E. FEINSTEIN

PART III: *Integrated Care for Medical Subspecialties and Behavioral Medicine in Primary Care*

19. Integrative Care Model for Neurology and Psychiatry: Non-Epileptic Seizures Project *351*
LYNNE FENTON, BRIAN ROTHBERG, LAURA STROM, ALISON M. HERU, AND MESHA-GAY BROWN

20. Women's Mental Health Across the Reproductive Lifespan *367*
NOA HEIMAN, ABBY SNAVELY, AND LIZA FREEHLING

21. Assessing and Treating Sexual Problems in an Integrated Care Environment *386*
KENNETH M. POLLOCK AND ALAN M. ALTMAN

22. Wellness: An Integrated Care Approach *409*
MEEGAN LIPMAN, JACQUELINE CALDERONE, JOEL YAGER, AND WWMARYANN WAUGH

23. Integrated Chronic Pain and Psychiatric Management *430*
ROBERT M. MCCARRON, AMIR RAMEZANI, IAN KOEBNER, SAMIR J. SHETH, AND JESSICA PALKA

24. Death and Dying: Integrated Teams *443*
ANNE A. BREWER AND JOSEPH V. CONNELLY

PART IV: *Psychosocial Treatments in Primary Care and Medical Specialty Clinics*

25. Health Coaching in Integrated Care *459*
MARILYN S. FEINSTEIN AND ROBERT E. FEINSTEIN

26. Crisis Intervention in Integrated Care *497*
SCOTT A. SIMPSON AND ROBERT E. FEINSTEIN

27. Best Practice for Family-Centered Health Care: A Three-Step Model *514*
JOANNA STURHAHN STRATTON, KATHERINE BUCK, AND ALISON M. HERU

28. Group Interventions in Integrated Care Settings *527*
BRIAN ROTHBERG AND HILLARY D. LUM

Index *541*

FOREWORD

by Robert Freedman, MD

Integrated care has become the focus of much of the planning for mental health and primary care in the future. Primary care physicians have learned that a substantive number of their patients view mental health needs as a major issue, and mental health practitioners have learned that a significant number of patients needing their help can best be treated in primary care settings. Early successful models relied on research funding or personal connections between primary care and mental health providers or both. Now the lessons of those models need to become part of general medical practice.

This book provides a comprehensive overview and guide to existing and innovative evidence-based integrated care models. It covers developments in multidisciplinary teams, describes the future of health care financing, telemental health, and evolutions in the development of the primary care medical home. This paves the way to discuss integrative care approaches to the evaluation and treatment of the major psychiatric disorders and other prevalent behavioral issues seen in medical practices. Where there are established models of care, they are described. Where there are gaps in our knowledge, the authors offer their expertise and experiences.

Strategies and pathways for integrated care take into account what has been learned about the capabilities of both primary care practices and mental health providers skilled in the management and treatment of specific mental illnesses. This combination of perspectives, integrating the medical home with psychiatric practice, is the unique value of this book. This book can be read as a user guide, a "how to" book, designed for multidisciplinary team members working in new integrated health care environments. It can be read as a specific guide, for primary care and mental health professionals, medical staff, medical students, and residents, for the evaluation, diagnosis, and brief treatment that can be offered within medical settings.

Feinstein, Connelly, and Feinstein, the editors, do not hesitate to address the full spectrum of mental disease and some behavioral health conditions. Personality disorders, for example, are often the most difficult for any mental health provider to treat. They are even more difficult for the primary care provider, whose first impulse is to do as much for the patient as possible. When this good-hearted approach fails, many primary care providers become immersed in the angry fallout and do not appreciate that they are dealing with an illness. The pathology of personality disorders is presented in terms that fit the primary practice setting. Narcissism manifests as idealization of the doctor and denigration of the staff; obsessionalism presents as the patient's excessive requests to review the medical record; attempts to fraudulently gain disability reveal antisocial behavior; and splitting the nursing staff becomes the hallmark of borderline personality disorder. Countertransference is introduced early in the discussion. Simultaneously, the authors discuss how to set up teams and therapies within the primary care setting rather than remaking the primary care doctor into a psychiatrist or reflexively recommending referral to a psychiatric clinic. From formation of teamlets of two individuals, to family and group psychotherapy, the guidance of how to proceed is clear and direct.

The ultimate use of this book may be as a terrifically practical reference, one that both primary care and mental health professionals can refer to as clinical situations arise. The book is most valuable for helping clinicians frame what they are doing, review the pathology, and then provide optimal treatment from the perspective of an integrated, patient-centered, medical home.

Robert Freedman, MD
Professor of Psychiatry
Department of Psychiatry
University of Colorado School of Medicine
Aurora, CO

FOREWORD

by Paul Summergrad, MD

Patients and their families bring the totality of their lives to all health care settings, not just the immediate illnesses or pain that cause them to seek care. Not all settings and circumstances, however, are equally conducive to open-ended and longitudinal evaluations. The person in an emergency department with severe and life-threatening injuries needs immediate interventions to prevent death. Specialists evaluating a patient with a newly discovered lesion will be focused on the procedures they are performing. However, in most of health care, as in much of life, the boundaries between disease and the experience of sickness, between the careful elucidation of symptoms and putting patients at ease so they can relate what they are concerned about, is not so clear. And it is especially in the longer-term care of patients in primary and specialty outpatient settings that issues of when and how we integrate these psychological, psychiatric, and general medical aspects of care become paramount.

It is especially in this domain that *Integrating Behavioral Health and Primary Care* is such an important addition to our thinking about these problems. Edited carefully by Feinstein, Connelly, and Feinstein, this book brings a wealth of expertise and clinical wisdom from a distinguished group of contributors. Beginning with what we know—evidence-based and other models of integrated care—the authors are careful to outline approaches that have been demonstrated to work in specific settings. They then do what physicians and others have always had to do: work within the limitations of what we know to nevertheless help those who are suffering.

It is a particular strength of this text that the editors are willing to begin with known models and algorithms. They apply them especially to primary care settings for common adult disorders and expand that effort into specialty and subspecialty medical outpatient settings. These latter areas have less often been studied but are nevertheless important for ongoing care. Indeed, many medical and surgical specialties are undergoing their own work to understand how they can best care for patients in primary care–centered health systems, especially as payment and quality systems evolve.

Integrating Behavioral Health and Primary Care will be an important and wise guide for those who are working at these uncertain boundaries and for the leadership who, working with caregivers, will need to continue to evolve the systems of care for which they are responsible. Most importantly, it will be of importance to patients and families who may never be aware of it but who rely on their doctors, nurses, social workers, and others to provide humane, whole-person, and expert care when much, and at times all, is truly on the line.

Paul Summergrad, MD
Dr. Frances S. Arkin Professor and Chairman
Department of Psychiatry
Professor of Medicine
Tufts University School of Medicine
Psychiatrist-in-Chief
Tufts Medical Center
Boston, MA

PREFACE

Our first book, *Primary Care Psychiatry and Behavioral Medicine: Brief Office Treatment and Management Pathways*,[1] was written in 1999. While well received, the book was written at a time when the practicalities of our vision of integrated care turned out to be aspirational ... not yet widely researched, easily implemented, or financially supported, except as grant-funded initiatives. Eighteen years later, a vision of multiple approaches to integrated care is emerging, from the confluence of collaborative care evidence-based research, the passing of the Affordable Care Act, federal sponsorship of integrated care demonstration projects, and potential changes in reimbursement models. Widespread adoption of integrated care and reverse integrated care (primary care integration into mental health settings) is in the design phase to meet the Institute for Healthcare Improvement's triple aim: (1) improve the patient experience of care (including quality and satisfaction), (2) improve the health of populations, and (3) reduce the per capita cost of health care.

While the core principles of integrated care are well known, a path to operationalize these principles for a variety of mental health, addictive disorders, and behavioral medicine problems has yet to be firmly established. In addition, integrating behavioral health with physical health and many medical specialties is in its infancy, with some notable exceptions, such as integrated cancer, cardiovascular, and transplantation services. These considerations have led us to focus on practicality, accessibility, and the creativity of our authors, offering pathways to be used by a wide array of professionals and practices working in integrated care. The book describes both successful integrated behavioral and physical care models and clinical care based on these models. The chapter authors were asked to use the basic principles of integrated care, discuss successful models that may not be widely known, and examine the utility of applying these existing models and principles, in territory where there is little research on "how" to take care of some mental health and behavioral health conditions seen frequently in primary care and integrated care environments. We asked the chapter authors to consider that medical practices will have a basic, common, integrated staff model: primary care or specialist provider(s) in a practice with front desk staff, medical assistant(s), nurse(s), nurse practitioners, behavioral health specialist(s), health coaches, consulting psychiatrist, and care coordinator(s) or case manager(s). We also encouraged our authors to be aspirational in making expert recommendations or suggestions on the potential for delivery of integrated care for specific disorders or problems, when no clear evidence for how to do this exists. Many of the authors also considered how they could best use health coaches, pharmacists, nutritionists/dietitians, educators, and other allied health professionals, and how to deal with the needs for specialized training required for core staff. In addition, all authors were asked to consider what kind of mental health treatments can be delivered, when to refer out, and how to collaborate with community resources. Most chapters were co-written by a primary care physician or medical specialist and a mental health professional. All chapters were reviewed and edited several times by a psychiatrist, a family physician, and a social worker/health coach. The tensions in writing the chapters were the same tensions in developing integrated care practices: fostering the collaboration between disciplines and between specialists and generalists. We asked the mental health professionals to distill and simplify complex clinical approaches. We asked the primary care physicians and specialists to go beyond the biomedical view to the widest practical views of biopsychosocial and prevention-oriented care that could be delivered in an integrated care environment.

The ultimate aim of this book is to reduce the suffering of our patients, particularly the still underrecognized and undertreated pain of mental and emotional suffering. By expanding the biopsychosocial principles of patient care from the individual practitioner to the system level, and by fully integrating care between the traditional medical and mental health specialties, we hope the health care system will more effectively address the tremendous burden this suffering has on our patients.

The book is divided into four sections:

Part I: Models of Integrated Care provides an overview and introduction to the principles of integrated care, which can be applied in many different settings. One size will never fit all, as the approaches to care are highly dependent on local needs and practice conditions, culture, and financing. This section focuses on five highly successful integrated practices, in addition to considering team-based care, financing, telebehavioral health, and the use of mental health outcomes.

Part II: Integrative Care for Psychiatry and Primary Care reviews the most common mental health problems treated in primary care. It is loosely based on the American Psychiatric Association's *Diagnostic and Statistical Manual of Mental Disorders*, fifth edition (DSM-5). These chapters review the basics of the most common psychiatric disorders and describe a team and population approach as well as the use of a patient registry and outcome measurements. Chapter authors discuss relevant team-based health care and treatment approaches that can be offered in integrated care environments. One of the many unique features of this section is our effort to suggest a longitudinal approach to patient care, moving beyond problem identification, differential diagnosis, and acute brief treatment. Our yearlong critical pathways and summary tables emphasize a practice-based continuity approach.

Part III: Integrated Care for Medical Subspecialties and Behavioral Medicine in Primary Care focuses on two models of integrating behavioral health care: (1) integrating wellness with behavioral health and (2) integrating psychiatry and neurology. Other chapters are "Women's Mental Health Across the Reproductive Lifespan," "Assessing and Treating Sexual Problems in an Integrated Care Environment," "Integrated Chronic Pain and Psychiatric Management," and "Death and Dying: Integrated Teams."

Part IV: Psychosocial Treatments in Primary Care and Medical Specialty Clinics describes brief office-based counseling and psychosocial treatment approaches. We believe psychosocial treatment in integrated care can be offered, although to date this treatment has been rarely taught to *teamlets* within a practice. A teamlet is a dyad of a mental health practitioner with any other health professional(s). We cover crisis intervention, a greatly underused individual and family form of mental health counseling, as an eclectic treatment with wide applications. We describe health coaching, stages of change, motivational interviewing, and use of cognitive-behavioral approaches with mindfulness-based stress reduction for assistance with lifestyle changes. We describe the use of family approaches and group interventions in integrated care, most helpful when trying to improve the patient experience and the quality of care. In addition, these approaches are particularly useful when treating a population of patients with specific problems who are in need of lifestyle change, prevention, and improving patient adherence to medical care.

Our hope is that this book is practical, office-based, and comfortably accessible for use by students, residents, faculty, and the wider scope of mental health professionals, primary care providers, and medical specialists.

Please note that the editors have no financial or proprietary interest in any products or programs discussed in the book. In addition, although the editors are comfortable that everything included in the book is based on the latest evidence-based information currently available, robust discussion and occasional disagreement occurred about some of the content. We hope that the book will generate some of the same thoughts and discussion among its readers. Please let us know your reactions or comments about our work, as this kind of dialog was the energy source of the book and will ultimately help us determine the book's usefulness.

Robert E. Feinstein, MD
Joseph V. Connelly, MD
Marilyn S. Feinstein, ACC, LCSW, USPTA

REFERENCE

1. Feinstein RE, Brewer AA, eds. Primary Care Psychiatry and Behavioral Medicine: Brief Office Treatment and Management Pathways. New York: Springer; 1999.

ACKNOWLEDGMENTS

We were delighted to work with all our authors/contributors from all over the United States and Canada. We are especially appreciative of the good-natured and productive dialog that emerged with the principal authors during the editorial process. Our authors seemed to understand the combination of our evidence-based approach, combined with creative and often aspirational suggestions that make this book unique. By the end of the process, the mental health professionals were sounding like primary care/specialist physicians, and vice versa. This was not really surprising, as ultimately integrated care requires patient care delivered from both perspectives.

We thank Robert Freedman, MD, Former Chair at University of Colorado School of Medicine, for his foreword and for leading a remarkable Department of Psychiatry, producing many of the distinguished faculty chapter authors. His support of us writing this book was invaluable.

We appreciate the support of Paul Summergrad, MD, Chair at Tufts University School of Medicine, and thank him for writing the foreword to the book.

We also thank Lori Raney, integrated care guru, colleague, and friend.

Judith Burks, our cyberspace editor from Louisiana, was exceptionally helpful. She reviewed the book (via email no less) for style, format, and consistency. Her kind style, encouragement, expertise, and efficiency made it a tremendous pleasure editing this book.

We deeply appreciate the creativity, hard work, diligence, and controversial discussions we had with many of the chapter authors whose contributions to the book have been invaluable.

Finally, we thank Oxford University Press for believing in our work and ultimately making this publication possible.

Robert E. Feinstein, MD
Joseph V. Connelly, MD
Marilyn S. Feinstein, ACC, LCSW, USPTA

PERSONAL ACKNOWLEDGMENTS

(Robert E. Feinstein, MD)

I would like to thank my mother, Florence Feinstein (deceased), who encouraged me with her unfailing belief in me. She helped me work through my ambivalence about medical school, convincing me that ultimately my psychological talents would be a valuable asset for helping to relieve the suffering of psychiatric patients. Also, my father, Harold R. Feinstein, MD (deceased), was a beloved and dedicated family physician who may never have fully appreciated his major contributions to my life and his patients' lives and care. In his memory, I have really enjoyed over 30 years of many collaborative efforts with family-medicine physicians and internists. Integrated care continues to refresh my affinity for this fertile partnership. I would also like to thank the large cadre of psychiatrists and psychologists in my extended family for their support and endless encouragement. An extra-special thanks is owed to my wife, co-editor Marilyn. I deeply appreciate her book chapter, good cheer, sense of humor, encouragement, patience, and detailed editorial assistance. Her help and support for the entire project was an absolute necessity to produce this work.

I especially want to thank Joseph V. Connelly, MD, my other co-editor. We worked together for almost 10 years in the 1990s in Stamford, Connecticut, and continue our collaboration to this day. He is an amazing person, clinician, and educator, and is most valued for his friendship. Like my father, he is a role model for several generations of family physicians for delivering biopsychosocial-cultural care. His hard work and editorial acumen, living and breathing in primary care, kept me grounded to produce a practical book for integrated care.

Robert E. Feinstein, MD

PERSONAL ACKNOWLEDGMENTS

(Joseph V. Connelly, MD)

To give full credit where credit is due, this work is the brainchild of Dr. Robert Feinstein. His extraordinary vision, creativity, passion, and drive are responsible for this book—from its conception to its birth. It has been an honor and a privilege to collaborate with Rob and Marilyn. In addition to being an outstanding editor, Rob is a brilliant and gifted clinician and teacher. Over our almost 30 years of being colleagues and friends, there has rarely been an interaction where I did not learn something new. I learned so much from working with Rob on this book that I am confident it will be of value to other primary care physicians who aspire to give the best care to their patients.

I had a long-term patient born to a very poor family on a Caribbean island, before moving to the mainland United States. Here she lived a humble and simple life to the age of 104. She was, despite her lack of formal education, a very wise woman. Almost every visit, whether in my office, her home, or eventually a nursing facility, she would say, "I never say that I'm lucky, I always say that I'm blessed." In this vein, I would like to acknowledge the blessings I have received—from my profession, patients, colleagues, friends, and ultimately the source of all blessings, my creator—that made my work on this book possible. My family—grandchildren, children and their spouses, parents, and most particularly, my beloved wife Melinda—deserve a special acknowledgment for their good-natured tolerance and support through the countless evening, weekend, and vacation hours that I spent working on this book.

Joseph V. Connelly, MD

PERSONAL ACKNOWLEDGMENTS

(Marilyn S. Feinstein, ACC, LCSW, USPTA)

It has been a distinct pleasure collaborating on this book as both an editor and chapter author. Joseph V. Connolly, MD's knowledge and experience in Primary Care was invaluable and helped us maintain a focus on using practical psychological and psychiatric interventions in the integrated care environment. He has a keen sense for shaping chapter content, and at the same time, honoring individual writing styles.

I owe a deep sense of gratitude to my mother, Tybie, who has been my greatest coach, and is a wonderful role model. A member of The United States Table Tennis Hall of Fame, she was given the Lifetime Achievement Award, as the only American woman to win two World Championships in table tennis. Tybie is self-taught, and exemplifies self-directed learning, by analyzing and emulating the greatest players. Finally, I lovingly appreciate the leadership of my husband, Rob. His vision of possibility is inspiring, demonstrated not only in his work with patients, creative teaching, warmth and humor, but his interest in shining the light on others, and advocating for their excellence. His stewardship is not unlike a great conductor, who skillfully show-cases the talents of his colleagues, and inspires them to play the music, and not just the notes.

Marilyn S. Feinstein, ACC, LCSW, USPTA

CONTRIBUTORS

Catherine A. Alder, JD, MSW, LSW
Aging Brain Care
Sandra Eskenazi Center for Brain Care Innovation
Eskenazi Health
Indianapolis, IN

Alan M. Altman, MD, IF, FACOG
Past President ISSWSH (International Society for the Study of Women's Sexual Health)
Consultative Gynecologist for Menopause and Female Sexual Dysfunction, Aspen, CO
Former Assistant Clinical Professor of Obstetrics, Gynecology and Reproductive Biology
Harvard Medical School
Boston, MA

Ellen Anderson, MD, MHSC, MCFP
Clinical Assistant Professor
Department of Family Medicine
University of British Columbia
Sooke, British Columbia

Mary Guerriero Austrom, PhD
Department of Psychiatry
Indiana Alzheimer Disease Center
Indiana University Center for Aging Research
Indiana University School of Medicine
Indianapolis, IN

Malaz A. Boustani, MD, MPH
Indiana University Center for Aging Research
Center for Health Innovation and Implementation Science
Indiana University School of Medicine
Regenstrief Institute, Inc.
Indianapolis, IN

Anne A. Brewer, MD, MPH
Medical Director, Palliative Care
Stamford Hospital
Stamford, CT

Mesha-Gay Brown, MD
Department of Neurology
University of Colorado School of Medicine
Aurora, CO

Katherine Buck, PhD, LMFT
Licensed Psychologist
John Peter Smith Family Medicine Residency
Fort Worth, TX

Jacqueline Calderone, MD
Departments of Psychiatry and Family Medicine
University of Colorado School of Medicine
AF Williams Family Medical Center
Helen and Arthur E. Johnson Depression Center
University of Colorado Anschutz Medical Campus
Aurora, CO

Sophie Collins, MD, MSc
Addiction Medicine Fellow
Department of Family Medicine
University of Colorado School of Medicine
Aurora, CO

Colleen Conry, MD
Department of Family Medicine
University of Colorado School of Medicine
Aurora, CO

Joseph V. Connelly, MD
Chairman, Department of Family Medicine
Stamford Hospital
Stamford, CT
Assistant Clinical Professor
Columbia University College of Physicians and Surgeons
New York, NY

Robert D. Davies, MD
Department of Psychiatry
University of Colorado School of Medicine
Aurora, CO

Frank V. deGruy III, MD
Chair, Department of Family Medicine
University of Colorado School of Medicine
Aurora, CO

Brian A. Fallon, MD, MPH, MEd
Department of Psychiatry
Columbia University Medical Center
New York, NY

Marilyn S. Feinstein, ACC, LCSW, USPTA
Associated Certified Coach
International Coaching Federation
Licensed Clinical Social Worker
Elite Pro, United States Tennis Association
Centennial, CO

Robert E. Feinstein, MD
Department of Psychiatry
University of Colorado School of Medicine
Aurora, CO

Lynne Fenton, MD
Department of Psychiatry
University of Colorado School of Medicine
Aurora, CO

Colleen T. Fogarty, MD, MSc
Department of Family Medicine
University of Rochester School of Medicine & Dentistry
Rochester, NY

Liza Freehling, WHNP-BC
Generations ObGyn
Aurora, CO

Alexis A. Giese, MD
Departments of Psychiatry and Family Medicine
University of Colorado School of Medicine
Aurora, CO

Isabelle Guillemet, MD
Department of Psychiatry
University of Colorado School of Medicine
Aurora, CO

Noa Heiman, PhD
Department of Psychiatry
University of Colorado School of Medicine
Aurora, CO

Alison M. Heru, MD
Interim Chair, Department of Psychiatry
University of Colorado School of Medicine
Aurora, CO

Bonnie T. Jortberg, PhD, RD, CDE
Department of Family Medicine
University of Colorado School of Medicine
Aurora, CO

Nicole Joseph, MD
Denver Health Medical Center
Department of Medicine
University of Colorado School of Medicine
Aurora, CO

Nick Kates, MB.BS, FRCPC, MCFP(Hon)
Chair, Department of Psychiatry and Behavioural Neurosciences
Michael G. DeGroote School of Medicine
McMaster University
Hamilton, Ontario

Parinda Khatri, PhD
Cherokee Health Systems
Knoxville, TN

Ian Koebner, MSc, MAOM, L.Ac
Department of Anesthesiology and Pain Medicine
University of California, Davis School of Medicine
Sacramento, CA

Michael A. LaMantia, MD, MPH
Department of Medicine
Robert Larner, MD College of Medicine at the University of Vermont
Burlington, VT

Alla Landa, PhD
Department of Psychiatry
Columbia University Medical Center
New York, NY

Shandra Brown Levey, PhD
Department of Family Medicine
University of Colorado School of Medicine
Aurora, CO

Meegan Lipman, MD
Department of Psychiatry
University of Colorado School of Medicine
Aurora, CO

L. Charolette Lippolis, DO, MPH
LCL Wellness, LLC
Evergreen, CO

Elizabeth Lowdermilk, MD
Denver Health Medical Center
Department of Psychiatry
University of Colorado School of Medicine
Aurora, CO

Hillary D. Lum, MD, PhD
Division of Geriatric Medicine
Department of Medicine
University of Colorado School of Medicine
Aurora, CO

Corey Lyon, DO, FAAP
AF Williams Family Medicine
Family Medicine Residency Program
University of Colorado School of Medicine
Aurora, CO

Marina Makous, MD
Departments of Psychiatry/Medicine/
Family Medicine
Columbia University Medical Center
New York, NY

Laura Martin, MD
Medical Director, Center for Dependency,
Addiction, and Rehabilitation (CeDAR)
Department of Psychiatry
University of Colorado School of Medicine
Aurora, CO

Robert M. McCarron, DO
Department of Anesthesiology
and Pain Medicine
Department of Psychiatry
and Behavioral Sciences
University of California,
Davis School of Medicine
Sacramento, CA

Susan H. McDaniel, PhD
Departments of Psychiatry and Family Medicine
University of Rochester School
of Medicine & Dentistry
Rochester, NY

Philip S. Mehler, MD, FACP, FAED
Department of Medicine
University of Colorado School of Medicine
Eating Recovery Center
Denver Health Medical Center
Denver, CO

Patricia Pade, MD
Program Director, Addiction Medicine Fellowship
Department of Family Medicine
University of Colorado School of Medicine
Aurora, CO

Jessica Palka, BS
Department of Psychiatry
and Behavioral Sciences
University of California,
Davis School of Medicine
Sacramento, CA

Gregg Perry, MD
Psychiatric Services
Cherokee Health Systems
Knoxville, TN

Kenneth M. Pollock, PhD
Department of Psychiatry
New York Medical College
Valhalla, NY
Department of Psychiatry & Behavioral Sciences
Albert Einstein College of Medicine, Montefiore
Medical Center
Bronx, NY

Michael R. Privitera, MS, MD
Department of Psychiatry
University of Rochester School of Medicine &
Dentistry
Rochester, NY

Amir Ramezani, PhD
Department of Anesthesiology and Pain
Medicine
University of California, Davis School of
Medicine
Sacramento, CA

Tziporah Rosenberg, PhD, LMFT
Departments of Psychiatry
and Family Medicine
University of Rochester School
of Medicine & Dentistry
Rochester, NY

Brian Rothberg, MD
Department of Psychiatry
University of Colorado School of Medicine
Aurora, CO

Lisa V. Rubenstein, MD, MSPH
VA Greater Los Angeles
UCLA David Geffen School of Medicine
UCLA Jonathan and Karin Fielding School of Public Health
RAND Corporation
North Hills, CA

Christopher D. Schneck, MD
Department of Psychiatry and Family Medicine
University of Colorado School of Medicine
Helen and Arthur E. Johnson Depression Center
Behavioral Health Director
University of Colorado Hospital HIV Clinic
Aurora, CO

Bruce J. Schwartz, MD
Department of Psychiatry & Behavioral Sciences
Albert Einstein College of Medicine, Montefiore Medical Center
Bronx, NY

Jonathan Shedler, PhD
Department of Psychiatry
University of Colorado School of Medicine
Aurora, CO

Samir J. Sheth, MD
Department of Anesthesiology and Pain Medicine
University of California, Davis School of Medicine
Sacramento, CA

James H. Shore, MD, MPH
Department of Psychiatry
University of Colorado School of Medicine
Depression Center Helen and Arthur E. Johnson
University of Colorado Anschutz Medical Campus
Aurora, CO

Scott A. Simpson, MD, MPH
Department of Psychiatry
University of Colorado School of Medicine
Denver Health Medical Center
Denver, CO

Abby Snavely, MD
Department of Psychiatry
University of Colorado School of Medicine
Aurora, CO

Gillian Stein
Montefiore Medical Center
Bronx, NY

Joanna Sturhahn Stratton, PhD, LMFT, Licensed Psychologist
Division of Counseling and Family Therapy
Regis University
Denver, CO
University of Colorado School of Medicine
Aurora, CO

Laura Strom, MD
Department of Neurology
University of Colorado School of Medicine
Aurora, CO

Adam Trosterman, MD
Department of Medicine
Division of Internal Medicine
University of Colorado School of Medicine
Aurora, CO

Debbie Voyles, MBA, HOM
Executive Director of UCHealth Telhealth Program
University of Colorado Hospital
Aurora, CO

Maryann Waugh, MEd
University of Colorado School of Medicine
University of Colorado Anschutz Medical Campus
Colorado Access
Aurora, CO

Scott Wetzler, PhD
Department of Psychiatry and Behavioral Sciences
Montefiore Medical Center
Bronx, NY

Alison R. Yager, MD
Department of Pediatrics
Kaiser Permanente
Aurora Centrepoint Clinic
Aurora, CO

Eileen D. Yager, MD
Department of Pediatrics
University of Colorado School of Medicine
Integrative Pain and Symptom Management Clinic
Children's Hospital Colorado
Aurora, CO

Joel Yager, MD, FAED
Department of Psychiatry
University of Colorado School of Medicine
Aurora, CO

INTEGRATING BEHAVIORAL HEALTH AND PRIMARY CARE

PART I

Models of Integrated Care

1

Conceptual Framework for Integrated Care

Multiple Models to Achieve Integrated Aims

ALEXIS A. GIESE AND MARYANN WAUGH

BOX 1.1

KEY POINTS

- **Integrated care is a conceptual framework that can be implemented using a variety of styles and models.**
- **Care integration relies on a biopsychosocial understanding of health and wellness.**
- **Effective integration builds on common elements including team-based information sharing and decision making, care coordination, a population-based approach to care, attitude shifts in mind–body distinctions, addressing stigma, administrative support (including new payment methods), and stepped access to specialty care.**
- **Successful integration models are flexible and locally tailored.**
- **Integration design should be built based on the needs, goals, and culture of the specific local patient population and the capability of the workforce.**
- **Systematic evaluation and outcomes monitoring is key to learning, adapting, and sustainability.**
- **Business and clinical models must be built in parallel, often through incremental stepped changes**

INTRODUCTION

This chapter proposes an underlying conceptual framework for integrated behavioral health care and associated key elements that transcend most integrated care models. A overview of these key elements are described in Box 1.1. Because integrated care programs and services vary widely and new variants frequently arise, it is helpful to conceptualize what is at the heart of integrated care, state its rationale, and establish a framework for evaluating it. This approach is intended to stimulate a deeper exploration of the critical and active components of integrated care transformation and stimulate providers, practices, payers, and health care systems to thoughtfully develop their own integration strategies and contribute to the ongoing innovation of new models of care.

"Integrated care" as a term is inconsistently defined and variously and informally used by many speakers, writers, and practitioners. The Substance Abuse and Mental Health Services Administration (SAMHSA) defines integration in its broadest sense as the bringing together and coordination of myriad health care components.[1] The Agency for Healthcare Research and Quality, in its Lexicon for Behavioral Health and Primary Care Integration, defines it as

> The care that results from a practice team of primary care and behavioral health clinicians,

> working together with patients and families, using a systematic and cost-effective approach to provide patient-centered care for a defined population. This care may address mental health and substance abuse conditions, health behaviors (including their contribution to chronic medical illnesses), life stressors and crises, stress-related physical symptoms, and ineffective patterns of health care utilization.[2]

In practice, "integration" has been used to refer to everything from traditional psychiatric consultation, to co-location of psychologists, to any setting with shared health values of treating the whole person.[2] This chapter focuses on the integration of behavioral health care with primary care. and with a variety of other types of medical care and settings. See Figure 1.1 to review the terminology frequently used when describing integrated care.

CONCEPTUAL BASIS FOR INTEGRATING BEHAVIORAL HEALTH CARE

Integrated care is not a specific structure, process, or clinical model. Practitioners and practices that want to provide integrated care need to embrace a framework of health and health care delivery that encompasses the full range of physical, psychological, social, spiritual, preventive, and therapeutic factors necessary for a healthy life, not just add new services or providers. Practices need to better align their culture of care, become more holistic in their approach, and redefine goals and outcomes. Table 1.1 reviews key resources that provide additional information about integrated care.

BIOPSYCHOSOCIAL MODEL OF HEALTH AND ILLNESS

The biopsychosocial model of health and illness is critical to the integrated care framework. In 1977, Engel began to promote an integrated view of human health based on the recognition that psychological and social factors are strong determinants of health and illness.[3] The (still relatively new at the time) biomedical model and the corresponding training model for physicians led to important scientific and technical advances in medicine. However, the biomedical model also contributed to an increasingly narrow view of health as being merely the absence of disease and a treatment emphasis on biologically based, technologically sophisticated, high-cost medical tests and interventions. The biopsychosocial model, in contrast, lays out a broader definition of health as a state of physical, mental, and social well-being and encourages providers to take a holistic and humanistic approach to care.[3,4] As described in a paper posted by the Word Health Organization,

> Psychosocial factors affect the onset and course of almost all chronic physical disorders. Neuroendocrine, immunological, and other physiological mechanisms may mediate the effects of psychological factors on physical processes. Psychological, behavioral, and social factors interact with pathological processes in the development and course of physical disorders. They also have substantial effects on consultation and compliance with treatment.[3]

A conceptual view of the patient through this lens includes behavioral health as a part of overall health, rather than a separable domain that requires a separate framework and treatment setting.

EXPANDED DEFINITION OF BEHAVIORAL HEALTH

Also inherent in the biopsychosocial construct is an expansion of the definition of behavioral health. In the traditional biomedical or disease model, behavioral disorders are defined by symptoms, deficits, and diagnosable conditions. This paradigm is reinforced in diagnostic nomenclature, reimbursement requirements (e.g., covered diagnoses, medical necessity), research design, and clinical training. Integrated care, in contrast, conceptualizes behavioral health as a key component of overall health, encompassing biological, psychological, behavioral, and sociocultural factors that affect health and mental wellness, as well as formally diagnosable disorders. A 1993 study found that about half of U.S. deaths were premature, and of those premature deaths, over 80% were attributed to three human behaviors: tobacco use, diet, and exercise.[5,6] More recent statistics show that the U.S. life expectancy continues to fall in relation to international life expectancy.[7] While deaths due to all causes combined (cancer, stroke, heart disease, unintentional injuries, and diabetes) have decreased between 1969 and 2013, decreases have slowed for heart disease, stroke, and diabetes. The death rate for chronic obstructive pulmonary disease (COPD) actually increased during this period.[8] This indicates a persistent impact of behavior upon medical health. While numerous studies have demonstrated improved

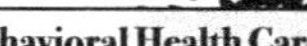
Illustration: A family tree of related terms used in behavioral health and primary care integration
Patient-Centered Care
"The experience (to the extent the informed, individual patient desires it) of transparency, individualization, recognition, respect, dignity, and choice in all matters, without exception, related to one's person, circumstances, and relationships in health care" –or "nothing about me without me" (Berwick, 2011).
Integrated Care
Tightly integrated, on-site teamwork with unified care plan as a standard approach to care for designated populations. Connotes organizational integration involving social and other services. "Altitudes" of integration: 1) Integrated treatments, 2) integrated program structure; 3) integrated system of programs, and 4) integrated payments. (Based on SAMHSA).
Coordinated Care
The organization of patient care activities between two or more participants (including the patient) involved in care, to facilitate appropriate delivery of healthcare services. Organizing care involves the marshalling of personnel and other resources needed to carry out required care activities, and often managed by the exchange of information among participants responsible for different aspects of care" (AHRQ, 2007).
Collaborative Care
A general term for ongoing working relationships between clinicians, rather than a specific product or service (Doherty, McDaniel & Baird, 1996). Providers combine perspectives and skills to understand and identify problems and treatments, continually revising as needed to hit goals, e.g. in collaborative care of depression (Unützer et al., 2002)
Shared Care
Predominantly Canadian usage – PC & MH professionals (typically psychiatrists) working together in shared system and record, maintaining 1 treatment plan addressing all patient health needs. (Kates et al., 1996; Kelly et al., 2011)
Co-located Care
BH and PC providers (i.e. physicians, NPs) delivering car in same practice. This denotes shared space to one extent or another, not a specific service or kind of collaboration (adapted from Blount, 2003)
Integrated Primary Care or Primary Care Behavioral Health
Combines medical and BH services for problems patients bring to primary care, including stress-linked physical symptoms, health behaviors, MH or SA disorders. For any problem, they have come to the right place – "no wrong door" (Blount). BH professional used as a consultant to PC colleagues (Sabin & Borus, 2009; Haas & deGruy, 2004; Robinson & Reiter, 2007; Hunter et al, 2009).
Behavioral Health Care
An umbrella term for care that addresses any behavioral problems bearing on health, including MH and SA conditions, stress-linked physical symptoms, patient activation and health behaviors. The job of all kinds of care settings, and done by clinicians and healthy coaches of various disciplines or training.
Patient-Centered Medical Home
An approach to comprehensive primary care for children, youth and adults – a setting that facilitates partnerships between patients and their personal physicians and when appropriate, the patient's family. Emphasizes care of populations, team care, whole person care – including behavioral health, care coordination, information tools and business models needed to sustain the work. The goal is health, patient experience, and reduced cost (Joint Principles of PCMH, 2007).
Mental Health Care
Care to help people with mental illnesses (or at risk) – to suffer less emotional pain and disability – and live healthier, longer, more productive lives. Done by a variety of caregivers in diverse public and private settings such as specialty MH, general medical, human services, and voluntary support networks. (Adapted from SAMHSA)
Substance Abuse Care
Services, treatments, and supports to help people with addictions and substance abuse problems suffer less emotional pain, family and vocational disturbance, physical risks – and live healthier, longer, more productive lives. Done in specialty SA, general medical, human services, voluntary support networks, e.g. 12-step programs and peer counselors. (Adapted from SAMHSA))
Primary Care
Primary care is the provision of integrated, accessible health care services by clincians who are accountable for addressing a large majority of personal health care needs, developing a sustained partnership with patients, and practicing in the context of family and community. (Institute of Medicine, 1994)
Thanks to Benjamin Miller and Jürgen Unützer for advice on organizing this illustration.

FIGURE 1.1: Lexicon for behavioral health and primary care integration: Concepts and definitions developed by expert consensus. AHRQ Publication No. 13-IP001-EF. Rockville, MD: Agency for Healthcare Research and Quality, 2013. http://integrationacademy.ahrq.gov/sites/default/files/Lexicon.pdf.

TABLE 1.1. INTEGRATED CARE WEB RESOURCES

Substance Abuse and Mental Health Services Administration (SAMHSA)	The SAMHSA-HRSA Center for Integrated Health Solutions (CIHS) has a wealth of online information regarding a variety of integration options and emerging research and evaluation for specific integration models. http://www.integration.samhsa.gov/integrated-care-models
University of Washington Advancing Integrated Mental Health Solutions (UW AIMS Center)	A center dedicated to improving the health of populations by advancing the research and implementation of Collaborative Care, a specific model of integrated care developed at the University of Washington to treat common and persistent mental health conditions such as depression and anxiety. The AIMS Center was founded by Jürgen Unützer, an internationally recognized psychiatrist and health services researcher. https://aims.uw.edu
U.S. Department of Health and Human Services, Health Services Administration (HRSA)	The primary federal agency for improving access to health care by strengthening the health care workforce, building healthy communities, and achieving health equity. http://www.hrsa.gov/publichealth/clinical/behavioralhealth/

health behavior outcomes related to health education and increased self-efficacy, outcomes are highly dependent on levels of patient engagement. Patient engagement, in turn, represents a complex interaction of behavior driven by psychosocial factors and environmental factors, including the environment of the health care system and practice.[5] With human behavior so highly correlated to mortality, the biopsychosocial approach is critical to modifying risks and preventing disorders at a population level.

The conceptualization of health as not just the absence of disease, but rather the state of positive functioning, supported by prophylaxis (prevention, protection, and resistance), is relatively new in the behavioral health arena compared to physical health care applications. Researchers argue, however, that a well-defined theoretical construct of mental resilience, the maintenance of positive functioning despite stressors, supports the integration of social and natural sciences by taking into account both psychosocial and biological models of mental health pathways.[9] This, in turn, supports the use of multicausal models of mental health and increases the role of activities and conditions that increase resilience. The biopsychosocial conceptualization of behavioral health contributes to the expanding recognition of the multiple determinants of overall human health. These include everything from genes to cultures, while additionally acknowledging mediating and transactional developmental processes.[9] The biopsychosocial, patient-centered framework gives rise to an expanded definition of behavioral health and defines several components of behavioral health relevant to clinical delivery design in an integrated care setting.[10] These are summarized in Table 1.2.

INTEGRATED CARE AND THE TRIPLE AIM

The Institute for Healthcare Improvement (IHI) developed the Triple Aim framework in 2007 as a three-dimensional approach toward transformation of the health care system to better meet the needs of individuals and society.[11] The Triple Aim is the simultaneous pursuit of improved patient experience of care, improved population health, and reduced per capita health care costs. Integrated behavioral health care is both conceptually aligned with the Triple Aim and essential to the required systems transformation needed to achieve its intended outcomes.

Patient Experience of Care

The IHI operationally defined patient experience of care using the Institute of Medicine's six dimensions: safe, effective, patient-centered, timely, efficient, and equitable care. Integrated care is particularly well aligned with this and potentially functions as an important driver to improve the quality of behavioral health services that most patients receive. The majority of behavioral health

TABLE 1.2. BEHAVIORAL HEALTH FOR CLINICAL INTEGRATED CARE DELIVERY

Behavioral Health Components	Clinical Delivery Examples
Behavioral health promotion	• Patient education and increased awareness regarding behavior as part of overall health • Opportunities for patient skill-building for improved resilience
Behavioral health impact/comorbidity with chronic conditions such as diabetes and obesity, and related treatment adherence	• Patient education regarding treatment adherence • Patient self-management skills • Clinical use of motivational interviewing • Clinical awareness of cultural factors impacting behavior and treatment adherence
Prevention, early detection, and intervention for behavioral health disorders	• Routine screening for substance use, high-risk behaviors, and depression, as well as grief, loss, trauma, and psychological stress • Prevention and intervention for insufficient coping strategies • Intervention/referral to address social and environmental risk factors and inadequate personal resources
Treatment of diagnosable mental disorders and/or substance use disorders	• Expanded options for treatment in a range of settings • High degree of coordination using team-based care

services are currently provided in primary care and other settings by medical generalists with insufficient resources to provide evidence-based care. Moreover, the majority of persons with behavioral health conditions receive no treatment or inadequate treatment in medical settings.[11,12]

Patient-centeredness is at the foundation of the integrated care constructs. Problems and solutions are understood in terms of the patient's point of view, preferences, culture, and experience, and patients are equally valued members of their care team.[13] The patient-centered perspective of integrated care emphasizes patient autonomy and shared decision making between providers and patients. These concepts, already integral to specialty behavioral health care training and practice, also influence how behavioral health is integrated into delivery in other medical settings. Care that is integrated cannot simply physically relocate providers from one health system into another without also including some of the critical components of the patient-centered care model. Integrated care has the potential to improve patient safety and treatment efficacy by bolstering the quality of behavioral health services provided to patients.[14] Integrated care also advances timeliness and efficiency by offering more convenient access and more efficient delivery approaches for behavioral health services, which are historically both difficult to access and lacking sufficient capacity.[15–17] Studies have demonstrated low rates of patient follow-through for persons screened and referred by primary care to specialty behavioral health. A study of commercially insured adolescents found that only 18% of those referred for behavioral health treatment actually completed at least one treatment session within 180 days of referral.[15] Follow-up rates for adults are estimated to be less than 50%.[16]

Population Health Approach

Integrated care has an important role to play in improving population health, which encompasses shared accountability for broadly defined health outcomes.[10,12] Improving health for an entire population shifts the health care system from a diagnose-and-treat-disease model to a whole-health continuum focus. Instead of being responsible only for treating sick persons, the health care system becomes responsible for the health and well-being of all persons through wellness promotion, prevention, early detection, and early intervention. Successful gains in population health dictates a whole-person approach. Accordingly, the Centers for Medicare and Medicaid Services Innovation Center's mission includes promoting "better health by encouraging healthier lifestyles in the entire population, including increased physical activity, better nutrition, avoidance of behavioral risks, and wider use of preventive care."[10]

Reducing Overall Health Care Costs

Integrated care is also a key strategy in reducing overall health care costs. The interaction of health behaviors, behavioral health disorders, and psychological and social factors on health care costs is well documented.[17–19] There is also growing evidence demonstrating that successful approaches to integrating behavioral health result in better clinical outcomes[17,20,21] and have the potential to reduce overall health care costs.[18,19,22] See Chapter 6: Financing Integrated Care Models for a detailed discussion about new financial models for mental health reimbursement and reducing costs.

Integrating Care into the Existing Care Systems

Integrated care is not constrained to a specific model or practice. Most published reports address collaborative care of depression in primary care settings in adult populations. These studies were implemented in relatively specific clinical settings: research or grant-funded projects, academic medical centers, or vertically integrated health care delivery systems.[19,20,23–25] There is relatively less systematic information regarding the science and critical components of these programs to guide implementation efforts.[11,12,25] In real-world implementations, there are numerous local variables such as policy environments, financial resources/funding models, staff expertise, time and interest, local practice patterns, health care ecosystems, regional culture, and populations that have major effects on implementation design, feasibility, fidelity, success, and sustainability. While most clinical settings attempt to adopt or, at least, to borrow from established or evidence-based models, complete fidelity is seldom achieved. Innovation and creativity are almost always required to adapt integration efforts into specific real-world environments. Variations in integrated care practice are as diverse as the settings in which they are embedded.

Thus, in a health care environment that places a priority on evidence-based practices, integration stands in contrast as a conceptual framework. Speaking to this unique positioning as evidence-based in concept but diverse in application is a quote from a Milbank report to the Canadian Collaborative Mental Health Initiative: "there are almost as many ways of 'doing' collaborative mental health care as there are people writing about it."[26] Those who would like to pursue integrated care initiatives are confronted with a vast number of disparate interventions to consider. The complex process of identifying how and what intervention to implement is made even more difficult because most integrated care interventions are implemented as hybrids and often blend one or more elements of different models. Depending on the specific implementation, a model may represent partial or full integration. This creates the imperative that each health care system, practice, or provider embarking upon or seeking to advance integrated care starts with a conceptual framework, adapts it to the unique features of the setting and population, and systematically evaluates its outcomes. In this manner, the system operates in parallel to the evolving approach to its patients: holistic, adaptive, and individualized.

While this local, organic process is both necessary and creative, it comes with associated challenges and risks. Varied models of implementation make it more difficult to compare program outcomes and efficacy, select appropriate models or starting points, and invest in the necessary groundwork to customize to local settings. Many evidence-based integrated care models described in the literature might be seen as requiring prohibitive expenditures of practice and system time, effort, training, and financial investment. Just as daunting may be the notion of creating and implementing de novo or customized models for each system of care. Additionally, the mechanisms to fund integrated care and achieve the expected offsets in health care costs are not always clear (and certainly not guaranteed) at the outset.[18]

LEVELS AND CATEGORIES OF INTEGRATED CARE

Most attempts to differentiate conceptual models of integration define graduated levels of integrated care based on care processes, workflow, and location/configuration of providers. Table 1.3 summarizes these proposed models.

These conceptual-level models may be useful to compare and measure integration progress but also have limitations. One limitation is that levels and models described to date are mostly applicable to behavioral health services integrated into primary care settings and may not be as applicable in other configurations (such as primary care services provided in a behavioral health clinic). Another limitation is that there is a lack of consistent literature findings associating proposed levels of integration with clinical effectiveness or other outcomes, despite an inherent assumption that higher levels of integration are better. A 2008 review of mental health integration and coordination efforts in the United States essentially concluded that more research is needed.[31] While the reviewers found an overall pattern of improved behavioral and physical health outcomes related to integrated as opposed to usual care, particularly for patients with depression, they noted widely varied outcomes and no correlation between outcomes and the extent of integration or the structure of integration processes. They found only one model, Improving Mood-Promoting Access to Collaborative Treatment (IMPACT), with consistent depression symptom severity improvements.[32] More recent studies confirm positive outcomes associated with various levels of integration. For example, one recent study identified reductions in both mood disorder symptoms and the frequency of medical visits associated with behavioral health consultative services delivered in primary care settings.[33] Another recent meta-analysis found positive symptom and reduced cost associated with collaborative chronic care models for the treatment of chronic mental illness across care settings.[34] The need for additional research and evaluation that addresses the level and type of integration across care models and care settings remains.

COMMON CORE ELEMENTS OF INTEGRATED CARE MODELS

As the body of research and evaluation findings builds a burgeoning array of integration models and configurations, there arises a need to describe and study common elements of effective integrated care efforts. As Kwan and Nease stated,

> In order to justify wide-scale system changes towards integrated behavioral health care, conclusive and consistent evidence is needed to convince policy and decision makers (including payers) of the value of collaborative care compared to the status quo. Such evidence includes an understanding of the models and their attributes that are feasible, sustainable, affordable, and effective.[20]

While not extensive, existing literature does suggest some common elements that are associated with most integrated care models, with varying levels of supporting evidence for each. Kwon and Nease described common elements grouped by structure, processes, and attitudes.[20] A 2015 study found five key organizing constructs that influenced the integration of primary care and behavioral health.[35] A 2010 meta-analysis identified 10 common elements necessary for health systems integration.[14] Many of their proposed components represent conceptual constructs rather than a specific set of structures, processes, or personnel. Ten key integrated care constructs are summarized below at a conceptual level and may be useful in considering both pragmatic and cultural aspects associated with meaningful integration.

Attitudes, Beliefs, and Culture Change

Integrated care requires a practice-wide acceptance of the biopsychosocial model and the mind–body connection and a commitment to building a new, shared culture, not a host culture with a foreign visitor or two cohabiting strangers. Attitudes of superiority of one's background, discipline, or clinical approach over another lead to professional self-interest, limited communication, and mistrust, which are all obstacles to integration even in optimal structural and financial situations.[14] The attitude toward patients must also align with integration efforts. Providers must be dedicated to caring for the whole person despite the limits of personal expertise and experience, which in turn calls for humility and challenges traditional authority. A true attitude shift is likely to require appropriate organizational support for culture change. This involves engaging and preparing all providers for change, and training for and encouraging a team-based approach to holistic, patient-centered, culturally competent, whole-person care.[20]

Counteracting Stigma

Integration demands that providers and practices address and reduce stigma directed at mental health patients and issues within their particular contexts. Stigma includes patients' internalized self-stigma and (perhaps unconscious) stigma among providers toward persons with behavioral health issues. While there is some evidence that the general public in the United States has improved its understanding of mental health problems and recognition of the need for treatment, there remains social distancing from persons who experience behavioral health challenges. Recent research finds that stigma persists but does not yet

TABLE 1.3. CONCEPTUAL CONSTRUCTS OF STEPPED INTEGRATION

Author/Source	Construct	Description
Doherty, McDaniel, & Baird (1996)[27]	Five levels of integration	Level 1—Minimal collaboration Level 2—Basic collaboration at a distance Level 3—Basic collaboration onsite Level 4—Close collaboration with some system integration Level 5—Close collaboration approaching an integrated practice
SAMHSA (2013) "A Standard Framework for Levels of Integrated Healthcare"[1]	Six levels of integration	Coordinated Care Level 1—Minimal collaboration Level 2—Basic collaboration at a distance Co-Located Care Level 3—Basic collaboration onsite Level 4—Close collaboration with some system integration Integrated Care Level 5—Close collaboration approaching integration Level 6—Full collaboration in a transformed/merged practice
Collins, Hewson, Munger, & Wade Milbank Report (2010)[26]	Eight qualitatively different practice models of care integration	1. Improving collaboration between separate providers 2. Medical-provided behavioral health care 3. Co-location 4. Disease management 5. Reverse co-location 6. Unified primary care and behavioral health 7. Primary care behavioral health 8. Collaborative system of care
Waxmonsky, Auxier, Romero, & Heath (2014) Integrated Practice Assessment Tool (IPAT)[28]	Six assessed levels of integration to match SAMHSA's Standard Framework	Level 1—Minimal collaboration Level 2—Basic collaboration at a distance Level 3—Basic collaboration onsite Level 4—Close collaboration with some system integration Level 5—Close collaboration approaching integration Level 6—Full collaboration in a transformed/merged practice
American Academy of Child and Adolescent Psychiatry, Martini et al., (2012)[29]	Levels of complexity and Best Principles for Integration of Child Psychiatry into the Pediatric Health Home	1. Preventive services and screening 2. Early intervention and routine care provision 3. Specialty consultation, treatment, and coordination 4. Intensive mental health services for complex issues
Alakeson, Frank, & Katz (2010)[30]	Primary care services in behavioral health settings	Flexible definition of a medical home; stepped, integrated care provision in specialty settings to support patient choice, preference, and needs

provide sufficient evidence for pragmatic mitigation methods. Integrated care plays a potentially critical role toward the solution. As Goffman reminded us early on (in 1963),

> stigma is fundamentally a social phenomenon rooted in social relationships and shaped by the culture and structure of society. If stigma emanates from social relationships, the solution to understanding and changing must similarly be embedded in changing social relationships and the structures that shape them.[36]

Organizational Support

The complex and numerous steps involved in building an integrated care system require substantial support from the administrative and policy levels of the host organization. Integrated care must be aligned with and reflective of the organization's mission and vision and should be implemented within a well-articulated operational strategy.[37] Studies within integrated Veterans Health Administration (VHA) primary care settings found that leadership is critical for successful integration. Leadership actions such as adequately allocating resources, resolving conflicts, defining job duties, supporting providers, and identifying clinical champions of change have been significantly associated with positive outcomes in VHA integration efforts and evaluations.[38] The VHA often uses clinical champions for new program and policy implementation as well. These champions are often respected clinicians who act as a resource and help drive change by disseminating relevant information to patients and staff and by providing staff support.[38] See Chapter 7: Integrating Physical and Mental Health Care in the Veterans Health Administration: A Path to the Future, for a detailed discussion.

The SAMHSA-HRSA Center for Integrated Health Solutions, in a discussion of sustainability, notes that organizations invested in sustaining integration form "change teams" to champion and advance integration efforts in their clinics. They also include integration-related goals and work processes in new employee orientation and incorporate supervisory review of physical health and behavioral health goals into standard team meetings. Integration then becomes a component of clinic policies, job descriptions, performance reviews, and even confidentiality agreements.[39]

Commitment, Flexibility, and Change Tolerance

Successful integration efforts have in common a willingness to embrace change. Practices generally need to have a culture that welcomes change, is willing to tolerate missteps and interruptions, is curious and actively engaged in learning, and is able to make iterative adjustments to both practice and policy. Systems change studies have identified the importance of allowing for professional flexibility in developing and maintaining this desired practice culture. Practices that actively engage their providers in practice-level decision making and empower providers to take individual initiative in identifying and addressing challenges have more successful change processes.[38]

Patient-Centered Care

The Institute of Medicine has made a patient and family-centered approach a priority in improving health experiences and outcomes. This includes improved care coordination and access, improved access to personal health records and health/disease information, and patient self-management support.[40] In addition to being a more humanistic and ethical approach, patient-centered care also increases patient autonomy, engagement (which is a critical component to behavioral change), and treatment adherence and is associated with improved intervention outcomes.[41]

Team-Based Care

Closely aligned with the notion of patient-centered care, team-based medical care has been linked to more coordinated care, streamlined medical services, quality improvement measures, and positive employee, organizational, and patient outcomes.[42] A team approach means that complementary sets of individual expertise contribute toward a shared vision for patient health and wellness without gaps and overlaps. Team-based care embraces shared decision making, which in turn incorporates a more comprehensive patient view, shared information, and common patient-centered goals. Team-based care represents a fairly sharp distinction from traditional medical care, in which patients are "referred" to "consultants" or other services; too often, the burden of organizing the providers, summarizing medical findings and recommendations, falls to the patient and results in inefficiency, duplication, gaps, errors, and conflicting goals and plans.[32]

Population-Based Approach

A population-based approach not only addresses patients with current symptoms and problems but also proactively identifies those in the population who may be at risk but do not seek care.[43] This includes screening processes for potential risk factors, resources for surveillance and results interpretation, and strategies for prevention and early detection/intervention. Integrated care integrates these efforts across the physical health and behavioral health perspectives. Two complementary types of integration, horizontal and vertical, allow primary care practices to provide this type of holistic care.[43] Horizontal integration embeds a "generalist service delivery model" of behavioral health into primary care, based on the assumption that most members of a primary care population can benefit from some generalized and brief psychosocial service. Vertical integration complements these broad, population-wide strategies that are primarily prevention-focused with targeted, specialized behavioral health services delivered only to specific and well-defined subgroups of primary care patients. Vertical integration strategies are comprehensive strategies for frequent utilizers or high-cost patient populations, including those with anxiety, depression, substance use disorders, and certain high medical utilizers, often patients with comorbid chronic behavioral and physical health needs.

Stepped Care

A key feature of successful integration is the ability to manage patients along a continuum of behavioral health needs. While horizontal integration is adequate for a large portion of primary care patients, those with more complex or persistent needs will be better served with additional specialty consultation, brief treatment, or more intensive ongoing specialty behavioral health services. A standalone (often part-time) behavioral health professional in a primary care or other medical clinic, unconnected to a continuum of care, is insufficient. Well-coordinated and timely access to psychiatrists, other specialty behavioral health services, and community supports is needed to adequately address all levels of need.[43,44] Specialty consultation ideally includes a psychiatrist who provides indirect care through caseload supervision and consultation/coaching for primary care providers as well as some direct care. Smooth coordination and linkage to higher levels of care (and back) are also critical. Research suggests that individual patient outcomes, especially for moderate and severe depression, are better when specialty care is part of treatment.[24,45] Patients with higher needs may benefit by enrollment in a more formal integration program (i.e., IMPACT, Life Goals) that is primary care-based but includes more structured behavioral health visits focused on patient education, self-management skills, medication compliance, and ongoing feedback to the primary care providers.[23]

Adapting Behavioral Health Services, Tools, and Personnel

Successful integration efforts do not merely transpose conventional behavioral health practices into primary care or other medical settings. While such co-located models do exist and may offer some advantages to patients and providers, they are insufficient to achieve the goals of integration as outlined above. In most models of integrated care in a primary care practice, services by behavioral health specialists occur in conjunction with primary care visits. Services are on demand or readily available, including immediate brief assessments and interventions. When behavioral and health screens identify potential risks or immediate concerns, behavioral health staff members provide evidence-based brief interventions such as motivational interviewing, problem-solving therapy, and behavioral activation.[44] To the extent possible, most patients continue to have the behavioral health condition addressed in the host setting. Behavioral health professionals have a key role in supporting that care as members of a team. Integration models require tools that are adapted for the setting, such as brief screening tools rather than comprehensive intake assessments. See Chapter 10: Automated Mental Health Assessment for Integrated Care: The Quick PsychoDiagnostics Panel (QPD Panel) Meets Real-World Clinical Needs, for a comprehensive brief mental health screening tool. Successful behavioral health personnel are those who are flexible, team-oriented, good communicators, and efficient.[4,43]

Outcomes Measurement

Another core element that allows population-level management of behavioral health is a process to document and monitor patient progress and outcomes and proactively pursue care opportunities for individual patients and for cohorts.[44] Registries, clinical datasets, and cost assessments are increasingly used in primary care and other settings to evaluate and improve care. In contrast, behavioral health settings have been less data-driven and more process-focused. Successful integrated care efforts involve a commitment to ongoing, data-driven evaluation and a shared responsibility for improving care and outcomes.[44]

APPLYING THE CONCEPTUAL FRAMEWORK AND COMMON ELEMENTS TO CREATE NEW MODELS

Primary care settings, especially vertically integrated health systems, Federally Qualified Health Centers, and academically affiliated settings, have been the early focus for integrated care. It is essential that this work continues. While there is less evidence for integrated care in other settings and populations, the conceptual framework and common elements are adaptable for use in many other spheres. Primary care offers certain advantages and drivers that are not common to all settings: large panel sizes, relatively long-term engagement with patients, higher baseline levels of interest and skills regarding behavioral health, and potential options for novel payment mechanisms. Other settings may borrow from the relatively robust literature from the primary care arena but must adapt clinical models and financial platforms to fit their specific needs and limitations. Alternative models and strategies are needed to expand and sustain integrated care

BOX 1.2

SUMMARY OF RECOMMENDED TREATMENT APPROACHES AND RELEVANT EVIDENCE

Strength of recommendation taxonomy (SOR A, B, or C)

- **A large number of U.S. deaths are premature; of those premature deaths, the majority are attributed to human behaviors (tobacco use, diet, and exercise). Creating lifestyle change will foster improved population health. (SOR A)[5,6,47,48]**
- **A well-defined theoretical construct of mental resilience, the maintenance of positive functioning despite stressors, supports the integration of social and natural sciences by taking into account both psychosocial and biological models of mental health pathways. (SOR B)[9,49]**
- **The majority of persons with behavioral health conditions, in medical settings, receive no treatment or inadequate treatment. (SOR A)[11,12]**
- **After traditional primary care referral to behavioral health, rates of follow-through are low. A study of commercially insured adolescents found that only 18% of those referred to, and agreeable to, behavioral health treatment actually completed at least one treatment session within 180 days of referral.[15] Follow-up rates for adults are estimated at less than 50%. (SOR B)[16]**
- **The interaction of health behaviors, behavioral health disorders, and psychological and social factors on health care costs is well documented. (SOR A)[17–19]**
- **There is also growing evidence demonstrating that successful approaches to integrating behavioral health result in better clinical outcomes (SOR A)[17,20,21] and have the potential to reduce overall health care costs. (SOR A)[18,19,22]**
- **More research is needed to describe the efficacy of mental health integration and coordination efforts in the United States. (SOR C)[31]**
- **Positive symptom and cost outcomes are associated with collaborative chronic care models for the treatment of chronic mental illness across care settings. (SOR B)[34]**
- **Research has identified 10 common elements necessary for health systems integration: (1) attitudes, beliefs, and culture change, (2) counteracting stigma, (3) organizational support, (4) commitment, flexibility, and change tolerance, (5) patient-centered care, (6) team-based care, (7) adapting behavioral health services, tools, and personnel, (8) stepped care, (9) population-based approach, and (10) outcomes measurement. (SOR C)[14]**

more broadly, such as technological solutions (e.g., telehealth services) for providing integrated care in a cost-efficient manner that drives practice transformation.[46] The chapters that follow describe a wide range of integrated care approaches that are variously adapted to primary care, pediatric, obstetrics/gynecology, specialty medical, rural, and other settings. Understanding the underlying conceptual framework of integrated care and its common key elements and applying them to their own unique systems will help practitioners and systems design their own solutions. It is recommended that health care systems define their specific problems and desired outcomes from the start, starting with the patients, and align all goals and incentives with the Triple Aim. In so doing, practices and providers will learn experientially and model the holistic individualized transformation of their systems in parallel with the transformation of the care those systems provide. An evidence-based summary of some of the essential elements of integrated care are described in Box 1.2.

REFERENCES

1. Heath B, Wise Romero P, Reynolds K. A Standard Framework for Levels of Integrated Healthcare. Washington, DC: SAMHSA-HRSA Center for Integrated Health Solutions, 2013. http://www.integration.samhsa.gov/integrated-care-models/A_Standard_Framework_for_Levels_of_Integrated_Healthcare.pdf. Accessed June 6, 2016.
2. Peek CJ and the National Integration Academy Council. Lexicon for Behavioral Health and Primary Care Integration: Concepts and Definitions Developed by Expert Consensus. AHRQ Publication No. 13-IP001-EF. Rockville, MD: Agency for Healthcare Research and Quality, 2013. http://integrationacademy.ahrq.gov/sites/default/files/Lexicon.pdf. Accessed June 6, 2016.
3. Engel GL. The clinical application of the biopsychosocial model. Am J Psychiatry. 1980;137(5):535–544.
4. Tomas MR, Giese AA, Waxmonsky JA. Transitioning to psychiatric service delivery in the medical setting. In Summergrad P, Kathol RG, eds. Integrated Care in Psychiatry: Redefining the Role of Mental Health Professionals in Medical Settings. New York: Springer Science+Business Media, 2014:14.
5. Adams JR. Improving health outcomes with better patient understanding and education. Risk Manag Healthcare Policy. 2010;3(1):61–72.
6. McGinnis JM, Foege WH. Actual causes of death in the United States. JAMA. 1993;207(18):2207–2212.
7. Kulkarni SC, Levin-Rector A, Ezzati M, Murray CJ. Falling behind: Life expectancy in US counties from 2000 to 2007 in an international context. Popul Health Metr. 2011;9(1):1–12.
8. Ward E, Siegel R, Jemal A. Temporal trends in mortality in the United States, 1969–2013. JAMA. 2015;314(16):1731–1739.
9. Davydov MD, Steward R, Ritchie K, Chaudieu I. Resilience and mental health. Clin Psychol Rev. 2010; 30(5):479–495.
10. Stoto MA. Population Health in the Affordable Care Act Era. Washington DC: Academy Health, 2013.
11. Case J. A Primer on Defining the Triple Aim. Institute for Health Care Improvement, 2014. http://www.ihi.org/communities/blogs/_layouts/ihi/community/blog/itemview.aspx?List=81ca4a47-4ccd-4e9e-89d9-14d88ec59e8d&ID=63. Accessed June 10, 2016.
12. Levey SMB, Miller BF. Behavioral health integration: An essential element of population-based healthcare redesign. Transl Behav Med. 2012;2(3):364–371.
13. Institute of Medicine, Committee on Quality of Health Care in America. Crossing the Quality Chasm: A New Health System for the 21st Century. Washington DC: National Academy Press, 2001.
14. Suter E, Oelke ND, Adair CE, Armitage GD. Ten key principles for successful health systems integration. Healthcare Quarterly. 2009;13(Spec No):16–23.
15. Hacker K, Arsenault L, Franco I, et al. Referral and follow-up after mental health screening in commercially insured adolescents. J Adolesc Health. 2014;55(1):17–23.
16. Kessler R. Mental health care treatment initiation when mental health services are incorporated into primary care practice. J Am Board Fam Pract. 2012;25(2):255–259.
17. Trendwatch American Hospital Association. Bringing Behavioral Health into the Care Continuum: Opportunities to Improve Quality, Costs and Outcomes, 2012. http://www.aha.org/research/reports/tw/12jan-tw-behavhealth.pdf. Accessed June 5, 2016.
18. Mauer BJ, Jarvis D. The business case for bidirectional integrated care: Mental health and substance use services in primary care settings and primary care services in specialty mental health and substance use settings. California Integration Policy Initiative 2010;943:206–230.
19. Melek SP, Norris DT, Paulus J. Economic Impact of Integrated Medical-Behavioral Healthcare: Implications for Psychiatry. Denver, CO: Milliman, Inc., 2014.
20. Kwan BM, Nease DE. The state of the evidence for integrated behavioral health in primary care. In Talen MR, Burke Valeras A, eds. Integrated Behavioral Health in Primary Care: Evaluating the Evidence, Identifying the Essentials. New York: Springer Science+Business Media, 2013:65–98.
21. Gerrity M, Zoller E, Pinson N, et al. Integrating Primary Care into Behavioral Health Settings: What Works for Individuals with Serious Mental Illness. New York: Milbank Memorial Fund, 2014.

22. Nielsen M, Gibson A, Buelt L, et al. The Patient-Centered Medical Home's Impact on Cost and Quality, Annual Review of Evidence 2013–2014. Patient-Centered Primary Care Collaborative, 2015. https://www.pcpcc.org/resource/patient-centered-medical-homes-impact-cost-and-quality-annual-review-evidence-2013-2014. Accessed June 16, 2016.
23. Strosahl K. New dimensions in behavioral health/primary care integration. HMO Prac. 1994;8(4):176–179.
24. Unutzer J, Katon W, Callahan CM, et al. Collaborative care management of late-life depression in the primary care setting: A randomized controlled trial. JAMA. 2002;288(22):2836–2845.
25. Katon W, Unutzer J, Wells KB, Jones L. Collaborative depression care: History, evolution and ways to enhance dissemination and sustainability. Gen Hosp Psychiatry. 2010;32(5):456–464. doi:10.1016/j.genhosppsych.2010.04.001.
26. Collins C, Hewson DL, Munger R, Wade T. Evolving Models of Behavioral Health Integration in Primary Care. New York: Milbank Memorial Fund, 2010.
27. Doherty WJ, McDaniel SH, Baird MA. Five levels of primary care/behavioral healthcare collaboration. Behavioral Healthcare Tomorrow. 1996;5(5):25–28.
28. Waxmonsky JA, Auxier A, Romero PW, Health B. Integrated Practice Assessment Tool, 2014. http://www.integration.samhsa.gov/operations-administration/IPAT_v_2.0_FINAL.pdf. Accessed June 6, 2016.
29. Martini R, Hilt R, Marx L, et al. Best principles for integration of child psychiatry into the pediatric health home. Am Acad Child Adolesc Psychiatry. 2012;52(1):1–5.
30. Alakson V, Frank RG, Katz RE. Specialty care medical homes for people with severe, persistent mental disorders. Health Affairs. 2010;29(5):867–873. doi:10.1377/hlthaff.2010.0080.
31. Butler TM, Yellowlees PM. Cost analysis of store-and-forward telepsychiatry as a consultation model for primary care. Telemed e-Health. 2012;18(1):74–77.
32. Butler M, Kane RL, McAlpine D, et al. Integration of Mental Health/Substance Abuse and Primary Care. Evidence Reports/Technology Assessments, No. 173. Rockville, MD: Agency for Healthcare Research and Quality, 2008. http://www.ncbi.nlm.nih.gov/books/NBK38632/. Accessed June 16, 2016.
33. McFeature B, Pierce TW. Primary care behavioral health consultation reduces depression levels among mood-disordered patients. J Health Disp Res Prac. 2011;5(2):36–44.
34. Woltmann E, Grogan-Kaylor A, Perron B, et al. Comparative effectiveness of collaborative chronic care models for mental health conditions across primary, specialty, and behavioral health care settings: Systematic review and meta-analysis. Am J Psychiatry. 2012;169(8):790–804. doi:10.1176/appi.ajp.2012.11111616.
35. Cohen D, Balasubramanian B, Davis M, et al. Understanding care integration from the ground up: Five organizing constructs that shape integrated practices. J Am Board Fam Med. 2015;28(Suppl):S7–S20. doi:10.3122/jabfm.2015.S1.150050.
36. Pescosolido B. The public stigma of mental illness: What do we think, what do we know, what can we prove? J Health Soc Behav. 2013;54(1):1–21. doi:10.1177/0022146512471197.
37. Porter ME, Lee TH. Why strategy matters now. N Engl J Med. 2015;372(18):1681–1684. doi:10.1056/NEJMp1502419.
38. Guerrero EG, Heslin KC, Chang E, et al. Organizational correlates of implementation of colocation of mental health and primary care in the Veterans Health Administration. Administration and Policy in Mental Health. 2015;42(4):420–428.
39. Reynolds K. Sustainability: Making Integrated Care Stick. 2013. http://www.integration.samhsa.gov/about-us/e-solutions. Accessed August 24, 2015.
40. Davis K, Schoebaum SC, Audet AM. A 2020 vision of patient-centered primary care. J Gen Intern Med. 2005;20(10):953–957. doi:10.1111/j.1525-1497.2005.0178.
41. Fortney JC, Jeffrey MP, Kimbrell TA, et al. Telemedicine-based collaborative care for posttraumatic stress disorder: A randomized clinical trial. J Am Med Assoc Psychiatry. 2015;72(1):58–67. doi:10.1001/jamapsychiatry.2014.1575.
42. Propp KM, Apker J, Aabava Ford WS, et al. Meeting the complex needs of the health care team: Identification of nurse-team communication practices perceived to enhance patient outcomes. Qual Health Res. 2010;20(1):15–28. doi:10.1177/1049732309355289.
43. Strosahl K. Building integrated primary care behavioral health delivery systems that work: A compass and a horizon. In: Cummings N, Cummings J, Johnson J, eds. Behavioral Health in Primary Care: A Guide for Clinical Integration. Madison, CT: Psychosocial Press; 1997:37–58.
44. Raney LE. Integrating primary care and behavioral health: The role of the psychiatrist in the collaborative care model. Am J Psychiatry. 2015;172(8):721–728. doi:10.1176/appi.ajp.2015.15010017.
45. Katon W, Robinson P, Von Korff M, et al. A multifaceted intervention to improve treatment of depression in primary care. Arch Gen Psychiatry. 1996;5(10):924–932.
46. Waugh M, Voyles D, Thomas MR. Telepsychiatry: Benefits and costs in a changing healthcare environment. Int Rev Psychiatry. 2015;2(6):558–568. doi:10.3109/09540261.2015.1091291.
47. Centers for Disease Control and Prevention. Up to 40 percent of annual deaths from each of five leading US causes are preventable. 2014. http://www.cdc.gov/media/releases/2014/p0501-preventable-deaths.html. Accessed January 4, 2016.

48. Committee on Population; Division of Behavioral and Social Sciences and Education; Board on Health Care Services; National Research Council; Institute of Medicine. Measuring the Risks and Causes of Premature Death: Summary of Workshops. Data from Major Studies of Premature Mortality. Washington DC: National Academies Press, 2015. http://www.ncbi.nlm.nih.gov/books/NBK279981/. Accessed June 6, 2016.
49. Friedli L. Mental Health, Resilience and Inequalities. World Health Organization (WHO) Regional Office for Europe, Copenhagen, Denmark, 2007.

2

Integrated Health Care at Cherokee Health Systems

PARINDA KHATRI, GREGG PERRY, AND FRANK V. deGRUY III, MD

BOX 2.1

KEY POINTS

- **Serving patients is our mission. Patients always point the way.**
- **Integrated behavioral health care is always rendered according to the principles of primary care.**
- **Work from careful financial models, but doing the right thing is always more important than making money.**
- **Contracting is a high-stakes game. Develop contracts that reward doing the right thing.**
- **Overcommunicate.**
- **Risk taking is encouraged. Try things.**
- **Developing the care model takes work. Just showing up is not enough.**
- **Close oversight is essential for high quality.**
- **Respond to problems quickly.**
- **Keep at it until the problem is solved. Persevere.**
- **Continuously reinforce successful changes.**
- **Extensive onboarding is expensive but worth it.**
- **Have fun.**

INTRODUCTION

History

From humble beginnings as the Mental Health Center of Morristown, Tennessee, in 1960, Cherokee Health Systems (CHS) has grown into a comprehensive health services organization throughout the Appalachian Mountain region of east Tennessee. Over the past 50 years, the need for quality health care in this region has fueled not only CHS's dramatic geographic growth but also the expansion of their deeply integrated scope of services. The range of staff expertise now includes behavioral health services and a highly original and effective network of medical, dental, pharmacy, social, and public health services. CHS's unique effectiveness, and the particular ways that they employ behavioral clinicians, can be better understood by first briefly tracing their history, then examining their current structure and organizational culture. An overview of the key elements of CHS's strategies can be found in Box 2.1.

For the first 15 years of its existence, CHS emphasized mental health services, first as the Mental Health Center of Morristown, then as the Cherokee Guidance Center, then as the Cherokee Mental Health Center. By 1980, school-based psychology services were established and primary care circuit rider outreach services had begun. In 1982, supervised housing was established for clients who needed structure and supervision, and the following year Cherokee's services merged with the Blaine Medical and Dental Board with the goal of bringing primary care to underserved populations. In 1984, the first Cherokee primary care clinic was established in Blaine, Tennessee.

This early move from behavioral health care into primary care can be understood as an inflection point in CHS's history and a defining element of its unique character to this day. In 1987, representatives from the federal government asked CHS to manage an existing health center. Later that year CHS opened a primary care office in Knoxville. Over the next few years, the organization continued to open additional integrated practices and in 1993 changed its name to Cherokee Health Systems to reflect its comprehensive mission of integrated primary and behavioral health care. Over the next seven years, all of Cherokee's clinics became integrated, after which additional services were added, including pediatrics and care for vulnerable populations (e.g., migrant health clinics and homeless clinics).

A significant event occurred in 2006 with the opening of a discount pharmacy in the Loudon County Clinic, Tennessee. The provision of affordable and available pharmacy services has become a hallmark of CHS and represents an additional dimension of comprehensiveness. The following year, in 2007, the Knox County Health Department transitioned their primary care services into CHS's Center City location, thereby incorporating public health resources into the fabric of care; that year also saw CHS become the East Tennessee Area Health Education Center (AHEC), thereby establishing an educational and workforce role. With the help of United Way funding, CHS developed a priority for the provision of comprehensive health care services for the uninsured in Knox County—a mission they have subsequently expanded to all sites.

By 2008, CHS had opened 18 school-based health clinics using telemedicine technology. Telemedicine has subsequently been a conspicuous, even a defining, feature of all of CHS's clinical programs, and in the next year CHS piloted two telepharmacy programs.

For the past eight years CHS has continued to expand its footprint throughout east Tennessee, from rural Appalachia to inner-city Knoxville, offering sustainable, comprehensive integrated health services to those most in need—the uninsured, the vulnerable, the homeless, refugees, the poor, and the sick. Such success is rare in this country. CHS has repeatedly been recognized nationally for the excellence of their telemedicine programs, for their contributions to the health of the needy in Tennessee, and as an exemplar for successful integrated services.[1]

Structure

Last year CHS rendered almost half a million services to 64,300 patients; 16,672 of these were new patients. They accomplish this in 51 integrated clinic settings and 21 school clinics. Table 2.1 lists CHS's clinical staff. The organizational structure of CHS is straightforward, as illustrated in Figure 2.1. In addition, each clinic has a clinical leader and a clinic manager.

Mission and Strategic Priorities

CHS's mission is "To enhance the quality of life of area residents through a comprehensive service delivery system that promotes mind and body wellness. To provide effective, collaborative and cooperative clinical, educational, preventive, community and management services in the context of financial stability and strength." Table 2.2 lists CHS's strategic priorities.

For more than 50 years, CHS has striven to serve all the people in east Tennessee, particularly those with insufficient health insurance and the medically underserved. Populations currently served include disadvantaged minority and urban

TABLE 2.1. STAFFING OF THE CHEROKEE HEALTH SYSTEMS

Roles	Number of Employees
Psychiatrists	9
Psychiatric nurse practitioners	9
Psychologists	54
Licensed clinical social workers	67
Primary care physicians	21
Primary care nurse practitioners/physician associates	41
Community workers	37
Pharmacists	11
Dentists	2
Cardiologists	1
Nephrologists	1
Obstetrician/gynecologists	1

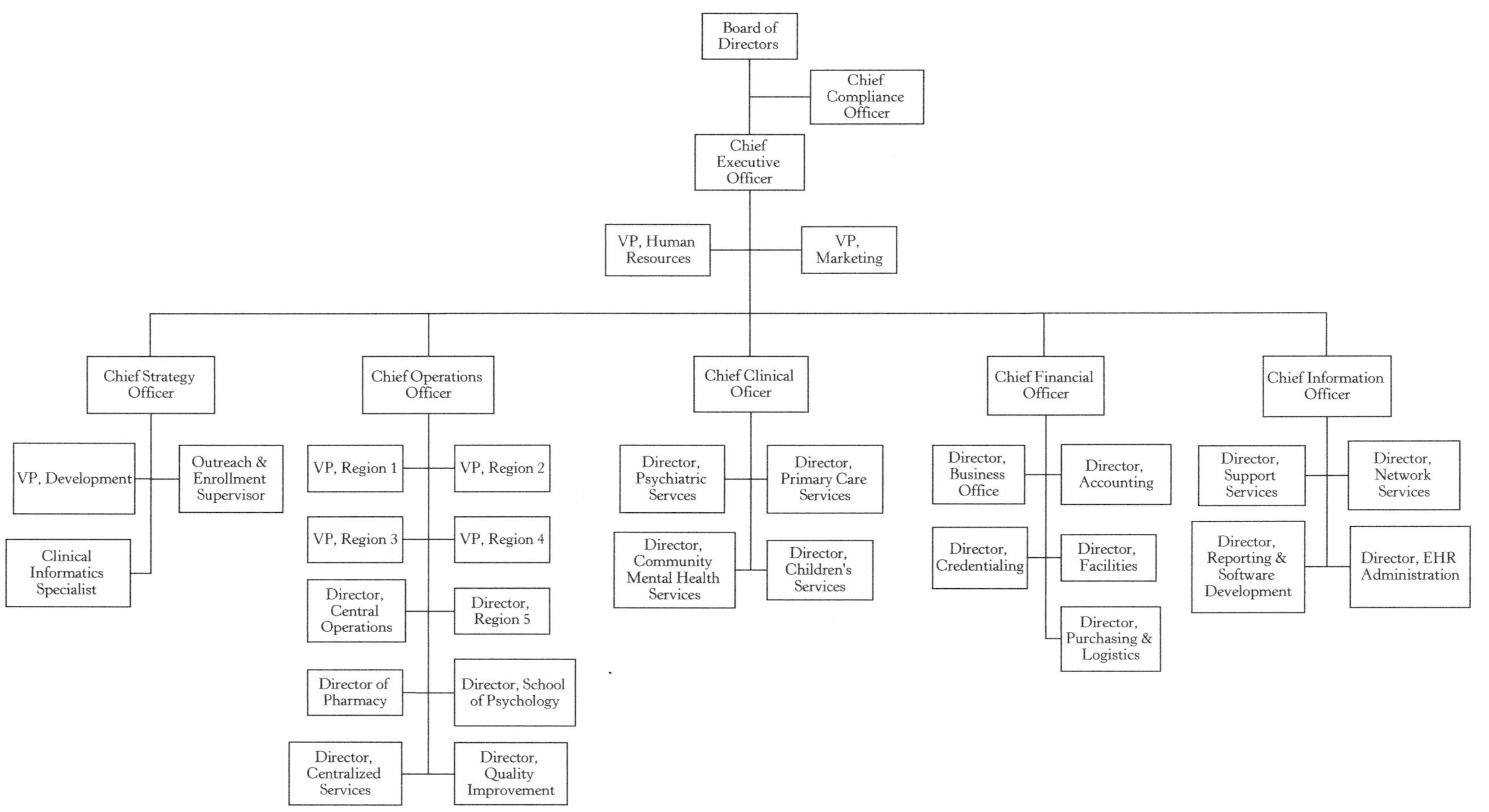

FIGURE 2.1: Organizational Structure of Cherokee Health Systems.

TABLE 2.2. CHEROKEE HEALTH SYSTEM STRATEGIC PRIORITIES

- Blending behavioral health and primary care
- Outreach to underserved populations
- Training of health care professionals
- Population-based care
- Telehealth applications
- School-based health services
- Safety-net preservation
- Value-based contracting

residents, refugees, homeless persons, and a growing Latino community. CHS has evolved into a nationally recognized leader in the training of clinicians in integrated care and the practice of integrated care. CHS is designated as a Federally Qualified Health Center (FQHC), reflecting the organization's commitment to serve the underserved, and indeed has further expanded those efforts through securing FQHC designation to serve special populations (e.g., migrant farm workers, the homeless, public housing residents).

The majority of CHS's patient population is low-income, rural, uninsured or underinsured, with complex medical conditions. These factors alone make the provision of comprehensive care challenging. Despite CHS's strong presence in east Tennessee, a shortage of health care professionals still exists in rural counties and low-income areas of Knox County. Accessing care can be a significant challenge. Even those with established primary or behavioral care struggle to keep appointments, understand their conditions, adhere to medication regimens, or make recommended changes in health behaviors. Geography, financial restrictions, lack of social support, lack of transportation, inclement weather, and psychiatric and medical problems prevent community residents from routinely participating in quality care. Low education and health illiteracy further reduce the likelihood that individuals will proactively care for their health. Whether patients face a few or many of these barriers, CHS endeavors to minimize their negative effects by offering comprehensive and integrated care services throughout east Tennessee. Telehealth, case management support, in-house pharmacies, and a wide range of physical and behavioral health treatment services are offered to meet patients where they live and, as in CHS's motto, "together, enhance life." To make treatment possible for those with limited financial resources, CHS offers a sliding-scale fee, special billing arrangements, medication samples, and support with pharmaceutical Patient Assistance Programs. Inability to pay is *never* a barrier. Community health coordinators, or case managers, are also available to help patients navigate barriers to treatment and to offer additional motivation for established treatment goals. To these ends, community health coordinators collaborate with homeless shelters, subsidized housing programs, food pantries, and other nonprofit community organizations who share the CHS mission.

As an AHEC, CHS is also committed to enhancing access to quality health care, particularly primary and preventive care, by improving the supply and distribution of health care professionals. CHS has an American Psychological Association–accredited psychology internship program and a postdoctoral fellowship program in psychology sponsored by the Association of Psychology Postdoctoral and Internship Centers. CHS not only trains graduate students in psychology doctoral programs (at the University of Tennessee and East Tennessee State University) but also offers clinical training to graduate social work students, undergraduate and graduate students in nursing, graduate pharmacy and nutrition students, and medical residents. In addition to a formal training relationship with the University of Tennessee's Department of Psychology, CHS has served as the outpatient placement site for family medicine residents from the University of Tennessee Medical Center and offers a training rotation for the University's behavioral medicine fellow. CHS also has training relationships with the University of Tennessee's departments of social work, nutrition, nursing, and pharmacy. Nursing students from Carson Newman University and King University also rotate through CHS clinics for training. Graduate students in pharmacy from South College are also trained through clinical placements with CHS. CHS has also participated in the Tennessee School Psychology Internship Consortium. Thus, CHS trains a multidisciplinary workforce in the principles and practice of comprehensive integrated primary care.

Values and Critical Success Factors

CHS attends to the clinical environment, organizational culture, principles of operation, and details of leadership, explicitly, repeatedly, and aggressively. Employees and volunteers can readily describe CHS's ethos, values, and core operating principles.

This common consciousness is thought by CHS's leaders to facilitate effective care, rewarding work, sustainability, and a dedicated workforce—to contribute, in other words, to their success. These environmental features of CHS are not captured by descriptions of team composition or workflows; they will be described on their own terms here in hopes of giving a feel for the environment in which these clinics operate. See Table 2.3 for a sample of what a visitor can hear in the halls and read on the walls from Cherokee's patients, supporters, and staff.

THE STRUCTURE AND LOGIC OF TEAM-BASED CARE

Guiding Principles

Integrated behavioral health care is always rendered as part of and according to the principles of primary care. This is a fundamental principle at CHS. That is, the behavioral clinicians, as members of a primary care team, are available as first-contact clinicians (accessible), are responsible for any problem

TABLE 2.3. CHEROKEE MISSION AND VISION: HEARD IN THE HALLS, READ ON THE WALLS

Our Vision: We will create a system of care that blends primary care and behavioral health, and as a result, we will improve the quality of life for our patients.

Our Mission: We are a mission-driven organization. Our clinical mission drives everything we do; it *always* has priority:

- Patients are at the center of everything we do.
- Access is a right, and we will strive to offer equal access for everyone.
- Health disparities are wrong, and we will eliminate them.
- We go where the grass is browner.
- We value wellness over health care.
- We believe in personal responsibility.
- We will create a common culture of values, behaviors, assumptions, and rules.
- Trusting each other is vital to our collective success. We practice trust.
- A group of people who have a family spirit can do amazing things together.
- Put others first. Big egos won't work, and don't belong here.
- People matter above all. There is healing power in relationship. We must connect with patients and each other in meaningful ways.
- Communities matter. Health is won and lost in the community. We will measure, account for, and use community factors, and will think population health.
- Our care will be synergistic. We will be greater than the sum of primary care plus behavioral health, by working well together.
- Over-communicate. Communicate continuously. Practice effective communication, accurate transmission of information—with patients and each other.
- We will adopt a culture of integration in all aspects of our organization.
- Integration serves our mission, but it is not our mission.
- Persistence pays off. Never give up on doing the right thing.
- We will measure our outcomes and results, and make them known to everyone.
- Stewardship is critical. We must do more with less.
- We will be fanatical, creative, and unrelenting about efficiency.
- We work from careful financial models, but doing the right thing is always more important than making money. "Do the right thing and the money will follow."
- The status quo is dangerous, so we need to be ready to change.
- Risk-taking is encouraged. Take the initiative and try things. Search for solutions. "Ready, fire, aim." Learn what works and adjust quickly. Experiment and fail fast.
- Fast, imperfect implementation trumps slow, careful planning.
- Have fun.

a patient may have (comprehensive), will organize and integrate all elements of care (coordinated), and will render this care in the context of a longitudinal partnership (continuous). Behavioral clinicians are obviously not able to meet these requirements alone, but they are personally responsible, as members of a patient's team, for ensuring that the care their team offers is in accordance with these principles of primary care.

Clinical Team Members and Their Clinical Functions

Primary Care Clinicians

Primary care clinicians (PCCs) assess and treat acute and chronic health problems with assistance from behavioral health consultants (BHCs) (generally clinical psychologists, who are also responsible for organizing primary care) or a behavioral health specialist (BHS) (generally psychiatrists or psychiatric nurse clinicians, who are pressed into service for special mental health problems), as indicated. PCCs organize a coherent, comprehensive care plan for a patient. They participate in preventive health interventions and population health initiatives.

Behavioral Health Consultants

BHCs, generally psychologists, assess and treat the behavioral dimension of all health problems and concerns. They communicate with prescribers to clarify diagnoses and unify treatment plans. They render behavioral interventions and treatments. They monitor symptoms and functioning and communicate, via the electronic health record (EHR) and other modalities as described later, concerns and progress to the medical providers.

Specialty Medical Providers

CHS has a limited number of medical specialists available as salaried staff; specialties include obstetrics/gynecology, cardiology, and nephrology. Other medical specialists are available by referral. Specialists respond to medical questions, concerns, and problems as requested, according to their expertise.

Psychiatrists

Psychiatrists and psychiatric nurse practitioners constitute the majority of the BHS workforce. While the psychiatric nurse practitioners are autonomous specialist clinicians, their care is supervised by the psychiatrist who directs psychiatric services. Psychiatrists clarify mental health diagnoses and offer psychotropic medication recommendations. They communicate with co-prescribers regarding medication concerns. They serve as specialty mental health clinicians, and sometimes temporarily assume full responsibility for the primary care of extremely symptomatic or unstable patients. Psychiatrists use telepsychiatry extensively for consultations with other clinicians and provide direct care for patients. The entire population of patients served by CHS is regarded as a primary care population, including those with severe, persistent, disabling mental illness, those in mobile crisis units or hospitals, and those whose defining health problems are psychiatric or involve abuse of substances. These patients require and receive the most expert care from fully trained psychiatrists, but this care is rendered in the context of comprehensive, integrated, team-based *primary care* that includes all the team members described in this section.

The psychiatrists' goals are, above all, to ensure that the psychiatric care that is rendered in all of CHS's settings is of the highest quality and is continuously improving. The psychiatrists are directly responsible for much, but not all, of this psychiatric care. It is the psychiatrists' responsibility to ensure that the PCCs and BHCs are rendering high-quality psychiatric care within the limits of their competence, and that their competence is continuously expanding. Psychiatrists ensure that the psychiatric medications prescribed for and dispensed to CHS's patients meet all criteria for clinical appropriateness and evidence-based care.

Nurses

Nurses identify and triage problems during visits and telephone consultations. They administer behavioral health screening tools. They coordinate with multidisciplinary staff to manage clinic workflow and coherent delivery of multiple services in a single visit.

Patient Services Representatives

Patient services representatives coordinate the scheduling of appointments. They obtain releases for information from outside agencies and coordinate the services with them.

Clinical Pharmacists

Clinical pharmacists dispense medications and educate patients and clinicians about their use and side effects. They develop and maintain an affordable, relatively comprehensive clinical pharmacy for patients.

Health Coaches

Health coaches are typically registered nurses who provide guidance and support for chronic care management and care coordination for the most medically complex patients. For example, recently hospitalized patients will meet with a health coach during a clinic visit following hospital discharge. A health coach helps run group medical visits for patients with diabetes and severe and persistent mental illness. See Chapter 25: Health Coaching in Integrated Care.

Community Health Coordinators

Community health coordinators work within the integrated team to help patients access social service resources, outreach into the community, and build self-sufficiency skills. About half their time is spent outside the clinic—in the community, in homes, under bridges, in the jails, and elsewhere.

Features of the Clinical Encounter

Visits and other encounters are not strictly structured according to a prearranged schedule, although careful attention to scheduling is a conspicuous feature of clinical care. Encounters are planned, but extreme flexibility is part of that planning. Time, content, site of service, and which team members are pressed into play are all adjusted according to the patient's needs as they arise before and during an encounter. While it is true that individual team members have specific job descriptions and particular areas of expertise, mature team members frequently "bleed" into each other's territory. General care delivery is shared across a team, and individuals take up each other's responsibilities and tasks when it is easier or more efficient and makes sense to do so. Behavioral health clinicians, either a BHC or less frequently a BHS, are pressed into service whenever behavioral problems show up, whether it is in the middle of an encounter arranged for an acute or chronic medical problem, during an unscheduled visit, on a telephone call for an accident or for a family crisis. Clinical encounters at CHS are typically characterized by the involvement of more than one clinician, by explicit attention to coordinating services among clinicians, by *very* high levels of flexibility, and by communication and documentation across multiple modalities (e.g., face to face, telephone, telehealth, and EHR). Encounters are also typically characterized by the mobilization of community-based resources that foster patient access (e.g., transportation, home visits). PCCs have office schedule templates that consist of new visits and return visits of predetermined length, with time built into daily schedules for huddles, ad hoc communication about unanticipated problems, and care plan coordination meetings. Time is monitored and adjusted on a continuous basis so that workflow remains efficient and all important tasks can be addressed. The behavioral clinicians are scheduled even more flexibly than the PCCs, with half or less of their time organized into short (usually 15 minutes) appointment slots with most of the remainder unscheduled, so they are available for consultation as needed, during and between visits, without delay.

Structure of the Clinical Model

The fundamental approach to care at each CHS clinic, as well as of the system as a whole, is to help the entire population. All the people living in and around their catchment area, whether or not they are established patients, have the opportunity to become healthier. CHS does this by providing health care to all residents who want it and by partnering with others (e.g., other health care professionals, public health, the criminal justice system, schools, food banks) in the community dedicated to improving health. This is a population health approach. Everyone working at CHS has a direct responsibility to strive to improve the health of their population. This means that all clinicians must respond to anyone who reaches out for help with his or her health, either directly and personally, or by finding a partner in their system equipped to do so, or by finding community resources equipped to do so. Every patient has a primary care team, as described below, and every team contains three or four primary care clinicians, a BHC (usually a psychologist), a consulting psychiatrist or psychiatric nurse practitioner available part-time, and others as specified below. A given panel of patients is shared by this team, who also share the health goals for this population of patients. The support staff works out the clinical workflow for this panel of patients together and shares a common physical space. This primary care team is responsible for co-management and care coordination of *all* the health-related problems that occur within this panel of patients. They share clinical documentation through a common record and plan treatment together.

Structure of Psychiatric Care

Psychiatric care is implemented using six strategies:

1. Patients are granted fast-track direct access to a psychiatrist for consultation and stabilization, as needed.
2. A psychiatrist is always immediately available to the primary and BHCs by telephone or telemed access for consultation.
3. Patients can be triaged directly to a psychiatrist for specialty psychiatric care.
4. Patients' care plans are discussed in concert with the psychiatrist at treatment team discussions.
5. The psychiatrists can co-manage patients with their primary care or behavioral care team members.
6. Psychiatrists educate and train the other clinicians via precepting sessions, formal didactics, continuing medical education sessions, and clinical case presentations.

Psychiatrists have other responsibilities as well: to supervise psychiatric nurse practitioners, to lead behavioral teams, to develop protocols and critical pathways, and to implement new guidelines and recommendations. It should be noted that the psychiatric team has developed a set of guidelines, ranging from arrangements for a telepsychiatry consultation to recommendations about the use of antidepressant medications or the management of attention-deficit/hyperactivity disorder. The implementation of these guidelines requires that the psychiatrist has competence as a leader of a team within a complex adaptive system, familiarity with the workflow of patients through the clinic system, and acquaintance with the roles and competencies of the other team members who are participating in the implementation effort.

With respect to system strategies for managing population health, CHS's approach is multimodal. The clinical leadership team (directors of primary care, psychiatry, community mental health, integrative services) works together to build and sustain a model of care that prioritizes access, clinical quality, and efficiency for the individuals and families in the communities served. From an operational perspective, the administrative team helps to bring clinical analytics to support this approach (e.g., data on access, clinical quality metrics, and complexity assessments based on biological, psychological, and social factors). No one discipline or service develops an independent management strategy.

PSYCHIATRIC TREATMENT PATHWAYS AND THE PRACTICE OF INTEGRATED CARE AT CHS

A set of clinical pathways has emerged that fits the needs of the CHS patient population and that makes use of the front-line PCCs and BHCs, who provide about 80% of the behavioral health care.

Pathway A: The Patient Is Managed in Primary Care

The patient may have an appointment with the PCC and a behavioral issue will emerge. The PCC will consult with the BHC, who will see the patient. If necessary, at this point, the BHC will consult a psychiatrist for diagnostic clarification, medication recommendations, or management advice. The psychiatrist may or may not see the patient via telehealth but will make recommendations at the point of care to the BHC, who will discuss these recommendations with the PCC. These recommendations will be incorporated into the patient's care plan, and ongoing behavioral management will occur concurrently with the PCC, the BHC, and the psychiatrist.

Pathway B: The Patient Is Managed Briefly by the Psychiatrist, then Returned to Primary Care with a Care Plan

The protocol begins as Pathway A, but the psychiatrist may decide that the patient would be best served by several psychiatric visits. This is arranged by direct face-to-face contact or telepsychiatry, with ongoing communication with the PCC and the BHC, until the patient is stable. After the patient is stabilized, the patient is returned to the primary care setting for continuity follow-up care, with ongoing psychiatric consultation as needed.

Pathway C: The Patient Is Managed by the Psychiatrist Long Term

This pathway begins as Pathway B does, but the psychiatrist decides that ongoing psychiatric care is indicated. In this case, the patient can be seen directly by the psychiatrist as long as necessary. The psychiatrist will continuously consult with the PCC for ongoing medical monitoring if necessary. For a review of 2013 calendar year data of BHC/psychiatric consultation in primary care across all CHS sites, see Box 2.2.

BOX 2.2

DATA ON BEHAVIORAL HEALTH CONSULTANTS/PSYCHIATRIC CONSULTATION IN PRIMARY CARE ACROSS ALL CHEROKEE SITES (2013)

- **Of patients who had contact with a behavioral health consultant (BHC), 71% involved documented collaboration with another discipline or provider (e.g., psychiatry, primary care clinician).**
- **Of patients who had contact with a BHC, 6% involved consultation with a psychiatric provider (psychiatrist or psychiatric nurse practitioner).**
- **Of patients who saw a BHC, 4% required a face-to-face visit with a psychiatric provider.**
- **Of patients who had contact with a BHC, 59% were also taking psychotropic medications.**

Box 2.2 data indicate that there is a high level of collaboration between BHCs and other providers, and that BHCs consult with psychiatric providers on less than 10% of the patients they see. When they do consult, only a small percentage actually see a psychiatric provider face to face, even though over half of all BHC patients are taking psychotropic medications. These data support the efficiency of a model that relies primarily on embedded BHCs to triage and manage psychiatric issues in primary care, with psychiatric consultation structured so that most patients' psychiatric problems and medications are managed in the primary care setting. Psychiatrists are precious resources in the CHS system, and the efficient use of the full range of their expertise across the roles described permits a very large number of patients to benefit from their care.

Special Place for Telepsychiatry

Over the past 17 years, CHS has developed an active and nationally recognized telehealth program to provide access to care for underserved communities. For example, in 2009, CHS was awarded the Honors Program Laureate for TeleHealth by Computer World. All CHS clinics are wired with high-speed communication lines and telemedicine equipment. CHS can provide telemedicine services for both primary care and behavioral health visits utilizing Polycom video infrastructure and AMD Global Medicine telemedicine instruments. CHS's telehealth equipment includes Polycom High Definition Video Codecs, AMD Stethoscopes, AMD Camera Illumination Systems, AMD Ear Nose and Throat Scopes, AMD General Exam Cams, and 32 high-definition monitors. Additional equipment includes a Polycom Video Bridge, Polycom video border proxies, and Polycom Real Presence desktop clients.[2]

CHS provides ongoing telehealth services for primary care, psychiatry, and behavioral health to most of its clinics in both rural and inner-city communities. Currently, 10 providers (psychiatrists, psychiatric nurse practitioners, family nurse practitioners, primary care physicians, and psychologists) offer care via telemedicine, with reports of high patient satisfaction. CHS also provides school-based telemedicine healthcare to 21 schools in rural east Tennessee and physically operates school-based clinics in two schools in rural communities. CHS's mobile crisis team uses telehealth services at local hospitals in Jefferson County, Cocke County, and Claiborne County to conduct crisis assessments and interventions. Similarly, telehealth services also support aftercare planning. Cherokee community health coordinators bring telehealth equipment directly to patients being discharged from Ridgeview Psychiatric Hospital to facilitate interviews with CHS clinicians so that posthospitalization treatment continues seamlessly. Finally, clinical pharmacists offer medication counseling at the time of prescription fulfillment in remote clinics via telehealth.

CHALLENGES IN IMPLEMENTING THE MODEL

Recruiting Health Professionals

Because of normal retirement and other turnover, and especially because of CHS's dramatic expansion, Cherokee is continually recruiting clinicians. Each discipline poses specific challenges and difficulties, based on national and local workforce production, pay and benefits, the fit between professional training and actual job requirements, the quality of life in east Tennessee, and a host of other variables. All health care positions require active recruiting; few clinicians spontaneously seek employment at CHS, even though job satisfaction is very high for almost all clinicians once acculturated and established in the system. Some clinicians are much more difficult to recruit and retain than others. From least to most difficult to recruit, the list looks like this: family nurse practitioners, psychologists, social workers, family physicians, psychiatric nurse practitioners, psychiatrists, and dentists. While it is beyond the purview of this chapter to speculate on national workforce production or the particulars of psychiatric training, CHS has extensive direct experience recruiting, hiring, onboarding, acculturating, and training over 35 psychiatrists and hundreds of other clinicians to work in its system.

All clinicians at CHS are salaried, and these salaries are somewhat lower than comparable positions in private practice or government positions such as the Veterans Administration. Most applicants, irrespective of discipline, understand that CHS is a safety-net organization, and salaried positions below median community levels are not unexpected.

As previously described, CHS's population-health model and team-based approach to care are not necessarily standard practice across the nation, but recruits in some disciplines have less trouble than others accepting and adjusting to this model of care. More and more frequently family nurse practitioners, psychologists, social workers, and family physicians are emerging from their training programs with exposure to the principles of population health and the practice of team-based care and are relatively comfortable accepting practice under such conditions. Psychiatrists across more than a score of training programs have little or no experience working in a setting where access, comprehensiveness of care, longitudinal responsibility for patients, coordination of whole-person care, collaboration (e.g., shared documentation, communication, and co-management) with a range of clinicians from different disciplines, and population health are a priority; substantial additional training is frequently necessary for psychiatrists. Dentists do not even know what these concepts mean and always require extensive additional training. For this reason, all new hires at CHS undergo a 16-week onboarding process before seeing and billing for their first patient. During this four months of additional training, they shadow all members of the care team, learn the roles and functions of each, follow patients through the system, study clinical workflows and billing practices, and generally acculturate to CHS's unique team-based shared-care model. New clinicians do not bill for any services until this 16-week onboarding experience is completed.

CHS believes that it is possible to leverage psychiatrists and extend the reach of psychiatric expertise to many more patients who need accurate diagnosis and appropriate management by operating in partnership with primary care teams, and by addressing even the most advanced psychiatric conditions in the context of a primary care model of practice. Psychiatrists who have consultation-liaison experience or psychiatric emergency expertise or who have worked in reverse integrated-care settings (primary psychiatric services with embedded primary care) generally have some sense of how to work in this setting, have some exposure to medical settings, and sometimes have been exposed to collaborative problem solving, but this does not adequately prepare clinicians with the breadth and depth of teaching skill, professional communication, co-management, flexibility, and interprofessional collaboration required for primary care consultation, nor does it obviate the need for extensive onboarding to acquire familiarity with this demanding and deeply complex kind of primary care and psychiatric practice. The principal difference with this approach is that treatment is rendered by a team, with the most relevant members of the team seeing the patient on an as-needed basis.

The flexibility required in primary care consultation is a novel demand for most of the psychiatrists who begin working at CHS. Some of these new hires have difficulty giving up a more orderly practice structure with a fixed and predictable schedule (e.g., with a preset number of follow-ups per day, a fixed number of new patients per day, return visits for medication management every 4 to 6 weeks). Psychiatrists at CHS must be available at the point of care, at the time of need, for the PCC, the BHC, and the patient. This produces a schedule that is highly variable and unpredictable both in times of availability and in content from one day to the next; the actual schedule rarely goes according to plans. It also means that CHS psychiatrists sometimes juggle several patient issues at once. A new patient is more likely to be first encountered during a primary care visit, during which a quick assessment and initial plan is formulated, either in person, by telephone, or via telepsychiatry. "Just schedule a new patient appointment" is not an acceptable response to the primary care team.

Psychiatrists' patient panels are quite large; schedules are not fixed, as they need to flex according to problems that arise unexpectedly; and the context—other social and medical considerations in which psychiatric problems are solved—is consistently broader and more complex than customary solo psychiatric practice. In other words, the consulting psychiatrist working as part of a primary care team will accept that all patients on the primary care panel are also on his or her panel, whether the psychiatrist has previously seen them or not. If a patient has a need that he or she can best meet, the psychiatrist will help meet that need when it first arises. Furthermore, it means that as a fully vested member of a primary care team, the psychiatrist will be responsible to all team members and generally does not work alone with the door closed. It should be noted that these conditions pertain to all members of the primary care team, and some members have more difficulty adjusting to these conditions than others.

The Skill Set of the Psychiatrist Needs to Be Extremely Broad

As previously described, the psychiatrist must not only diagnose and manage psychiatric problems but must also synthesize a breadth of information to ensure that the work is done in the context of other medical problems and family and social issues, and do this quickly and sometimes with incomplete or changing information. It also means that the psychiatrist's scope of practice will include prevention, at-risk intervention, and co-management of a patient's comprehensive health and wellness. The psychiatrist will share responsibility for this panel's *overall* health and functioning. Thus, tobacco cessation, obesity management, and support for chronic health problems like diabetes will be part of the expected scope of psychiatric practice. Finally, teaching will be a core element of the job. This means recognizing the level of readiness of other team members to take on psychiatric issues, such as comfort level with prescribing antidepressants, and facilitating learning at the top edge of this zone of professional development. Each case discussed, each conversation, each encounter is an opportunity to transmit information to other team members and to share "pearls" for practice.

THE KEYS TO SUCCESS

The successful integration of clinicians into a team, exercising all the skills described, does not occur automatically. CHS's ability to create teams that address this population's health needs have been the subject of much reflection and study and can be summarized by the following principles and quotations from CHS staff.

Leadership

Leadership occurs at the level of the chief executive leaders, the service line directors, and the clinical teams. The upper echelon of leaders seems to operate according to the principles of complex adaptive leadership,[3] although these principles have been acquired through empirical application—trial and error—and not as a matter of a priori strategic planning or design. For example, the chief executive officer describes his principal functions as speaking the vision, finding resources, recruiting talent, and then staying out of their way. Speaking the vision means not only describing what CHS will be and will do for the people in east Tennessee, but describing what integrated care looks like there. The chief financial officer (CFO) understands the details of clinical operations, negotiates complex contracts, and knows what it takes to accomplish successful clinical care, but also advocates for the primacy of the mission: "Accomplish the mission, and the money will follow." At the level of the clinical teams, a culture of reciprocal responsibility and accountability, flexible problem solving, and shared success prevails: "We never do this solo. We always approach problems as a team."

Close Oversight

All components of care, and operations, are under continuous, constructive scrutiny: "Our care is usually excellent, but can always be better. We will make it better together." CHS has built systems that ensure close clinical and operational oversight. For example, there are clinical quality improvement programs in place that involve peer review; a systematic review of outcomes data across disease and whole-patient outcomes; and cost reports. Every clinician gets an emailed report by 7 a.m. with a list of patients coming in that day, with any care gaps. Patient registries are used for specific diseases, and clinician and clinic dashboards are regularly produced and pushed to clinicians, clinics, and system leaders.

Continuous Reinforcement

Finding a solution to a problem is only the first step to solving the problem. The solution must be refined and consolidated by ongoing reinforcement, or previous patterns will return. Just as described by Lencioni,[4] teams that function well hold each other accountable for their outcomes. The most mission-concordant outcomes are measured and reported behind every problem that is solved, and this measure of success (or lack thereof) is reinforcing. There are no financial rewards for success.

Creative Approach to Problem Solving

"Problems are always coming at us out of left field, and we are used to having to think out of bounds to solve a problem, so we will shed attachments to a specific way of doing things." CHS describes itself as in a continuous state of alpha and beta testing, and staff members are trained to bring two or three possible solutions to every problem-solving conversation. Rapid-cycle problem solving, with many mistakes and failures, is a normal pathway to a solution. All members of the team are encouraged to participate in solving problems, and those doing the actual work are expected to have the best ideas about how to solve problems around that work. CHS lives on very thin margins, and a constant awareness of this fact imbues problem solving with a certain sense of urgency and importance.

Respond to Problems Quickly and Iteratively

Things are always going wrong—it's the nature of complex systems. "We try to act fast, recognizing that there is no perfect solution, and knowing that we are OK with failing and going to plan B, C, or D, as needed." Clinical teams have mini-huddles every day before patient care begins and weekly treatment team problem-solving meetings. These meetings are critical. Also, shared clinical space facilitates deeper communication and better problem solving. The EHR is also a medium for regular problem solving.

Persistence

"Most people would call our persistence delusional, given the setbacks we have faced. We *never* give up on trying to solve important problems." The entire organization takes inspiration from senior leadership on this point, where persistent pressure on the state legislature or the city council, sometimes for years on end, eventually wins a change in a bus stop or telepharmacy laws. The entire organization is accustomed to and tolerant of a high failure rate and views each failure as containing an important lesson. Part of the onboarding acculturation is to reassure new employees that they will not be penalized for trying and failing to solve a problem. It is considered more of a failure to not try to solve a problem.

Recruit for Fit, and Don't Take Those Who Don't Fit. Release Those Who Cannot Adapt

"If you want a private office with your name on the door, this is not the place for you." "If you aren't comfortable having every element of your care under scrutiny and shared by all your team members, this is not the place for you." "If you are uncomfortable with unpredictability, this is not the place for you."

Grow Our Own

It is not possible to hire clinicians who have been trained to practice according to the conventions at CHS. Therefore CHS has developed a 16-week extensive and protracted onboarding process, previously described. "We have had to train psychiatric providers, including psychiatric nurse practitioners, to provide fast, flexible consultation to primary care."

Detailed and Ever-Changing Job Descriptions

While the work requires flexibility and creative problem solving, the job descriptions are detailed. This is a reflection of the respect for a disciplined, close understanding of workflow and the relative contributions various team members make to successful workflow. Job descriptions are developed in collaboration with CHS's human resources office and the discipline director or clinic leader. They are updated as necessary. CHS clinicians and clinics are covered by the Federal Tort Claims Act,[5] and therefore the standards for credentialing, privileging, peer review, patient safety, and clinical quality control are stringent. The Bureau of Primary Care, in particular, is very strict about job descriptions, scope of practice, credentialing, and privileging.

Do Whatever It Takes to Make It Work

"We will revise job descriptions, create new job categories, tear out walls, advocate for legislative changes—whatever it takes to do our work better. Nothing is off limits." Problems are solved at the lowest possible level; for example, minor workflow problems might be solved by the staff person who

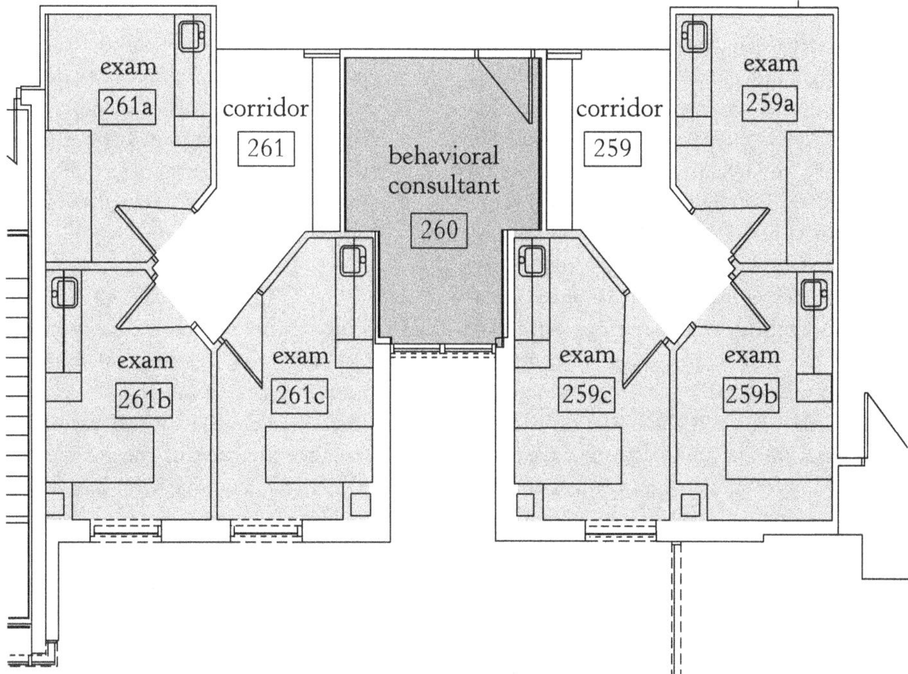

FIGURE 2.2: Patient care workspace with embedded behavioral health consultant.

rooms a patient or by the scheduling clerk. More substantial problems, such as relocating a child waiting room or adding a new clinical service, might require that midlevel or senior-level leadership gets involved. These problems are addressed in the leadership setting to which they rise, if not solved closer to the ground.

Four Breakthrough Innovations

A few dramatic innovations deserve emphasis.

Telehealth

The ability to leverage technology for clinical consultation and patient care across 13 counties has been an absolute game changer. CHS has been an early adopter of this technology and has invested in state-of-the-art equipment and methods.

Developing Behavioral Health Clinicians Trained to Support Psychiatric Consultation in Primary Care

This is a very high-profile agenda item that has received much attention and investment. Behavioral resources, particularly psychiatric resources, are precious; they are continuously scrutinized and optimized to maximize their value and effectiveness.

Electronic Health Record

All team members have access to a useful and shared EHR (NextGen[6], with major modifications and add-ons) via laptops, telephones, and clinical workstations. Team members conduct high-bandwidth conversations and consultations via the EHR. The EHR also connects to outside entities. This has been very expensive to create and maintain.

Pay Attention to the Physical Workspace

Much thought goes into the physical relationship of patients to their clinicians,[7] and of clinicians to each other and to other nonclinical staff. Space is constantly being adjusted and remodeled to optimize team functioning and efficient workflow. PCCs and BHCs are always scheduled together, and the clinical space is arranged so that they can easily see one another and immediately discuss patients together. Figure 2.2 illustrates a typical patient care workspace for two PCCs and a BHC.

FINANCING

A high proportion of CHS's patients are financially disadvantaged, have complex health problems, or both. This requires a highly disciplined approach to the financial management of the organization. CHS's mission-driven philosophy shapes not only the approach to the design of clinical services, but also the approach to finances. With the guiding mantra of "Do the right thing and the money will follow," CHS's leadership has positioned the organization to negotiate contracts that favor its chosen model of care. As a FQHC and licensed Community Mental Health Center, CHS is eligible for enhanced reimbursement for patients with TennCare (Tennessee's equivalent of a state Medicaid program). However, with a large uninsured and underinsured population of patients, and the ever-changing health care climate, CHS has had to be imaginative, aggressive, thoughtful, and persistent in order to maintain financial strength with their comprehensive model of care. The organization has effectively executed a successful funding model that prioritizes clinical goals through a combination of strategies, including (1) a deliberate organizational expansion to increase negotiating power with payers; (2) seeking global, risk-based funding streams (in contrast to fee for service), such as capitation, percent of premium, and case rates, to allow for flexibility in clinical practices; (3) consistent and obsessively vigilant management of internal costs and efficiency; (4) data tracking to quantify the value of an integrated model of care on cost and quality of care; and (5) close collaboration between the CFO, financial staff, and clinicians to structure funding in alignment with clinical practice goals. Having a CFO who understands integration has been critical in effectively building a financially sustainable model of care.

Here are several examples of CHS's approach to finances:

- CHS's CFO, after learning of the frequent provider-to-provider consultations to support patient care, searched for billing codes that would capture this valuable clinical activity. He was able to find a care coordination "G-Code" that he subsequently included in several major payment contracts. Thus, rather than directing clinicians to focus solely on billable visits, he focused on finding an alternative funding model to support collaboration between providers.
- CHS has calculated that the efficient use of BHCs in the course of "ordinary" pediatric well-child care visits enables the PCCs to see about one additional patient per hour; even in a fee-for-service system, this generates sufficient revenue to carry the entire cost of the BHCs' salaries.
- CHS negotiated, for over a year, with state lawmakers to win the ability to conduct prescription counseling via video, thus vastly improving the efficiency and reducing the cost of prescription dispensing across their network of practices, even while improving the quality of patients' education about their medication.

CONCLUSION

CHS is the dominant health care provider in east Tennessee and has enjoyed steady growth for 30 years. It is a deeply integrated, comprehensive care system that continuously revises its services and structure in accordance with the needs of the people it serves. CHS has a unique team-based, population health approach that produces high-quality care for vulnerable populations. The standard training that health professionals receive does not prepare them for practice at CHS, and extensive onboarding is necessary to acculturate them to this kind of care. While CHS's clinical care is driven by standard evidence-based guidelines, the overall approach to care, the constitution of teams, and the evolving clinical structure have been developed in response to the local needs and problems that have emerged over time, and not by an empirical literature.

REFERENCES

1. A Guidebook of Professional Practices for Behavioral Health and Primary Care Integration. Observations from Exemplary Sites. AHRQ Publication No. 14-0070-1-EF, 2015. https://integrationacademy.ahrq.gov/sites/default/files/AHRQ_AcademyGuidebook.pdf. Accessed April 15, 2016.
2. http://www.amd.com/en-us. Accessed June 4, 2016
3. Uhl-Bien M, Marion R, McKelvey B. Complexity leadership theory: shifting leadership from the industrial age to the knowledge era. Leadership Quarterly. 2007;18(4):298–318.
4. Lencioni P. Overcoming the Five Dysfunctions of a Team. A Field Guide for Leaders, Managers, and Facilitators. San Francisco: Jossey-Bass, 2006.
5. U.S. Department of Health and Human Services Health Resources and Service Administration Website. Federal Tort Claims Act. http://www.bphc.hrsa.gov/ftca/about/index.html. Accessed June 6, 2016.
6. NextGen Healthcare Information Systems. https://www.nextgen.com/. Accessed June 6, 2016.
7. Gunn R, Davis MM, Hall J, et al. Designing clinical space for the delivery of integrated behavioral health and primary care. J Am Board Family Practice 2015;28(Supplement 1):S52–S62.

3

Canadian Approach to Integrated Care

NICK KATES AND ELLEN ANDERSON

BOX 3.1

KEY POINTS

- **The past 20 years have seen a significant expansion in collaborative activities between primary care and mental health.**
- **Providers, planners, and funders are now considered to be an integral part of an integrated practice. An increasing number of family physicians have mental health professionals and psychiatrists working as part of the team.**
- **A collaborative model has been used to address the needs of many diverse and traditionally underserved populations.**
- **There are many adjustments any mental health services can make to work more collaboratively with primary care.**

INTRODUCTION

Canada has a federal government with limited responsibilities for health care (mainly health education and health care for the military, prisoners, and First Nations). Most health care is delivered by its 10 provinces and three territories, each of which has its own health care system and priorities, within a common framework laid down by the Canada Health Act. Proclaimed in 1964 and reaffirmed in 1984, The Canada Health Act identifies the five principles on which Canada's health care system is based: accessibility, universality, portability, public administration, and comprehensiveness. Each province's health care is funded on a cost-shared basis, although the contribution of the federal government has shrunk from 50%, when Medicare was established in 1964, to less than 20%. In most provinces, health care consumes about 40% of total provincial spending.

The Canadian health care system is committed to "cradle to grave," 24/7 integrated physical and mental health care developed from within a primary care home.[1] Consequently, primary care is the place where the majority of mental health and substance use care is delivered, often without the involvement of specialized mental health providers. As in most other countries, up to 70% of individuals with a mental health or addiction problem in Canada will receive no treatment over the course of a year, although over 80% of these individuals will visit their family physicians in the same timeframe. This suggests that primary care is the best and perhaps the only place to detect many of these problems and to initiate treatment.

For almost 20 years, mental health and primary care services and providers have been rethinking their relationship, how they work together, and the roles each can play in a better-integrated and coordinated system. The goals are to improve access to care, maintain quality, and ensure that individuals reach the services they need when they need them.

In 1997, the Canadian Psychiatric Association (CPA) and the College of Family Physicians of Canada (CFPC) published a joint position paper to promote collaboration between the two sectors.[2]

This position paper made the case that psychiatrists and family physicians need to improve collaboration and outlined principles to guide integrated care (or shared care as it was previously named). This paper also highlighted examples of ways to improve collaboration, emphasized the importance of training future practitioners in these models, and outlined the benefits of collaboration for underserved communities and populations. The two organizations then set up a conjoint national working group to oversee the implementation of the ideas in the position paper. This working group continues to meet regularly to promote system change with the ongoing support of the CPA and the CFPC.

In the 19 years since that first report, psychiatrists and other mental health providers have routinely collaborated with primary care colleagues. Provincial Ministries of Health Primary Care and Mental Health planners are working together, developing and funding integrated projects, either as single entities or as part of a more comprehensive provincial strategy. These projects include the Centres de Santé et de Services Sociaux in Quebec, Family Health Teams in Ontario (FHTs), Primary Care Networks in Alberta, and the Practice Support Program in British Columbia. These programs have all demonstrated improvements in access to services, reduced waiting times, and high levels of patient satisfaction with the services provided.

A major boost for multiple collaborative care projects was provided by two Federal Primary Care Innovation Funds at the beginning of the 21st century. One of these projects was the Canadian Collaborative Mental Health Initiative (CCMHI), which brought together 12 national organizations representing providers, consumers, and family members. By 2006, the CCHMI had laid down a conceptual framework for collaborative care, completed a comprehensive review of the existing literature, and developed web-based toolkits to guide the implementation of Collaborative Mental Health Care (CMHC) in general settings and for specific populations. This period also saw an expansion of collaborative partnerships, bringing together a broader range of health professionals, including nurses, psychologists, social workers, pharmacists, and occupational therapists. Of significance, these partnerships also included consumers and families, which was an important step in the greater acceptability of CMHC across the health care system.

Other changes have supported the growth of collaborative care:

1. Provinces have introduced changes in their billing tariffs to support telephone consultations between psychiatrists and family physicians.
2. The Canadian Medical Protective Association (professional insurance organization) has acknowledged that informal case discussions (corridor or curbside consultations) should be encouraged, as long as accepted standards of care for each discipline are followed.
3. In 2010, the Royal College of Physicians and Surgeons of Canada made training in collaborative care a routine requirement for all psychiatry residents, while the College of Family Physicians of Canada has introduced a new "Triple C" (Comprehensive education, Continuity of education, and Centered in family medicine) curriculum that emphasizes the integration of mental health care as a core practice into every family physician's practice.
4. In 2014, the Canadian Medical Association, in partnership with the Canadian Psychiatric Association, the Canadian College of Family Physicians, and the Mental Health Commission of Canada, produced a paper using the CanMEDS framework to outline mental health core competencies that all physicians, in all specialties, should acquire during their training.[3]

In 2011, these collaborative activities and changes led the CPA and CFPC to produce a second position paper[4] which presented the following: (1) summarized the evidence regarding the success of CMHC, (2) noted the key components of effective collaboration, (3) highlighted examples of successful models in Canada and elsewhere, (4) presented a framework for an integrated mental health and primary care system, with suggestions for ways to improve collaboration, and (5) pointed out the importance of additional and broader system changes to support collaborative care. These changes included academic departmental support of collaborative care experiences for residents in their training programs, provincial governments funding new projects, and developing billing tariffs that support collaborative activity, and national and provincial professional associations promoting collaboration among their members.

CANADIAN APPROACH TO COLLABORATIVE CARE

For a summary and overview of the Canadian framework for collaborative care see Table 3.1.

A Definition of Collaborative Mental Health Care

The 2011 position paper[4] proposed the following widely accepted definition for collaborative mental health care: "an evolving partnership between two or more stakeholders (including patients and families) characterized by common goals or purpose; recognition and respect for strengths and differences; shared and effective decision making; clear and regular communication, to help ensure that all patients reach the right service, from the right provider, in the right location, at the right time."

Guiding Principles of Collaborative Mental Health Care Initiatives

Whatever the setting or focus, successful projects invariably share a number of features. In order for an initiative to thrive, it needs to be based upon principles which guide effective collaborative partnerships, rather than transplanting an external model from the outside. Among the key principles, the relationship between individual providers requires mutual respect and support, recognition of each other's strengths and limitations, and the need for ongoing personal contact between providers working in different settings. Coordination between services should be centered on the needs of patients and their families, regular two-way communication between providers, a willingness on the part of all partners to make adjustments, sharing the responsibility for care, an agreement between services on the goals of the initiative, and ensuring that models of care respond to local needs and demands.[4]

TABLE 3.1. THE CANADIAN FRAMEWORK FOR COLLABORATIVE CARE

1. A shared definition of collaborative care.
2. Common principles to guide any collaborative project.
3. A shared vision of the potential roles of primary care and mental health services within an integrated system.
4. Four kinds of activity that will improve collaborative practice:
   i. Activities and strategies that any mental health service can implement
   ii. Approaches that will increase the skills and capacity of primary care and primary care providers
   iii. The integration of mental health services within primary care settings
   iv. Visits to mental health services by primary care providers
5. Agreement on the need for broader system changes to support integration

Kates N, Mazowita G, Lemire F, et al. The evolution of collaborative mental health care in Canada: A shared vision for the future. Joint position paper of the Canadian Psychiatric Association and the College of Family Physicians of Canada. Can J Psychiatry 2011;56(5):11–110. http://www.cfpc.ca/uploadedFiles/Directories/Committees_List/Collaborative%20mental%20health%20care-2011-49-web-FIN-EN.pdf. Accessed May 15, 2016.

A Shared Vision of the Roles of Primary Care and Mental Health Services in an Integrated System

As most primary care practices look after a discrete population and have ongoing relationships with their patients, the family physician's office is often the first point of contact for someone with mental health or addiction problems. Primary care, with appropriate support, is well positioned to deliver services beyond the scope of traditional mental health services. Collaborative practices can foster integration of physical and emotional care (especially for individuals with complex conditions), provide preventive interventions and mental health promotion, and facilitate earlier detection of mental health and addiction problems. Practices can initiate treatment, provide monitoring after an episode of care, thereby preventing further relapses, and can help coordinate and navigate other needed systems of care.

In order for primary care to assume a broader role in mental health care, mental health services need to make adjustments in how they support these roles. Primary care providers need to offer rapid access to mental health and substance use consultation, and reassessment for acute problems, even when there are delays in accessing long-term psychiatric care. In addition, mental health services need to provide targeted individual and programmatic care for selected individuals or groups of patients who cannot be managed in primary care. This targeted care is essential for patients requiring substance abuse rehabilitation programs or more specialized mental health treatment. In addition, mental health providers need to provide ongoing support and training for primary care providers in person, by telephone, via tele-behavioral health, or by using web-based applications. Finally, mental health services need to provide advice and consultation for population health, community management, and assistance with resource development.

Activities and Strategies to Improve Collaboration with Primary Care Colleagues

Mental health and primary care providers can develop strategies that improve communication, working relationships, provide consultation, and coordinate care which can easily be introduced at little or no cost.

Improving Communication Between Providers

The foundation of all collaborative partnerships is effective communication between providers who know, understand, and respect each other. Providers should know each other personally and understand the abilities and limitation of each other. Partners can simplify intake procedures and inclusion or exclusion criteria for referrals. They can develop protocols for communicating with each other, when a patient is admitted to a service or develop a process for initiating and managing medications or other treatments. Primary care and mental health providers can jointly plan for discharge and decide on appropriate referrals to other needed services.

Mental health professionals need to rapidly transmit concise, clear, and practical reports for a family physician to follow. This might include information about prescribed medications, changes in treatment, or specific guidance on use of community resources. Patients and/or their family members need to understand and retain a summary of their care plan to foster communication with the entire system of care. Mental health providers need to follow up with the family physician a week and a month after discharge to determine whether mental health connections have been made and how the care plan is working.

Mental Health Consultation with Primary Care

While traditional face-to-face consultation with a patient remains a central activity for a mental health provider, family physicians can also access helpful advice about their patients. through telephone consultations[5], e-mail communication, tele-behavioral health consultations, or communication via an electronic medical record.

To improve access to mental health care, when mental health appointment wait times are longer than 3 months, mental health providers can set up a rapid consultation service which offers a quick consultation and initial treatment/management advice to a family physician. The patient can remain on the mental health waiting list for ongoing care, as required. Such a rapid consultation may involve two mental health visits: (1) a visit with a nurse or social worker, conducting an initial assessment and (2) a brief, focused visit with a psychiatrist. Following the second visit, a report can be sent to the family physician, outlining key diagnoses and management strategies which also should include a clear interim treatment plan. The mental health team can continue to provide telephone or consultation advice/support to the family physician until the patient can gain full access to the appropriate mental health or addiction services, or until the problem has resolved. Collaborative care may also include discussion among the family physician, mental health professional, and patient or family member about active management of symptoms while a patient is on a waiting list. "What to do while waiting" can be integral to improving a patient's well-being and long-term outcome.

Treatment planning is an important part of both the rapid consultation and effective communication. Plans need not be lengthy, nor redundant with information from previous records. An effective plan includes a succinct, integrated impression of the patient's situation; a detailed, practical, point-by-point treatment plan; and when necessary, a contingency plan.

Coordination of Care

Individuals with mental health and/or addiction treatment needs, often face difficulties arising from service fragmentation and difficulty in in transitioning from one service or sector to another. To increase the ease and coordination of care, the following is recommended: (1) regular communication and decisions about responsibility for each part of the care plan, (2) support with guidelines for referrals and transition of care, (3) an individualized treatment plan that is brief, focused, practical, and accessible to the patient, and (4) the creation of a discharge planning checklist with specific steps routinely followed by all providers in a service. Review Table 3.2 for an example of an inpatient discharge plan.

A mental health provider may call patients at 1, 3, 6, and 12 months after completion of an episode of care to see how they are doing. Cases should be kept open so that a patient who is experiencing problems can be quickly reassessed to prevent further deterioration. If, on the other hand, the patient is doing well and the plan is working, the case can be closed. A mental health provider can also arrange the last appointment, before a mental health discharge from the office of the family physician, to ensure that everyone knows the plan and his or her responsibility for ongoing care.

Building the Capacity and Capability of Primary Care Providers to Manage the Mental Health Problems of Their Patients

Initiatives in the primary care setting can be geared towards increasing the skills and comfort of family physicians and all other primary care providers in recognizing and managing mental health and substance abuse problems, thereby expanding the number of patients being seen, and the range of services being delivered. Teaching about mental health and addictions can be accomplished by formalized continuing medical education (CME) workshops, presentations, or conferences. CME is most effective when it is brief, practical, and taught interactively using a case-based or problem-focused approach. Topics addressed can be chosen by family physicians and should be relevant to the immediate realities of primary care. Presenters should include family physicians and specialists who also offer a follow up session one month later.[7]

TABLE 3.2. INPATIENT DISCHARGE CARE PLAN

- Contact the family physician at admission to discuss possible follow-up plans.
- Contact the family physician when a firm discharge date is envisaged.
- Discuss the follow-up plan with the family physician and determine which roles the family physician could take.
- Develop a written plan for post-discharge care, including medications.
- Give a copy of the plan to the patient.
- Fax, email, or send through an electronic medical record a copy of the care plan to the family physician on the day of the patient's discharge.
- Prepare a succinct and relevant discharge summary immediately after discharge, and get it to the family physician as soon as possible.
- Call the patient a week after discharge to ensure the plan is understood and is being implemented.
- Call the family physician a month after discharge to ensure the plan is being implemented.

Mental health specialists visiting the primary care setting expand the opportunities for learning and build on these CME principles. In-office consultations (around active and current cases) that are brief, focused, and immediately helpful are appreciated. A specific training program for a group of primary care providers or other members of the collaborative team may focus on the treatment for a specific problem, assist with population management, or help with the development of groups (see Chapter 28: Group Interventions in Integrated Care Settings) and can cement effective collaboration and bring new skills to the primary care practice.

Mental health providers can introduce the use of standardized screening instruments, management guidelines, and books geared toward patient self-management strategies, as well as links to readily useable and downloadable online materials, interactive resources for patients, and information on community programs, all contained within a single accessible web-based location. These materials can be used by the family physician both for his or her own information and as resources for patient discussions and teaching.[8]

Example: British Columbia's Practice Support Program Mental Health Module

The Practice Support Program: Adult Mental Health Module (AMH), a joint initiative of Doctors of British Columbia (BC) and the BC Ministry of Health, is a training and support program for physicians and their medical office assistants (MOAs). The program is designed to improve clinical skills, practice management, and to enhance delivery of mental health patient care. The AMH offers a series of modules that include screening and assessment tools and three supported self-management approaches. The three modules include: (1) Bounce Back, a program that combines DVDs and workbooks for individuals with depression with or without anxiety, (2) an Antidepressant Skills Workbook, which teaches specific skills to improve overall well-being, and (3) The Cognitive Behavioral Interpersonal Skills (CBIS) manual,[9] which forms the core of the AMH. CBIS provides an organized, guideline-based system for physicians. This system aids in patient assessment as well as development of treatment strategies that incorporate self-management processes to empower patients to be active partners in their mental health treatment. The manual is also featured in the Canadian Medical Association's national e-learning anti-stigma course for physicians, in partnership with the Mental Health Commission of Canada.

Practice support (PSP) learning modules[9] are designed to teach the use of common screening scales, a diagnostic assessment interview tool, a tool for organizing patient issues, a cognitive-behavioral skills program, and the use of a patient self-management workbook. These learning modules are typically taught in three half-day group-learning sessions, offered locally in communities throughout the province. Each group session is followed by an action period of approximately 8 to 12 weeks, during which PSP participants test what they have learned in their own practices. MOAs are specifically targeted to receive the 2-day Mental Health First Aid training offered by the Canadian Mental Health Association to increase their confidence in dealing with patients they will see in their practices.[10]

During action periods, participants receive in-practice support to ensure they get as much benefit as possible from the learning sessions and have the guidance they need to incorporate newly acquired tools and processes into their everyday practice workflow.

The Child and Youth Mental Health (CYMH)[7,11] module offers similar screening and assessment tools designed for children and youth. Module training, tools, and resources encourage and support collaboration of the various practitioners in the multi-sectoral team who provide care for these young patients. Family physicians who complete the CYMH module training, learn how to work together with child and adolescent psychiatrists, pediatricians, child and youth mental health clinicians, and school counselors in their local communities. To date, over 1,600 family physicians have participated in the module. This model has been adopted by Nova Scotia, and has also been introduced in a variety of other jurisdictions. Evaluation has shown significant improvements in the skills and confidence of primary care providers in managing these problems, with these improvements being maintained over a 12-month period.[12]

Common Models for Integrating Mental Health Services Within Primary Care Practice Settings and Establishing Teams

Different levels of integration of mental health services into primary care include the following:

1. Co-location of mental health and primary care; contacts or case sharing is usually incidental rather than planned.
2. Mental health professionals visiting primary care to provide educational presentations, complex case discussions or review, or a one-off clinical consultation or visit.
3. Mental health professionals coming to primary care for the final mental health discharge visit with a patient, so the family physician is actively involved in the follow-up plans and the patient is clear about the roles of all the providers.
4. Regular visits by a mental health team as an outreach activity of a mental health service.
5. Full integration of mental health providers as part of the primary care team.

For a description of levels of integrated care in the United States see Chapter 1: Conceptual Framework for Integrated Care: Multiple Models to Achieve Integrated Aims.

Most Canadian programs have adopted an approach that is similar to the Collaborative Care model developed by Wayne Katon and his colleagues in Seattle, Washington.[13,14] The collaborative care model utilizes a care manager/therapist/counselor, who may be a nurse, a social worker, and less frequently a psychologist, as well as a consulting psychiatrist; both mental health professionals are integrated within the primary care practice. The counselors can fill multiple roles and can facilitate the psychiatrists integration in the primary care setting. Such programs emphasize evidence-based practices, often introduced by the psychiatrist or mental health counselor with a population focus. Collaborative programs may address the needs of all patients being seen in a primary care practice, or may focus on specific populations, such as individuals with depression or anxiety, children and youth, older patients, or individuals with psychosis or addiction issues.

Most Canadian programs follow one of three approaches:

1. Visits by mental health providers working in a mental health program for a brief "one-off

event," such as a clinical consultation, an educational event, a case review, or for a patient's final primary care visit when a patient is about to be discharged from a mental health service.

2. A "shifted" outpatient clinic, in which mental health professionals (MHPs) either individually or as a team visit the primary care setting for a specific number of half-days, usually as part of an outreach program of a mental health service.
3. The full integration of MHPs as part of the primary care team, as in the Hamilton Family Health Team Mental Health Program.

Evidence for the Benefits of Collaborative Care

Convincing evidence has accrued from Canadian projects[4] and from the international literature[12] of the short and long term benefits of collaborative partnerships, measured by symptom and functional improvement of patients, reduced disability days, increased workplace tenure, increased quality-adjusted life years, and increased compliance with medication. These benefits have also been identified for youth, seniors, people with addiction problems, and indigenous populations.

There is also evidence that collaborative programs are cost-effective[15] and can lead to reductions in health care costs, through a more efficient use of medications, reduced use of other medical services (especially for people with chronic medical conditions), more efficient use of existing resources,[14] and a greater likelihood of a more rapid return to the workplace.

Collaborative care also improves the passage of individuals through the mental health system, by creating a better-coordinated continuum of care, making flow between services easier, enabling the sharing or shifting of resources as needed, ensuring mutual accountability, and strengthening linkages with other sectors.[16,17]

Key Components of Effective Programs

Collaborative programs include multiple linked components, combined with a redesign of existing processes of care.[4,14] The key components employ screening of patients with chronic medical conditions for depression or anxiety, enhanced patient education or access to educational resources, and/or brief psychological therapies for those with a problem. Other key components focus on increasing the skills of primary care providers and changing the way care is delivered. Collaborative programs may introduce evidence-based guidelines for treatment, will monitor progress after treatment is started, treat a specific problem or diagnosis, and often utilizes telephone follow-up or other forms of consultations. In addition, changing the methods of systems/care delivery is usually required to support and get the most out of collaborative interventions. Systemic changes may include employing systematic (proactive) follow-up of patients after treatment is initiated or completed, supporting patient self-management, inviting feedback from patients and families regarding the effectiveness of interventions, and providing rapid access to essential services. Team-based care and clarity in the roles of different providers are also keys to better outcomes.

Whitebird et al[18] reviewed two programs: Improving Mood-Promoting Access to Collaborative Treatment (IMPACT) in Seattle and Minnesota's Depression Improvement Across Minnesota, Offering a New Direction (DIAMOND) Program. Table 3.3 lists the nine identified factors that led to effective collaboration.[18]

Integrating Primary Care Providers Within Mental Health Services

Individuals with severe and persistent mental illnesses have an increased risk of developing chronic conditions such as diabetes, vascular disease, and respiratory problems. Patients often have more than just one medical problem. Many of these individuals have trouble accessing timely primary care, which can contribute to the chronicity of these conditions and reduced life expectancy. In some instances, this leads to the use of emergency departments for primary care services. Some psychiatrists may provide treatment for the physical as well as the psychiatric disorders, including prescribing, although many psychiatrists do not feel they possess the skills to safely manage medical problems.

With increasing frequency, a primary care provider may be added into a mental health service, sometimes referred to as "reverse shared care" or "reversed integrated care." The provider can be a family physician or an advanced practice nurse, whose role is to assess the physical health problems of patients using a mental health service, initiate medical treatment, monitor progress, and refer on to more specialized medical care, if required. The primary care physician (PCP) is usually present for

TABLE 3.3. WHITEBIRD'S NINE FACTORS LEADING TO EFFECTIVE COLLABORATION

- An engaged psychiatrist who is available to all team members and responsive to patient needs.
- A strong family physician champion who actively promotes and supports the project.
- Supportive organizational leadership that understands and supports the goals of the project.
- Buy-in by primary care providers who support the model and are willing to make adjustments.
- Funding is not an obstacle, with adequate resources for the program to function.
- A strong care manager who understands the model and is a good fit with the practice.
- The care manager's role and expectations are clear and regularly reviewed.
- The care manager is onsite and is accessible and available, with adequate working space.
- Warm handoffs with referrals, case discussions, and reports conducted face to face.

Whitebird RR, Solberg LI, Jaeckels NA, et al. Effective implementation of collaborative care for depression: what is needed? Am J Manag Care 2014;20(9):699–707.

half a day every 1 to 2 weeks, and can also be available by phone, between visits. In these settings, the PCPs need to bring the full range of their usual clinical skills in chronic and acute disease management. They also need additional expertise in planned proactive care, motivational interviewing, trauma-informed care, supported self-management, and care planning.

The Hamilton Family Health Team Mental Health Program: Integrating Mental Health Services in Primary Care

The Hamilton Family Health Team (HFHT) Mental Health Program,[19] established in 1994, became part of the Hamilton Family Health Team in 2006. Family Health Teams are Ontario's model of transformed primary health care, emphasizing comprehensive, round-the-clock care; prevention and health promotion; chronic disease management; and team-based care. The HFHT, located in the city of Hamilton, a community of 500,000 people in southern Ontario, serves approximately two-thirds of the population of the city. The HFHT is the largest in the province, and includes 170 family physicians, most of whom are in small (one- or two-person) practices. In total, there are 86 practices, each of which will have, in addition to the family physician(s), a nurse and other health professionals, such as pharmacists or dietitians, as well as a counselor and a visiting psychiatrist.

The mental health counselor is usually a nurse or social worker, experienced in outpatient mental health, and in working with people with severe and persistent mental illness. The counselor ratio is approximately one full-time equivalent (FTE) for every 7,000 patients or 1.5 days per family physician per week. In other words, solo physicians will have a counselor in their offices for two or three half-days a week; a four-physician practice will usually have one full-time counselor. For psychiatrists, the ratio is half a day per month per family physician, which means a four-person practice will have a psychiatrist in the office for half a day per week. Counselors and psychiatrists are well integrated within the practice, participate in team meetings and social events, and will use the same electronic medical records as the rest of the primary care team.

Although most psychiatrists and counselors are used to seeing adults rather than children, in primary care they see patients of any age. In addition to the adult mental health program, the HFHT has also recruited three child and youth mental health workers and a child psychiatrist, as well as three addiction specialists. Because of the size of the HFHT and the number of individuals with these problems, rather than delivering much direct care, these child and addiction teams have focused more on running psycho-educational or other support groups. They also provide information on community resources, assist with system navigation, and provide consultation advice and support (in person, by phone, or using other electronic methods) to the general primary care clinicians working in the program. All counselors may see a selective small number of complex cases for a consultation. The roles and tasks of members of the HFHT are described in Table 3.4.

Data from the Program's Evaluation

The Hamilton program has significantly improved access to mental health services.[19] Today, family physicians refer approximately 11 times as many individuals for a general mental health assessment as they did before the program began and this improvement has been maintained over 20 years. The program has reduced both the number of mental health inpatient admissions and the length of stay for patients in the caseload of physicians in the program. It has also demonstrated continuing and significant improvement in measures of both mood, using the Center for Epidemiological Studies Depression (CES-D)[20] scale, and overall functioning, using the Short Form-8 (SF8).[21]

The Hamilton Program patients have given the service high ratings. They appreciate the shorter wait times, convenience of being seen closer to home, feel less stigma, and that their physical and emotional care is better coordinated. There is also a high level of satisfaction on the part of counselors, psychiatrists, and family physicians. Family physicians feel the program has increased their comfort and confidence in assessing and managing a broad range of mental health problems in their offices. The program has become a prototype for other family health teams in Ontario and elsewhere.

Competencies for Mental Health Providers Working in Primary Care

For successful collaboration, mental health personnel need to remember they are "guests" in someone else's home. They need to be both respectful and flexible, and understand that in primary care, their working conditions and practice styles will differ from a mental health setting. They need to be open to learning about new ways to practice, and avoid assuming that primary care must adapt to incorporate them and their skills. They must also be willing to learn about the demands of primary care and its possibilities and limitations in delivering comprehensive mental health care.

Building personal contacts is a key to successful partnerships; counselors and psychiatrists are more successful when they invest time in getting to know their primary care colleagues. Often the informal contacts, brief conversations, and "hallway discussions" are the most helpful for family physicians.

Mental health professionals also need to be able to unpack their skills and adapt them to the demands of primary care. For example, it may be unrealistic for a counselor to devote 16 weeks to a single patient for cognitive-behavioral therapy (CBT) if the goal is to promote access and patient flow. In contrast, short-term approaches to CBT and solution-focused therapy have demonstrated their efficacy within five sessions.[22]

Mental health professionals need to be willing to see a wide range of problems and populations, including children, teens, and seniors. They must possess the skills to deliver interventions, individually tailored to the skills and interests of each family physician, and provide education that is specific, focused, brief, and problem/case-based to fit with the timeframe of a family physician's day. Mental health providers need to write succinct notes without repeating known history, develop and document a treatment plan, and suggest contingencies in case the plan does not work. The well developed collaborative model reveals a shared relationship between providers and team members that recognizes complementary knowledge, expertise, and conceptual models.

The Hamilton Program meets all of Whitebird's nine criteria for a successful integrated program. The counselor is always onsite and well integrated within the team. Expectations are spelled out by the central program team, laying down the program's framework and ensuring that the FHT leadership remains aware and supportive of the project's goals. Face to face referrals and case feedback, preferred by the family physicians foster physician buy-in and champions of the program.

Successes and Challenges

Successes

The Hamilton Program has been extremely successful in its primary goal, improving access to mental health care, and in providing opportunities for earlier detection and intervention, as well as relapse prevention. It has also been able to expand the range of available services in primary care, both through the activities of the mental health team and through an increase in the confidence and skills of family physicians in managing mental health problems. Developing groups to meet the needs of a variety of different populations has also expanded the range of available services in an effective and efficient manner.

The program has also been successful in using case-based learning to increase the skills and competence of participating family physicians, through discussion about individual patients and through more formally organized CME workshops, presentations, or conferences geared to the demands of primary care.[23] Because the mental health practitioner is present in the primary care setting, new opportunities for learning open up, building on these three principles.

Any case being seen or discussed in consultation presents educational opportunities. While usually brief and focused on the case at hand, often the formulations, treatment decisions, and management

TABLE 3.4. ROLES AND TASKS OF MEMBERS OF THE HAMILTON FAMILY HEALTH TEAM

Counselors

- Conduct assessments (children, adolescents, adults, families).
- Deliver short-term therapies; average 6.5 visits (supportive, behavioral, social activation, solution-focused/interpersonal therapy, and cognitive-behavioral therapy) in a "shared care" model.
- Run groups (e.g., stress management for women, self-esteem, depression education, marital counseling).
- For selected cases, serve as a case manager or care coordinator.
- Assist individuals and families in navigating the system and accessing community and other resources.
- Support family physicians through case discussion, providing information on resources, and providing ongoing care in a shared care model.
- Establish and enhance links between primary care and mental health services.
- Treat or advise predominantly about depression; anxiety; situational problems; trauma; addictions; workplace, stress, family, or marital issues; finances or housing problems.
- Participate in other program activities as appropriate.

Psychiatrists

- Support the family physician and counselors.
- Provide psychiatric consultation.
- Where necessary, offer follow-up visits to complete an assessment or assist in the stabilization of an individual (50% of patients are seen more than once, the average being 2.1 total visits).
- Be available to see individuals (and with their families, as needed) with enduring problems on an intermittent/as-needed basis.
- Provide addiction advice and management.
- Assist the family physician with medication management.
- Advise the team on best practices in the treatment and management of individuals (and with their families, as needed) with mental illness.
- Be available to discuss cases and provide advice on medication, management, or available resources (usually brief case-based, curbside consultations or "huddles").
- Offer more structured, case-based educational sessions for the primary care team.
- Back up the team by phone, email, or other forms of communication.
- Encourage a population health approach.

Family Physicians

- Continue to deliver integrated physical, mental health, and addiction care, including prescribing medication.
- Participate in brief mental health discussions and a daily "huddle."
- Available to discuss cases with the counselor and psychiatrist as needed.
- Offer agenda for mental health learning topics needed by the practice.

Other Team Members

- Medical office assistants: provide relevant background information on people being seen, including observation about their behavior in the waiting area or on the phone.
- Pharmacists: review psychotropic medications, contribute to discussions of patients with complex conditions, requiring multiple medications.
- Practice nurses: manage patients with chronic or complex conditions, make referral to community agencies.
- Dietitians: provide nutrition counseling for people with mental health problems/taking psychotropic medications, screen for eating disorders and other mental health issues.

TABLE 3.4. CONTINUED

Central Management Team
The Central Management Team consists of the program medical lead, manager, three administrative supports, one of whom assists with program evaluation, and leads for specialized programs (child, addictions, group) who also work in the practices. • Program administration. • Links with the Ontario Ministry of Health and Long-Term Care (the program's funder). • Recruitment and preparation of counselors and psychiatrists. • Evaluation of the counselors, including career development. • Program evaluation. • Helping to solve problems that arise in a practice. • Building partnership with community organizations. • Overseeing any additional research projects. • Assisting practices with the logistics of housing the mental health team. • Providing educational resources and information on community programs to the practices.

strategies can be generalized to other cases, For example, it is an educational opportunity for the family physician when the mental health provider gives reasons for choosing a particular antidepressant for a senior or explains differences in the ways that depression can present in adolescents. This kind of shared training can be reinforced through regular (usually monthly) meetings to discuss or review cases that are in the family physicians caseload, or cases they are finding challenging.

The mental health team is also able to provide links to readily useable online materials (e.g., a book with self-management skills for someone who is depressed) and can offer in-office educational presentations on a specific topic chosen by the primary care team. As well as being case-based, these can also teach new skills, including brief therapies that can be used in primary care, the introduction of standardized approaches, such as screening instruments, management guidelines, or information on community programs. The program also makes sure these are accessible either through individual electronic medical records or via a single accessible web-based location. Through the recommendations and advice of the psychiatrist and mental health counselors, evidence-informed guidelines are introduced into primary care.

The Hamilton Program has also helped practices build linkages with the rest of the health care system, better integrating primary mental health within the local mental health and addiction system, and also in building partnerships with community agencies and local schools. In some cases, the primary care practice is visited by community agency staff, such as child protection workers or community nurses. These linkages are often facilitated by the mental health counselors, who are able to assist with program information and with system navigation.

Overall, the Hamilton Program has provided a model for other programs in Ontario, in Canada, and internationally, whose leaders have come to Hamilton to learn from the program's experience and see how it functions on a day-to-day basis. It has also provided an invaluable training experience for psychiatry residents and other learners who are interested in making this type of practice a part of their careers.

Challenges

The Hamilton Program has also faced some challenges. Many of these relate to its size and the logistics of supporting activities in over 80 unique clinical settings. Finding space for the counselors (along with other allied health professionals working in that practice) can also be difficult in smaller practices.

As the program has expanded, recruitment of psychiatrists to meet the needs of all the practices, particularly with the large number of solo physician practices in the program, has been a challenge. Most psychiatrists work only part-time (one to three half-days a week) in the program, and while the total psychiatry complement required is only five FTEs, this often requires as many as 15 psychiatrists interested in working in the program.

With such a large number of counselors involved in the program (close to 75, many of whom also work part-time), maintaining consistent standards of practice can also be a challenge. Consequently, it has not been easy to introduce standardized evidence-informed treatment approaches within all practices, or to introduce progress and outcomes measures used by every counselor.

Shifting from an individually focused model to integrating population approaches with individual treatment, something many practices are slowly moving toward, is an additional challenge.

Implementing a Collaborative Project

Any collaborative project needs to be a joint endeavor from the outset, rather than one party approaching the other with predetermined ideas for the project. Shared ownership increases acceptance, and enables all parties to contribute their ideas and understanding to the eventual program. Partners need to begin by talking about the problems from their respective frames of reference, and work to understand the root causes of these problems. They can then identify their needs and discuss possible solutions. At this point, they may be ready to agree on specific goals for the project, but they may also need to bring these back to their own organizations to make sure there is buy-in from everyone involved. Each partner needs an opportunity to contribute additional suggestions when shaping the direction of the project. The importance of starting with a shared common purpose cannot be overstated. Each organization will also identify a liaison person, who will work with his or her counterpart around implementation. The organization may also wish to set up a small steering committee to oversee the project, especially in its early stages. The next step is to clarify the details of the new initiative, define how it will work on a daily basis, and explore its potential implications for everyone involved. It should be evidence-informed and draw on the experiences of similar programs in other settings, while adapting the learning to the local context. Roles of key participants need to be clarified, expectations spelled out, and criteria for measuring the success of the project determined. It is important to identify the "champions" for the project. Implementation can be effective when gradually introduced, so the impact can be measured and, where necessary, adjustments made along the way. If multiple components are to be introduced, they should be introduced one at a time so that the impact of each can be assessed or measured before the next is put in place. The steering committee should continue to meet to adjust the project based upon lessons learned and look at how the initial gains can be maintained, built upon, and spread to other colleagues.

Advice to Others

Primary mental health care is not simply the delivery of mental health care in a primary care setting. The language, culture, time frame, and kinds of problems being seen in primary care differ from secondary care, and require mental health providers to be able to unpack their skills, approaches, and language and translate them to make them relevant to the world of primary care and general medical settings. MHPs working in primary care need to be able to adapt their skills and knowledge to the demands and realities of each individual physician or practice, rather than replicating the same thing in every office.

It is also impossible to overstate the importance of addressing children's mental health needs, and using the opportunities that arise in primary care to change the trajectory for children with multiple risk factors or who are coping with the consequence of adverse or traumatic events.

A practice always needs to examine whether staff are working at the highest scope of their training, because doing so will increase staff satisfaction as well as broaden the range of available services. One of the best ways to assess this is to ask primary care staff how they might raise their capabilities for delivering mental health care.

Organizationally, there needs to be a shared common purpose for any collaborative project, and agreed-upon goals. Clarity around program and service limitations, as well as a realistic understanding by all of what providers can and cannot accomplish are more likely to support successful change.

The importance of personal contacts and building relationships between staff, fostering an understanding of each other's strengths, limitations, and interests cannot be overstated. This is aided by physical proximity of co-location. The mental health team needs to be well integrated within the practice. A mental health clinician situated in an office somewhere in the practice, who receives referrals without opportunities for shared planning and goal setting, cannot be very effective. Even small distances between staff can significantly impact the degree of

BOX 3.2
SUMMARY OF RECOMMENDED TREATMENT APPROACHES AND RELEVANT EVIDENCE

Strength of recommendation taxonomy (SOR A, B, or C)

- **The Collaborative Care model developed by Wayne Katon and his colleagues in Seattle is an effective model of integrated care for the treatment of depression. (SOR A)[13]**
- **There is convincing evidence from Canadian projects and from the International literature as to the short- and long-term benefits of collaborative partnerships. (SOR A)[4,13,16,17]**
- **Collaborative programs are cost-effective and can lead to reductions in health care costs through a more efficient use of medications, reduced use of other medical services (especially for people with chronic medical conditions), a more efficient use of existing resources, and a greater likelihood of a more rapid return to the workplace. (SOR C)[15,16]**
- **Integrating primary care with mental health improves access to mental health care. (SOR A)[4,14,16,19]**
- **The Hamilton program has significantly improved and maintained access to mental health services. (SOR B)[19]**
- **Whitebird et al identified nine factors that lead to effective collaboration (see Table 3.4). (SOR C)[4,18]**
- **A collaborative-care approach can reduce length of stay on inpatient mental health units. (SOR B)[19]**
- **There are examples of short-term approaches to CBT and solution-focused therapy that have demonstrated their efficacy within five sessions. (SOR A)[22]**
- **Self-management support for depression in primary care is effective. (SOR C)[8]**

collaboration within a practice. Above all, patients and families always need to be at the center of care. Their views, lived experiences, opinions, and voices must always be included in the planning, implementation and evaluation process.

One of the keys to the sustainability of collaborative mental health care is to train learners to understand the principles and practices of working in collaborative models. All Canadian psychiatry residents now need to spend 1 to 2 months working in a collaborative care experience (usually in primary care, sometimes with a community agency), in which they will refine their collaborative skills and come to appreciate the role that primary care plays in delivering mental health care. Equally important in many ways is that the psychiatric residents will learn to consider and understand the role played by primary care and to involve the family physician for all their cases.

In most family medicine programs, training in behavioral health is integrated within the family medicine unit. At McMaster University, for example, the behavioral science half-day is divided into four parts, led by a family medicine tutor and a psychiatrist who model collaboration in their relationship and in the following ways: (1) a didactic session on topics of relevance to family medicine led by the two co-tutors, who each bring their own perspective, (2) discussion of cases seen by the residents, (3) a review of tapes (audio or video) of the residents interviewing patients, and (4) an opportunity to observe the psychiatrist conducting a consultation.

FUTURE STEPS

As collaborative care models become more accepted as mainstream practice in Canada, opportunities arise to take advantage of the potential these partnerships offer to address wider problems in the health care system. Collaborative care can reduce avoidable emergency department visits, foster earlier detection and intervention in mental health problems, and improving access and transitions between services.

There is also a gradual shift toward incorporating concepts from the quality improvement agenda into collaborative care, with an increasing focus on population health and patient-centered care. The latter also gives practices a chance to listen to the experiences of people using collaborative services and to redesign these services accordingly.

The integration of mental health workers in primary care can allow primary care teams to address a broader range of problems, such as managing individuals with complex medical conditions and multiple problems, and understanding the interactions between the different enduring conditions. Integration also enables the management of other significant problems in which primary care may be the only place where effective interventions can take place. Examples include: (1) examining the issue of poly-pharmacy, and reducing the number of medications a patient uses and (2) focusing on the needs of specific populations, such as seniors with early cognitive impairment, or, in the Hamilton Program, turning an adolescent's routine visit into a "well teen" visit.

Collaborative care has already demonstrated its potential to address populations who often underuse mental health services, including individuals residing in shelters or suffering with addictions. Collaborative care has also been adopted by Canada's military. We now need to look at how these models can meet the needs of other populations, such as refugees and other newcomers to Canada, individuals struggling with adverse childhood events, and seniors, as well as finding ways to reduce the stigma associated with the presence of a mental health problem.

There is also a need to create frameworks or networks that will promote the spread of ideas that have worked in one location to other practices and other parts of the communities or different parts of the province, to accelerate the uptake of these concepts by patients and providers.

REFERENCES

1. College of Family Physicians of Canada. A Vision for Canada: Family Practice—The Patient's Medical Home. Position paper. September 2011. http://www.cfpc.ca/A_Vision_for_Canada/#sthash.jMy-8TOn7.dpuf3. Accessed May 15, 2016.
2. Kates N, Craven M, Bishop J, et al. Shared mental health care in Canada. Can J Psychiatry. 1997;42(8, suppl):1–12.
3. Mental Health Core Competencies Steering Committee. Mental Health Core Competencies for Physicians, 2014. Ottawa, Ontario. http://www.royalcollege.ca/portal/page/portal/rc/common/documents/policy/mhcc_june2014_e.pdf. Accessed May 15, 2016.
4. Kates N, Mazowita G, Lemire F, et al. The Evolution of Collaborative Mental Health Care in Canada: A Shared Vision for the Future. Joint position paper of the Canadian Psychiatric Association and the College of Family Physicians of Canada. Can J Psychiatry. 2011;56(5):11–110. http://www.cfpc.ca/uploadedFiles/Directories/Committees_List/Collaborative%20mental%20health%20care-2011-49-web-FIN-EN.pdf. Accessed May 15, 2016.
5. Kates N, Crustolo A, Nikolaou L, et al. Providing psychiatric backup to family physicians by telephone. Can J Psychiatry. 1997;42(9):955–959.
6. Wagner E, Austin B, Davis C, et al. Improving chronic illness care: Translating evidence into action. Health Affairs. 2001;20(6):64–78.
7. Wienerman R, Campbell H, Miller, et al. Improving mental health care by primary care physicians in British Columbia. Healthcare Quarterly. 2011;14(1):36–38.
8. Bilsker D, Goldner EM, Jones W. Health service patterns indicate potential benefit of supported self-management for depression in primary care. Can J Psychiatry. 2007;52(2):86–95.
9. General Practice Services Committee. Adult Mental Health. http://www.gpscbc.ca/what-we-do/professional-development/psp/modules/adult-mental-health. Accessed May 10, 2016.
10. Ganshorn H, Michaud N. Mental Health First Aid: An Evidence Review. Mental Health Commission of Canada, August 2012. http://www.mentalhealthfirstaid.ca/EN/about/Pages/Evaluation.aspx. Accessed May 10, 2016.
11. Kallstrom L. GP learning session focuses on improving care for adolescent depression. BC Med J. 2010;52(2):96.
12. MacCarthy D, Weinerman R, Kallstrom L, et al. Mental health practice and attitudes can be changed! Perm J. 2013;17(3):14–17.
13. Katon W, Von Korff M, Lin E, et al. Collaborative management to achieve treatment guidelines: Impact on depression in primary care. JAMA. 1995;273(13):1026–1031.
14. Rainey L. Integrating primary care and behavioral health: The role of the psychiatrist in the collaborative care model. Am J Psychiatry. 2015;172(8):721–728.
15. Melek SP, Norris DT, Paulus J. Economic Impact of Integrated Medical-Behavioral Health: Implications for Psychiatry. Milliman American Psychiatric Association Report, 2013. http://www.psychiatry.org/File%20Library/Practice/Professional%20Interests/Integrated%20Care/Milliaman-APAEconomicImpactofIntegratedMedicalBehavioralHealthcare2014.pdf. Accessed May 16, 2016.

16. Collins C, Hewson DL, Munger R, Wade T. Evolving Models of Behavioral Health Integration in Primary Care. New York: Millbank Memorial Fund, 2010.
17. Butler M, Kane RL, McAlpine D, et al. Integration of Mental Health/Substance Abuse and Primary Care. No 173. AHRQ Publication No 09-E003. Rockville, MD: Agency for Healthcare Research and Quality, 2008. http://www.ahrq.gov/downloads/pub/evidence/pdf/mhsapc/mhsapc.pdf. Accessed May 10, 2016.
18. Whitebird RR, Solberg LI, Jaeckels NA, et al. Effective implementation of collaborative care for depression: What is needed? Am J Manag Care. 2014;20(9):699–707.
19. Kates N, MacPherson-Doe C, George L. Integrating mental health services within primary care settings. J Ambul Care Manage. 2011;34(2):174–182.
20. Radloff LS. The CES-D scale: A self-report depression scale for research in the general population. Appl Psych Meas. 1977;1(3):385–401.
21. Ware J, Kosinski M, Dewey J, Gandek B. How to Score and Interpret Single-Item Health Status Measures: A Manual for Users of the SF-8 Health Survey. Boston: Qualy Metric, 2001.
22. Churchill R, Hunot V, Corney R, et al. A systematic review of controlled trials of the effectiveness and cost-effectiveness of brief psychological therapies for depression. Health Technology Assessment. 2001;35(5):1–6.
23. Thistlethwaite JE1, Davies D, Ekeocha S, et al. The effectiveness of case-based learning in health professional education. A BEME systematic review. BEME Guide No. 23. Med Teach. 2012;34(6): 421–444.

4

Team-Based Integrated Primary Care

TZIPORAH ROSENBERG, COLLEEN T. FOGARTY, MICHAEL R. PRIVITERA, AND SUSAN H. MCDANIEL

BOX 4.1
KEY POINTS

- **Teams of interdisciplinary professionals expand access to primary and specialty care for patients who need and use the most care.**
- **Transdisciplinary professionalism promotes team collaboration for the benefit of patients and clinicians alike.**
- **The psychiatrist in primary care can have various collaborative roles, some unique and some that can overlap with other behavioral health professionals.**
- **Collaboration with other professionals requires both a shared mental health model and a common mission of biopsychosocial and culturally sensitive care of the patient and a synergism of professional expertise.**
- **Psychiatric consultations can take many forms and correspond with levels of integration with primary care. This occurs on a spectrum from minimal collaboration and some awareness of each other, to the highest level of integration that results in a collaborative treatment plan constructed by differing health care professionals, patients, and family members.**
- **The psychiatrist also provides consultation and education on patient-specific issues to the primary care clinician and other team members, including other mental health clinicians and clinical support staff.**
- **Clinical administrative support and leadership are critical to successful integrated behavioral health and primary care.**

INTRODUCTION

Experts from many fields, from dancer Twyla Tharp[1] to engineer Ian Mitroff[2] and organizational consultant Mary Uhl-Bien,[3] have described the move from focus on individuals to focus on teams in order to improve performance in endeavors as diverse as modern dance choreography, corporate business, and health care. Artist Twyla Tharp[1] thoughtfully articulates the "collaborative habit": "Collaboration may be a practice—a way of working in harmony with others—but it begins with a point of view." This point of view consists in the move from "me" to "us," from an arguably archaic, but also more traditional and familiar hierarchy, to something more akin to a team sport.

Scientist and organizational psychologist Eduardo Salas[4] and colleagues study the elements of successful teamwork in settings as diverse as aerospace, business, and health care. Teams are ubiquitous, and many endeavors are made more successful by invoking the power of multiple perspectives, frameworks, and worldviews. This phenomenon is perhaps timelier in no other field than health care. In this chapter we will describe the current range of teamwork in primary care vis-à-vis biopsychosocial care; that is, the full spectrum of biological, psychological, social, and cultural perspectives needed to fully care for all patients. We will discuss interprofessional care and integrated care, and provide focus on the emerging role for psychiatric specialty consultants in primary health care. An overview of the key elements of team-based integrated primary care is found in Box 4.1.

The Affordable Care Act has propelled a national shift toward population health in the United States. This shift, coupled with a decades-long evolution of the complexity in primary health care, has heightened the need for high-functioning teams in health care.[5] Population health aims to improve the health of an entire human population, with an explicit focus on reduction of health inequities or disparities attributable to social determinants of health, among other factors. Population health shifts the focus away from individual patients (characteristic of most mainstream medicine) and toward exploring barriers to our collective ability to maintain health as defined by "the capacity of people to adapt to, respond to, or control life's challenges and changes."[6] These factors require a different approach to how health care is provided, away from the traditional model of solo clinician. These new complexities require the development and deployment of teams of professionals, each of whom has specific skills, abilities, and interventions to offer, working at the highest level of their training, in complementary and collaborative ways. In primary care, these teams integrate behavioral health professionals such as psychiatrists, psychologists, therapists, and care managers skilled not only in direct patient care but also in supporting the primary care team members to extend their expertise and manage their patient encounters more efficiently.

In this chapter we will (1) discuss transdisciplinary professionalism; (2) discuss the differences between traditional mental health and primary care cultures, and their respective abilities to meet the needs of primary care patients and teams through transdisciplinary collaboration; (3) describe the interprofessional roles in an integrated primary care team with a focus on those filled by a psychiatrist; (4) discuss potential levels of collaboration between and among professionals, as well as the implications for patient care; (5) describe our own long-term experience with integrated primary care in the Department of Family Medicine at the University of Rochester; and (6) conclude with some discussion about the future of health care given the tremendous amount of change upon which this country is about to embark.

TRANSDISCIPLINARY PROFESSIONALISM

Collaboration within any team, but especially in health care, requires a way of thinking and working that the literature refers to as *transdisciplinary professionalism*.[7] This occurs when discipline-specific experts have working knowledge of other disciplines' roles. It allows inputs to be made with regard to other disciplines and uses this multidisciplinary expertise on all cases.[8] Transdisciplinary professionalism requires a shared approach to creating and carrying out patient care. Multiple health disciplines, drawing from their own expertise and working in concert, implement a biopsychosocial approach to the primary care provided for patients. At their best, these teams synthesize and extend discipline-specific expertise to create new ways of thinking and acting that improve patient care and achieve better health outcomes. For suggested ways of increasing transdisciplinary professionalism see Box 4.2.

DIFFERENCES BETWEEN PRIMARY CARE AND TRADITIONAL MENTAL HEALTH ENVIRONMENT: ADAPTING TO THE NEEDS OF PRIMARY CARE THROUGH TRANSDISCIPLINARY COLLABORATION

Building an integrated care team that can meet a full range of patient-care needs requires adaptation and divergence from "business as usual," both for primary care members and for mental health clinicians. The practice climates, cultures, and habits typical for each may clash at times, which can make collaboration challenging. For example, a primary care clinician (PCC) in a traditional model may believe that she does not "have time for depression" so therefore does not engage in screening or case finding, as she finds the biomedical concerns in her patients complex and time-consuming enough. Likewise, a mental health/therapist in a traditional model might believe that a patient's chest pain requires ongoing and repeated referral back to the PCC or specialty cardiologist when, in fact, adequate workup has demonstrated this symptom

BOX 4.2
WAYS OF INCREASING TRANSDISCIPLINARY PROFESSIONALISM

- **Understand each team member's role.**
  - **Participate in interprofessional education and training.**
  - **Shadow a "day in the life" of each health professional as part of orientation.**
- **Encourage questions (e.g., "There's no such thing as a stupid question").**
- **Use first names for everyone on team.**
- **Encourage feedback as an essential expectation of daily practice.**
  - **Teach "feedback sandwich" (positive feedback, followed by constructive criticism, then additional positive feedback) and other techniques to tactfully convey feedback.**
  - **Use "ground rules": remain calm, respectful, and honest.**
- **Be aware of issues regarding patient confidentiality while providing information to teammates that allows them to provide the best care for the patient.**
  - **Work within the rules of the Health Insurance Portability and Accountability Act (HIPAA) and need-to-know content relevant to team members.**
  - **Receptionists, patient care technicians, nurses, and health coaches should hear global outcomes as they are part of the team process.**
- **Be inclusive and transparent.**
  - **In team discussions, define terms to keep all engaged.**
  - **Maximize the opportunity for 360-degree input on patient care.**
- **Educate support staff on major treatment pathways.**
- **Educate support staff on major/common problems so that they can assist in detection or management:**
  - **Potential for suicide**
  - **Potential for violence**
- **Customer responsibility versus customer service balance**
- **Respect is at the core of all communication.**
  - **Self-management skills are important to deal with patient distress.**
  - **Receptionists represent the entire team; they are the "face" of the clinic—equal importance on the team, difference of role.**
  - **Receptionists have a crucial role in telephone contact with patient; ability to help solve problems related to the practice operations.**
  - **Receptionists' dual roles: Protect and advocate for the primary care clinicians (to reduce their occupational stress) while also advocating for the patient.**
  - **Respect families and help get their health care needs met.**

rests primarily in the psychosocial domain. Each domain regards time as a resource but operates at a completely different pace, rhythm, and flow than the other. Further, when it comes to information exchange, participants in each realm may delineate boundaries around health information and with whom to share it in very disparate ways. A traditionally separate physical space and medical record would make it difficult for these clinicians to communicate, and traditional privacy regulations represent barriers to communication. These important historical and cultural differences between primary care and mental health require understanding and flexibility in adapting to an integrated model.

Additionally, the process of adapting from our respective cultural homes toward a more integrated culture requires learning about traditional paradigms while simultaneously learning more about each other's training and clinical expertise. Clinical leadership that understands transdisciplinary professional collaboration is essential to create space to understand the differences and work toward creating a climate of mutual respect, mutual engagement, and collaboration on behalf of the patient.

INTERPROFESSIONAL ROLES IN INTEGRATED PRIMARY CARE TEAMS

Integrated care in the primary care setting can address the full spectrum of biopsychosocial and cultural needs of patients. All members of the team may take on roles that integrate behavioral/mental health care into primary care. While not all team members need be experts in the diagnosis, treatment, and management of mental disorders, each professional contributes meaningfully from his or her skillset in a manner that supports that management. See Table 4.1 for an expanded view of these roles, training, and expertise.

Primary Care Clinicians

Primary care biomedical clinicians, including physicians, advanced practice nurses, and physician assistants, focus on biomedical screening and prevention and management of chronic illnesses such as diabetes, asthma, and hypertension. They also address common mental health conditions such as depression, anxiety, somatoform disorders, attention-deficit/hyperactivity disorder, and substance use disorders. Integrated care expands the possibilities for broader care in areas that were the historical purview of "mental health" or "addiction" units and offers expanded treatment for depression, anxiety, chronic pain, alcoholism, and opiate addiction, as well as other mental health and substance abuse conditions. It provides brief behavioral counseling and other strategies to augment the patient's knowledge, management, and coping with chronic biomedical conditions.

Clinicians, Clinical Support Personnel, and Clerical Personnel

Team-based care, while distinct from the concept of integrated care, dovetails with integrated care in that the entire primary care delivery system is conceptualized and acts as a team with respect to the patient and family. Typical teams in the patient-centered medical home (PCMH) include clinicians, clinical support personnel, and clerical personnel. Clinicians, as noted above, include biomedically or psychosocially trained licensed providers such as physicians, psychologists, advanced practice nurses, physician assistants, marriage and family therapists, licensed social workers, health coaches, and psychiatrists/behavioral health consultants. In traditional fee-for-service mental health practice, these clinicians could usually serve as the "billing provider" for a given encounter. Fully integrated teams may or may not have access to a consulting psychiatrist, depending on the size of the practice and the local community.

Clinical support personnel, such as medical assistants, licensed practical nurses, registered nurses (RNs), health coaches, and care managers, provide assistance to patients to both extend and deepen the care provided. For example, the medical assistant or licensed practical nurse may obtain medical history, review and reconcile medications, input information, administer screenings (Patient Health Questionnaire [PHQ-9][9] and General Anxiety Screen [GAD-7][10] and others), and track progress and outcome measures in patient registries. RNs on the team may follow up on both biomedical and psychosocial concerns, for example reviewing abnormal laboratory tests, providing patient education, and assisting with patient self-management and goal setting. RNs may also follow up on mental health and substance use screenings, monitor patients' response to treatment over time as part of the clinical team, and add relevant information in registries and may participate in group medical visits around a particular topic, whether biomedical, like diabetes, or behavioral, like depression. Health coaches, relatively new to the integrated care team, often collaborate with the patient, family, and primary care providers to facilitate lifestyle change. See Chapter 25: Health Coaching in Integrated Care for further discussion of their roles and capabilities.

Care Managers

Care managers or care coordinators are also staff relatively new to the primary care team. The care manager, often RN trained, but alternatively with a social work background, is an important member of the team for patients who have multiple diagnoses or require substantial coordination of care. Care managers may have defined panels, such as patients who present to an emergency department or who are admitted to the hospital frequently; or they may be assigned to a patient based on a diagnosis, such as uncontrolled diabetes. Depression care managers (DCMs) and mental health care managers are care managers who focus specifically on patients who have depression or another mental health diagnosis. These staff may use standardized rating scales such as the PHQ-9, the GAD-7, and the Mood Disorders

TABLE 4.1. PROFESSIONAL ROLES IN INTEGRATED PRIMARY CARE

Profession	Training	Typical Role and Duties
Psychiatrist/ Psychiatric Nurse Practitioner (NP)	Physicians/NP with psychiatric training in diagnosis and treatment of patients with mental health and substance-related disorders	• Consultation on diagnosis and comorbid medical illnesses that contribute to psychopathology • Development of biopsychosocial treatment plans, including somatic therapies • Focused consultant to primary care clinician (PCC); clarify diagnosis and setting up psychiatric treatment plan • May initiate treatment or wait until patient sees PCC to initiate, depending on acuity and logistical issues of the patient • Provide consultation, education, some supervision of behavioral health specialists, other team members, and care managers • Help develop population health approach with the PCC • Organize practice registries for mental health and substance abuse
Psychologist	May have adult/child clinical, counseling, or health psychology doctorates. PhD (doctor of philosophy) has significant research and clinical training. PsyD (doctorate in psychology) focused on clinical practice.	• Provides behavioral health consultation • Brief psychotherapy (cognitive-behavioral therapy, problem solving, crisis intervention, motivational interviewing) • Intensive long-term psychotherapy • Work with families or groups • Health behavioral change • Adjustment to chronic medical conditions, consultation or intervention with complex cases • Leadership consultation • Team facilitation • Program development and evaluation • Supervise other behavioral health clinicians and/ or care managers
Primary Care Physician	Family medicine, general internal medicine, or pediatrics; some obstetrics and gynecology physicians may be the PCC for women	• First contact for a person with an undiagnosed health concern • May treat all age groups (family medicine) • Continuing care of varied medical conditions • Management and brief treatment of mental health conditions and addictions • Refer to specialists as needed • Lead quality and safety for the practice • Develop population health approach for prevention, wellness, physical and mental health conditions
Nurse LPN/LVN	Licensed practical (vocational) nurse: 1 year of courses and hands-on practice	• Check vital signs • Screen for mental health conditions • Collect health history, monitor clinical status of patients • Provide injections, wound care, collect samples • Supervise aides and patient care technicians

TABLE 4.1. CONTINUED		
Profession	Training	Typical Role and Duties
Nurse RN	Registered nurse: 3 or 4-year degree in nursing, associate degree or bachelor's degree in nursing	• Screenings, assessments, health promotion education, interpret patient data, and lab values • Administer medications and injections • Follow-up care for patient adherence • May run patient education groups or multiple family education • Coordinate care among wide variety of health care professionals
Advanced Practice Nurse	Master's-level preparation or doctor of nursing practice (DNP) and clinical practice requirements	**Nurse Practitioner** • Provide a wide range of primary and preventive health care services • Diagnose and treat common illnesses and injuries • Prescribe medication • Treat a panel of primary care patients, consulting with the PCC when necessary **Clinical Nurse Specialist** • Handle a wide range of physical and mental health problems • Help integrate care across continuum of patient, nurse, and system • Focus on disease management, health promotion, and prevention **Certified Nurse Midwife** • Provide well-woman gynecological and low-risk obstetrical care
Health Coach	May be RN, social worker, PhD, medical assistant, community health worker (i.e., promoter), health educator or have a health coach certification	• Coach patients about the knowledge, skills, and tools they need to become more actively engaged in their own care • Help establish health and wellness goals that are important to the patient, and help patients attain them through short-term goal setting and motivational interviewing, behavioral activation • Build patient self-efficacy around established health goals
Patient Care Technician/ Medical Assistant	Patient care technician or medical assistant program	• Patient care: obtain data, mental health/substance abuse screenings, vital signs, EKGs, phlebotomy, etc. within a regulated scope of practice • Manage flow and free clinicians to see more patients • May act as scribe with PCC for medical record documentation
Physician Assistant	Most programs are 26 months, similar to prerequisite courses that medical schools require	• Collect medical history • Perform physical exams • Diagnose and treat a variety of medical illnesses

(continued)

TABLE 4.1. CONTINUED

Profession	Training	Typical Role and Duties
Care Managers	Often a bachelor's-level or master's-level nursing or social work educational background	• Provide outreach to others in the health care system • Provide patient education • Provide follow-up from acute care services • Coordinate care with others in the care team • Coordinate care with the patient and family
Social Work	Either bachelor's level (BSW) or master's level (MSW; graduate school training)	• Provide care coordination • Provide case management, patient education, liaison with local agencies/resources to promote health and wellness • Licensed clinical master social workers may provide therapy and counseling.
Master's-Level Mental Health Clinicians	2–3 years of school, including didactics and clinical practicum	• Triage and distinguish those who can benefit from short-term intervention from those with serious mental illness who may require specialty care • Care managers for depression and other conditions • Provide warm handoffs • Collaborate with others in the care team • Provide primary care mental health services
Other Doctoral-Level Mental Health Clinicians	PhD in marriage and family therapy, counseling, or other related disciplines	• May provide direct clinical service for individuals, families, groups • May administer integrated mental health services • Provide clinical supervision • Offer quality improvement, data gathering and analysis for population health management
Receptionist	Various training and experience	• The first and often the last person to have contact with the patient • Presents the public face of the clinic • Begin the healing experience by displaying respect and compassion for patients
Administrator	College and sometimes a master's degree in business or a related field	• Allocate resources needed for patient care • Reduce organizational barriers to efficient care • Develop practice workflow and quality improvement • Facilitate development of electronic medical records

Questionnaire (MDQ)[11] for symptoms of hypomania or mania. In large primary care practices, a DCM may follow the patient from the initial diagnosis of depression and obtain follow-up PHQ-9 scores until a clinical remission is achieved. The DCM may reach out to the patient in person through contact at the office visit or a home visit, at a depression group visit, or via telephone, text messaging, telehealth, patient portal, or other web-based resources. The role of the DCM is to provide support to the patient as well as the rest of the care team to improve outcomes in depression care.

Traditionally clerical staff such as secretaries, unit clerks, and medical records staff did not have any primarily clinical responsibility. In the team-based model of care, they may facilitate and encourage patients in the following ways: providing appointment reminders; facilitating referrals; resolving difficulties to patient access, such as insurance counseling or transportation; and otherwise providing overall support to the patient in their role as the point of first contact into primary care. They may also have their own therapeutic relationships with patients who come to see them as a familiar and welcoming face of the practice, well beyond just the "front door" to get appointments.

The Role of the Psychiatrist in Primary Care: Patient Consultation, Clinician Education, and Population Health

The literature on the value of integrated behavioral health and primary care is robust and growing. Others have described several organizing principles around which successful integration is most likely to occur. Seaburn et al,[12] for example, outline key ingredients as follows: (1) development of mutually respectful relationships over time that are characterized by a flexible hierarchy and shared leadership and a common vision/purpose (i.e., patient-centered care); (2) a paradigm that allows blending and valuing of different professional perspectives; (3) communication that is appropriate to the task in terms of frequency, format, content, and delivery; and (4) a location that meets the needs of the patients and clinical team members (e.g., co-located vs. separately housed).

Relatively little, however, has been written about the role of psychiatrists in a primary care team. The psychiatrist in primary care can have a number of collaborative roles, some unique and some that can overlap with other behavioral health professionals. Typically the psychiatrist in primary care provides overall system consultation to ensure that up-to-date clinical protocols for screening, diagnosis, and treatment are appropriately used by the primary care teams. Additionally, the psychiatrist provides specific consultation for complex patients on the interaction and synthesis of biological, psychological, and social-cultural issues to arrive at a psychiatric assessment and treatment plan. Since other professionals available to PCCs can aptly address the psychological factors and social-cultural factors, the specific training of the psychiatrist allows for an integration of biomedical, psychiatric, and pharmacological management with psychosocial cultural determinants.

Collaboration between the PCC and psychiatrist has a spectrum of possible arrangements but is consistently characterized by both a shared mission of biopsychosocial and culturally sensitive care of the patient and a synergism of professional expertise.[13] Typically the psychiatrist may consult in a primary care practice part time, giving him or her a "specialist" role on the team, as opposed to those who are there full time. Funding time for psychiatric consultation is presently in flux with U.S. health care reform. Currently it ranges from traditional fee-for-service to bundled payment with salaried clinicians. The spectrum of options for psychiatric consultation ranges from noncollaborative to collaborative subtypes[13] and exists in a context shaped by the degree of integration of primary care and behavioral health services.

LEVELS OF INTEGRATION BETWEEN PRIMARY CARE AND BEHAVIORAL HEALTH

Doherty, McDaniel, and Baird[14] described collaborative care as a process, with the potential for evolution from one level to another over time and with concerted effort. Their classification system delineates not only the extent to which a practice actually engages in collaborative practice, but also its capacity to do so.

Doherty, McDaniel, and Baird's Taxonomy

Level 1: Minimally Collaborative; Separate Sites for Primary and Behavioral Health Care

Traditionally the dominant model of health care, primary care was considered a biomedical enterprise, and mental or behavioral health care functioned separately. In most places, these two domains functioned at separate facilities and in separate clinical systems—partly from the historical tradition since Cartesian dualism, and partly from state and federal statutes, and partly based on separate insurance reimbursement processes. The clinicians involved in caring for the same patient might or might not know about each other's care. Each clinician addressed his or her "piece" of the patient's care, often without awareness of the patient's other treatments and without communication with the other clinicians. Although this approach, described

BOX 4.3
CASE 1

Dr. Panges, a family physician at a federally qualified community health center (FQHC) practice, has many patients who need mental health treatment. The FQHC has no behavioral health professionals or services. Most of her patients prefer to attend a community mental health center several blocks away. She receives periodic communication in the form of therapist's or psychiatric clinician's notes; occasionally she is asked to complete a "physical assessment" form that the community mental health center requests to ensure their patients have a primary care clinician and are enrolled in biomedical care. Aside from this, there is little interaction with psychiatric care providers and primary care, and there is no specific method used for tracking patients.

in Box 4.3, sometimes still occurs, it is becoming less common in the face of increased recognition of the value of collaboration and the widespread use of electronic health records.

Level 2: Basic Collaboration with Primary and Behavioral Health Care Delivered in Parallel

In this level, PCCs practice in separate locations from mental health providers although they are both aware of the contributions of the other in their pursuit of health with their shared patients. These clinicians may exchange information from time to time. Standards of communication do not necessarily exist and may depend on the degree and nature of linkages between two systems of care. Clinicians from both "sides" have clearly defined non-overlapping responsibilities and roles, as described in Box 4.4.

Level 3: Basic Collaboration with Co-located Services

Primary care and behavioral health are housed in the same geographical space yet still maintain separate systems. They may maintain separate notes, document in distinct/separate formats, and bill through different systems. The co-location allows for some face-to-face collaboration, although this may be occasional at best. Proximity between behavioral health and primary care makes communication better overall and, likely, also more routine. Clinicians still use separate documentation systems, but

BOX 4.4
CASE 2

For 10 years Dr. Panges has been caring for a 60-year-old woman with a diagnosed bipolar disorder, treating her osteoarthritis, hypertension, and electrolyte disturbances caused by medications. The patient has faithfully attended her therapist's and psychiatrist's appointments for the same 10 years and has a stable mental health regimen of therapy and medications. At one visit, the patient informs Dr. Panges: "My psychiatrist tells me I'm stable. He'd like to know if you would be willing to prescribe my medications from now on. I don't need to see him anymore." Dr. Panges reviews the medications: oxcarbazepine, zaleplon, and bupropion. She agrees to take over these medications. The patient notifies her psychiatrist, who sends a psychiatric summary, and the primary care physician assumes the responsibility for prescribing the psychiatric medications. Ideally, the psychiatrist should send a treatment summary letter to the primary care clinician and/or communicate via the electronic health record if this is available. Alternatively, in the busy practice world, the patient may communicate the medication plan to the primary care practitioner.

BOX 4.5

CASE 3

The FQHC engages with the nearby community mental health center to provide a part-time on-site therapist for short-term counseling and intervention. The therapist works 1.5 days per week at the primary care office. The primary care clinician can refer patients to the therapist, who uses a separate medical record from the parent agency and also uses the FQHC record for brief communication with the referring clinician. The therapist notifies the referring clinician when the referred patient has made an appointment, kept (or broken) the appointment, and is discharged from care. The therapist also shares the initial treatment plan, progress reports, and the discharge plan, and occasionally asks the clinician to secure a consultation for medications from a consulting psychiatric prescriber offsite. Some clinicians provide "warm handoffs" (i.e., they introduce the patient to the behavioral health professional) at the time of the primary care appointment, but many just make a "cold" referral. Barriers to warm handoffs include part-time clinicians practicing on days opposite the therapist, clinicians being "too busy" to provide a warm handoff, or the therapist's appointments with other patients.

communication becomes more regular due to close proximity, especially by phone or email, with an occasional meeting or curbside consultation to discuss shared patients. Referral of patients between practices is facilitated because both practices are in the same location. Functionally this arrangement may look like a loosely defined team, though the individual clinicians make most decisions about patient care independently and notify each other as these changes. Box 4.5 describes a case managed in this manner.

Level 4: Close Collaboration in a Partially Integrated System

Primary care and behavioral health services are coordinated at multiple levels, including through some shared systems (e.g., scheduling or a shared electronic health record). Treatment plans for conditions like depression and diabetes are co-created and include both biomedical and psychosocial interventions. The team members understand the importance of those from other disciplines and seek to understand the other's professional expertise and culture. Face to face meetings to discuss shared patients are more common. Box 4.6 describes the way in which a case might be handled in a partially integrated system.

Level 5: Close Collaboration in a Fully Integrated System

Health care professionals from all disciplines share and have far more in common than they are separate. These commonalities include practice location, vision for patient-centered care, integrated systems that support patient care, and a commitment to knowing and valuing those from other disciplines. Hallmarks of this collaboration, described in the example in Box 4.7, include a shared health record, shared clerical and reception staff, shared reception areas, co-located and/or shared offices, and team members who routinely reference and include each other with patients, for the benefit of the patients. There are high levels of collaboration and integration between behavioral health and PCCs. The clinicians begin to function as a true team, with frequent in-person contact or telebehavioral health consultations, as well as written communication. The team members actively seek system solutions as they recognize barriers to care integration for a broader range of patients. However, some issues, like the availability of an integrated medical record, may not be readily available. Clinicians understand the different roles and operate more as an integrated health care team. Team members are changing their practices and the structure of care to better achieve patient goals by using the integrated care team.

Level 6: Full Collaboration in a Transformed/Merged Practice

The highest level of integration involves the greatest amount of practice change. This level was not described initially by Doherty and colleagues and represents an ideal for primary health care that may be elusive for many. See Chapter 2: Integrated

BOX 4.6

CASE 4

The FQHC has long realized a need to offer onsite behavioral health services. The agency grows to several clinical locations, one of which has a small behavioral health unit onsite. The unit accepts referrals. Despite having onsite space and a shared medical record, the no-show rate for new mental health patients is approximately 50%, which is much higher than the no-show rate among those seeing their primary care clinician. The psychiatric nurse practitioner consults (via mobile phone or telebehavioral health) with the primary care clinician or via the electronic medical record; she is readily available to the primary care practitioner for medication questions and emergencies.

The FQHC expands the behavioral health services by providing a licensed clinical social worker therapist for one day per week at Dr. Panges' location. Dr. Panges happens to have the same clinical day as the therapist and quickly begins referring her patients for behavioral health counseling. Often she and the therapist are able to accomplish a warm handoff, and the show rate for these patients is close to 75%. Several of Dr. Panges' patients have connected well with the therapist, and Spanish-speaking patients have become comfortable with some of the medical interpreters available on staff. The therapist and Dr. Panges exchange updates via "telephone encounters" as well as onsite "curbside updates" when they are both in the office. Medication consultation occurs with the doctoral-level nurse practitioner prescriber (via telephone or telebehavioral health), directly with Dr. Panges, or with the therapist and the nurse practitioner, who then messages Dr. Panges.

Health Care at Cherokee Health Systems for a description of a successful, fully integrated system of care. Full collaboration between PCCs and behavioral health clinicians has allowed antecedent system cultures (whether from two separate systems or from one evolving system) to merge into a fully transformed practice. Clinicians and patients view the operation as a single health practice or system treating the whole person, as in the practice described in Box 4.8. The principle of treating the whole person is applied to all patients, not just targeted groups. It is also likely that a practice attaining this level of collaboration offers regular staff trainings about common mental health and

BOX 4.7

CASE 5

At a local residency practice for family physicians, the university-based behavioral health service is co-located and integrated within the primary care practice. The patients can see their primary care clinician in the same building as their family therapist. Family therapists or psychologists are assigned to each of seven family medicine teams. Registered nurse care managers assist with complex care coordination, and the behavioral health clinicians function clinically in patient care as well in a consultative role on the teams, to ensure that teams are functioning smoothly. The psychiatrist consults through a combination of electronic chart review, in-person assessments, telebehavioral health, ad hoc inquiries via messaging through the electronic health record, and resident training. Resident physicians collaborate with medical assistants, licensed practical nurses, and faculty to conduct rapid-cycle tests of change targeting practice quality improvement.

BOX 4.8

CASE 6

The local residency practice has become fully integrated, with a shared system for appointments and an open medical record. Nurse care managers have become the first contact for biopsychosocially complex patients and can arrange or make appointments. The care managers can freely consult with either the primary care clinician, the patient's behavioral health clinician, or a health coach. The psychiatrist is readily available for curbside consults, psychiatric emergencies, or difficult/complex cases. The patient's care flows easily between team members. Communication with team members is in person or via phone, email, electronic medical record, or telebehavioral health. Psychiatrists and the primary care clinician work with the team to develop patient registries and population management strategies. Team meetings are regular occurrences so that all members of the team (including the receptionist and medical assistant staff) know about the integrated care plan, and they are welcome to contact any and all members of the team.

substance abuse issues; uses stepped care, patient registries, and other algorithmic methods to track and optimize clinical outcomes; offers group and/or family visits (See Chapter 28: Group Interventions in Integrated Care Settings and Chapter 27: Best Practice for Family-Centered Health Care: A Three-Step Model); and engages in regular mini-team and whole-team meetings.

Psychiatric Consultation as a Parallel to Levels of Integration

As described above, integrated care teams may include a wide variety of behavioral health members. However, local resources may drive the actual personnel who fulfill given roles in the primary care team. In most areas of the United States, psychiatrists may be scarce within a given geographical region and are in high demand by PCCs given the illness burden of mental health concerns. Just as Doherty and colleagues described the range of possible integration and collaboration, so too can we articulate a range of ways in which PCCs may work specifically with a psychiatric consultant that vary by time, degree of involvement, and complexity.

Informal Consultation: "Curbside" or "Hallway" Consultation

In an integrated team with a psychiatric clinician available, that clinician could be a PCC, psychiatrist, physician assistant, or advanced practice nurse with specialty psychiatric training. The scope of training would be at the specialist level and would enhance, not duplicate, the treatment that the primary care team could provide. In a model of informal consultation, the PCC asks the consulting psychiatrist's advice about a patient's care without requesting a formal visit with the consultant. This consultation can occur in the hallway between cases (with attention to preserving confidentiality) or can be by telephone, email, telebehavioral health, or other technological method.[12] (See Chapter 9: Telehealth in an Integrated Care Environment). The PCC hears the consultation suggestions and then considers whether and how to implement care and treatment with the patient. There is no consultant note or other formal documentation.

Formal Indirect Consultation Through the Care Manager

In systems that have a psychiatric consultant, there is often a psychiatric care manager, who may be a psychiatric social worker, psychologist, or nurse. With the IMPaCT (Improving Mood Promoting Access to Collaborative Treatment) model of integrated care, the DCM plays an important role tracking depressed patients with, for example, the PHQ-9. These data can alert the PCC and the psychiatrist about those patients with severe depression, or depression that is not improving discovered by DCM monitoring.[15]

In large practices, the care manager may focus exclusively on depression. In these practices the DCM extends the care of both the PCC and the psychiatric consultant. The DCM can identify patients newly diagnosed with depression and build a registry of these patients to track outcomes. The

DCM provides an important conduit for the PCC to consult with the psychiatrist. In our practice, the DCM reviews active cases with a lead PCC, family therapist, and psychiatrist. In other practices, a designated medical assistant, nurse, or care manager may serve this role. In these periodic case consultation meetings, the team reviews the patient panel, with particular attention to patients who may be highly impaired, are not improving, or need psychiatric consultation. With complex cases exceeding the capacity of the integrated primary/behavioral health team, a seasoned/senior PCC or psychiatric consultant can provide evidence-based treatment suggestions regarding further diagnostic evaluations, medications, and/or psychotherapy, sometimes triaging to a specialty level of mental health care when needed. The PCC, the DCM, and the psychiatric consultant all document in the patient's primary care chart. In large practices that employ a patient registry for patients with depression, interventions, progress, and clinical outcomes can be documented for ease of access and for quality monitoring. Clinicians and care managers monitor the patient's progress through use of outcomes measures.

Formal Direct Consultation

The PCC, DCM, or other team member selects these consultation cases. These frequently represent patients followed by the PCC, who will continue in the integrated practice after a consultation with the psychiatrist. With these patients, the psychiatrist will assist with more accurate diagnosis and evidence-based treatment recommendations as requested or needed by the PCC. If the PCC is not comfortable caring for the mental health needs of the patient, then these patients should be referred directly to mental health clinicians for diagnosis and treatment within the practice, while the psychiatrist is available for consultation.

Some models require that tests and medications be suggested by the consulting psychiatrist but ordered by the PCC.[16] A prescheduled follow-up appointment with the PCC immediately after the psychiatrist visit is important for this model to work. However, in our experience, situations arise where wisdom and sensitivity to the patient's current clinical severity should prevail. For example, the PCCs may anticipate so many barriers to the patient's return for follow-up in such a short timeframe (e.g., barriers in the patient's work schedule, transportation problems, heavy demands on the PCC's schedule, financial barriers like copayments) that they ask the psychiatrist to order any necessary tests or write for an initial prescription. In large multiclinician primary care practices, one PCC on the team may initiate the psychiatric consult, while another is expected to follow the patient.

The psychiatrist's experience with complex dual diagnosis patients, for example substance abuse with severe panic disorder with agoraphobia, provides crucial expertise to assist PCCs with management options. In this scenario, many PCCs would be appropriately cautious and reluctant to prescribe benzodiazepines. The psychiatrist could recommend or prescribe a selective serotonin reuptake inhibitor and a limited number of benzodiazepines per month to minimize the possibility of addiction. Here the psychiatrist could initiate the treatment, provide psychoeducation to the patient, and develop a plan that the PCC can continue, with the agreement of the patient and psychiatrist as a team.

With this arrangement, PCCs (who in the past might find themselves "stuck" managing psychiatrically complex patients who refused to see a psychiatrist) are now in a position to provide primary care and ongoing complex mental health care with the support of the consulting team psychiatrist. In the integrated team model with a psychiatric prescribing consultant, PCCs and patients benefit as the patient can see the psychiatrist for a one-time consultation in the same clinical space or via telebehavioral health, and the PCC can then assume care of a complex medication regimen initiated by the psychiatrist after the patient has stabilized.

Electronic Record Consultation: "E-Consults"

A designated PCC, DCM, or other care manager maintains a registry of patients diagnosed with depression, other mental health diagnoses, or substance use conditions, and ensures that the consulting psychiatrist reviews these patients periodically. Care managers or DCMs, or health coaches, may also manage the PCC's request for a psychiatrist's initial consultation or follow-up. The psychiatrist reviews the case presentation, including relevant rating scales, and initial medications and can provide further psychopharmacological suggestions to the PCC. A PCC who has experience with psychopharmacology can provide treatment on straightforward cases. Psychiatric consultation suggestions delivered through the e-consult appear in the patient's chart and are routed to the patient's PCC, who can decide whether and when to implement the interventions for the patient. Although liability risk increases for the psychiatric or mental health consultant across the continuum from curbside/hallway (more limited liability), to formal indirect, to formal direct consultation (greater liability), the liability risk for the whole practice decreases with collaborative models because better outcomes have been shown to occur in over 80 randomized controlled trials.[17]

Patient-Specific PCC Education

Psychiatric consultations are a form of transferring expertise and increasing the fund of knowledge PCCs need to effectively manage the mental health issues of their patients. The psychiatrist or other mental health professionals can educate the PCC on patient-specific issues, including differential diagnosis, psychotherapy recommendations, psychotropic medication choices, and stepped care for depression, other psychiatric disorders, and substance misuse. Providing the rationale behind differential diagnosis and various treatments builds knowledge and confidence in the PCC's ability to care for the patient's psychiatric problem(s). The mental health team can track and contribute new evidence-based developments from the literature in mental health, which would be difficult for a full-time PCC to follow closely.

The psychiatric consultant should clearly and specifically document the rationale for findings and recommendations, as in this example:

> After careful review of patient's history, old records, and collateral history, it is clear that the patient did not have a bipolar disorder. Rather, she had a major depression/unipolar disorder, recurrent, with euthymic periods alternating with depression for the past several weeks. In the depressed period, she was irritable, had low tolerance for irritating events, got angry easily, and then cycled back to normal moods again.

This formulation logically leads to the "plan" or "recommendations" that follow. A typical plan consists of a concise, culturally sensitive, biopsychosocial assessment and detailed recommendations. For example, a typical set of recommendations may read as follow:

1. Check thyroid stimulating hormone (TSH), complete blood count (CBC) with differential, vitamin B12, folate levels. Rule out common medical mimics of depression. If TSH is ≥ 3.5 mU/L consider thyroid workup.
2. Consider antibodies to thyroid given depressive symptoms and high normal TSH.
3. Repeat B12 if B12 is ≤ 300 pg/ml as neuropsychiatric symptoms can occur with levels less than 300 even though she may have a hematologically normal B12.
4. After 3–4 days on the sertraline as subsequently described, discontinue Depakote slowly over the next few weeks, decreasing the dose by about 25% per week. Reduction of dose on a gradual basis is still important for better patient adjustment to tapering of the drug. Also, waiting 3–4 days after starting sertraline before starting the Depakote will be more likely to sort out side effects of the new medication versus withdrawal effects of the old medication.
5. Begin sertraline at a 50-mg dose, one-half pill for two days, then one pill per day thereafter. Target dose with her would be about 100 to 150 mg per day. Increase from 50 mg at 2 weeks if either no or partial response.
6. See the patient within the next 2 weeks, then approximately every 3–4 weeks until the major depressive episode has been stabilized.
7. Continue to follow PHQ-9 at visits.
8. Consider escitalopram or venlafaxine XR next, given the severity of her symptoms, if sertraline is insufficiently effective.
9. Coordinate with patient's psychotherapist to address her depressive symptoms and develop a conjoint treatment plan.
10. Consider encouraging patient to return to her home church to help with behavioral activation as well as to strengthen her connection with her faith community again.

Collaboration and Connection with Rest of Mental Health Team

The electronic record also gives the option of two-way communications between all members of the integrated health care team. All members of the team should be aware of the diagnosis and treatment recommendations and should be able to report and track progress and outcomes in a patient registry. In some cases, the original team plan may have been to treat the mental health problems on site. However, numerous clinical factors may be uncovered by team members necessitating a referral out of the practice for consultation or follow-up by a psychiatric specialist, psychopharmacologist, psychologist/behaviorist, family therapist, or other clinician. At times, referrals will need to be made to an emergency department for psychiatric evaluation for dangerousness or grave disability, for hospitalization or partial hospitalization, or to a community mental health center or other community support services.

Communication in Shared Care Models

Inherent in the most successful levels of integration and consultation, communication plays a crucial role so all parties know their roles have value, they are clear on what is expected of them as it relates to the functions and roles of others, and all team members maintain a shared vision for the collaborative work. The electronic health record can function as a convenient bridge among collaborative partners provided that there is a shared expectation for the form and function of such communication. Typical expectations might include a standard format or label, such as "mental health communication." Standards for regular communication such as communication upon initial consultation with the PCC should be established. Standard notes or note templates with recommendations from the consulting psychiatrist or a note from the PCC to update changes of status are useful. In-person, telephone, or telebehavioral health conversations should be facilitated when there are specific risks of harm for the patient (e.g., an urgent suicidal or violent patient, or a question of urgent medicolegal practice). Another reason for telephone/telebehavioral health consultation might be that the PCC or psychiatrist is confused about a presentation and needs the opportunity to "think out loud" about the care of the patient with a colleague who is literally "on the same team." Less formal opportunities for communication also exist in day-to-day practice when sharing office space or passing other team members in the hallways. These informal communications shape the collaborative relationships needed to do the work of collaborative care by developing and maintaining interprofessional rapport.

Ways of Maximizing Efficiency of Team Members' Time

As with any resource, optimal use results in the best outcome. For example, if the psychiatric consultant has limited time available to support the PCC's practice, a well-formulated consultation question, when referring the patient, provides the start to a more efficient consultation compared to the historical standard "evaluate and treat," or no question or formulation, or simply a working diagnosis communicated to the psychiatric consultant. Similarly, "knowing your question" is a useful strategy when any team member needs consultation from any other. Examples include when a mental health therapist needs to understand about the complications of diabetes, a nurse needs support from a mental health colleague about phone triage for a patient in a domestic violence situation, or a PCC wonders how marital difficulties may affect his patient's adherence to a new medication. Membership in a high-functioning team dictates that team members are well aware of the roles, expertise, and functions of others such that these consultations or feedback requests can be well timed and appropriately directed. This becomes even more important as resources (like a psychiatrist's time) become scarcer.

ENGAGING THE CLINICAL-ADMINISTRATIVE TEAMS TO SUPPORT INTEGRATED CARE

A team culture of clinicians and administrators is critical to enhancing care, improving workflow, and reducing occupational stress.[18] In health care today, more than in the past, hospital and health care leaders are not generally physicians, nurses, or other clinically trained individuals. Yet in their leadership capacity, they have the potential to affect the quality of care provided to many more individuals than any single clinician could. Incorporation of administrative leaders into even granular issues that are involved in the care of patients is essential. The opportunity for leaders to be involved helps them to better understand the implications of higher-level decision making on day-to-day patient care issues.

ROCHESTER INTEGRATED PRIMARY CARE: AN EXAMPLE

The Pursuit of Integration Begins

At the University of Rochester Department of Family Medicine, we have had an integrated behavioral health service in some form since 1986. Prior to this, our Department Chair, Tom Campbell, MD, and Associate Chair, Susan McDaniel, PhD, a family physician and psychologist respectively, noticed a striking degree of difficulty for local psychiatrists or mental health therapists in communicating about patients referred to them by family resident physicians. Notwithstanding the efforts Dr. McDaniel made visiting community practices and clinics, in an effort to attempt to create something more akin to Level 2: Basic Collaboration at a Distance, no change occurred. In retrospect, we would call the original state Level 1: Minimal (or No) Collaboration while noting that many, including the departmental leaders, clearly saw the limitations.

Based on this experience, the department hired a mental health clinician to work onsite, to provide support to the primary care team, to begin to teach the residents, and to establish standards for collaborative practice. When this experienced marriage and family therapist joined the department, the problem of sparse communication around mental health referrals and mutual patients disappeared, as did the misunderstandings between members. The close contact between this therapist and referring clinicians represented Level 3: Basic Collaboration Onsite. Within one year's time, the number of referrals increased so rapidly that two more doctoral-level marriage and family therapist faculty members joined the group. The levels of communication, shared scheduling, and charting represented an organic shift to Level 4: Close Collaboration with Some System Integration. As part of this ongoing collaborative evolution, the department also first contracted with a part-time psychiatric consultant who both taught residents as part of their psychiatry rotations and consulted for the Department of Family Medicine for more challenging patients. Together, this team of on-site mental health providers represented one of the first models of collaborative care in a primary care setting.

Evolution into Co-located Yet Integrated Clinics

Since the late 1980s, the department's family medicine and behavioral health services have evolved toward greater levels of collaboration and integration. Local statutes had prevented the primary care practice from billing for mental health services provided on site. To ameliorate this, in 2005 the behavioral health service successfully applied to become a satellite of a New York State Office of Mental Health–regulated service, housed in the tertiary hospital's outpatient psychiatry division. The structures that replaced the early model in many ways replicated more traditional, noncollaborative mental health outpatient clinics (e.g., a return to formal referral structure, new templates for documentation, and standardized protocols aligned with hospital clinic and the Office of Mental Health). In spite of these processes and procedures, the co-location and values for collaborative care remained, and the transition facilitated a valuable connection to the larger service in the Department of Psychiatry. This connection enabled ready access to psychiatric support, consultation, and ongoing management for those patients who were most in need and who still preferred to receive the bulk of their care from the primary care clinic. So, even though the structural change could have resulted in barriers to collaboration, the closer connection to the Department of Psychiatry created an evolution toward Level 5: Close Collaboration Approaching an Integrated Practice; that is, a full-spectrum primary care practice integrating behavioral health clinicians, with ready access to a higher level of psychiatric services, including partial hospitalization and emergency/crisis support, as needed by patients, while maintaining some ability to meet the real-time, primary care–based psychosocial needs of patients and PCCs.

At the same time, the dual identity and affiliations across two departments have generated some additional challenges with establishing a cultural "norm" (between and among other behavioral health clinics who operate in a far more traditional manner) and, to some degree, flexibility to tailor our clinical offerings to the specific needs of our primary care stakeholders.

Toward Higher Levels of Integration: Electronic Records and Team-Based Care

Since the adoption of an electronic health record in 2006, all clinical services document in the same system. A shared record has improved the ability to share care and provide asynchronous methods of communication in addition to traditional face to face methods. Behavioral health notes maintain a special security level, and all PCCs are permitted routine access to these notes.

However, in 2007, another significant shift had an even greater impact. That year, our residency was selected by TransforMED as one of 14 programs nationwide to pilot an innovation in residency education. The P4: **P**reparing the **P**ersonal **P**hysician for Practice project aimed to "inspire and examine innovation in Family Medicine education and training" over a 6-year period.[19] Our department embarked on the evolution toward team-based care and ultimately toward designation as a National Center for Quality Assurance PCMH. Between 2007 and 2013, we transformed from a more "physician-centric," physician-led model of care and administration to one that is team-based, with shared leadership and improved ability to deliver high-quality, patient-centered care for our community of largely underserved families. The transition to team-based care was facilitated by the long history of the integration of behavioral health faculty and staff as team members.

Now, instead of individual PCCs working in their own individual practices, sharing at the clinical unit consists of teams composed of PCCs, clinical support staff, clerical support staff, and behavioral health faculty and staff all sharing a location. Clinical teams meet bimonthly to address staffing, patient care, office workflow, and other administrative concerns. Team meetings serve two functions: (1) to discuss the content of primary care practice and (2) to examine the process of team development and function. The behavioral health faculty member participates as a member of the team in his or her role as direct care provider. Based on their skill sets, in addition to patient care, the behavioral health faculty members also serve as consultants to the team on group process. This helps to address difficult relationships and resolve interpersonal conflicts and supports team members who are struggling, independent of their role (i.e., as medical assistant, nurse practitioner, physician).

Given that the practice is divided into seven teams, the department wanted to capture the successes and learn from the struggles of each team, as well as provide an opportunity for standardizing processes and learning across teams. To this end, the practice hosts monthly, practice-wide "team collaboratives." These hour-long meetings include all members of the practice (administrative support staff and all clinical team members). The aims of each collaborative are to focus on team functioning, team relationships, quality improvement, and patient engagement. A family therapist faculty member facilitates the team collaboratives. Each month he or she focuses on one skill/principle of patient-centered care, using small- and large-group teaching techniques, to activate the team members and stimulate learning. One explicit goal in each meeting is to enhance all members' sensitivity and skills to manage the challenges faced by our patients and their families, many of whom struggle with mental health and substance abuse issues in addition to other social determinants of health. Behavioral health faculty/staff, including psychiatric providers, have also taken on roles as practice consultants regarding adapting to the process of change, providing education to staff and clinicians about mental illness, managing safety and high-risk concerns, handling difficult clinical encounters, and conflict de-escalation.

Another hallmark of team-based care in our practice has been an expansion of the role of support staff to include more direct patient contact and engagement, more population health management responsibilities, and more opportunity to participate in assessment of all primary care patients. For example, medical assistants provide the initial assessment of patients' symptoms of depression and anxiety via the PHQ-9 and GAD-7. Their work in gathering data, as well as talking with patients about their concerns, enhances the diagnostic process and serves as an integral part of depression and anxiety management. These team members work closely with the PCCs for those visits and help to implement the collaborative plans designed with the patient/family and the clinician. Anecdotally, these clinical support staff members find that using such tools provides them with a greater role in patient care and provides important experience with the connection between mental health and physical health concerns in patients' lives.

The consulting psychiatrist plays a vital role in the primary care team, though perhaps less evident in the day-to-day, in-person contacts across clinical teams. The flexibility our consulting psychiatrist has to provide electronic consultations and prescheduled traditional patient consultations allows for a patient-centered approach to psychiatric care. The team clinical and clerical support staff learn about the differences between psychiatric consultation and psychotherapy and understand which patients may benefit from which intervention and when. Family medicine residents have opportunities to observe an expert conducting psychopharmacological assessments, and our faculty members enjoy having an established relationship with our consultant such that they are able, informally, to inquire about recommendations and briefly follow up on consults.

In what we now consider Level 6: Full Collaboration in a Transformed/Merged Practice, we have trained dozens of postdoctoral psychology fellows, marriage and family therapists, and residents in the value and practice of integrated care. We owe our success to several important elements: (1) establishing a common language; (2) expecting frequent communication (in person and asynchronous); (3) developing and nurturing a team of champions over time (not only at the inception of the concept in 1986, but through the last three decades as both departments sort out clinical domains, billing and regulatory infrastructure, and training needs); and (4) maintaining the leadership and staffing to sustain a flexible course with minimal drift.

Our integrated care clinic provided approximately 66,500 visits in the last year. Our behavioral health services as a whole had nearly 2,500 visits, 70 of which were in-person psychiatric consultations and the remainder outpatient psychotherapy assessments or follow-up appointments. Our consultant and the depression care team also entered 73 e-consultations during that same time period. Our experience reflects one example of the evolution of primary care over time, to create collaborative, then integrated and team-based care, providing culturally responsive biomedical and psychosocial care to patients over time.

FUTURE EVOLUTION OF TEAMS, TEAM CULTURE, AND INTEGRATED CARE

As the PCMH evolves (see Chapter 5: The Patient-Centered Medical Home) and more staff members work at the top of their scope of practice, we will see more provision of collaborative care by members of the team other than primary care and mental health professionals. Medical assistants or other nonlicensed, trained personnel will maintain responsibility for "panel management."[20] This refers to tracking a designated cohort of patients in a patient registry, whether by medical condition or some other identifier, to ensure that they receive the appropriate care and follow-up. These staff members, and perhaps others, may work closely with the DCM or other nurse, health coaches, and social work colleagues to provide outreach and follow-up to patients, including administering symptom screens; checking for medication adherence and side effects; and engaging in problem-solving, goal setting, and action planning for patients with mental health conditions.

Given the explicit focus of the PCMH on patient engagement, in addition to the care team, the patient and family must play a central role in their health care. As patient and family engagement evolves, teams will shift to incorporate improved processes to encourage and activate patients and families as full partners in care.

Finally, the National Committee for Quality Assurance[21] predicts that the "medical home" must continue to evolve to create "neighborhoods" of care so that integrated care teams and the systems that support them partner across clinical settings and institutions. Achieving this goal, as it relates to population health, will require partnerships between primary care, patient-centered specialty practices, and accountable care organizations, and will oblige all of us to fully embrace a team orientation.

CONCLUSION

In this chapter, we have provided a foundation for the "art and science" of team collaboration, together with some scenarios and reflections from our own practices. A brief summary of recommended approaches and relevant evidence is in Box 4.9.

BOX 4.9

SUMMARY OF RECOMMENDED TREATMENT APPROACHES AND RELEVANT EVIDENCE

Strength of recommendation taxonomy (SOR A, B, or C)

- **Collaborative care was associated with significant improvement in depression and anxiety outcomes compared with usual care in a Cochrane Review of 79 randomized controlled trials. (SOR A)[17]**
- **The IMPaCT (Improving Mood Promoting Access to Collaborative Treatment) model of integrated care, with a depression care manager to provide panel management for patients with depression and a consulting psychiatrist, demonstrated improved depression outcomes among depressed patients. (SOR A)[15]**

We anticipate that current trainees from a wide variety of disciplines will continue to work together with the primary care psychiatrist to develop integrated models of collaboration to better serve the biopsychosocial needs of patients into the future.

REFERENCES

1. Tharp T. The Collaborative Habit: Life Lessons for Working Together. New York: Simon and Schuster, 2009.
2. Mitroff II. Think like a sociopath, act like a saint. J Bus Strategy. 2004;25(5):42–53.
3. Uhl-Bien M, Marion R, McKelvey B. Complexity leadership theory: Shifting leadership from the industrial age to the knowledge era. Leadership Quarterly. 2007;18(4):298–318. doi:10.1016/j.leaqua.2007.04.002.
4. Salas E, Rosen MA, Burke C. The making of a dream team: When expert teams do best. In Ericsson KA, Charness N, Hoffman RR, Feltovich PJ, eds. The Cambridge Handbook of Expertise and Expert Performance. New York: Cambridge University Press, 2006:439–453.
5. Bodenheimer T. Coordinating care-a perilous journey through the health care system. N Engl J Med. 2008;358(10):1064–1071.
6. Frankish C. Health Impact Assessment As A Tool For Population Health Promotion And Public Policy. Vancouver, BC: University of British Columbia, Institute of Health Promotion Research, 1996.
7. McDaniel SH, Campbell T, Rosenberg T, Schultz S, deGruy F. Innovations in teaching about transdisciplinary professionalism and professional norms. In: Workshop Summary: Establishing Transdisciplinary Professionalism for Improving Health Outcomes. Institute of Medicine of the National Academies, 2014.
8. Direnfeld G. Understanding Collaborative Team Models. Interaction Consultants. www.yoursocialworker.com/s-articles/collaborative_team_models.doc. Published 2009. Accessed April 30, 2016.
9. Kroenke K, Spitzer RL, Williams JB. The PHQ-9: Validity of a brief depression severity measure. J Gen Intern Med. 2001;16(9):606–613.
10. Spitzer RL, Kroenke K, Williams JB, Lowe B. A brief measure for assessing generalized anxiety disorder. Arch Intern Med. 2006;166(10):1092–1097.
11. Hirschfeld RMA, Williams JBW, Spitzer RL, et al. Development and validation of a screening instrument for bipolar spectrum disorder: The Mood Disorder Questionnaire. Am J Psychiatry. 2000;157(11):1873–1875. doi:10.1176/appi.ajp.157.11.1873.
12. Seaburn DB, Lorenz AD, Gunn WB, Gawinski BA, Mauksch LB. Models of Collaboration: A Guide for Mental Health Professionals Working with Health Care Practitioners. New York: Basic Books, 1996.
13. Heath B, Wise Romero P, Reynolds, K. A Standard Framework for Levels of Integrated Healthcare. Washington DC: SAMHSA-HRSA Center for Integrated Health Solutions, 2013.
14. Doherty WJ, McDaniel SH, Baird MA. Five levels of primary care/behavioral healthcare collaboration. Behav Healthc Tomorrow.1996;5(5):25–27.
15. Unützer J, Katon W, Callahan C, et al. Collaborative care management of late-life depression in the primary care setting. JAMA. 2002;288(22):2836–2845.
16. Raney LE. Integrating primary care and behavioral health: The role of the psychiatrist in the collaborative care model. Am J Psychiatry. 2015;172(8):721–728.
17. Archer J, Bower P, Gilbody S, et al. Collaborative care for depression and anxiety problems. Cochrane Database Syst Rev. 2012;10(10).doi:10.1002/14651858.CD006525.pub2.
18. Merlino J. The responsibility matrix: A strategy for stronger physician/administrator partnerships. Becker's Hospital Review. http://www.beckershospitalreview.com/hospital-physician-relationships/the-responsibility-matrix-a-strategy-for-stronger-physician-administrator-partnerships.html. Published August 19, 2015. Accessed February 1, 2016.
19. Green L, Jones S, Fetter G, Pugno P. Preparing the personal physician for practice: Changing family medicine residency training to enable new model practice. Acad Med. 2007;82(12):1220–1227.
20. Bodenheimer T, Pham H. Primary care: Current problems and proposed solutions. Health Aff. 2010;29(5):799–805.
21. National Committee for Quality Assurance. The Future of Patient-Centered Medical Homes. http://www.ncqa.org/Portals/0/Public%20Policy/2014%20Comment%20Letters/The_Future_of_PCMH.pdf. Published 2014. Accessed February 1, 2016.

5

The Patient-Centered Medical Home

COLLEEN CONRY, SHANDRA BROWN LEVEY, AND BONNIE T. JORTBERG

BOX 5.1
KEY POINTS

- **The patient-centered medical home (PCMH) is a framework to provide patient-centered, comprehensive, coordinated, and accessible care.**
- **The PCMH is the hub of care, representing an interface of specialty care, behavioral health, hospitals, home health, nursing homes, and community services. Formal relationships with the medical neighborhood are essential.**
- **The PCMH has been shown to decrease costs and improve patient outcomes.**
- **Payment models to support the PCMH are beginning to be implemented and include fee-for-service, a monthly maintenance fee, and shared savings.**

INTRODUCTION

Patient-centeredness ... is the core; it is that property of care that welcomes me (as a patient) to assert my humanity and individuality. If we be healers, then I suggest that that is not a route to a point; it is the point.

—Don Berwick[1]

The Patient-Centered Medical Home (PCMH) is a multifaceted approach to providing health care that is based on the relationship between the patient and the provider. The concept of the PCMH began in 1967 with the American Academy of Pediatrics (AAP).[2] In this model, the PCMH concept meant having a central location for archiving a child's medical record. In 2002, the AAP expanded the PCMH concept to describe care that is accessible, continuous, comprehensive, family-centered, coordinated, compassionate, and culturally effective.[3]

In 2007, the American Academy of Family Physicians (AAFP), the AAP, the American College of Physicians (ACP), and the American Osteopathic Association (AOA) developed seven joint principles to describe the PCMH.[4] These joint principles have become the cornerstone of transformation of primary care practices. These principles, defining the main characteristics of the medical home, are as follows:

1. *Personal Physician:* each patient has an ongoing relationship with a personal physician trained to provide first contact and continuous and comprehensive care.
2. *Physician-Directed Medical Practice:* the personal physician leads a team of individuals at the practice level who collectively take responsibility for the ongoing care of patients.
3. *Whole Person Orientation:* the personal physician is responsible for providing for all of the patient's health care needs.
4. *Care is Coordinated and/or Integrated* across all elements of the complex health care system.

5. *Quality and Safety* for patient care.
6. *Enhanced Access to Care* is available through practice systems.
7. *Payment Reform* that appropriately recognizes the added value provided to patients who have a PCMH.[4]

Building on this work, the Agency for Healthcare Research and Quality (AHRQ) defined the medical home as encompassing five functions and attributes: (1) comprehensive care, (2) patient-centered care, (3) coordinated care, (4) accessible services, and (5) quality and safety.[5] AHRQ defines the medical home as not simply a place, but as a model of the organization of primary care that delivers the core functions of primary health care.[5] Also pertinent to the development of PCMH, the Institute for Healthcare Improvement developed the Triple Aim: improving the individual experience of care, improving the health of populations, and reducing the per capita costs of care for populations.[6]

BUILDING BLOCKS OF THE PCMH

In 2014, Bodenheimer et al[7] described the results of studying 23 "highly regarded practices," the researchers' experiences as practice facilitators in more than 25 practices, and a review of existing models and research on primary care improvement. Practices were selected for site visits, because they were innovative and had reputations for high performance in one or more of the Triple Aims. From these case studies and coaching experiences, the researchers used an iterative process to identify common attributes of high-performing primary care. They developed a set of building blocks, illustrated in Figure 5.1, that occurred with regularity among well-functioning practices. The 10 building blocks of primary care also embrace Starfield's four pillars of primary care,[8] elements of the joint principles, and PCMH recognition standards, and other core components of the PCMH.

Four building blocks emerge from this research: (1) engaged leadership, (2) data-driven improvement, (3) assignment of a patient to a provider, and (4) team-based care. Once these blocks are in place, practices are ready to move on to the patient–team partnership, population management, continuity of care, and finally to prompt access to care, comprehensive and coordinated care, and the development of a template for the future.

The researchers concluded that the 10 building blocks provide a practical conceptual model that can help practices in the journey toward becoming high-performing PCMHs. Even though the building blocks are not a universal roadmap, they provide an overview that assists practices to transform.

WHY THE MEDICAL HOME WORKS

The Patient-Centered Primary Care Collaborative (PCPCC) was founded in 2006 to advance an efficient health system built on a strong foundation of primary care and the PCMH.

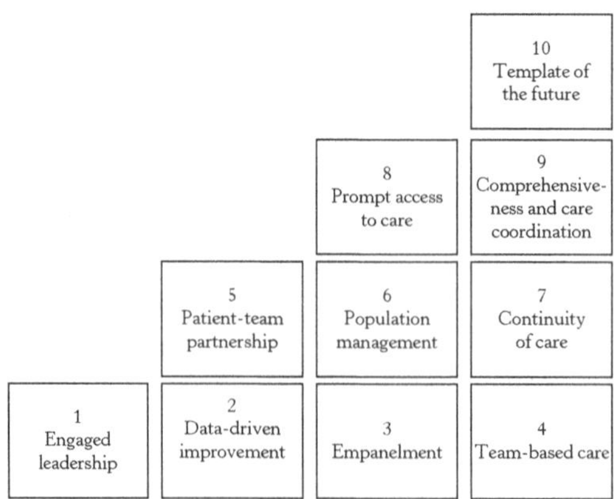

FIGURE 5.1: Building blocks of the PCMH Reprinted with permission from Bodenheimer T, Ghorob A, Willard-Grace R, Grumbach K. The 10 building blocks of high-performing primary care. Ann Fam Med. 2014;12(2):166–171.

The PCPCC works through stakeholder centers across the country to disseminate results and outcomes from medical home initiatives, advocate for public policy that advances and builds support for primary care and the medical home, and bring together health care experts, patients, and thought leaders to promote learning, awareness, and innovation of the medical home model. They created a framework shown in detail in Figure 5.2 that offers definitions, strategies, and potential impacts of the medical home.[9]

PRACTICE TRANSFORMATION

"I don't feel like a passive spectator anymore. I'm an integral part of my health-care team; we're working together to find long-term solutions to my health issues."

—University of Colorado patient

Becoming a PCMH is challenging, because it involves a very different way to operate a practice

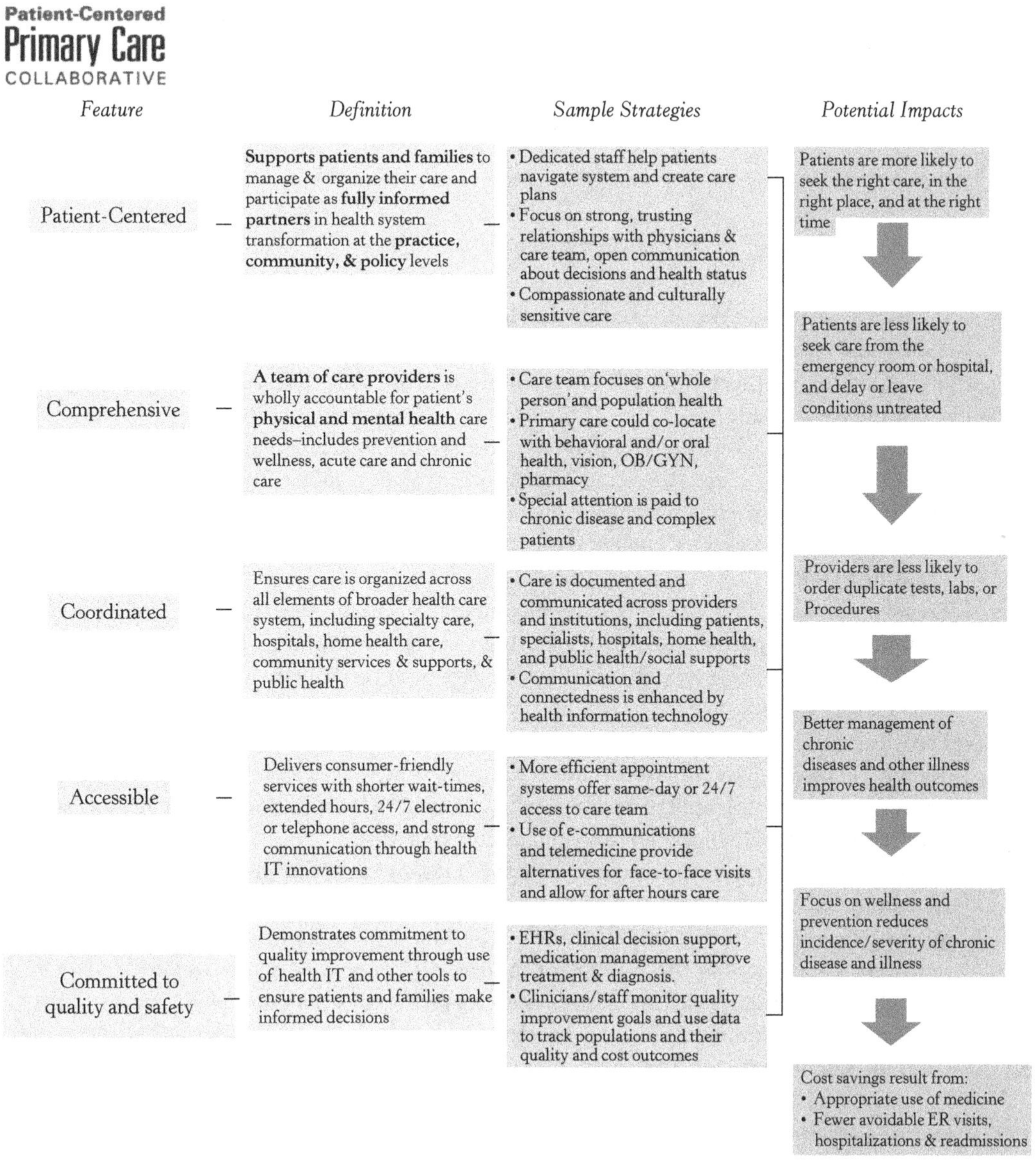

Patient-Centered
Primary Care
COLLABORATIVE

Feature	*Definition*	*Sample Strategies*
Patient-Centered	**Supports patients and families** to manage & organize their care and participate as **fully informed partners** in health system transformation at the **practice, community, & policy** levels	• Dedicated staff help patients navigate system and create care plans • Focus on strong, trusting relationships with physicians & care team, open communication about decisions and health status • Compassionate and culturally sensitive care
Comprehensive	**A team of care providers** is wholly accountable for patient's **physical and mental health** care needs–includes prevention and wellness, acute care and chronic care	• Care team focuses on 'whole person' and population health • Primary care could co-locate with behavioral and/or oral health, vision, OB/GYN, pharmacy • Special attention is paid to chronic disease and complex patients
Coordinated	Ensures care is organized across all elements of broader health care system, including specialty care, hospitals, home health care, community services & supports, & public health	• Care is documented and communicated across providers and institutions, including patients, specialists, hospitals, home health, and public health/social supports • Communication and connectedness is enhanced by health information technology
Accessible	Delivers consumer-friendly services with shorter wait-times, extended hours, 24/7 electronic or telephone access, and strong communication through health IT innovations	• More efficient appointment systems offer same-day or 24/7 access to care team • Use of e-communications and telemedicine provide alternatives for face-to-face visits and allow for after hours care
Committed to quality and safety	Demonstrates commitment to quality improvement through use of health IT and other tools to ensure patients and families make informed decisions	• EHRs, clinical decision support, medication management improve treatment & diagnosis. • Clinicians/staff monitor quality improvement goals and use data to track populations and their quality and cost outcomes

Potential Impacts

Patients are more likely to seek the right care, in the right place, and at the right time

↓

Patients are less likely to seek care from the emergency room or hospital, and delay or leave conditions untreated

↓

Providers are less likely to order duplicate tests, labs, or Procedures

↓

Better management of chronic diseases and other illness improves health outcomes

↓

Focus on wellness and prevention reduces incidence/severity of chronic disease and illness

↓

Cost savings result from:
- Appropriate use of medicine
- Fewer avoidable ER visits, hospitalizations & readmissions

FIGURE 5.2: Why the medical home works: a framework Reprinted with permission from Patient-Centered Primary Care Collaborative. Why the Medical Home Works: A Framework, 2013. https://www.pcpcc.org/resource/infographic-why-medical-home-works.

and care for patients.[10] It requires *transformation* of the primary care practice. Several health care reform efforts have focused on stimulating the PCMH transformation, providing guidance and funding to help practices make the wholesale changes required. These changes reach into the very philosophy of primary care, and touch every member and aspect of a practice, including patients.

Support from employers, insurers, state and federal agencies, and professional organizations have enabled numerous transformation projects in nearly every state. Early recommendations from the American Academy of Family Physicians' National Demonstration Project[10] are described in Box 5.2.

FORMAL ACCREDITATION

Three organizations have attempted to standardize the PCMH, with specific criteria to measure the medical "homeness" of individual practices. Recognition from these organizations has been useful to researchers attempting to measure the outcomes of practice transformation and to insurance companies willing to pay additional financial support for PCMHs. The National Committee for Quality Assurance (NCQA) is the most widely used certification process to transform primary care practices into medical homes.[11] NCQA's PCMH standards are aligned with federal "meaningful use" definitions. The American Board of Family Medicine, American Board of Pediatrics, and

BOX 5.2

STEPS TO TRANSFORMATION OF THE PRIMARY CARE PRACTICE

- **The PCMH requires a transformation that involves a continuous and unrelenting process of change and represents a fundamental re-imagination and redesign of practice.**
- **Implementing new technology is always more difficult and time-consuming than anticipated and envisioned.**
- **PCMHs employ markedly different approaches to patient care, which challenges physicians to reexamine their identities. Transformation involves a move from physician-centered care to a team approach in which care is shared among others.**
- **The magnitude and pace of change required to transform into a PCMH produces fatigue. Transformation occurs in fits and starts.**
- **Transformation to a PCMH is a developmental process. The strategic developmental approach that is required starts with ensuring a strong structural core and then implementing smaller changes that help to build the adaptive reserve. Only then can larger, more complex changes begin.**
- **Transformation is a local process and is highly dependent on initial conditions at the local practice, in the health care system, and at the community level. Practices with strong adaptive reserve were better able to develop and implement PCMH components that made sense in the context of their characteristics and circumstances.**
- **Successful transformation requires skills that are not taught to physicians in traditional education. To move toward success, practices must establish realistic initial expectations for the time and effort that will be needed to build better communications, trust, and relationships so that the adaptive reserve for change will be up to the challenges.**
- **Transformation requires a flexible and reflective technology plan for the practice.**
- **Successful transformation obligates practices to monitor change fatigue and think about holding periodic learning sessions so that participants can be reenergized and motivated.**
- **Practices transforming to a PCMH must accept the challenge to become a continuous learning organization, rather than relying solely on external expertise for "fixes."**

From Patient-Centered Primary Care Collaborative. Why the Medical Home Works: A Framework, 2013. https://www.pcpcc.org/resource/infographic-why-medical-home-works.

American Board of Internal Medicine all recognize certification as work toward ongoing specialty board certification.

The Joint Commission accredits ambulatory care organizations for PCMH[12] and is often used by hospitals or hospital systems that already receive Joint Commission accreditation. Similarly, the Utilization Review Accreditation Commission[13] recognizes PCMH achievement for hospitals and systems using their accreditation process. Different PCMH demonstration projects and insurance companies have required recognition or certification by one of these organizations in order to qualify to participate in projects or receive additional payments. In addition, some states have created their own PCMH criteria. While all of these organizations provide roadmaps to becoming a PCMH, true transformation requires significant change beyond just meeting a set of criteria.

TEAM-BASED CARE IN THE PCMH

"I like having a team of people working with me, and I like that you share in my care so I don't have to repeat myself, and things are more coordinated. It makes it easier knowing I have a team that is talking with each other."

—University of Colorado Patient

Team-based care includes other health care personnel along with primary care practitioners (PCP) in the health management of patients. There is mounting evidence that team-based care improves health.[14–16] Team-based care is a PCMH pillar, and will likely continue to grow as research continues to demonstrate that this approach can decrease costs and improve outcomes. A team-based approach to care allows PCPs opportunities to provide the care for which they are best suited, while other team members can assist with a variety of other patient needs. Depending on the particular makeup of the team, the way this looks in practice can vary significantly. In a more advanced PCMH, additional providers may include specialty care providers, advanced practice professionals, pharmacists, psychologists, psychiatrists, diabetes educators, nutritionists, social workers, health coaches, and care managers. The entire care experience is improved for patients and team members alike, when the team works together to determine patient preferences, goals, needs, and barriers to appropriate care; anticipates patient needs; collaborates on the care given; and communicates findings with appropriate follow up. This experience can result in high-quality care, and can lead to the accomplishment of shared goals within and across settings.[17]

For a high-functioning, healthy team to develop and thrive, it must be continuously developed and nurtured. According to Mitchell et al,[18] the most effective members of high-functioning teams in health care display honesty, discipline, creativity, humility, and curiosity. Team principles, processes, and design elements that facilitate team-based health care include shared goals, clear roles, mutual trust, effective communication, and measurable processes and outcomes, which are interwoven and dependent on each other.[18] In general, key features of effective teams also include building trust, mastering conflict, achieving commitment, embracing accountability, and focusing on results.[19]

Patient-centered care is essential for truly effective team functioning. When the patient is at the center, each team member understands his or her role on the team and in the care of the patient. When all team members have a voice, team-based care can function as it is intended. In addition, protected time for teams to meet for patient care discussions as well as to discuss the functioning of the team will help to maintain a healthy and highly functioning team unit. With the team-based care elements addressed, team members can enjoy working to the top of their scope, learn new skills, and develop more connected relationships with patients that will enhance the doctor–patient relationship. Physicians often report feeling a sense of relief and an increase in satisfaction when they can practice within the scope of their training. See Chapter 4: Team-Based Integrated Primary Care for additional discussion of teams.

PCMH SPACE

The primary care practice will need to redesign its physical space to suit the needs of a PCMH. In shifting toward team-based care, population management, and relationship-centered partnerships with patients, a PCMH must accommodate personnel from behavioral health, pharmacy, social work, and care management. New space design will help integrate additional health professionals as well as modified workflows.

One observational study of 19 practices located across the United States looked at practices that had successfully integrated behavioral health providers into primary care practices.[20] PCPs and behavioral health providers who were located in the same workspace had more face-to-face patient-care coordination than providers who were located in separate work areas (41.5% of observed encounters vs. 11.7%).[20]

These observations likely extend to other team members such as medical assistants, care managers, and pharmacists. Teams with ready access to each other are more prone to interface in real time around patient issues and truly share care. However, a balance between private workspace needed for focused work, spaces for direct patient care, and space for private discussions must be maintained. Practices with options for redesigning or building anew should carefully consider co-located spaces to foster team functioning and efficiency.

THE MEDICAL NEIGHBORHOOD

A key component of the PCMH is the coordination of care across the entire health care system, including specialty care, behavioral health care, hospitals, home health, nursing homes, and community services.[21] While primary care and the PCMH are the obvious hub for this coordination and communication, many other entities must be engaged in the care of the patient. In a white paper published by the AHRQ in 2011, Taylor et. al.[22] describe the medical neighborhood as a "PCMH and a constellation of other clinicians providing health care services to patients within it, along with community and social service organizations."[22] This neighborhood is not a geographical location but rather a "set of relationships revolving around the patient." Principles of a high-functioning neighborhood are outlined in Box 5.3.

Creation of a medical neighborhood requires changes in practice from both the PCMH and its

BOX 5.3

PRINCIPLES OF A HIGH-FUNCTIONING NEIGHBORHOOD

- **Clear agreement upon, and delineation of, the respective roles of neighbors in the system (e.g., through care coordination agreements between primary care clinicians and specialty physicians, agreement on care transitions, referral arrangements, referral and follow-up guidelines from professional societies)**
- **Shared clinical information needed for effective decision making and reduced duplication and waste in the system, supported by appropriate health information technology systems**
- **Care teams, typically anchored by the PCMH, that develop individualized care plans for complex patients**
- **Continuity of needed medical care when patients move between settings, with active communication, coordination, and collaboration among everyone involved in the patient's care, including clinicians, patients, and families**
- **A focus on the patient's preferences, perhaps with the dedicated primary care coordinator in the PCMH playing a key role in interfacing with other clinicians to ensure that patient preferences are incorporated into decision making**
- **Strong community linkages that include both clinical and nonclinical services (e.g., personal care services, home-delivered meals, school-based care, linkages with mental health and addiction services)**

From Gunn R, Davis MM, Hall J, et al. Designing clinical space for the delivery of integrated behavioral health and primary care. J Am Board Fam. 2015;28(Supplement 1):S52–S62 and American College of Physicians. The Patient-Centered Medical Home Neighbor: The Interface of the Patient-Centered Medical Home with Specialty/Subspecialty Practice: A Position Paper, 2010. https://www.acponline.org/system/files/documents/advocacy/current_policy_papers/assets/pcmh_neighbors.pdf. Accessed May 18, 2016.

neighbors. The PCMH must develop workflows that track referrals using patient registries. Further, when the PCMH requests a consultation, it must form a specific question, provide adequate patient history and test results, and inform the specialist of the type of relationship the PCP expects between the patient and specialist.

When the consultation request is received, the specialist must track the arrival of patients for consultation and report back to the PCMH. The specialist needs to tell the PCMH if the patient fails to come in for an appointment, should discuss with the PCP the relationship the specialist will have with the patient, and must inform the PCP in a timely fashion of the results of the consultation. In addition, specialists should avoid "lateral referral" to other specialists without first involving the PCP.

Implementation of the medical neighborhood varies widely. Historically, PCPs have had informal relationships with consultants, often based on shared hospitals for admission, insurance contracts, and personal relationships. With fewer PCPs caring for patients who are in the hospital, there may be less "curbside" consultation than in the past. Shared electronic health records make it much easier for physicians to quickly request and report consultations.

In an attempt to formalize the PCMH/medical neighborhood relationship, many practices have developed formal contracts outlining the responsibilities of each party. Often called compacts, these may be very short or quite detailed. Some large groups have integrated these compacts into their employment agreements or into the medical staff bylaws.

NCQA first published its Patient-Centered Specialty Practice Program in 2012,[23] reflecting the interwoven relationship with the NCQA's PCMH standards. Some specialty practices have achieved recognition from NCQA, but there is currently no economic imperative to do so.

Beyond the medical neighborhood, the accountable care organization (ACO) concept seeks to integrate the PCMH, specialty care, acute and post acute care, behavioral health care, pharmacy, and diagnostic services. Inherent in the ACO is the expectation that the organization takes financial risk for the entire care of populations. Community and social services, such as hospice, personal care services, transportation, and education, as well as state and local public health services, must be part of the entire neighborhood. Improved care coordination, with the PCMH as the hub, has the potential to improve health outcomes and decrease overall costs.

RESEARCH TO SUPPORT THE MEDICAL HOME

"I have never in my 66 years felt so well cared about and for. Every person I spoke to was genuinely caring and happy. Dr. L has a very special ability to look me in the eye and know on another level what I am telling her."

—University of Colorado Patient

The PCPCC publishes yearly reports on evidence supporting the PCMH. Multiple studies across the country continue to investigate PCMH outcomes, both economic and medical; a periodic review of the field is required in order to maintain an ongoing sense of the benefits of the PCMH model. The most recent PCPCC report (2014)[24] indicated that PCMH studies (Box 5.4) continue to demonstrate impressive improvements across a broad range of categories, including: cost, utilization, population health, prevention, access to care, and patient satisfaction, while a gap still exists in reporting impact on clinician satisfaction.

Rosenthal[25] evaluated several PCMH models to determine if earlier findings of improved outcomes and satisfaction are corroborated. The author used standard literature databases and websites of numerous professional organizations, government organizations, business groups, and private health organizations. Over 200 references, reports, and books about PCMH were evaluated. The studies of the PCMH outcomes that received an evidence rating of SOR A and SOR B are listed in Box 5.5. The author concluded that evidence from multiple settings and several countries supports the ability of the medical home to advance societal health.

PAYMENT FOR THE PCMH

A major criticism of the PCMH has been the increased cost of providing care coordination and enhanced population management. Although payment reform has not yet supported widespread adoption of team-based care, particularly with interdisciplinary team members, efforts are under way to help team-based care become a more routine experience and expectation for all involved. It is crucial that new models of payment include mechanisms to pay

BOX 5.4

STUDIES DEMONSTRATING THE EFFECTIVENESS OF THE PCMH

- **PCMHs decrease the cost of care, such as per member/per month costs, return on investment, and total cost of care (61% of peer-reviewed and 57% of industry-generated studies)**
- **PCMHs reduce the use of unnecessary or avoidable services, such as emergency department or urgent care visits (61% of peer-reviewed and 57% of industry-generated studies), inpatient admissions (31% peer-reviewed and 57% industry-generated studies), and hospital readmissions (13% of peer-reviewed and 29% of industry-generated studies)**
- **PCMHs improve population health indicators and increase in preventive services, such as better-controlled HbA1c, blood pressure, and LDL levels (31% of peer-reviewed and 29% of industry-generated studies) and increases in screening and/or immunization rates (31% of peer-reviewed and 29% of industry-generated studies)**
- **PCMHs improve access to care, such as improved overall access to primary care clinicians, as well as non–face-to-face visits (31% of peer-reviewed and 29% of industry-generated studies)**
- **PCMHs improve patient satisfaction, such as overall satisfaction, recommending the practice to family and friends, and satisfaction with provider communications (23% of peer-reviewed and 14% of industry-generated studies)**

From Rosenthal TC. The medical home: Growing evidence to support a new approach to primary care. J Am Board Fam. 2008;21(5):427–440.

for expanded team membership, acknowledging the critical role each team member provides. The current fee-for-service payment methodology does not account for these activities and structure, and most of the services have not been billable. The AAFP, AAP, and the ACP have recommended a payment strategy of (1) fee-for-service (per visit), (2) a monthly maintenance fee for practices contracting to provide medical home services, and (3) an additional bonus for reporting on quality performance measures.

BOX 5.5

SUMMARY OF RECOMMENDED TREATMENT APPROACHES AND RELEVANT EVIDENCE

Strength of recommendation taxonomy (SOR A, B, or C)

- **Patients who have a continuing relationship with a primary care physician have better health process measures and outcomes. (SOR A)[25]**
- **In primary care, patients present at most visits with multiple problems. (SOR A)[25]**
- **Multiple visits over time with the same provider create renewed opportunities to build management and teaching strategies tailored to individual progress and receptivity. (SOR B)[25]**
- **Minorities become as likely as nonminorities to receive preventive screening and have their chronic conditions well managed in a medical home. (SOR B)[25]**
- **Specialists generate more diagnostic hypotheses within their domain than outside and assign higher probabilities to diagnosis within that domain. (SOR B)[25]**
- **The more attributes of the medical home that a primary care practice demonstrates, the more likely patients are to be up to date on screening, immunizations, and health habits counseling, and the less likely they are to use emergency departments. (SOR B)[25]**

While such a structure has yet to be implemented, both the Centers for Medicare & Medicaid Services (CMMS) and private insurers are beginning to address the cost through different mechanisms. CMMS has added "transitions of care" and "care management services" billing codes for services that can be provided within a practice by non-physicians. Many insurers are beginning to provide a "care-coordination" payment to address the additional cost of care managers and chronic disease management. Some ACO strategies include shared-savings and pay-for-performance payments that increase the potential for additional revenue to the PCMH. Bundled payments for episodes of care aim to decrease certain disease costs. However, payment remains a challenge for the PCMH, since much of the cost savings occurs downstream via the reduction of admissions and emergency department visits, and often these savings are not attributed to the PCP or the PCMH. See Chapter 6: Financing Integrated Care Models for a detailed discussion.

Payment reform incentives have featured more prominently in PCMH initiatives, growing from just 26 in 2009 to 114 in 2013. During the same period, the number of patients covered by such initiatives increased from about five million to nearly 21 million. Even so, the payments and bonuses did not increase over that time.

PCMH AND EDUCATION

Training the future workforce in the principles of the PCMH is critical. In 2010, the primary care organizations (i.e., AAFP, AAP, ACP, AOA) jointly published their recommendations for the education of physicians planning to practice in a PCMH.[26] While primarily directed at medical student education, this document created a framework for early introduction to the principles of the PCMH. In 2013, the Family Medicine Residency Review Committee published a new set of residency training criteria.[27] This document does not specifically mention PCMH, but expects residents to be trained in a practice operating under the principles of the PCMH. Many residency programs have embraced the PCMH and are training new physicians not only to practice within a PCMH but also to lead the transformation of existing practices into PCMHs.

THE FUTURE OF THE PCMH

The PCMH is a concept and an outline for high-functioning primary care. It is neither a beginning nor an end, but a journey of change. Innovations continue across the country to enhance the care provided to patients.

Sinsky et al[28] outline five characteristics of successful PCMHs: (1) proactive planned care, with pre-visit planning and pre-visit laboratory tests (2) sharing clinical care within a team, with expanded rooming protocols, standing orders, and panel management (3) sharing clerical tasks with collaborative documentation (scribing), non-physician order entry, and streamlined prescription management (4) improving communication by verbal messaging and in-box management and (5) improving team functioning through co-location, team meetings, and workflow mapping. These characteristics describe care that is team-based with a focus on outcomes. Other models, such as the Care By Design practices at the University of Utah,[29] have developed similar advanced ways of using principles of Lean Management and other theories to create efficient flow, and high-level use of electronic medical records. Their model has shown improved physician satisfaction with practice. Practices at the University of Colorado Health have developed the APEX (Amazing Patient Experience) model, based on the Care By Design model, to improve patient experience, staff and provider satisfaction, and patient outcomes. In this model, medical assistants receive training to enhance skills they must have in order to (1) prepare patients for a physician visit through use of protocols and standard documentation of past medical history, (2) record medications and the review of systems, (3) identify care gaps for chronic disease management and prevention, (4) provide documentation assistance during the patient's visit with the physician; and (5) deliver post-examination care of the patient including lab draws, scheduling of appointments, and goal setting. Medical assistants also assist with "in-box management" to decrease the burden of paperwork on the physician. Initial outcomes have been very positive, with improved patient, staff, and provider satisfaction.

Going forward, other practices will innovate to enhance the care of patients in a patient-centered way, providing care not only in the traditional practice location but though telephone visits, electronic visits, workplace visits, and home visits. The PCMH will become a way of caring for patients, rather than a location.

REFERENCES

1. Berwick DM. What "patient-centered" should mean: confessions of an extremist. Health Aff (Millwood). 2009;28(4):w555–w565.

2. Council on Pediatric Practice (U.S.). Standards of Child Health Care. Evanston, IL: American Academy of Pediatrics, 1967.
3. The medical home. Pediatrics. 2002;110(1 Pt 1):184–186.
4. American Academy of Family Physicians (AAFP), American Academy of Pediatrics (AAP), American College of Physicians (ACP), American Osteopathic Association (AOA). Joint Principles of the Patient-Centered Medical Home, 2007. http://www.aafp.org/dam/AAFP/documents/practice_management/pcmh/initiatives/PCMHJoint.pdf. Accessed May 18, 2016.
5. Agency for Healthcare Research and Quality. Patient-Centered Medical Home Resource Center. https://pcmh.ahrq.gov/. Accessed October 12, 2015.
6. Berwick DM, Nolan TW, Whittington J. The Rriple Aim: care, health, and cost. Health Aff (Millwood). 2008;27(3):759–769.
7. Bodenheimer T, Ghorob A, Willard-Grace R, Grumbach K. The 10 building blocks of high-performing primary care. Ann Fam Med. 2014;12(2):166–171.
8. Starfield B. Is primary care essential? Lancet. 1994;344(8930):1129–1133.
9. Patient-Centered Primary Care Collaborative. Why the Medical Home Works: A Framework, 2013. https://www.pcpcc.org/resource/infographic-why-medical-home-works.
10. Nutting PA, Miller WL, Crabtree BF, Jaen CR, Stewart EE, Stange KC. Initial lessons from the first national demonstration project on practice transformation to a patient-centered medical home. Ann Fam Med. 2009;7(3):254–260.
11. National Committee for Quality Assurance. Patient-Centered Medical Home: Recognition Programs. http://www.ncqa.org/programs/recognition/practices/patient-centered-medical-home-pcmh. Accessed May 18, 2016.
12. The Joint Commission. Primary Care Medical Home Certification Program, 2013. http://www.jointcommission.org/accreditation/pchi.aspx. Accessed November 20, 2015.
13. URAC. The Patient-Centered Medical Home, 2016. https://www.urac.org/accreditation-and-measurement/accreditation-programs/all-programs/patient-centered-medical-home/. Accessed February 11, 2016.
14. Proia KK, Thota AB, Njie GJ, et al. Team-based care and improved blood pressure control: A community guide systematic review. Am J Prev Med. 2014;47(1):86–99.
15. Goodrich DE, Kilbourne AM, Nord KM, Bauer MS. Mental health collaborative care and its role in primary care settings. Curr Psychiatry Rep. 2013;15(8):1–12.
16. Carter BL, Rogers M, Daly J, Zheng S, James PA. The potency of team-based care interventions for hypertension: A meta-analysis. Arch Intern Med. 2009;169(19):1748–1755.
17. Naylor MD, Coburn KD, Kurtzman E. Inter-professional team-based primary care for chronically ill adults: State of the science. Unpublished white paper presented at the ABIM Foundation meeting to Advance Team-Based Care for the Chronically Ill in Ambulatory Settings, March 24–25, 2010, Philadelphia, PA.
18. Mitchell P, Wynia M, Golden R, et al. Core Principles & Values of Effective Team-Based Health Care. Discussion Paper, 2012. http://nam.edu/wp-content/uploads/2015/06/VSRT-Team-Based-Care-Principles-Values.pdf. Accessed October 6, 2015.
19. Lencioni P. Overcoming the Five Dysfunctions of a Team: A Field Guide for Leaders, Managers, and Facilitators. San Francisco: Jossey-Bass, 2005.
20. Gunn R, Davis MM, Hall J, et al. Designing clinical space for the delivery of integrated behavioral health and primary care. J Am Board Fam. 2015;28(Supplement 1):S52–S62.
21. American College of Physicians (ACP). The Patient-Centered Medical Home Neighbor: The Interface of the Patient-Centered Medical Home with Specialty/Subspecialty Practice. A Position Paper, 2010. https://www.acponline.org/system/files/documents/advocacy/current_policy_papers/assets/pcmh_neighbors.pdf. Accessed May 18, 2016.
22. Taylor EF, Lake T, Nysenbaum J, Peterson G, Meyers D. Coordinating Care in the Medical Neighborhood; Critical Components and Available Mechanisms. White Paper. AHRQ Publication No. 11-0064. Rockville, MD, June 2011.
23. National Committee for Quality Assurance. Patient-Centered Specialty Practice Recognition, 2013. https://www.ncqa.org/Portals/0/Newsroom/2013/PCSP%20Launch/PCSPR%202013%20White%20Paper%203.26.13%20formatted.pdf. Accessed November 20, 2015.
24. Patient-Centered Primary Care Collaborative. Results and Evidence. https://www.pcpcc.org/results-evidence. Accessed November 20, 2015.
25. Rosenthal TC. The medical home: growing evidence to support a new approach to primary care. J Am Board Fam. 2008;21(5):427–440.
26. American Academy of Family Physicians (AAFP), American Academy of Pediatrics (AAP), American College of Physicians (ACP), American Osteopathic Association (AOA). Joint Principles for the Medical Education of Physicians as Preparation for Practice in the Patient-Centered Medical Home, 2010. https://www.acponline.org/system/files/

documents/running_practice/delivery_and_payment_models/pcmh/understanding/educ-joint-principles.pdf. Accessed May 19, 2016.

27. Accreditation Council for Graduate Medical Education. ACGME Program Requirements for Graduate Medical Education in Family Medicine, 2015. http://www.acgme.org/acgmeweb/Portals/0/PFAssets/ProgramRequirements/120_family_medicine_07012015.pdf. Accessed May 19, 2016.

28. Sinsky CA, Willard-Grace R, Schutzbank AM, Sinsky TA, Margolius D, Bodenheimer T. In search of joy in practice: A report of 23 high-functioning primary care practices. Ann Fam Med. 2013;11(3):272–278.

29. University of Utah Health Care. The Next Phase in the Evolution of Health Care. http://healthcare.utah.edu/publicaffairs/spotlight/spotlight_461.html. Accessed November 20, 2015.

6

Financing Integrated Care Models

BRUCE J. SCHWARTZ, GILLIAN STEIN, AND SCOTT WETZLER

INTRODUCTION

The integration of medical and behavioral care holds a vast and largely untapped potential to reduce mortality, morbidity, and health care spending through improved care coordination and alignment of financial incentives. Historically, constraints on mental health coverage and a culturally embedded lack of communication between general medical physicians and their behavioral counterparts had created a fractured system of care. This system hinders the successful treatment of patients with comorbid medical and behavioral disorders, a population representing some of the most expensive patients in the health care system. In fact, individuals with comorbid behavioral health problems cost 2.5 to 3.5 times more to treat than those without. What is more, the majority of their spending goes to general medical services.[1] These data suggest that mental health issues are not being adequately addressed, and these individuals' physical health is suffering as a result.

Countless studies and reviews over the past two decades have demonstrated that providing behavioral services through integrated care models is cost effective.[2,3] More importantly, integrated care has been shown to be significantly beneficial from a clinical standpoint. As noted in one cumulative meta-analysis, "sufficient evidence had emerged by 2000 to demonstrate the statistically significant benefit of collaborative care."[4] Based on these demonstrations, various collaborative care models have been implemented. Yet despite this abundance of evidence and experience, financial support for these models remains problematic. Collaborative programs that do not rely on extrinsic research funds are few and far between. The complexity of funding integrated care reflects the "siloed" nature of our current health care system and the difficulty of developing a financially viable model of productivity and reimbursement.

In this chapter, we argue that the Mental Health Parity and Addiction Equity Act (MHPAEA) and the Affordable Care Act (ACA) offer a new opportunity to develop financial models for integrated care and provide a unique opportunity to achieve the triple aim: improving quality of care, increasing population-wide access to care, and reducing health care expenditures.[5] While the standard model of collaborative care focuses on improving access for individuals with mild to moderate mental illness within the general medical population, there may be limited financial gain if a higher-risk target population is not further specified. It is likely that the development of integrated physical and behavioral health care focused on the higher-cost medically ill patients with comorbid mental illness will lead to much larger increases in quality as well as much greater cost savings. Additionally, the viability of integrated care programs requires shifting from siloed reimbursement to a global budget. This chapter will outline a brief history of integrated care financing before describing the opportunities to replace traditional fee-for-service payment schemes. Ultimately, we will show that the financial sustainability of integrated care depends on narrow patient targeting, value-based incentives, and global budgeting.

CONSULTATION-LIAISON PSYCHIATRY

For most of the field's history, psychiatry has been split off from general medical care. Consultation-liaison (C-L) psychiatry, especially for medical inpatients, represented one of the only areas where there was collaborative interaction between mental health and medical providers. C-L services focus on behavioral disorders complicating the care of medical inpatients and were funded in response to a growing recognition that medical services required psychiatric input. C-L services are widespread in the United States, with 56 accredited psychosomatic fellowship programs in hospitals across the country.[6] Despite this longstanding need and prevalence, C-L services are not financially self-sustaining; they are so-called loss leaders.

At the crux of the issue lies the question of who is responsible for reimbursing psychiatric consultations in general medical inpatient settings. Many commonly used billing systems cannot route charges correctly when there is a psychiatric diagnosis or if the behavioral health benefit is "carved out," meaning behavioral health benefits are not covered by a typical insurance plan, and are instead provided through a contract with a separate behavioral health managed care entity. Behavioral managed care organizations often did not accept financial responsibility for these benefits, considering C-L consultations as part of the general medical benefit rather than a medically necessary piece of the behavioral benefit. Compounding the problem, the absence of strong mental health parity laws, prior to 2008, allowed insurers to reject claims for mental health services provided in medical inpatient settings. This practice stood in contrast to consultations conducted by other medical specialties. Further negatively impacting reimbursement, higher copays and deductibles could be applied to psychiatric consultations, depending upon the insurer. Finally, psychiatry remains a low-tech field, meaning there are no high-cost tests or procedures to help subsidize services as in other areas of medicine.

Compromising their fiscal viability even further, the reimbursement for C-L services disproportionately depends on one of the nation's lowest payers: Medicaid. Safety-net providers in inner cities treat a population that has much higher behavioral health needs, and Medicaid insures a majority of these patients. To put it another way, the prevalence of mental illness in the Medicaid population is estimated at 50%, whereas the prevalence in commercially insured primary care populations is 28%.[7] Consequently, other specialties see a better-insured population, which leads to higher rates of reimbursement, while C-L services are often needed most in underinsured communities. This confluence of factors has meant that C-L consultations are consistently underreimbursed.

Psychiatrists have also proven unable to develop economic productivity models that support C-L services. Psychiatric consultations of medical inpatients are highly time-intensive. Consultations are often extended due to the presence of complicating acute and chronic medical and behavioral issues. Moreover, consulting requires psychiatrists to be in ongoing communication with other physicians, as well as to assist and monitor nursing staff with the implementation of behavioral management strategies. As such, C-L psychiatrists simply cannot see as many patients in the course of the day as nonpsychiatric physicians, nor can they see as many patients as they can see in an outpatient mental health setting.

The funding of C-L services represents a particularly informative example for understanding the issues facing integrated care financing. Hospitals value C-L services because they can contribute to shortened length of stay and reduced cost-intensive observation (one-to-one) for these patients. In inpatient settings, hospitals can support these services financially—despite being low volume and low revenue—because insurers typically reimburse inpatient care with large per diem sums. Accordingly, related models of integrated care may be financially sustainable in a medical inpatient setting. Alternatively, C-L psychiatry has generally not been sustainable in a medical outpatient environment, where reimbursement is fee-for-service, discriminatory insurance practices are prevalent, and there is an inability to subsidize behavioral health care. In such settings, C-L services become too large of a financial loss, and hospitals cannot financially bear supporting them. Accordingly, few hospital-run outpatient settings have developed substantial integrated care services.

The few C-L services that do operate in outpatient settings are those embedded in highly specialized medical and surgical services, where they are either required for regulatory approval (e.g., bariatric surgery, transplant) or given special government funding (e.g., human immunodeficiency virus [HIV]). In these specialized services, consensus exists that the success of the medical/surgical care is inextricably tied to the patient's mental health. The success of a liver transplant, for instance, often requires psychiatric intervention for patients whose liver failure was associated with alcohol or substance abuse. In this population, behavioral modification is vital, as well as addressing underlying psychological factors that originally contributed to the patient's substance abuse or comorbid psychiatric disorders. Other specialty services, such as HIV/AIDS or hepatitis C treatment, also frequently offer C-L services, and receive enhanced funding.

Despite these exceptions, C-L psychiatry—the most widespread enactment of an integrated care philosophy to date—largely remains confined to medical inpatient care.

MANAGED BEHAVIORAL HEALTH ORGANIZATIONS

On the opposite end of the integration spectrum sit managed behavioral health organizations (MBHOs). The advent of MBHOs in the late 1980s cemented a growing conceptual and practical division between behavioral health and physical health. MBHOs operate as independent, contractual entities, functioning in nested arrangements with insurers. Behavioral health care is "carved out." Defining behavioral health benefits in such a way has severed any remaining ties between the two care systems. Moreover, it severed those ties at every level—conceptually, financially, and administratively. MBHO-contractual behavioral providers had no connection to general medical providers, and financial incentives grew to be completely misaligned.

MBHOs aimed to curb "medically unnecessary" behavioral health spending, permitting only a highly limited inpatient and outpatient benefit. They did so with astonishing success. How did carve-out companies achieve such large spending cuts? MBHOs aggressively regulated utilization levels. They were able to drastically decrease inpatient use of behavioral health services, a costly piece of the financial pie. They also focused on recruiting nonphysician outpatient providers, significantly shifting the behavioral health provider landscape. MBHOs emphasized services provided by licensed social workers as well as master's-level psychologists. These providers were much less expensive than psychiatrists. This not only filled the large gap left by a shortage of psychiatrists (largely a regionally dependent shortage) but also further solidified the division between behavioral health services and general medicine. Directing mental health care to nonmedical providers unaffiliated with the medical sector precludes the possibility of providing integrated care. Finally, MBHOs have no incentive to reimburse behavioral care for patients coping with medical disorders; they actually have incentives to deny such reimbursements and shift costs into the medical sector.

The fractured system of care that this arrangement fostered made it difficult to coordinate the care of patients with comorbid mental and physical disorders. Primary care physicians were rarely aware of behavioral health treatment of their patients and vice versa. Despite their financial success, carve-outs have had a major negative impact on integrated care. Carve-outs reduced costs, but they did so at the expense of adequate care, particularly for individuals with physical and mental health comorbidities. Consequently, low participation of psychiatrists in MBHOs provider panels and fundamental problems of insufficient manpower, low reimbursement, and maldistribution remain today.

The 2008 MHPAEA was passed in large part to address these excessive restrictions on care associated with MBHOs. Reimbursement parity between mental and physical health services has long been a major health care issue. Before the Mental Health Parity Act of 1996, for instance, lifetime and annual dollar limits for mental health benefits were prohibitively less favorable than those for medical/surgical benefits. MBHOs' cost-controlling tactics exacerbated this preexisting disparity, leading to greater inequality in available funds for mental health care. Employer-sponsored group health plans largely complied with the 1996 parity law, but only to restrict mental health benefits elsewhere in their plans. In May 2000, the U.S. General Accounting Office reported that 87% of compliant employer-sponsored plans contained at least one other design feature that restricted mental health benefits more than medical/surgical benefits. For example, 65% of plans restricted the number of covered outpatient office visits and hospital days for mental health treatment further than for other health treatment.[8] The MHPAEA responded to these stubborn limitations and expanded existing parity law. By specifically prohibiting such treatment limitations, the MHPAEA offers a novel opportunity to level the playing field and finance mental health services that have become restricted and isolated under MBHOs.

DE FACTO MENTAL HEALTH CARE PROVIDERS

In addition to emphasizing nonphysician providers, MBHOs' aggressive cost-cutting shifted the landscape of behavioral health care even further. Poor coverage, reduced access to specialty care, and the shortage of psychiatric physicians meant more patients had to turn to primary care for mental health services, particularly for prescriptions. Primary care physicians took up the necessity of providing first-line treatment for mental illness and became de facto mental health care providers.[9,10]

Present-day prescribing trends reflect this shift. In 2008, over 70% of adults being treated with antidepressants received their prescriptions from general medical providers.[11] Similarly, in a 2010 investigation of national ambulatory medical care, antidepressants were the third most frequently prescribed therapeutic drug during physician office visits.[12] A 2005 study of 12-month mental health treatment in the United States also found that primary care physicians treated the vast majority of those receiving treatment. Primary care physicians had become redefined as "gatekeepers" for access to specialty mental health care that was difficult to obtain, and therefore had to provide much of the care themselves.[13]

Despite offering a single point of access to care, this shift does not represent truly integrated care. The same researchers who found that primary care treatment had become the most common treatment profile for mental health also found that those in specialty mental health treatment were much more likely than those in general medical treatment to receive adequate treatment. Primary care as de facto mental health care is not an integrated care model; it is a lack of access model with primary care doctors filling the vacuum. Primary care physicians lack the time and specialty training to provide adequate mental health care for more severe mental disorders, and this in turn has the potential to impact patients' physical outcomes.

INTEGRATED CARE MODELS: AN OVERVIEW

Attempts to address these inadequacies have resulted in a proliferation of research into the potential benefits of integrated care. Poor physical outcomes and high utilization of health resources were increasingly being linked to behavioral comorbidities. In particular, researchers discovered a powerful connection between depression and poor control of diabetes mellitus.[14,15] Based on this association, the IMPACT model (Improving Mood: Promoting Access to Collaborative Treatment) was developed to study the potential benefits of collaborative care. In a randomized trial of 1,800 elderly patients, investigators found that a significant improvement in depressive symptomatology led to a significant improvement in diabetes status as compared with usual care. Collaborative care more than doubled the effectiveness of primary care depression treatment, such that 45% of those receiving collaborative care experienced a 50% reduction in depression symptoms, as compared to 19% of those receiving usual care.[16] A follow-up study confirmed these results and reported that one year after the withdrawal of IMPACT resources, IMPACT patients still fared significantly better on depression measures.[17] A more recent analysis of the multicondition collaborative care intervention program, TEAMcare, showed an increase in depression-free days, better-controlled diabetes mellitus and coronary heart disease (as measured by quality-adjusted life years), and lowered mean outpatient health costs as compared to usual care, when depression symptoms were targeted.[18] These studies demonstrated on a large, statistically significant scale that integrated care positively impacts both physical and mental health outcomes. Accordingly, consensus has grown over the past decade that integrated care is a necessary piece of the provision of quality health care.

The most effective integrated care models rely on team-based care management grounded in the philosophy of stepped care. Currently, a significant evidence base exists demonstrating that, as compared to usual care, these models reduce depressive symptoms and severity, increase rates of depression treatment, and improve patient satisfaction and quality of life.[19,20] In these models, primary care physicians collaborate with care managers, who are often nonmedical behavioral health providers, as well as psychiatrists. The stepped care model ensures maximum efficiency of resource allocation by beginning with the least intensive treatment options and intensifying care only for patients who are not responding. Most frequently, the psychiatrists' role is to provide decision support via indirect consultation. However, for cases with more complex disease presentations that require higher levels of care, psychiatrists will see patients face to face via direct consultation. In these cases, ultimate responsibility for the patient's care remains with the primary care provider, but the psychiatrist takes on a larger role within the team. Finally, if treatment targets remain unmet, patients will be referred to specialty mental health providers who will take over the direction and provision of mental health treatment.

Integrated care models all have documented benefits and drawbacks, often in equal measure. The most common benefits are increased diagnosis of mental illness, increased access to psychiatric care, and decreased medical costs resulting from such treatment. The most common drawbacks are the challenges of implementation, such as the complexity of integrating different medical records (particularly when confidentiality restrictions exist) and billing systems, the difficulty of overcoming cultural differences between providers and training them to work within the new system, and the fiscal demands of hiring an often-large number of new employees, such as care managers. Most importantly, psychiatrist consultants in primary care are much less productive than in other psychiatric settings, and when they do not see the patient, they are not eligible for reimbursement. Thus, it is impossible for psychiatrists in integrated care settings to generate sufficient reimbursement to support their salaries. Telemedicine and computer-based care may help defray implementation costs by allowing for greater productivity. These services may be of particular value in rural areas where behavioral health services face extreme workforce shortages.

It is important to note the existence of one major directional distinction among the variety of integrated care models. Integrated care and so-called reverse integrated care[21,22] both aim to enhance treatment outcomes, but the primary site of integration differs between the two. The former seeks to improve mental health treatment in general medical settings, while the latter focuses on general medical treatment within mental health settings, particularly for those with serious mental illness. These models reflect the segmented population in need of mental health services: those whose chronic medical illnesses are complicated by mild to moderate mental illness, and those whose physical health is compromised by severe mental illness. Reverse co-location represents a vital attempt to address the needs of the latter population, who face a serious lack of access to medical care. Nevertheless, this chapter focuses on bringing behavioral health services into primary care settings, and will therefore focus on the population with mild to moderate mental illness.

FINANCING INTEGRATED CARE

Fee-for-Service Models

Despite the advent of the MHPAEA, fee-for-service models for the reimbursement of integrated behavioral care are not sustainable. This is particularly true considering the lower productivity and lack of reimbursement for psychiatric consultations in primary care settings and the lingering carve-out of behavioral care. Among the barriers impeding fee-for-service reimbursement are restrictive billing code regulations. A large number of integrated care services are difficult to quantify, making fee-for-service billing challenging. Moreover, rules concerning who can provide reimbursable care, and in what setting, complicate implementation. For instance, care management billing codes are largely unrecognized by insurers, particularly when billing for behavioral health services within a medical setting. Furthermore, consultation between physicians is unlikely to be reimbursed. In collaborative care models requiring decision support from psychiatrists, if the psychiatrist does not actually see the patient he or she cannot bill for the service under typical fee-for-service arrangements. The time psychiatrists spend consulting on cases (a fundamental piece of most integrated care models) is not reimbursable. MBHOs have exacerbated this issue by requiring behavioral care to be provided by their network providers, who may or may not be co-located in primary care practices.

In 2017, the Centers for Medicare and Medicaid Services (CMS) has released a final rule for the Medicare Fee Schedule that includes a CPT code and a fee for Psychiatric Collaborative Care Management Services. The fee will be used to reimburse primary care practices for behavioral consultations provided by psychiatrists in the collaborative care model. The psychiatric collaborative care model is expected to be a coordinated team-based approach and include the psychiatrist, a behavioral health care manager, and the primary care clinician. Payment is expected to assist with the challenge of adequately funding behavioral collaborative care. At this time it is difficult to determine whether these payments will be sufficient to support and sustain these services.

Within the current siloed system, fee-for-service creates a major administrative burden on health care providers, who must manage a diverse set of contracts and billing regimes. Amidst a multitude of separate providers and health plans, all of whom might see varying pieces of the return on investment, where to place the onus of implementation remains unclear. For certain medical and surgical specialties, the introduction of health and behavior Current Procedural Terminology (CPT) codes somewhat addressed these complexities. Meant for patients with comorbid mental and physical illness, these codes allowed for the financial recognition that mental health services are essential in cases where a mental health disorder is not the primary diagnosis. Nevertheless, it has proved difficult to reliably acquire reimbursement under the health and behavior codes.[23]

Above all, inadequate fee-for-service reimbursement precludes meaningful incentives for cost savings in the health system. A fundamental part of the economic reasoning behind integrated care holds the following: Patients with physical and behavioral comorbidities use significantly higher levels of health care resources within the medical sector when compared to those without behavioral comorbidities. As such, effectively addressing these patients' behavioral health needs will lower health care costs in *the medical sector.* Health care costs in the mental health sector will necessarily increase, however, to effectively address behavioral needs (i.e., by implementing integrated care protocols). With carved-out fee-for-service reimbursement, mental health costs will simply grow, with no return on investment that can be used to retroactively fund such growth. The only way for decreased medical costs to underwrite increased mental health costs is for payment to be merged into a single system. In other words, the financial sustainability of integrated care depends on financial integration, such that incentives for the behavioral and physical health services are aligned and resources are shared.

Medical Cost Offset

Cummings, Dorken, Pallak, and Henke coined the term "medical cost offset" in 1990 to describe the idea that programmatic reduction of medical costs would result from mental health treatment, so much so that that these savings would more than pay for the cost of said mental health treatment.[24,25] While many studies have demonstrated the cost-effectiveness of collaborative care,[2–4] cost *savings* are much more important to study if medical cost offset is to make integrated care financially viable. In support of the cost offset hypothesis, many studies have concluded that integrated care offers potential savings ranging from $32 to $70 per member per month. In fact one study, looking at the cost effects of the IMPACT trial, actually concluded that integrated care led to over $3,000 in health care cost savings per patient over four years, even after accounting for higher implementation costs of the intervention.[26] A meta-analysis of 23 studies concluded that at the very least, collaborative care was cost-neutral, and it did in fact generate savings for most programs.[27] Investigators have posited various reasons to account for these savings, including decreased need for physical health services (particularly among patients with chronic medical conditions), decreased indulgence in unhealthy behaviors (e.g., drinking, smoking, and overeating), and decreased anxiety and somatization.

It is important to note that most of these cost-effectiveness studies did not include the costs associated with implementing integrated care. Moreover, if they did so, the authors often concluded that the return on investment made integration cost-effective at a level comparable with other widely accepted treatments because of substantial increases in treatment effectiveness. Nevertheless, integrated care did not *save* money in these studies. When looking at the cost offset hypothesis, we must remember that preventive care does not necessarily mean cost savings, at least in the near term. In the realm of physical care, it has been repeatedly shown that most preventive health care costs more than it saves.[28,29] One *New York Times* reporter eloquently paraphrased the issue: "Indeed, if it were somehow possible to wave a wand and turn people into thin nonsmokers who remembered to take their statins, this country's health care expenses would fall. But any effort to promote health has its own costs."[30] In other words, the cost offset model may underestimate the costs of providing more treatment. In particular, our intuitive sense that preventing future illness will save money ignores the fact that to prevent future illness, a significant number of people must be treated who never would have gotten sick, and that there are not significant savings to be achieved by intervening with the less severely ill.[31] Ultimately, from a financial standpoint, we must take care to differentiate between initiatives that are cost-effective and those that are actually cost-saving, regardless of the beneficial effects on quality outcomes.

High-Cost Patients

As it stands, then, untargeted integrated care programs can only generate moderate savings, if that. Preventing future negative outcomes for certain patients requires the treatment of a much larger number of individuals whose symptoms may never have worsened, regardless of the use of stepped care interventions. However, if we could clearly define a target population of high-cost patients for integrated care initiatives, we could minimize the amount of "unnecessary" treatment and maximize cost savings. Patient targeting could also help maximize the effective use of limited psychiatric manpower. A clearly defined target population for integrated care is the linchpin of financial sustainability for integrated care programs, and this population ought to represent the greatest potential for improved outcomes and cost savings. A 2001 study found that the most expensive 5% of patients account for over 50% of expenditures.[32] Evidence suggests that this extreme concentration of health care spending comes from the medical sector but stems in part from inadequate management of mental health.[33,34] New York State Medicaid data indicate that in 2011, only one in five Medicaid beneficiaries had behavioral health diagnoses, but they accounted for almost half of total Medicaid expenditures.[35] However, their higher expenses were not simply the result of expensive psychiatric care. Individuals with comorbid behavioral health problems typically cost 2.5 to 3.5 times more to treat than those without, but the majority of their spending goes to general medical services.[1] While the highest rates of readmission occur among patients with mental health/substance abuse (MH/SA) diagnoses, these readmissions are predominantly related to medical complications. Patients with behavioral diagnoses are costing the state more money, but for medical rather than behavioral reasons. In New York State, for instance, data from 2007 reveal that almost $520 million was spent on potentially preventable readmissions (PPRs) for specifically medical reasons. Of the $520 million, $370 million was spent on 35,056 PPRs for patients with MH/SA diagnoses, whereas $149 million was spent on 11,403 PPRs for those without an MH/SA diagnosis.[36] Untreated mental illness can lead to poor treatment adherence, an increased likelihood of engaging in unhealthy behaviors, somatization, and greater anxiety associated with higher frequency of seeking treatment, all of which increase health care costs, particularly in the general medical sector.

In light of these data, integrated care programs should target individuals with high-cost medical comorbidities. These patients represent the highest-cost subset of patients with both physical and mental illness. In targeting them for integrated care, the health care system will see the greatest return on investment, because these patients currently use care in an expensive and ineffective manner. As noted in a report prepared for the American Psychiatric Association (APA), high-severity comorbidities, such as chronic kidney disease, chronic obstructive pulmonary disease, hypertension, and circulatory conditions, are most likely to provide savings on a per-patient basis. Alternatively, high-incidence comorbidities, such as arthritis and asthma, are most likely to provide savings through the entire population.[33] Choosing which comorbidities to target will require a detailed analysis of provider capacity and patient populations in order to maximize this intersection of high severity and high incidence. Larger health care networks will likely benefit from taking a population-based approach that targets high-incidence comorbidities.

Financial Models for Integrated Care

The medical cost offset hypothesis requires not only patient targeting, but also transitioning from siloed reimbursement to a global budget. The ACA emphasizes quality measurement and value-based, prospective payments, offering the health care financing sector a novel opportunity for innovation in this realm. Recently, a number of new financial models have been developed to replace fee-for-service reimbursement. In the hopes of curbing unnecessary expenditures, these new models emphasize value-based payment over volume-based payment. In doing so, they call for a reshaping of the entire landscape of health care financing. While payment reform may appear to increase practices' administrative burdens, it can actually reduce this burden in the long term by reducing system complexity.[37] These new models attempt to align financial incentives across the board, controlling costs by encouraging cost-effective, collaborative medical care. Accordingly, these value-based payment plans are potentially ideal for financing integrated care. Financial integration not only reflects the ideological mission of integrated care but also creates a sustainable funding mechanism.

Pay-for-Performance (P4P)

One new idea has been to use pay-for-performance (P4P) incentives.[38,39] P4P incentives entail that a percentage of program funding is contingent on meeting several quality indicators, such as timely follow-up with patients after discharge from the hospital. P4P incentives based on quality targets that reflect the mission of integrated care programs (e.g., ensuring that patients taking psychotropic medications are treated according to systematic guidelines and with appropriate psychiatric oversight) can be used to generate higher rates of reimbursement for these services. In addition, such incentives applied to entire medical systems can encourage the development of integrated care programs in the first place. Administrators will be more likely to implement integrated care programs when quality standards are financially consequential since such programs are linked to better outcomes. However, it is important to note that many P4P incentives are linked to comparative quality metrics across provider systems. Risk-adjusted comparisons between providers or provider networks require large caseloads of patients in order to be statistically significant, which could make the use of P4P incentives problematic in rural or other underserved areas.

Bundled Payment and Capitation Plans

Prospective payment contracts, such as bundled payment plans and capitation plans, offer a more radical departure from current fee-for-service plans. Bundled payments, also known as case rates, involve fixed payments for episodes of care as negotiated by payers and providers and can be risk-adjusted for age, illness severity, and other characteristics that influence the projected cost of care. This system functions well within an integrated framework because it aligns incentives across various providers. Episodes of care are diagnosis-based and defined as a collection of care to treat a particular condition. As such, each episode may involve multiple specialized providers. Because payment is fixed for the episode, providers have an incentive to coordinate their efforts and maximize cost-effectiveness. The less money they require for services, the more money providers are able to then keep as "savings," giving providers the opportunity to reinvest in the system of care. In an integrated care setting, as long as providers can accurately predict how many patients they will treat and thereby project revenue, they can ensure that expenses remain within the budget.

Capitation plans function similarly but on a much larger scale, such that providers receive a lump sum to provide all care for an individual. The capitation model was somewhat more prevalent in outpatient settings during the middle to late 1990s but gained such a negative reputation among providers that it fell out of favor by 2000. First and foremost, these models failed because the majority of them limited capitation to outpatient costs alone. This eliminated the opportunity for outpatient providers to create savings by reducing inpatient hospitalizations. A second major problem concerned perverse incentives. In making providers assume risk, capitated payments turned providers into insurers, focusing their attention on more than just providing optimal care.[40] Making matters worse, capitation was used in systems where mental health care was carved out, which meant that incentives were not truly aligned. As providers became aware of a need to control provision of services, this misalignment often led to inadequate referral, mistrust, decreased collaboration, and cost shifting into the mental health sector.[41] Finally, another major issue at the time was the inability of all but large provider networks to sufficiently control financial risk by spreading it over a large number of patients.

Today, the popularity of capitation models is seeing a resurgence. One particular success story comes from the DIAMOND project (Depression Improvement Across Minnesota, Offering a New Direction), which has organized and studied the implementation of collaborative care in provider systems across Minnesota. DIAMOND has done remarkably well using capitated reimbursements, specifically the payment of flat monthly fees for each patient in the program. Each participating health plan negotiates a fee with each participating clinic, and this fee covers the initial and follow-up care manager contacts, weekly consultations, and psychiatrist case reviews for up to 12 months.[42] The DIAMOND project demonstrated that capitated models create value in paying for integrated behavioral care. Moreover, they were able to avoid many pitfalls seen in the 1990s by integrating funding streams and using quality targets—similar to those used by P4P incentives—which likely helped health plans avoid adopting a rigid corporate focus on cost reduction.

Despite the DIAMOND project's success, capitated payment models do have certain drawbacks. The relative novelty of these models makes it difficult to set payment levels that will successfully underwrite the cost of providing integrated care while maintaining budget neutrality. Additionally, some providers worry that this type of reimbursement will lead to reduced standard reimbursement levels, or downward rebasing, once savings have been achieved. If true, this could decrease provider reimbursement in the long term, despite achieving high-quality care. With regard to risk sharing, many health insurers and health care scholars have voiced concerns about actually increasing inefficiency and costs by turning efficient providers into inefficient insurers.[43]

Shared Savings Model

An alternative to case rates and capitation is the shared savings model. This model has the potential to fund integrated care by using fee-for-service reimbursement and a risk-adjusted projected global budget. Shared savings models build off the accountable care organization (ACO) framework. ACOs are designed as collaborative, patient-centered institutions that finance integrated care by supporting necessary services that are nonbillable.[44] They also allow provider groups to assume higher levels of financial risk and reward than currently available in other models.[45] In a shared savings model, providers contract with a payer to provide care for a patient population, setting predetermined benchmarks for cost and quality that must be met over a set period of time. If the ACO can provide care at a lower cost than the predetermined threshold, it shares in these savings with the payer.

Like P4P, capitation, and bundled payments, a shared savings model provides incentives for quality and cost control by transferring a portion of the risk onto health care providers and tying that risk to quality metrics. A common concern voiced by critics of all prospective health care budgeting posits that these plans encourage low-volume care. In other words, rather than moving from volume-based to value-based, we would be moving from a high-volume-reward system to a low-volume-reward system. Quality benchmarks should ameliorate this possibility, although many available quality measures have limited analytic capacity beyond an appraisal of isolated, superficial markers. A shared savings plan helps to further combat this harmful potentiality, better than other models, through its underlying fee-for-service reimbursement mechanism. Providers can focus more energy on patient care than on how much of their capitated budget has been used. Consequently, shared savings models are often perceived as better able to maintain physician autonomy with regard to medical decision making.

In summary, shared savings and global budgets provide the greatest opportunity for funding integrated care, making it financially possible to implement these programs that have been proven to effectively address all three dimensions of the triple aim. The success of these financial models requires specific targeting of high-cost patients, particularly those with a substantial behavioral comorbidity, with higher premiums to reflect the higher morbidity of this population. Furthermore, bundled payments, capitation rates, or shared savings arrangements ought to be based on an actuarial analysis of the patient population to be served, tailoring each contract to reflect the realities of care provision in a given setting. Value-based arrangements that integrate funding streams across physical and mental health care provision not only provide incentives for quality care but also create reliable funding mechanisms for integrated programs designed to provide such care.

The Montefiore Story

In recent decades, Montefiore Medical Center has emerged as a leader in the integrated care movement, in part because of the use of a population-based approach and negotiated value-based arrangements with payers. Montefiore serves a low-income, minority population in the Bronx. With over 31% of residents living below the poverty line, this population has complex health and health care needs. To address these needs within the increasingly challenging health care financing environment, Montefiore began very early to develop integrated approaches to health service delivery. In 1995, Montefiore established an integrated provider association (IPA) and a behavioral care IPA. These programs worked to align the medical center, its physicians, and various health plans. Soon after, Montefiore established the Care Management Organization and University Behavioral Associates. To finance these programs, Montefiore negotiated value-based agreements with insurers. A majority of these agreements were fully capitated, while others were shared savings arrangements that used an IPA or ACO as the contracting entity. As of today, approximately 395,000 patients are covered by these risk arrangements.

These financial arrangements have allowed Montefiore to develop high-risk programs (e.g., Managed Addiction Treatment Services [MATS]) that target the most needy and expensive patients and prioritize care management. For instance, MATS reduced total Medicaid expenditures for substance use treatment by 56%.[46] Using case management to improve outpatient follow-up, MATS was able to substantially reduce unnecessary inpatient detoxifications. While MATS was not an integrated care project, it showed that targeting the highest-cost, highest-need patients was effective. Montefiore's existing and continuing investment in technological infrastructure has aided in this high-risk endeavor. Computerized monitoring systems to track the progress of their patients, with effective, time-sensitive data analysis, allow care managers to successfully direct patients' care, particularly in the implementation of stepped care protocols. Information technology systems also alert care managers when a targeted patient enters the emergency department, allowing high-cost emergent care to be controlled more efficaciously.

With this care management infrastructure in place as well as a large primary care system, with an accordingly large pool of patients for appropriate risk adjustment and management, Montefiore is an ideal site for integrated care innovation. In 2012, the use of a co-location model was studied in a naturalistic and qualitative case study that focused on financial sustainability.[5] The study followed three psychiatrists working at four primary care sites, two of which were certified as federally qualified health centers (FQHCs). Several reimbursement models were used. FQHC reimbursement was cost-based, and the other two sites, despite not being FQHCs, relied largely on full-risk capitated payments. Annual projected revenue depended on psychiatrists' experience and productivity levels but was sufficient for all three to be sustainable as full-time providers. The study did find that high no-show rates contributed to financial difficulties, as well as the need for social work staff to assist in specialty MH/SA referrals. Ultimately, however, this first foray into co-located care found that co-location was financially sustainable under certain conditions and able to effectively identify and treat psychiatric comorbidities.

In light of Montefiore's organizational familiarity with integrated care, the Centers for Medicare & Medicaid Services (CMS) designated the health system a Pioneer ACO Program in January 2012. The payment model for Pioneer ACOs was fee-for-service, but organizations able to achieve significant shared savings by year 2 had the opportunity to move toward a population-based payment structure with full financial risk. Pioneer ACOs were held to cost and quality benchmarks. Montefiore's program was the ACO with the best financial performance in years 1 and 2, saving Medicare over $23 million each year.[47] According to the shared savings arrangement of the Pioneer ACO program, Montefiore received $14 million and $13.41 million of the savings in years 1 and 2 respectively. These funds were then reinvested in Montefiore's health care system. The Pioneer ACO continues to do well at Montefiore, with a recent CMS analysis reporting gross savings of 3.6% for 2014.

Funding for Montefiore's integrated care efforts has relied on multiple funding streams, including extrinsic grants and budgetary expansions derived from shared savings projections. Based on these funding streams, today 10 psychiatrists and one psychologist work in 20 primary care sites, and these settings are in the process of adding seven more behavioral providers. These integrated care efforts have recently expanded due to a large Health Care Innovation Award from the Center for Medicare and Medicaid Innovation. The grant's goal is to develop the Bronx Behavioral Health Integration Project (Bronx-BHIP), which strives to increase the availability of behavioral health services by using an integrated care model. Notably, Bronx-BHIP is using this grant to test the utility of a capitated reimbursement methodology. To implement this case-based payment model, Montefiore is collaborating with several health plans. It remains too early to draw meaningful conclusions from the data, but it is hoped that Bronx-BHIP will provide a real-world example of how to successfully implement integrated care in a larger hospital setting.

Allowing Montefiore to further expand integrated care programs is New York's new Medicaid Delivery System Reform Incentive Payment (DSRIP) program to combat rising health care costs. This $6.4 billion program aims to reduce avoidable hospital use by 25% over the course of five years. DSRIP functions as a quality performance payment incentive for providers. Performing provider systems applying to participate in DSRIP were required to choose a behavioral health project involving integrating care. This condition reflects an acknowledgment by the state that a majority of avoidable, costly hospital readmissions involve behavioral patients. In other words, DSRIP illustrates a governmental recognition of the importance of integrating care. DSRIP funds will be used to fund the transformation of primary care practices to integrated care models, thereby helping neutralize deficits associated with implementation.[48] DSRIP will act as a bridge to value-based contracting and shared savings financing, reflecting the state government's belief in the value of integrated care and, more importantly, in the necessity of cost savings to fund this care. Notably, DSRIP will expand coverage for the dual-eligible population. DSRIP encourages providers to include dual eligibles in value-based payment models, particularly managed care plans, which will remove significant barriers and care discontinuities facing the most vulnerable Medicaid and Medicare patients.[49]

Despite the fact that some of the funding is grant-based, Montefiore is hopeful that the health system can sustain these programs from savings accrued through its value-based arrangements. The savings produced by this Pioneer ACO as well as by MATS reinforced this hope, demonstrating that value-based, shared savings arrangements can lead to program profitability.

CONCLUSION

A summary of the evidence supporting new financial models for integrated care is described in Box.6.1. Implementing an integrated care program poses a substantial financial risk, but not doing so poses one equally as grave. Investing in integrated care can dramatically improve the quality and outcomes of primary care. Moreover, in reaching for the triple aim, integrated care programs have the potential to positively impact overall health care spending. However, simply expecting a cost offset to make integrated programs pay for themselves may be overly optimistic. Novel reimbursement models are necessary to create financially stable programs. The ACA represents a meaningful new regulatory framework within which these models can be developed. Bundled payments, capitation, and shared-risk plans are all potential funding mechanisms for integrated care. It is our opinion that the strongest financial model will be one that targets individuals with higher-severity, high-frequency medical comorbidities and relies on a carefully crafted reimbursement scheme based in global budgeting.

Ultimately, despite the importance of ensuring financial viability, we cannot forget that the collaborative care model was developed to address the unavailability of quality mental health care. The historical underfunding for behavioral health will require enforcement of mental health parity. Reduction of costs should be a secondary concern.

BOX 6.1

EVIDENCE FOR FINANCIAL MODELS OF INTEGRATED CARE

Strength of recommendation taxonomy (SOR A, B, or C)

- **A cumulative meta-analysis showed "sufficient evidence had emerged by 2000 to demonstrate the statistically significant benefit of collaborative care."[2] (SOR A)**
- **The IMPACT model of collaborative care more than doubled the effectiveness of primary care depression treatment, such that more than twice as many patients experienced a significant reduction in depression symptoms compared those receiving usual care.[15] (SOR A)**
- **TEAMcare, a multicondition collaborative care intervention program, showed an increase in depression-free days, better-controlled diabetes mellitus and coronary heart disease (as measured by quality-adjusted life years), and lowered mean outpatient health costs as compared to usual care, when depression symptoms were targeted.[17] (SOR A)**
- **Stepped care models reduce depressive symptoms and severity, increase rates of depression treatment, and improve patient satisfaction and quality of life.[18–22] (SOR A)**
- **A meta-analysis of 23 studies concluded that at the very least, collaborative care was cost-neutral, and it did in fact generate savings for most programs.[30] (SOR A)**
- **A clearly defined target population for integrated care is the cornerstone of financial sustainability for integrated care programs, and this population ought to represent the greatest potential for improved outcomes and cost savings. (SOR C)**
- **Integrated care programs should target individuals with high-cost medical comorbidities. By targeting them for integrated care, the health care system will see the greatest return on investment. (SOR C)**
- **The DIAMOND Project (Depression Improvement Across Minnesota, Offering a New Direction) is a capitated model that creates value in paying for integrated behavioral care. Each participating health plan negotiates a fee with each participating clinic, and this fee covers the initial and follow-up care manager contacts, weekly consultations, and psychiatrist case reviews for up to 12 months.[48] (SOR B)**
- **P4P incentives entail that a percentage of program funding is contingent on meeting several quality indicators. P4P can be used to generate higher rates of reimbursement for integrated care services and to encourage the development of integrated care programs in the first place.[44,45] P4P incentives do, however, rely on risk-adjusted comparisons between providers or provider networks, which require large caseloads of patients in order to be statistically significant. (SOR C)**
- **Bundled payments, or case rates, involve fixed payments for episodes of care that can be risk-adjusted for age, illness severity, and other characteristics that influence the projected cost of care. Because payment is fixed for the episode of care, bundled payments align incentives across various providers, encouraging coordination and efficiency. In an**

integrated care setting, if providers can accurately predict how many patients they will treat and thereby project revenue, they can ensure that expenses remain within the budget.[50] (SOR C)

- Capitation plans involve a global budget for the provision of all care for an entire population. In systems where mental health care is not carved out, capitation has the potential to align incentives across various providers and increase the efficiency and cost-effectiveness of care. Certain drawbacks to capitated payment models are the difficulty of setting sufficient payment levels, the possibility of downward rebasing, and decreased provider efficiency as physicians are turned into insurers.[51] (SOR B)
- The shared savings model has the potential to fund integrated care by using fee-for-service reimbursement and a risk-adjusted projected global budget. A shared savings model provides incentives for quality and cost control by transferring a portion of the risk onto health care providers and tying that risk to quality metrics, as with P4P, bundled payments, and capitation models. With shared savings providers can focus more energy on patient care than on how much of their limited budget has been used. Shared savings models are thus perceived as able to maintain physician autonomy with regard to medical decision making.[52] (SOR B)
- Shared savings and global budgets provide the greatest opportunity for funding integrated care, making it financially possible to implement these programs that have been proven to effectively address all three dimensions of the triple aim. (SOR C)
- The Montefiore Model involves the use of a population-based approach and negotiated value-based arrangements. A majority of these value-based arrangements are fully capitated, while others were shared savings arrangements that use an IPA or ACO as the contracting entity. As of today, approximately 395,000 patients are covered by these risk arrangements. In 2012, CMS designated Montefiore Medical Center a Pioneer ACO. The payment model for Pioneer ACOs was fee-for-service, but organizations able to achieve significant shared savings by year 2 had the opportunity to move toward a population-based payment structure with full financial risk. Pioneer ACOs were held to cost and quality benchmarks. Montefiore's program was the ACO with the top financial performance in years 1 and 2, saving Medicare over $23 million each year.[53] (SOR B)

As one author put it, "although research into cost-benefit results is likely to be a strong driving force, it is also important to consider the integration of psychiatry and medicine because it addresses patients' problems most comprehensively and sensibly."[47]

REFERENCES

1. Melek SP, Norris DT, Paulus J. Economic Impact of Integrated Medical-Behavioral Healthcare: Implications For Psychiatry. Denver, CO: Milliman Inc., 2014.
2. Simon GE, Katon WJ, Von Korff M, et al. Cost-effectiveness of a collaborative care program for primary care patients with persistent depression. Am J Psychiatry. 2001;158(10):1638–1644. doi:10.1176/appi/ajp/158.10.1638.
3. Katon W, Russo J, Lin EHB, et al. Cost-effectiveness of a multicondition collaborative care intervention: A randomized controlled trial. Arch Gen Psychiatry. 2012;69(5):506–514. doi:10.1001/archgenpsychiatry.2011.1548
4. Gilbody S, Bower P, Fletcher J, Richards D, Sutton AJ. Collaborative care for depression: A cumulative meta-analysis and review of longer-term outcomes. Arch Intern Med. 2006;166(21):2314–2321. doi:10.1001/archinte.166.21.2314
5. Berwick DM, Nolan TW, Whittington J. The triple aim: Care, health, and cost. Health Affairs. 2008;27(3):159–769. doi:10.1377/hlthaff.27.3.759
6. Psychosomatic Medicine Programs Academic Year 2015–2016 United States. Accreditation Council for Graduate Medical Education. https://apps.acgme.org/ads/Public/Reports/ReportRun?ReportId=1&CurrentYear=2014&SpecialtyId=139&IncludePreAccreditation=false&ReportId=1&Curr

entYear=2014&SpecialtyId=139&IncludePreAccreditation=false. Accessed August 31, 2015.

7. Weiss M, Schwartz BJ. Lessons learned from a colocation model using psychiatrists in urban primary care settings. J Primary Care Community Health. 2012;4(3):228–234. doi:10.1177/2150131912468449
8. U.S. General Accounting Office. Mental Health Parity Act: Despite New Federal Standards, Mental Health Benefits Remain Limited, May 2000. http://www.gao.gov/new.items/he00095.pdf Accessed September 17, 2015.
9. Regier DA, Goldberg ID, Taube CA. The de facto US mental health services system: A public health perspective. Arch Gen Psychiatry. 1978;35(6):685–693. doi:10.1001/archpsyc.1978.01770300027002
10. Norquist GS, Regier DA. The epidemiology of psychiatric disorders and the de facto mental health care system. Annu Rev Med. 1996;47(1):473–479. doi:10.1146/annurev.med.47.1.473
11. Mojtabai R, Olfson M. National patterns in antidepressant treatment by psychiatrists and general medical providers: Results from the National Comorbidity Survey Replication. J Clin Psychiatry. 2008;69(7):1064–1074.
12. National Ambulatory Medical Care Survey: 2010 Summary Tables. CDC/NCHS. 2010. http://www.cdc.gov/nchs/data/ahcd/namcs_summary/2010_namcs_web_tables.pdf. Accessed August 17, 2015.
13. Wang PS, Lane M, Olfson M, Pincus HA, Wells KB, Kessler RC. Twelve-month use of mental health services in the United States: Results from the National Comorbidity Survey Replication. Arch Gen Psychiatry. 2005;62(6):629–640. doi:10.1001/archpsyc.62.6.629
14. Ludman EJ, Katon W, Russo J, et al. Depression and diabetes symptom burden. Gen Hosp Psychiatry. 2004;26(6):430–436. doi:10.1016/j.genhosppsych.204.08.010
15. Egede LE, Zheng D, Simpson K. Comorbid depression is associated with increased health care use and expenditures in individuals with diabetes. Diabetes Care. 2002;25(3):464–470. doi:10.2337/diacare.25.3.464
16. Unützer J, Katon W, Callahan CM, et al. Collaborative care management of late-life depression in the primary care setting: A randomized controlled trial. JAMA. 2002;288(2):2836–2845. doi:10.1001/jama.288.22.2836
17. Hunkeler EM, Katon W, Tang L, et al. Long-term outcomes from the IMPACT randomized trial for depressed elderly patients in primary care. BMJ. 2006;332(7536):259–263. doi:10.1136/bmj.38683.710255.BE
18. Katon W, Russo J, Lin EHB, et al. Cost-effectiveness of a multicondition collaborative care intervention. Arch Gen Psych. 2012;69(5):506–514. doi:10.1001/archgenpsychiatry.2011.1548
19. Katon W, Unützer J, Wells K, Jones L. Collaborative depression care: History, evolution and ways to enhance dissemination and sustainability. Gen Hosp Psychiatry. 2012;32(5):456–464. doi:10.1016/j.genhosppsych.2010.04.001
20. Archer J, Bower P, Gilbody S. Collaborative care for people with depression and anxiety. Cochrane Database Syst Rev. 2012;(10):CD006525. doi:10.1002/14651858.CD006525.pub2
21. Maragakis A, Siddharthan R, RachBeisel J, Snipes C. Creating a "reverse" integrated primary and mental healthcare clinic for those with serious mental illness. Primary Health Care Research & Development. 2015(Nov 20):1–7. doi:10.1017/S1463423615000523
22. Collins C, Hewson DL, Munger R, Wade T. Evolving Models of Behavioral Health Integration in Primary Care. New York: Milbank Memorial Fund, 2010. http://www.milbank.org/uploads/documents/10430EvolvingCare/EvolvingCare.pdf. Accessed December 2, 2015.
23. Duke DC, Guion K, Freeman KA, Wilson AC, Harris MA. Commentary: Health & behavior codes: Great idea, questionable outcome. J Pediatr Psychol. 2012;37(5):491–495. doi:10.1093/jpepsy/jsr126
24. Cummings NA, Dorken H, Pallak MS, Henke C. The Impact of Psychological Intervention on Healthcare Utilization and Costs. San Francisco: Biodyne Institute, 1990.
25. Blount A, Kathol R, Thomas M, et al. The economics of behavioral health services in medical settings: A summary of the evidence. Professional Psychology: Research and Practice. 2007;38(3):290–297. doi:10.1037/0735-7028.38.3.290
26. Unützer J, Katon WJ, Fan M-Y, et al. Long-term cost effects of collaborative care for late-life depression. Am J Managed Care. 2008;14(2):95–100.
27. Melek SP, Norris DT, Paulus J. Economic Impact of Integrated Medical-Behavioral Healthcare: Implications for Psychiatry. Milliman American Psychiatric Association Report. Denver, CO: Milliman, Inc., April 2014.
28. Sanger-Katz M. No, giving more people health insurance doesn't save money. *New York Times*, August 5, 2014. http://www.nytimes.com/2015/08/06/upshot/no-giving-more-people-health-insurance-doesn't-save-money.html?_r=0. Accessed August 10, 2015.
29. Cohen JT, Neumann PJ. The Cost Savings and Cost-Effectiveness of Clinical Preventive Care. The Robert Wood Johnson Foundation, Research Synthesis Report No. 18. September 18, 2009. http://www.rwjf.org/content/dam/farm/reports/issue_briefs/2009/rwjf46045/subassets/rwjf46045_1. Accessed August 10, 2015.
30. Leonhardt D. Free lunch on health? Think again. *New York Times*, August 8, 2007. http://www.nytimes.com/2007/08/08/business/08leonhardt.html. Accessed August 10, 2015.

31. Laupacis A, Sackett DL, Roberts RS. An assessment of clinically useful measures of the consequences of treatment. N Engl J Med. 1988;318(26):1728–1733. doi:10.1056/NEJM198806303182605
32. Berk ML, Monheit AC. The concentration of health care expenditures, revisited. Health Affairs. 2001;20(2):9–18.
33. Simon GE, Von Korff M, Barlow W. Health care costs of primary care patients with recognized depression. Arch Gen Psychiatry. 1995;52(10):850–856. doi:10.1001/archpsych.1995.03950220060012
34. Henk HJ, Katzelnick DJ, Kobak KA, Greist JH, Jefferson JW. Medical costs attributed to depression among patients with a history of high medical expenses in a health maintenance organization. Arch Gen Psychiatry. 1996;53(10):899–904. doi:10.1001/archpsyc.1996.01830100045006
35. Behavioral Health in the Medicaid Program—People, Use, and Expenditures. Report to Congress on Medicaid and CHIP. Medicaid and CHIP Payment and Access Commission, June 2015. https://www.macpac.gov/wp-content-uploads/2015/06/Behavioral-Health-in-the-Medicaid-Program%E%80%94People-Use-and-Expenditures.pdf. Accessed August 19, 2015.
36. Lindsey M, Patterson W, Ray K, Roohan P. Statistical Brief #3: Potentially Preventable Hospital Readmissions Among Medicaid Recipients with Mental Health and/or Substance Abuse Health Conditions Compared with All Others: New York State, 2007. NYSDOH, Division of Quality and Evaluation, Office of Health Insurance Programs. https://www.health.ny.gov/health_care/managed_care/reports/staistics_data/3hospital_readmissionsmentahealth.pdf Accessed September 17, 2015.
37. Cutler D, Wikler E, Basch P. Reducing administrative costs and improving the health care system. N Engl J Med. 2012;367(20):1875–1878. doi:10.1056/NEJMp1209711
38. Bremer RW, Scholle SH, Keyser D, Know Houtsinger JV, Pincus HA. Pay for performance in behavioral health. Psychiatr Services. 2008;59:1419–1429.
39. Unutzer J, Chan Y, Hafer E, et al. Quality improvement with pay-for-performance incentives in integrated behavioral health care. Am J Public Health. 2012;102(6):e41–e45.
40. Frakt AB, Mayes R. Beyond capitation: How new payment experiments seek to find the "sweet spot" in amount of risk providers and payers bear. Health Affairs. 2012;31(9):1951–1958. doi:10.1377/hlthaff.2012.0344
41. Goldberg RJ. Financial incentives influencing the integration of mental health care and primary care. Psychiatr Services. 1999;50(8):1071–1075. doi:10.1176/ps.50.8.1071
42. Initiative Features Fixed Monthly Payments to Primary Care Clinics for Providing Depression Care Bundle, Allowing Many Patients to Achieve Good Outcomes. Agency for Healthcare Research and Quality. https://innovations.ahrq.gov/profiles/intiative-features-fixed-monthly-payments-primary-care-clinics-providing-depression-care. Last updated August 13, 2014. Accessed August 19, 2015.
43. Cox T. Exposing the true risks of capitation financed healthcare. J Healthc Risk Manag. 2011;303(4):34–41. doi:10.1002/jhrm.20066
44. Schwartz BJ, Blackmore MA, Wetzler S, Chung H. Psychiatrist's changing role in a reformed delivery system: Adding value in accountable care organizations. In Summergrad P, Kathol RG, eds. Integrated Care in Psychiatry: Redefining the Role of Mental Health Professionals in the Medical Setting. New York: Springer Science+Business Media, 2014:69–85.
45. Next Generation ACO Model. Centers for Medicare & Medicaid website. http://innovation.cms.gov/initiatives/Next-Generation-ACO-Model/. Last updated August 6, 2015. Accessed August 10, 2015.
46. Montefiore Medical Center Community Service Plan 2014–2017. https://www.montefiore.org/documents/communityservices/Montefiore-2014-2017-Community-Services-Plan.pdf. Accessed August 31, 2015.
47. Medicare Pioneer ACO Model Performance Year 1 and Performance Year 2 Financial Results. Centers for Medicare & Medicaid Services, October 2014. http://innovation.cms.gov/Files/x/PioneerACO-Fncl-PY1PY2.pdf. Accessed August 17, 2015.
48. A Path Toward Value-Based Payment: New York State Roadmap for Medicaid Payment Reform. NYS Medicaid Redesign Team, June 2015. https://www.health.ny.gov/health_care/medicaid/redesign/dsrip/docs/vbp_roadmap_final.pdf. Accessed August 19, 2015.
49. Value-Based Payment Reform in New York State: A Proposal to Align Medicare's and NYS Medicaid's Reforms, July 2015. https://www.health.ny.gov/health_care/medicaid/redesign/dsrip/docs/vbp_draft_medicare_alignment_paper.pdf. Accessed September 10, 2015.
50. Korda H, Eldridge GN. Payment incentives and integrated care delivery: Levers for health system reform and cost containment. Inquiry. 2011;48(4):277–287. doi:10.5034/inquiryjrnl_48.04.01
51. Wetzler S, Schwartz BJ, Sanderson W, Karasu TB. Academic psychiatry and managed care: A case study. Psychiatr Serv. 1997;48(8):1019–1026.
52. Berwick DM. Launching accountable care organizations—The proposed rule for the Medicare shared savings program. N Engl J Med. 2011;364(16):e32–e35. doi:10.1056/NEJMp1103602
53. Medicare Pioneer ACO Model Performance Year 1 and Performance Year 2 Financial Results. Centers for Medicare & Medicaid Services, October 2014. http://innovation.cms.gov/Files/x/PioneerACO-Fncl-PY1PY2.pdf. Accessed August 17, 2015.

7

Integrating Physical and Mental Health Care in the Veterans Health Administration

A Path to the Future

LISA V. RUBENSTEIN

BOX 7.1

KEY POINTS

- **It is not possible to achieve optimal care goals for chronic physical conditions at a patient population level without integrating mental health and physical health care, particularly for patients at highest risk of preventable adverse outcomes.**
- **Organizational readiness for integrated care needs to be promoted by strong leadership through a commitment to frequent interaction and coordination between mental health specialists and primary care.**
- **Both adequate staffing for integrated care and integrated mental health and primary care medical record systems are major facilitators for integrated care programs.**
- **Population-based mental health care requires reshaping of traditional mental health services to meet patient and physical health care provider needs in a stepped care approach.**
- **Key target conditions for VA integrated programs in primary care include depression, anxiety, and alcohol misuse. All 3 conditions are prevalent in primary care, and can be improved through brief primary care–based interventions.**
- **Target problems that require shared responsibility between primary care and mental health include: pain, disruptive patients, poor adherence, and other vulnerabilities. These are conditions that may or may not require mental health medications or psychotherapy, but for which mental health perspectives may be critical for management.**
- **The organizational structure of integrated care models must reflect mental health specialty, primary care, and administrative leadership perspectives, and can be documented in strategic plans, memoranda of understanding, and/or interservice agreements. Achieving meaningful agreement on integrated care model implementation within a given organizational context requires thoughtful development and monitoring.**
- **Monitoring and improvement of integrated mental health and primary care programs can be enhanced by clinically meaningful, population-based measures that reflect program goals.**
- **Appropriate training for VA integrated mental health staff, primary care providers, and other team members is essential with particular focus on depression, anxiety, and alcohol misuse. Training must also include a focus on the skills needed for developing coordinated, integrated care plans for complex patients that reflect both medical and mental health needs.**

VETERANS AFFAIRS DRIVERS FOR THE DEVELOPMENT OF INTEGRATED PHYSICAL AND MENTAL HEALTH CARE

Since its inception in the 1930s, mental health care has been a major Veterans Affairs (VA) mission. Through its support of the joint mission of caring for veterans with physical and mental health conditions, the VA has developed and/or evaluated many of the mental health–related research, education, and patient care innovations that are common across many health systems today. The VA's new mission of fully integrating mental and physical health care, however, is recent, and still in the implementation process. See Box 7.1 for an overview of the development of integrated physical and mental health care in the VA.

The VA Primary Care Context as a Driver for Integrated Mental and Physical Health Care

The history of VA primary care has influenced primary care/mental health integration efforts. The VA was constituted as an acute care system for wounded war veterans. Over the years after World War II, individual VA facilities provided urgent and ambulatory care to an increasingly broader group of veterans based on complex eligibility formulas. At that time, laws and regulations governing VA facilities prohibited provision of comprehensive primary care. Legal barriers notwithstanding, by 1993, 38% of VA facilities provided some level of primary care.[1] A 1994 congressional directive legalized this trend, followed by the 1996 Veterans Healthcare Eligibility Reform Act that essentially mandated availability of primary care for enrolled veterans. Over the subsequent decade, as primary care continued to evolve, the need for a more advanced patient-centered primary care model suitable for meeting the complex medical and mental health needs of veterans became apparent. It also became clear that the focus on comprehensive primary care management would raise the stakes for achieving primary care/mental health care integration.

The VA currently manages over 150 hospitals with associated emergency care, nursing homes, specialist care, and primary care. Primary care is delivered through over 900 hospital or community based primary care practices, each linked to a medical center hub (usually but not always located in a hospital).[2] As of 2008, all primary care sites with at least 5,000 patients are required to have at least one full-time equivalent mental health professional on site—either a psychiatrist, a psychologist, or a mental health–trained social worker.[3] In general, the VA mental health specialty workforce also includes mental health–trained nurse practitioners, clinical nurse specialists, and physician assistants. All providers and facilities function within a single medical record and within a multilevel local, regional, and central (Washington DC-based) management system.

The majority of VA patients with or without mental health conditions receive most of their care in the primary care setting. All veterans who visit the VA are assigned to a single primary care provider (physician, nurse practitioner, or physician assistant). Since 2010, when the VA implemented a patient-centered medical home model (Patient Aligned Care Teams [PACT]),[4–6] each primary care provider is linked to a "teamlet" consisting of a nurse care manager, a licensed practical nurse or health technician, and a clerk. Each teamlet manages a continuity panel of 1,200 patients who have visited primary care at least once in the past 24 months; non-visitors are continuously removed from the panel. Each five or six teamlets are linked to a larger team that includes a social worker, pharmacist, dietitian, coach, and an integrated mental health specialist or team. By 2013, this staffing model was about 60% implemented across primary care practices. National continuity-of-care performance measures show that on average about 70% of all in-person clinician visits occur with the patient's assigned primary care provider, excluding mental health specialist visits.[7] In the past, patients with schizophrenia or bipolar disorder might receive little or no continuity primary care. As a result of these changes, nearly all such patients now visit their continuity primary care providers. The team-based organization of primary care provides a strong basis for leveraging mental health specialty resources through integrated primary care teams. In addition, the team- based model creates an imperative to integrate ever more fully, because the best efforts of mental health specialists alone cannot meet the needs of the now more fully detected mental health conditions of the full primary care population.

During the period preceding implementation of primary care in the 1990s, all VA care, including mental health care, aimed to focus on being a safety net for very ill and impoverished patients unable to receive needed care in the community. Mental health care in particular, like most non–private practice mental health care at the time, focused on serious mental illness, with substantial resources committed to inpatient care. Mental health specialty resources were predominantly directed at severe major depression, posttraumatic stress disorder (PTSD), bipolar disorder, and schizophrenia. Mental health outpatient care was also geared to serious persistent mental illness, and was often intensive, long term, and difficult to access. There was little routine interaction between mental health specialists and physical health providers. For example, mental health patients, might never see a primary care provider outside of an emergent health need.

As primary care and the capabilities and ease of use of psychiatric medications expanded during the 1990s, the limitations of the prevailing mental health care models both within and outside the VA began to become apparent. For example, research showed that most depressed patients in primary care were not detected[8] and most of those detected did not complete even minimally appropriate treatment.[5,9] The clinical consequences of provider reluctance to treat, and of patients' tendencies to become poor consumers (apathetic, withdrawn) as a direct result of their depressive states, began to be recognized. In addition, research and clinical experience identified the critical importance and effectiveness of treating major depression and its sequelae: job loss, family dissolution, or deteriorations in physical health which could be prevented.[9] Within the VA, mental health specialists found it difficult to reconcile the new awareness of veteran population needs with a mental health system intensively focused on a much smaller group of persistently mentally ill patients.

Mental Health Policy as a Driver for Integrated Care

The national political context of the past two decades has further influenced VA mental health care. As a publicly supported system, the VA has added impetus to respond to political demands and legal developments. In the United States prior to the 1990s, insurers considered most mental health care optional, and coverage for less than catastrophic mental illness was severely limited. As the full physical and functional status impacts of depression were identified (e.g., in the World Health Organization's identification of depression along with cardiac disease as having the largest contributions worldwide to poor overall quality of life),[10] health care organizations began to realize that a more proactive approach to mental health was needed. Mental health consumer organizations began exerting political pressure, focusing in part on legal parity for mental health with physical health conditions. The Mental Health Parity Act of 1996[11] and the Mental Health Parity and Addiction Equity Act of 2008[12] focused on parity in group health plans, while the Affordable Care Act of 2010[13] extended parity to individual insurance plans, and by 2016 to include small group plans. Meanwhile, the long-term consequences of the Vietnam War on veterans' long-term mental health outcomes were recognized, and the impacts of the recent Gulf, Iraq, and Afghanistan conflicts became increasingly evident. The following were fundamental drivers for changes in the VA mental health care models: (1) a veteran population with higher mental health needs than typical managed care populations and (2) the VA's accountability for providing for mental and physical health care throughout the lifespan of all eligible veterans.

Increasing legal developments related to equity have also affected both mental and physical health care. Congress, for example, has legal authority over the VA and can exert pressure for reform of VA services, as can the President of the United States (who appoints and can fire VA leadership). It has become increasingly possible to document disparities in access to care related to race, age, education, and other demographic characteristics. In this context, the VA has striven to ensure that not only do all veterans attending a given setting receive equitable mental and physical health care, but also that individuals living in different types of areas, such as inner-city or rural areas, receive equitable care.

New developments related to equity may also shape future VA mental and physical care integration. Legal developments related to lesbian, gay, bisexual, and transgender active military have raised awareness of equity for these groups. For example, currently the VA is a major provider of care for transgender individuals. Furthermore, the Veterans Access, Choice and Accountability Act of 2014,[14] provides funds for contracting with non-VA providers for veterans living at a distance from a VA primary care practice, or when needed care is not available from VA and may also impact equity of access to mental health care. While evidence suggests that most enrolled depressed veterans receiving any mental health care do so through the VA, rather than from non-VA providers,[15] this may not always be the case. Overall, as a government-sponsored organization, the VA will need to continue to monitor its mental and physical health services for fairness. This will likely create additional pressures affecting integrated care initiatives.

Health Outcomes and Costs as Drivers for Integration

In most if not all health care systems, a small proportion of patients account for the majority of costs. In the VA, a fraction of veterans (5%) account for almost half (47%) of VA costs at any given time. These costs, in turn, are driven mainly by hospital admissions (half of all costs), most of which are for medical rather than mental health conditions. However, nearly half (48%) of these high-cost patients, carry a major mental health diagnosis.[16] Having a mental health diagnosis, particularly depression or substance abuse, strongly predicts future admission or emergency department use for ambulatory care–sensitive conditions, such as diabetes.[17] Consequently, looked at from the physical health viewpoint, more holistic approaches to mental health care among the physically and mentally ill are essential for avoiding acute health deteriorations that result in emergency department use, hospitalization, and death. Looked at from the mental health care point of view, seriously mentally ill patients are subject to a variety of physical health complications, including those due to psychiatric medications. These physical health complications can benefit from resources predominantly available through primary and medical sub-specialty care.[18]

Furthermore, mental health conditions are often potentially treatable. If we consider potential for improvement or illness resolution, mental health conditions rise still higher on the priority list. The need for hospitalization of a kidney transplant or heart attack patient who is adherent and receiving appropriate care is unlikely to change. On the other hand, treatment of depression in a diabetic may avoid future costs for this physical illness.

Mental Health Comorbidities as a Driver for Integration

In addition to physical health comorbidities, many veterans with one mental health condition are also afflicted by one or two additional mental health diagnoses. Co-occurring mental health diagnoses, such as substance abuse, PTSD, and depression, are common among veterans,[19,20] and may require an integrated approachs across various mental health as well as physical health specialists. Furthermore, despite its early mental health start, the VA was unprepared for the onslaught of veterans with substance abuse and mental health problems generated by the Vietnam War.[21] In the absence of legal VA primary care, and with limited mental health specialty resources, many Vietnam War veterans did not receive the care they needed. These patients still remain the bulk of veterans treated in either primary care or mental health specialty. Veterans of later wars, particularly those of the past decade, have received quicker mental health and primary care treatment; this may reduce the long-term consequences experienced by earlier veteran cohorts.

While uncomplicated depression (without suicidal plans or major mental health comorbidities) can clearly be successfully treated in primary care practices with care management support and minimal mental health backup, this may not be the case for complicated depression. Among veterans, for example, a third of primary care patients screening positive for depression also have significant PTSD symptoms. Substance abuse, dysthymia, and suicidal ideation or plans are also frequent. Among these complex patients, availability of a care manager alone may not be enough to improve outcomes;[20] the availability of true collaborative care through an integrated primary care/mental health team may be essential. Additionally, a patient with depression plus schizophrenia or PTSD, might develop congestive heart failure at a level that requires intensive engagement with primary care. The availability of an integrated mental health program in primary care may be critical for such a patient, even though typical collaborative care guidelines might classify such a patient as too severely mentally ill for primary care–based collaborative care.[22]

The complexity of the veteran population also means that a higher skill and comfort level among primary care clinicians, as well as availability of mental health specialty access are likely necessary for successful treatment of these patients. Skill and comfort with providing mental health–directed care among primary care providers is promoted by better collaboration and communication with mental health specialists,[23] and is unlikely to occur in the absence of fully integrated mental health care in primary care settings.

Preservation of Mental Health Access as a Driver for Care Management in Primary Care

At the population level (using any likely calculation of need for mental health care in primary care), if mental health conditions are treated only by mental health specialists, many patients will remain untreated. In the past, relatively few patients in the VA, often with serious mental illness diagnoses, consumed the majority of mental health specialty resources. Most of these patients were frequently seen over a long period of time. Review of patient panels in VA mental health, revealed that these patients were often stable, insofar as they required the same dose of an antipsychotic over years, without episodes of de-compensation. As a result, preserving access to mental health specialists for more acute needs requires a deeper look into mental health specialty access than simply adding capabilities for depression care. For example, if only 10% of primary care patients required mental health medications or treatments for a new depression episode in a given year,[24] the average primary care practice panel in the VA would generate 120 mental health referrals, each of which would require at least four visits over the next six months. Even if follow-up were mostly delivered through mental health–based nurse care managers, the mental health load generated by a VA group practice of, for example, 20,000 patients would quickly exceed supply, even with generous mental health specialty staffing. This calculation only covers depression; adding other mental health conditions would quickly swamp existing resources. Consequently, it is essential for primary care providers to participate in guideline-concordant care for depression and other mental illnesses while preserving mental health specialist access for the cases for which this access is most cost effective. This is not dissimilar from preserving access to cardiologists, by predominantly delegating chronic care to primary care providers. Care management by nurse care managers in a collaborative care environment can leverage primary care teams, while providing strong links to mental health specialists. Proactive nurse care management for depression is a foundational element of the VA's integrated mental health approach.[3,25]

Crossover Conditions and Engagement Behaviors as Drivers for Integration

In addition to the classical mental health diagnoses, there are conditions for which neither mental health specialists nor primary care providers have primary responsibility. Crossover conditions include: mild to moderate substance abuse, poor adherence to medical treatments, personality disorders, somatization, insomnia, stress management, and treatment of chronic pain. Among patients with these conditions, mental, physical, and social issues often intertwine, requiring a long-term bio-psycho-social-cultural approach. Management of such patients is often complicated by difficulties providers experience in trying to engage them in effective self-care. Achieving appropriate care for patients with these conditions may require sophisticated coordination between mental health specialists (e.g., psychiatrists, psychologists, and substance abuse specialists), social workers, nurses, clerks, and primary care providers, in a team-based model.

Prevention as a Driver for Integrated Care

Prevention is the key to a fully operationalized biopsychosocial-cultural approach to care. Few organizations to date, including the VA, have yet succeeded in fully implementing this approach. Work on reducing homelessness, for example, highlights the extent to which linking community resources to clinical care can improve outcomes.[26] Integrating mental and physical health care is a key component for maximizing preventive biopsychosocial-cultural care.[2,27]

Integrated mental and physical health care substantially expands opportunities for prevention. Rather than waiting for a patient to develop a severe mental health condition to initiate preventive care, primary prevention in primary care settings can help avoid the development of serious mental health conditions. For example, VA efforts directed at newly discharged military, aim to reduce or prevent the development of chronic combat-related PTSD by early intervention for new traumatic events. Early depression treatment may serve as primary prevention for some chronic diseases, such as heart disease. Secondary prevention aims at early detection and treatment of serious mental health conditions to avoid downstream negative consequences, and strives to return a person to his or her original quality of life and functioning. Early detection and treatment of depression, through screening in primary care, can prevent job loss and other social consequences.[28] Tertiary prevention aims to reduce the consequences of chronic mental illness, often through helping the individual address complex illness management challenges. Integrated mental health specialists can work with primary care providers to prevent negative physical consequences of mental health medications, and promote adherence and engagement in care.

TABLE 7.1. VA MENTAL HEALTH QUALITY MEASURES RELEVANT TO PRIMARY CARE/MENTAL HEALTH INTEGRATION

Measure	*Description*
Adequate antidepressant treatment for a new episode of depression	% of patients newly started on an appropriate antidepressant who receive 84 days of continuous treatment, or who receive 180 days of continuous treatment.
Any psychotherapy for depression	% of patients with a depression diagnosis, who had a psychotherapy visit for depression.
Adequate psychotherapy for depression	% of patients treated for a depression diagnosis who had at least 3 psychotherapy visits in six weeks.
Site level primary care/mental health integration penetration rate	Proportion of patients in a primary care practice site, seen for a primary care/mental health integration in a face-to-face encounter.

Trafton JA, Greenberg G, Harris AH, et al. VHA mental health information system: Applying health information technology to monitor and facilitate implementation of VHA Uniform Mental Health Services Handbook requirements. Med Care. 2013;51 (3 Suppl 1):S29–36.

VA Performance Measurement as a Driver Toward Integrated Care

VA performance measures have been a major driver for the development of equitable, population-based mental health care delivery. Initially instituted during the 1990s, based on rigorously designed medical record review,[1] outpatient performance measures now focus on a highly developed electronic measurement system. While including and contributing parallel measures to those used by the National Committee for Quality Assurance, the VA performance measure and monitoring system now spans an even wider variety of conditions and issues, only the most critical of which are mandated and generate performance-related pay. Critical measures are further supported by clinical reminders, which in turn generate data on performance measure adherence. Performance pay initially went to regional leadership; now, however, physicians can also earn some additional income related to overall performance measure adherence. Measure results can be electronically accessed through local and national dashboards.

Mental health care measures have been part of the performance measure system since its inception, and are a resource for promoting primary care/mental health integration. While more than 200 VA mental health measures exist, most are not used as performance measures. Several performance measures particularly relevant to primary care/mental health integration are shown in Table 7.1.[29]

Screening for depression for all primary care patients was mandated during the 1990s, followed later by screening for alcohol and for PTSD. Yearly computer-generated screening reminders for all three conditions appear in the electronic medical record for every primary care patient, and can be completed by nurses (most commonly) or physicians. Currently a positive depression screen using the Patient Health Questionnaire-2 (PHQ-2)[30] mandates a follow-up suicide assessment by the primary care provider, and includes a requirement to urgently see a mental health specialist, if active suicidality is documented. Positive screening for depression, PTSD, or alcohol misuse is found in more than 20% of the VA's primary care population. As primary care providers have become increasingly aware of the prevalence of these conditions, it has become unacceptable not to have prompt access to mental health specialist support when acutely needed, or reasonable access for less acute but still important issues.

BARRIERS AND RESOURCES FOR VA PHYSICAL AND MENTAL HEALTH INTEGRATION

The VA's Capabilities for Adopting and Testing New Care Models in Mental Health

The VA can have a key role among U.S. health care organizations as a test for integrated care. As a government sponsored managed health care system, the

VA can bypass reimbursement challenges that have hampered development of integrated care in other settings. Additionally, the VA (with its mission to be a learning health care system and its cadre of embedded health service researchers) is well positioned to test the large-scale feasibility of research-based care models, such as integrated care. Because the VA is a large integrated system across 50 states, the results from evaluation of implementation of integrated care models are likely to reflect feasibility and effectiveness under routine care conditions. The VA is not able to promote approaches that cannot be widely spread, or that require boutique-level resources. For mental health in particular, the VA has the added advantage of a longstanding mission for providing mental as well as physical health care. This mission drives VA research and education, adding capabilities and impetus for state-of-the-art models of mental health care as a focus for the VA's commitment to functioning as a learning health care system.

The VA's Integrated Electronic Medical Records as a Resource for Integrated Care

The VA's computerized patient record system (CPRS) is a key resource for achieving integrated physical and mental health care. Outpatient primary care, mental health, and specialty care notes, as well as emergency department, inpatient, and long-term care notes, appear chronologically in each patient record. Telephone visits and secure email messages are chronologically visible. Laboratory, pharmacy, consultation requests, radiology, and other procedure notes are available by accessing separate tabs. Notes from other VA sites the patient has attended can be accessed, as well as straightforward medical information resources for providers and patients. For example, it is easy to identify all mental health related medications ever used or currently taken, and look up any questions about their appropriateness or side effects. In this way, CPRS provides continuity mental health and primary care providers with substantial resources for development of an integrated care plan, or for communication regarding any questions that arise. CPRS and its associated data storage and analysis structures also support electronic mental health related performance or improvement measures that can provide a full population view of mental health diagnoses and the care provided for them.

Many worried about whether the inclusion of mental health assessments and notes, along with those from primary care and other services, would threaten mental health provider-to-patient communication. Inclusion of these notes, however, has not resulted in major veteran complaints or mental health provider issues, despite the open note capabilities that enable veterans to view notes online. Under some circumstances, mental health specialists are allowed to keep limited private notes, but basic assessment, monitoring, and treatment plans must be documented in a patient's electronic medical record.

Evaluation of communication between mental health and primary care suggests that the medical record is the preferred method of communication between mental health specialists and primary care, supplemented by telephone calls and meetings.[31] Electronic consultation requests can include substantial information related to appropriate triage, and if appropriate, can be responded to electronically. Mental health patients may see different mental health social workers, addiction specialists, trainees, psychologists, or psychiatrists, and may attend a variety of groups. They may also interact with mental health focused pharmacists and dietitians. Each veteran attending mental health specialty care is therefore assigned to one primary mental health treatment coordinator, who may be a psychiatrist, psychologist, or social worker.

CPRS has limitations. So far, it has not been possible to develop an electronic integrated care plan. It has been difficult to develop care management software that is intrinsic to CPRS, due to inherent limitations in the system's capabilities. New care management software (the Patient Care Assessment System) has recently been released, but not yet fully tested. Future developments in these areas may pave the way for further integrated care advances.

VA Research and Education as Resources for Integrated Care

The VA's research and education contributions to mental health care are substantial. For example, the VA has conducted the majority of research on PTSD. The VA was among the first to support the development of the PhD degree for psychologists. The availability of research trained teams to participate in program improvement has made it possible to investigate areas of need, develop new measures, and rigorously develop and test new mental health care models tailored to the VA.

The VA's training programs span disciplines, including internal medicine, nursing, psychology, psychiatry, social work, addiction medicine, health services, quality improvement research, and informatics. Trainees from all of these disciplines, as well as clinical pharmacists and dietitians, have participated in integrated program development, and have expanded the system wide and non-VA impacts of VA's integration initiatives.

IMPLEMENTING INTEGRATED MENTAL AND PHYSICAL HEALTH CARE

All of the drivers, barriers, and facilitators discussed above influenced the development of an approach to integrated mental health care, including the existence of VA tested models for depression, alcohol abuse care, and for integrating mental health specialists. In addition, detailed study of military returnees from Iraq and Afghanistan documenting their mental health needs provided a tipping point toward integrated care.[32]

The Primary Care-Mental Health Integration (PC-MHI) initiative, officially initiated by directive in 2007,[3] was preceded by a 2006 large voluntary demonstration project focused on implementing integrated care models for depression. The 2007 directive mandated adoption of one of three previously VA tested models of mental health care which include: (1) Translating Initiatives in Depression into Effective Solutions (TIDES),[33,34] (2) the Behavioral Health Laboratory model,[35] or (3) the White River Junction co-located mental health care model.[22] The directive further mandated that all primary care sites with at least 5,000 patients have a mental health specialist on site. By 2009, nearly all VA health care systems had adopted one or more of these models; the large majority, however, focused on co-located care.[36] Evidence suggests that co-located care often simply meant positioning a mental health specialist in primary care. This limited approach did not reflect the full White River Junction model, which included patient self-administered assessments, health technician support, and an integrated, collaborative mental health team situated in primary care space. Co-located care, while not fully evidence-based, was relatively easy to implement and was easily accepted by mental health specialists and primary care providers.

Accompanying these directives, the VA Office of Mental Health initiated an educational and management initiative that widely engaged, and continues to engage, a broad group of primary care providers and their integrated mental health specialists.[37,38] The Michigan-based PC-MHI initiative team continues to monitor and evaluate the program, and to encourage research on new improvements and measures. The team conducts monthly nationwide teleconferences and supports training efforts for integrated care, in coordination with the VA's Employee Education System. Educational and training efforts have been supported in part through ongoing engagement of embedded researchers, as clinical program experts and implementation scientists.[39,40]

During the years after 2007, the limitations of depression as a disease-oriented focus to integrated care began to emerge. While the mounting evidence on the importance and effectiveness of depression care management was most compelling, given the prevalence of the condition in primary care and extensiveness of prior research, alcohol misuse and abuse approaches were a close second. In addition, the concept of a fully integrated approach, versus implementing, for example, care management silos for individual conditions, such as depression, alcohol misuse, or anxiety, began to develop. The greater prevalence of co-morbid mental health conditions among veterans with depression, with the accompanying greater resistance to treatment, made care management approaches without full mental health specialty backup less sufficient and likely less effective for the typical depressed patient in primary care.

Despite the attractiveness of fully integrating mental and physical health care, efforts to achieve integration in the VA quickly encountered resistance. In order to preserve access to their time, integrated mental health specialists had to adopt a very different style of care. They provided fewer visits per patient, thereby leveraging primary care providers for providing follow-up care whenever possible. In addition, they proactively engaged patients through needs detected by their primary care providers. While this approach was familiar to, providers such as cardiologists or consultation-liaison psychiatrists, most mental health specialists were accustomed to a different, non–population based model that saw the patient as the primary driver for seeking mental health care. The integrated care paradigm also demanded a more fluid approach to acute mental health care needs. While primary care providers were well trained in cardiology, their comfort in detecting and acting on urgent mental health issues was low, leading to both over/under detection. Availability of curbside consultation and treatment of psychiatric emergencies had to be ensured for the program to be perceived as successful by primary care. All of these requirements were often complex to implement due to the extensive involvement of VA sites in mental health training programs.

Additionally, the evolution of integrated care required workforce changes. The VA mental health specialty workforce had primarily focused on psychiatry. Data on the effectiveness of cognitive-behavioral therapy for depression in primary care, and frequent patient preference for therapy over medication demanded greater availability of psychologists and mental health trained social workers, in addition to psychiatrists, in primary care. New directives focused on ensuring greater availability of group therapies. Finally, primary care patients and providers began to promote new supportive mental health group approaches that could be educational, could serve as a lead-in to other mental health care, or could engage the patient in holistic approaches to relaxation, meditation, or yoga. Once the scope of addiction issues in primary care began to become apparent, the inability of small, segregated substance abuse and alcohol programs to meet the veteran population's needs quickly became apparent. All of these activities required adjustments of the VA mental health workforce.

Cultural issues between mental health and primary care perspectives and training also became apparent. Mental health specialists initially resisted the idea that primary care providers and teams (e.g., nurse care managers) could treat mental health conditions, despite the extensive evidence that primary care providers prescribe the large majority of psychiatrically active medications.[41] As continuity VA primary care providers and teams became a reality in the patient-centered medical home model, the strong relationships between patients and their primary care providers challenged relationships with mental health providers for patients with serious mental illness, who also needed to regularly be seen for their chronic physical health conditions. This conflict provoked resistance, based on mental health specialty concepts of who could do what. On the primary care side, many primary care providers resisted prescribing mental health medications, or being viewed as treating mental health conditions. These providers wanted to refer all patients with mental health issues to mental health specialists, despite the clear evidence that this was an ineffective approach, due to limitations in the availability of mental health specialists and the no-shows for mental health appointments by patients referred from primary care. The strong incentive for a mental health specialist was to see the same patient for a long time, rather than to take in new patients, while the incentive for primary care was to abdicate responsibility for mental health conditions through a referral that might or might not be completed.

Communication and collaboration styles further limited robust development of integrated care. Mental health specialists often resisted the idea of allocating time to supervising nurse care managers as a bridge with primary care providers, despite the availability of methods for accounting for the workload. In part, this resistance reflected the differences between mental health and physical health care plans. For a cardiologist, a shared care plan is typical with primary care. For example, the cardiologist's order might be "continue current medications unless the blood pressure drops below 100/60, if so, hold the medication and notify cardiology." For a psychiatrist, saying to a primary care provider "continue the current antipsychotic unless the patient develops worrisome hallucinations, a significant decrease in functioning, or other new symptoms" was not a familiar approach. Differences in appointment structures, responsiveness to email or secure messaging, and telephone management were also documented. Often a mismatch emerged between mental health specialty and primary care perceptions of their roles around conditions that could not easily be assigned to one group or the other, and were difficult to manage. The predominant mismatch was around pain, although disruptive patients in general, and those with personality disorders, caused particular stress in the mental health specialty–primary care relationship.

Finally, issues frequently arose around who owned or who was responsible for an integrated program—mental health specialty or primary care. The two services were historically independent, with leadership for mental health positioned at the local health care system (medical center), regional, and VA Central Office levels. Integrating leadership for mental health care in primary care proved challenging, raising a wide variety of workforce, space, and role issues. Despite these issues, integrated care has continued to progress and is now seen by most providers and staff as a normal primary care requirement.

A VISION FOR THE FUTURE FOR PRIMARY CARE/MENTAL HEALTH INTEGRATION

To begin to address the variety of issues not resolved through the foundational directives for developing integrated approaches, in 2012, the Offices of Mental Health and Primary Care convened a 12 member strategic planning committee, composed of mental health and primary care experts. These experts met for a year and through a series of surveys with discussion of results and confirmation of final conclusions, came to consensus on a set of recommendations for future program development. Several members of the committee participated in a later publication that further elucidated some of the recommendations.[2] The committee proposed the following mission statement for the PC-MHI initiative: "To provide high quality, collaborative mental and behavioral health care to improve the health of both individual Veterans and the Veteran population as a whole."[42,43] Box 7.2 and Box 7.3 provide a summary of committee results.

As a vision, the PC-MHI initiative should aim "to achieve seamless integration between mental health care provided through VA's Patient Aligned Care Teams (PACT), and care provided through the full spectrum of VA Mental Health Services. Overall, PC-MHI should ensure high quality, accessible mental health care that meets the needs and preferences of all primary care patients with mental health concerns."[43] To achieve these results, a stepped care approach would be needed, such that more intensive, longer term mental health services would be accessible outside of primary care for those who needed them. Care management for depression and anxiety, and availability of brief interventions for alcohol misuse, should be foundational elements of the initiative.

The committee agreed that PACT, when fully developed, together with PC-MHI, should provide the majority of the mental health care needed by primary care patients with mental health conditions of low to moderate complexity, shown to respond to brief, evidence-based interventions. For primary care patients with more complex mental health conditions or those needing specialized resources, PC-MHI would expect to link to the appropriate additional mental health services, based on a service agreement between primary care and mental health specialty services.

Target Conditions for Management Through Integrated Care in Primary Care

The committee agreed that the target conditions for PC-MHI should be depression, anxiety, and alcohol misuse. The designation of anxiety incorporates positive screening for PTSD; many veterans have symptoms of PTSD without meeting full criteria. The PC-MHI leadership role for these conditions

BOX 7.2
PC-MHI MISSION AND VISION

Mission: **To provide high-quality, collaborative mental and behavioral health care to improve the health of both individual Veterans and the Veteran population as a whole.**

Vision: **The VA Primary Care–Mental Health Integration (PC-MHI) initiative aims to achieve seamless integration between mental health care provided through VA's Patient-Aligned Care Teams (PACT) and care provided through the full spectrum of VA Mental Health Services.**

- **When fully developed, PACT, together with PC-MHI, will provide the majority of the mental health care needed by primary care patients with low-to-moderate complexity mental health conditions that have been shown to respond to brief, evidence-based interventions.**
- **PC-MHI care for these conditions will be measurement based, proactive, and guideline concordant.**
- **For primary care patients with higher-complexity mental health conditions or those needing specialized resources, PC-MHI will link to appropriate additional mental health services.**
- **PC-MHI will ensure high-quality, accessible mental health care that meets the needs and preferences of all primary care patients with mental health concerns.**

Report on Integrating Mental Health Into PACT (IMHIP) in the VA. VA Office of Patient Care Services, 2013. http://www.hsrd.research.va.gov/publications/internal/IMHIP-Report.pdf. Accessed May 2, 2016.

BOX 7.3

RECOMMENDATIONS FOR ACHIEVING THE PC-MHI VISION

Each VA facility appoints division-level (primary care site) PC-MHI leaders (one from PACT, one from Mental Health) to jointly manage the initiative at their site. These individuals should have sufficient authority, support from higher levels of leadership, and appropriate dedicated time to accomplish their leadership roles. Recommendations include:

1) **The PC-MHI initiative shows evidence of ongoing monitoring of PC-MHI goals and problems locally and nationally. This will require a national gap analysis and national implementation of quality measures for target PC-MHI conditions.**
2) **PC-MHI leaders, in collaboration with PACT and Mental Health, *design care pathways and flow* for target mental health conditions into a seamless, flexible, and patient-centered approach using stepped-care principles.**
3) **Local Mental Health Specialty, PACT and PC-MHI sign and regularly review/update *inter-service collaboration agreements* specifying (a) the services that will be provided for mental health conditions in primary care, (b) the staff who will be allocated to PC-MHI for how much time to provide these services, and (c) which mental health conditions will be primarily managed in PACT/PC-MHI and which in Mental Health Specialty.**
4) ***Standardized electronic tools for providing symptom measure based care* for depression, alcohol misuse, and anxiety, and for monitoring local PC-MHI program quality and productivity need to be in place.**
5) **National Mental Health Specialty and Primary Care leadership develop *appropriate training for both integrated mental health staff and PACT providers and team members*, with particular emphasis on incorporating *alcohol misuse* into the curricula. Local PC-MHI leaders systematically ensure appropriate training for site PACT providers and care managers through national programs and engage in supportive educational activities.**

Report on Integrating Mental Health Into PACT (IMHIP) in the VA. VA Office of Patient Care Services, 2013. http://www.hsrd.research.va.gov/publications/internal/IMHIP-Report.pdf. Accessed May 2, 2016.

should include: (1) ensuring veteran access to appropriate primary care based, guideline-concordant treatment, (2) monitoring PACT and PC-MHI performance on relevant quality measures, and (3) training and supervision of PACT providers and care managers in identifying, assessing, and providing stepped care for the target conditions. In addition, the PC-MHI leadership role should include collaborating with primary care and other specialists to support primary care management of stress, sleep disorders, pain, obesity, tobacco use, and other behaviorally sensitive problems, impacting health and wellness.

The rationale for the three target conditions focused first on their prevalence. These three conditions account for the large majority of mental health diagnoses in primary care. While exact estimates vary, about 12% of veterans in primary care screen positive for major depression,[24] about 5% to 12% screen positive for PTSD,[44] almost 4% screen positive for social anxiety disorder,[45] and about 20% to 25% screen positive for alcohol misuse.[46,47] In addition, primary care based treatments can prevent consequences of low to moderate level depression, anxiety, and alcohol misuse. Anxiety-related conditions, such as PTSD, may require additional specialized services. On the other hand, patients with generalized anxiety or PTSD-related anxiety symptoms without fully diagnosable PTSD, may benefit from short-term treatment in primary care.

The committee highlighted that treating mental health conditions in the primary care setting can preserve veteran access to more intensive mental health care, when needed. Brief, primary care based interventions, delivered in coordination with mental health providers, are effective for treating most primary care patients with depression, anxiety, or alcohol misuse. If treatment is not provided in early stages, unnecessary suffering can occur, and both the mental and physical health care for these patients becomes complex and difficult. The committee thought detection of patients with mental health concerns is typically best achieved through primary care, while initial assessment, engagement, and reassessment should involve PC-MHI. This initial assessment might occur through a PC-MHI care manager or provider, or through PC-MHI oversight of PACT care managers.

Evaluation of Integrated Primary and Mental Health Care

While no study has definitely evaluated the effects of the fully integrated model, economic evaluation suggests a new pattern of mental health care that may reflect effects of PC-MHI. Both a national cross-sectional evaluation of PACT outcomes,[48] and a regional evaluation of a longitudinal cohort followed for four years,[49] independently found that since implementation of PACT, the rate of face-to-face visits to mental health specialty providers has significantly decreased. Decreased rates may reflect increased use of non–face-to-face visits, greater adoption of shorter-term PC-MHI modalities, or more engagement of primary care clinicians in treatment. During this period, the VA hired increased numbers of mental health specialists, and received an influx of new patients. The reduced visit rate was not accompanied by worsening of mental health performance measures, or more frequent adverse outcomes among patients with mental health conditions.

Few primary care population based studies of the quality of care for the three PC-MHI conditions have been conducted. An evaluation of depression care quality in nine geographically diverse regions (Veterans Integrated Service Networks), based on validated longitudinal electronic measures of guideline-concordant depression care, showed that 8% of veterans visiting primary care per year are newly diagnosed with depression.[50] Over 70% of veterans diagnosed with a new depression episode complete minimal appropriate treatment, defined as at least 60 days of appropriate antidepressant medicine or at least four psychotherapy visits during the following year. Over 90% of veterans with co-occurring depression and PTSD complete treatment. Future evaluation may discover whether or how often treatment has resulted in resolution of depression symptoms, or improved quality of life, and the extent of involvement of integrated mental health in the treatments delivered. Studies of quality of care for alcohol misuse in primary care are ongoing, with results not yet available. We know of no studies in process on the quality of care for anxiety, other than studies of misuse of anxiety medications.

Eventually, evaluation of integrated care should extend outside of the primary care setting to treatment delivered to patients in VA inpatient units, specialty settings, the community, and long-term care. However, quality of care evaluation conducted in these additional settings is scarce, and consensus on approaches to promoting integrated care outside of the primary care setting has not yet been achieved. We hope that establishing integrated primary care will be a foundation for these future developments.

Organizing Integrated Physical and Mental Health Care Within Care Systems

While research studies can allocate key staff to a particular project, care settings must build on prior mental health and primary care research to develop feasible, sustainable management approaches to integrated care.

In the case of managed care settings, these approaches must aim to provide equitable access to care at a population level, such that any patient screened positive for depression, anxiety, or alcohol misuse has a strong likelihood of receiving appropriate care. Finally, the roles of those involved must be defined and managed. Table 7.2 summarizes the lessons learned, based on the VA experience about the key elements and activities for promoting integrated care within a complex health care system.

One of the challenges in implementing integrated care has been achieving integrated leadership. PC-MHI leadership must have the ability to garner resources, including space and staff for the program, and, in concept, must involve both primary care and mental health specialty leaders. In practice, leaders or champions for the initiative at local sites, have sometimes been primary care and sometimes mental health; strong collaboration between leaders from the two areas has, however, been crucial for success.

Primary care settings are increasingly complex. PC-MHI staff members work closely with PACT providers, generalist nurse care managers, pharmacists, social workers, coaches, and other PACT team members. In addition, PC-MHI staff

TABLE 7.2. LEARNING FROM VETERANS AFFAIRS INTEGRATED MENTAL HEALTH INITIATIVES

Key Integrated Program Elements	Activities
Executive and disciplinary leadership support/believe in integrated care	• Systematic strategic planning involving key stakeholders • Memoranda of understanding or inter-service agreements, that include staffing arrangements, as well as program goals • Education of top leaders and middle managers • Engagement of all stakeholder disciplines • Veteran patient engagement
Ongoing communication and collaboration between mental health and primary care	• Integrated mental health and physical health electronic records • Inter-service agreements • Physical co-location
Clear local leadership roles for primary care and for mental health	• Designated primary care and mental health leaders with clear roles at the primary care practice site level • Engagement of all relevant disciplines in local program planning and operation (e.g., nursing, psychology, social work)
Adequate staffing of integrated care	• Identification of primary care/mental health integration team members with adequate designated time commitments to integration, including nurses and clerks
Standardized yearly mental health screening in primary care	• Computer reminders for depression, suicidality among depressed patients, and alcohol misuse • Reminders are typically administered by licensed professional nurses or health care technicians; may be administered by mail, computer kiosk, or computer tablet.
Guided (stepped) patient flow based on need	• Standardized initial assessment of patients who screen-positive or are referred prior to triage, to primary care follow-up or to an integrated mental health care modality or visit; integrated mental health specialist guidance prior to referral to specialized mental health resources
Structured, prospectively timed follow-up	• Follow-up templates suitable for use by nurses, social workers, or health technicians • A computerized diary system for prospectively planning follow-up telephone calls or visits
Ongoing training of both mental health specialists and primary care providers	• Regular national cyber-seminars, training consultant assistance, and coaches • Educational materials and tools • Group case consultations directed at local primary care sites • Electronic consultation availability
A fast-paced multimodal mental health delivery style	• Brief treatments in the integrated program with referral to intensive mental health or to supported primary care follow-up • Primary care–based multimodal psychology groups (e.g., relaxation and meditation) as support, and as gateways to more intensive treatments, if needed • Development of integrated care plans dealing with multiple comorbidities and goals rather than a single condition
High integrated program access	• Routine first visit appointments available within one to two weeks • Availability of "curbside" quick consultations with primary care providers, often when a patient is at a primary care visit • Immediate availability of mental health backup for psychiatric emergencies as perceived by primary care
Ongoing measurement and evaluation	• National program resources, including electronic measures • Local program-tailored evaluation measures

coordinates closely with the full range of non–PC-MHI mental health specialty services, including psychiatry, psychology, chemical dependency, vocational rehabilitation, and others, to meet the needs of patients requiring long-term or specialized treatments. Finally, supportive and therapeutic integrated care groups, physically based in primary care, sometimes with the inclusion of alternative care modalities, such as tai chi or yoga, have become an increasingly valued part of many PC-MHI programs.

In the VA, PC-MHI staffing is guided by national standards. Within these standards, exact PC-MHI staffing patterns at individual sites vary. For example, generalist nurse care managers may be integrated into PC-MHI care, sites may engage specially trained care managers working at a distance, and co-located mental health providers themselves may provide measurement-based care and proactive follow-up. Clerical and nursing support for PC-MHI providers may be provided by primary care or by mental health specialty personnel. Telephone and

BOX 7.4

SUMMARY OF RECOMMENDED TREATMENT APPROACHES AND RELEVANT EVIDENCE

Strength of recommendation taxonomy (SOR A, B, or C)

- **VA implemented a patient-centered medical home model are called patient-aligned care teams (PACT); PACT outcomes included reduced mental health specialty and primary care face-to-face visits, and increased non–face-to-face encounters.[48,49,52] (SOR B)**
- **Standardized primary care screening and mental health assessment: Research documented that about half of depressed patients in primary care were not detected, and that over-diagnosis in primary care is also prevalent.[53] (SOR B)**
- **Prompt treatment of depression: Research further identified the critical importance and effectiveness of treating major depression prior to its full potential results, such as job loss, family dissolution, or deteriorations in physical health, occurred.[26,54] (SOR C)**
- **Integrated mental health treatment of high-risk primary care patients: Addressing mental health issues is key to success.[16,17] (SOR C)**
- **Translating Initiatives in Depression into Effective Solutions (TIDES) took a multilevel, interdisciplinary approach (evidence-based quality improvement) toward implementing collaborative care, and then spreading the model. TIDES tools, policies, procedures, and training approaches were developed in partnership between researchers and national, regional, and local depression quality improvement leaders and stakeholders.[25,33,34] (SOR C)**
- **The Behavioral Health Laboratory model is a method for providing integrated care that uses computer-assisted telephone-based assessment and, if indicated, care management for primary care patients referred for suspected depression or alcohol misuse.[35] (SOR C)**
- **The White River Junction model is a method for providing co-located, integrated mental health care that uses in-person tablet-based comprehensive assessment of primary care patients with behavioral health needs, followed by integrated mental health care.[22] (SOR C)**
- **The Michigan-based Primary Care–Mental Health Integration (PC-MHI) initiative supports policy development, communications, data and measurement, technical assistance, and training and education. Local PC-MHI programs can access the initiative from anywhere in the country, including its technical support capabilities, predominantly virtual training activities, and formal mentoring program.[37] (SOR C)**
- **Rates of completion of minimal appropriate treatment with antidepressants or psychotherapy are high among patients diagnosed with depression across the VA primary care population.[50] (SOR C)**

videoconference care play different roles depending on local conditions.

Education for Integrated Primary Care and Mental Health Care

A discussion of PC-MHI would not be complete without mentioning the training needs generated. Primary care providers already provide a majority of the psychoactive medications prescribed to veterans, yet evidence suggests that as many as a third of primary care clinicians are uncomfortable treating depression, the most common mental health condition in primary care.[51] It is likely that even fewer are comfortable treating other serious mental illnesses or addiction. On the mental health side, clinicians are often uncomfortable with the integrated role, including the emphasis on short-term, team-based care, and the partnership role of supporting treatment through primary care clinicians. In addition, mental health specialists, perhaps with the exception of psychiatrists, rarely have the full range of training in management of mental health issues in relationship to the need to ensure the best possible physical health care. For example, primary care clinicians may benefit from consultation on issues, such as co-occurring personality disorders, disruptive behavior, poor adherence, and others unlikely to be cured by mental health treatments, but that may require management in primary care. Finally, evidence-based group treatment is a critical component of integrated care; psychiatrists may not be trained in these treatments, and even psychologists and social workers may require additional group training to function effectively in the primary care setting. Additional development of educational programs for mental, social, and physical health care providers and trainees aimed at partnership or team roles is critical for achieving integrated care goals. See Chapter 4: Team-Based Integrated Primary Care. In addition, training in how to effectively engage patients in care (e.g., through motivational interviewing), will be needed to achieve full impact, particularly on vulnerable, high-risk patients. See Chapter 25: Health Coaching in Integrated Care.

NEED FOR FUTURE RESEARCH

The preceding sections provide ample opportunity for further investigation, including evaluations of the effectiveness of the current VA PC-MHI model. However, guidelines for delivery of integrated care across many other conditions are also needed, and are described in other chapters in this *book*. Current disease-by-disease guidelines provide insufficient support for guiding care that may require integration of depression treatment with co-occurring smoking, PTSD symptoms, family system issues, substance abuse issues, or patient treatment preferences, as well as chronic physical diseases. Finally, achieving maximum benefit from integrated primary care and mental health specialist depression treatment in the VA system will require increased development and testing of methods for integrating care plans across mental and physical health care providers. Review Box 7.4 for a summary of treatment approaches and relevant evidence supporting the VA approach.

DISCLAIMER

The views expressed in this article are those of the authors and do not necessarily reflect the position or policy of the Department of Veterans Affairs or the United States government.

REFERENCES

1. Yano EM, Simon BF, Lanto AB, Rubenstein LV. The evolution of changes in primary care delivery underlying the Veterans Health Administration's quality transformation. Am J Public Health. 2007;97(12):2151–2159.
2. Pomerantz AS, Kearney LK, Wray LO, Post EP, McCarthy JF. Mental health services in the medical home in the Department of Veterans Affairs: factors for successful integration. Psychol Serv. 2014;11(3):243–253.
3. VHA Handbook 1600.01: Uniform Mental Health Services in VA Medical Centers and Clinics. Washington, D.C.: Veterans Health Administration, Department of Veterans Affairs; 2008.
4. Team-Based Care—PACT. http://www.va.gov/health/services/primarycare/pact/team.asp. Accessed April 2, 2016.
5. Hepner KA, Rowe M, Rost K, et al. The effect of adherence to practice guidelines on depression outcomes. Ann Intern Med. 2007;147(5):320–329.
6. Klein S. The Veterans Health Administration: Implementing Patient-Centered Medical Homes in the Nation's Largest Integrated Delivery System. Issue Brief (Common Fund). 2011;16(1537):1–20.

7. Yoon J, Cordasco KM, Chow A, Rubenstein LV. The relationship between same-day access and continuity in primary care and emergency department visits. PloS One. 2015;10(9):e0135274.
8. Borowsky SJ, Rubenstein LV, Meredith LS, Camp P, Jackson-Triche M, Wells KB. Who is at risk of nondetection of mental health problems in primary care? J Gen Intern Med. 2000;15(6):381–388.
9. Wells KB, Schoenbaum M, Unutzer J, Lagomasino IT, Rubenstein LV. Quality of care for primary care patients with depression in managed care. Arch Fam Med. 1999;8(6):529–536.
10. Moussavi S, Chatterji S, Verdes E, Tandon A, Patel V, Ustun B. Depression, chronic diseases, and decrements in health: Results from the World Health Surveys. Lancet. 2007;370(9590):851–858.
11. Pacula RL, Sturm R. Mental health parity legislation: Much ado about nothing? Health Serv Res. 2000;35(1 Pt 2):263–275.
12. Cunningham PJ. Beyond parity: Primary care physicians' perspectives on access to mental health care. Health Aff (Millwood). 2009;28(3):w490–w501.
13. Barry CL, Huskamp HA. Moving beyond parity—mental health and addiction care under the ACA. N Engl J Med. 2011;365(11):973–975.
14. Shulkin DJ. Beyond the VA crisis—becoming a high-performance network. N Engl J Med. 2016; 374(11):1003–1005.
15. Liu CF, Bolkan C, Chan D, Yano EM, Rubenstein LV, Chaney EF. Dual use of VA and non-VA services among primary care patients with depression. J Gen Intern Med. 2009;24(3):305–311.
16. Zulman DM, Pal Chee C, Wagner TH, et al. Multimorbidity and healthcare utilisation among high-cost patients in the US Veterans Affairs Health Care System. BMJ Open. 2015;5(4):e007771.
17. Yoon J, Yano EM, Altman L, et al. Reducing costs of acute care for ambulatory care-sensitive medical conditions: The central roles of comorbid mental illness. Med Care. 2012;50(8):705–713.
18. Iyer SP, Young AS. Health screening, counseling, and hypertension control for people with serious mental illness at primary care visits. Gen Hosp Psychiatry. 2015;37(1):60–66.
19. Waltz TJ, Campbell DG, Kirchner JE, et al. Veterans with depression in primary care: Provider preferences, matching, and care satisfaction. Fam Syst Health. 2014;32(4):367–377.
20. Campbell DG, Felker BL, Liu CF, et al. Prevalence of depression–PTSD comorbidity: Implications for clinical practice guidelines and primary care-based interventions. J Gen Intern Med. 2007;22(6):711–718.
21. Kulka RA, Schlenger WE, Fairbank JA, et al. Trauma and the Vietnam War Generation: Report of Findings from the National Vietnam Veterans Readjustment Study, Vol. 18. Philadelphia: Brunner/Mazel; 1990.
22. Pomerantz AS, Shiner B, Watts BV, et al. The White River model of colocated collaborative care: A platform for mental and behavioral health care in the medical home. Fam Syst Health. 2010;28(2):114–129.
23. Foy R, Hempel S, Rubenstein L, et al. Meta-analysis: Effect of interactive communication between collaborating primary care physicians and specialists. Ann Intern Med. 2010;152(4):247–258.
24. Yano EM, Chaney EF, Campbell DG, et al. Yield of practice-based depression screening in VA primary care settings. J Gen Intern Med. 2012;27(3):331–338.
25. Collaborative Care for Depression in the Primary Care Setting. A Primer on VA's Translating Initiatives for Depression into Effective Solutions (TIDES) Project. VA Health Services Research and Development Service, Office of Research and Development, Department of Veterans Affairs; 2008. http://www.hsrd.research.va.gov/publications/internal/depression_primer.pdf. Accessed May 2, 2016.
26. Wells KB, Jones L, Chung B, et al. Community-partnered cluster-randomized comparative effectiveness trial of community engagement and planning or resources for services to address depression disparities. J Gen Intern Med. 2013;28(10):1268–1278.
27. Johnson-Lawrence V, Zivin K, Szymanski BR, Pfeiffer PN, McCarthy JF. VA primary care-mental health integration: patient characteristics and receipt of mental health services, 2008–2010. Psychiatr Serv. 2012;63(11):1137–1141.
28. Wells KB, Sherbourne C, Schoenbaum M, et al. Impact of disseminating quality improvement programs for depression in managed primary care: a randomized controlled trial. JAMA. 2000;283(2):212–220.
29. Trafton JA, Greenberg G, Harris AH, et al. VHA mental health information system: Applying health information technology to monitor and facilitate implementation of VHA Uniform Mental Health Services Handbook requirements. Med Care. 2013;51(3 Suppl 1):S29–S36.
30. Kroenke K, Spitzer RL, Williams JB. The Patient Health Questionnaire-2: Validity of a two-item depression screener. Med Care. 2003;41(11):1284–1292.
31. Chang ET, Wells KB, Young AS, et al. The anatomy of primary care and mental health clinician communication: a quality improvement case study. J Gen Intern Med. 2014;29(Suppl 2):S598–S606.
32. Cerully J, Smith M, Wilks A, Giglio K. Strategic Analysis of the 2014 Wounded Warrior Project Annual Alumni Survey: A Way Forward. Santa Monica, CA; 2015.
33. Chaney EF, Rubenstein LV, Liu CF, et al. Implementing collaborative care for depression treatment in primary care: a cluster randomized evaluation of a quality improvement practice redesign. Implement Sci. 2011;6(121):1–15.
34. Rubenstein LV, Chaney EF, Ober S, et al. Using evidence-based quality improvement methods for translating depression collaborative care research into practice. Fam Syst Health. 2010;28(2):91–113.

35. Oslin DW, Ross J, Sayers S, Murphy J, Kane V, Katz IR. Screening, assessment, and management of depression in VA primary care clinics. The Behavioral Health Laboratory. J Gen Intern Med. 2006;21(1):46–50.
36. Chang ET, Rose DE, Yano EM, et al. Determinants of readiness for primary care-mental health integration (PC-MHI) in the VA Health Care System. J Gen Intern Med. 2013;28(3):353–362.
37. Post EP, Van Stone WW. Veterans Health Administration primary care–mental health integration initiative. N C Med J. 2008;69(1):49–52.
38. Zivin K, Pfeiffer PN, Szymanski BR, et al. Initiation of Primary Care–Mental Health Integration programs in the VA Health System: Associations with psychiatric diagnoses in primary care. Med Care. 2010;48(9):843–851.
39. Rubenstein LV, Mittman BS, Yano EM, Mulrow CD. From understanding health care provider behavior to improving health care: The QUERI framework for quality improvement. Quality Enhancement Research Initiative. Med Care. 2000;38(6 Suppl 1):I129–I141.
40. Ritchie MJ, Dollar KM, Kearney LK, Kirchner JE. Research and services partnerships: Responding to needs of clinical operations partners: transferring implementation facilitation knowledge and skills. Psychiatr Serv. 2014;65(2):141–143.
41. Mojtabai R, Olfson M. Proportion of antidepressants prescribed without a psychiatric diagnosis is growing. Health Aff (Millwood). 2011;30(8):1434–1442.
42. VA Office of Mental Health. Primary Care–Mental Health Integration (PC-MHI) Functional Tool, version 1.0, 2012. http://www.mentalhealth.va.gov/coe/cih-visn2/Documents/Clinical/Operations_Policies_Procedures/PC-MHI_Functional_Tool_v10_090712.pdf. Accessed July 16, 2013.
43. Report on Integrating Mental Health Into PACT (IMHIP) in the VA. VA Office of Patient Care Services; 2013. http://www.hsrd.research.va.gov/publications/internal/IMHIP-Report.pdf. Accessed May 2, 2016.
44. Ramchand R, Schell TL, Karney BR, Osilla KC, Burns RM, Caldarone LB. Disparate prevalence estimates of PTSD among service members who served in Iraq and Afghanistan: Possible explanations. J Trauma Stress. 2010;23(1):59–68.
45. Kashdan TB, Frueh BC, Knapp RG, Hebert R, Magruder KM. Social anxiety disorder in Veterans Affairs primary care clinics. Behav Res Ther. 2006;44(2):233–247.
46. Bradley KA, Rubinsky AD, Sun H, et al. Prevalence of alcohol misuse among men and women undergoing major noncardiac surgery in the Veterans Affairs health care system. Surgery. 2012;152(1):69–81.
47. Hoggatt KJ, Williams EC, Der-Martirosian C, Yano EM, Washington DL. National prevalence and correlates of alcohol misuse in women veterans. J Subst Abuse Treat. 2015;52:10–16.
48. Hebert PL, Liu CF, Wong ES, et al. Patient-centered medical home initiative produced modest economic results for Veterans Health Administration, 2010–12. Health Aff (Millwood). 2014;33(6):980–987.
49. Yoon J, Chow A, Rubenstein LV. Impact of medical home implementation through evidence-based quality improvement on utilization and costs. Med Care. 2016;54(2):118–125.
50. Farmer MM, Rubenstein LV, Sherbourne CD, et al. Depression quality of care: Measuring quality over time using VA electronic medical record data. J Gen Intern Med. 2016;31(Suppl 1):36–45.
51. Chang ET, Magnabosco JL, Chaney E, et al. Predictors of primary care management of depression in the Veterans Affairs healthcare system. J Gen Intern Med. 2014;29(7):1017–1025.
52. Jackson GL, Powers BJ, Chatterjee R, et al. Improving patient care. The patient-centered medical home. A systematic review. Ann Intern Med. 2013;158(3):169–178.
53. Mitchell AJ, Vaze A, Rao S. Clinical diagnosis of depression in primary care: A meta-analysis. Lancet. 2009;374(9690):609–619.
54. Wells K, Sherbourne C, Schoenbaum M, et al. Five-year impact of quality improvement for depression: Results of a group-level randomized controlled trial. Arch Gen Psychiatry. 2004;61(4):378–386.

8

Aging Brain Care

A Model of Integrated Care for Dementia and Depression

CATHERINE A. ALDER, MARY GUERRIERO AUSTROM, MICHAEL A. LAMANTIA, AND MALAZ A. BOUSTANI

BOX 8.1

KEY POINTS

- **Fragmented care can be especially problematic for older adults with cognitive impairment and late-life depression because these conditions complicate the management of comorbidities.**
- **The Aging Brain Care (ABC) program provides a structure for integrating interventions for dementia and depression into the primary care environment and coordinating care across multiple providers, settings, and community resources.**
- **The ABC program incorporates and integrates the common features of the IMPACT and PREVENT evidence-based collaborative care models while also attending to the implementation barriers.**
- **Scalability of the program was accomplished using innovative processes to develop and train a new workforce of direct care workers modeled on the concept of task shifting.**
- **The program was successfully converted to a population health management program with the support of the Enhanced Medical Record—Aging Brain Care (eMR-ABC), a web-based care coordination software.**
- **Early performance data suggest the ABC program has made substantial progress toward improving the health outcomes of patients with dementia and late-life depression.**

INTRODUCTION

While fragmented care is a problem across the entire health care delivery system, it is especially problematic for vulnerable older adults suffering from dementia and late-life depression. Most older adults have multiple chronic conditions. In addition to depression and dementia, hypertension, diabetes, and cardiovascular disease are common comorbid conditions. Patients may seek help from their primary care physicians and specialists in managing one or more of these conditions. However, communication among these physicians is often lacking or inadequate. The primary care physician, faced with the task of managing multiple chronic conditions, must prioritize comorbidities posing the most immediate threat to the patient's physical health and well-being, and the patient's cognitive and depressive symptoms are often not assigned the highest priority. This approach not only fails to recognize the potential negative impact of dementia and depression on both the patient and family, but also fails to appreciate the complex interrelationships among cognitive, emotional, social, and physical health. Cognitive impairment and mood disorders complicate the management of comorbid conditions by interfering with the patient's ability to monitor and report symptoms, adhere to the prescribed medication regimen, and otherwise comply with the plan of care.

To reduce fragmentation, each medical provider must adopt a more holistic view of health care, recognizing the potential impact of any one action on the patient's overall health. Communication and collaboration among all providers, as well as the patient and family caregiver, is critical to developing a plan of care that takes into account not only the patient's medical needs but also the patient's cognitive and emotional status and the social supports available to assist with care management.

The Aging Brain Care (ABC) model described here provides a structure for integrating evidence-based interventions for dementia and depression into the primary care environment. An overview of the key elements of the ABC model is contained in Box 8.1. By extending the delivery of care beyond the clinic into the homes and communities of patients and their caregivers, ABC offers patient-centered services aimed at coordinating care across multiple providers, settings, and community resources.

BACKGROUND

Scientists at the Indiana University Center for Aging Research (IUCAR) have dedicated much of the last 30 years to developing, testing, and implementing models of integrated care. Two such models were tested and validated in clinical trials conducted in a primary care practice within Eskenazi Health (formerly Wishard Health Services), a safety-net hospital serving a diverse population of vulnerable adults in Indianapolis, Indiana.

The IMPACT (Improving Mood–Promoting Access to Collaborative Treatment) depression care model was shown to be effective in reducing patients' symptoms of depression as well as improving physical function, health-related quality of life, and satisfaction with care.[1] The critical component of this model was the expansion of the care team to include a care coordinator who partnered with the patient's primary care physician to provide personalized, patient-centered depression care including both antidepressant medications and problem-solving therapy within the primary care setting.[1]

Inspired by the success of the IMPACT model, IUCAR scientists designed the PREVENT (Providing Resources Early to Vulnerable Adults Needing Treatment for Memory Loss) intervention with a goal of improving care for dementia within the primary care setting by using the same personalized, patient-centered, collaborative care approach.[2] The PREVENT model also included a care coordinator, equipped with a toolbox of nonpharmacological interventions for both the patient and the caregiver, who served as a liaison connecting the patient and caregiver to the primary care provider, expert consultants, and community resources.[2] The PREVENT trial was shown to be effective in reducing not only the behavioral and psychological symptoms of the patient but also the burden on the informal caregiver.[2]

THE HEALTHY AGING BRAIN CENTER

In late 2007, building on the positive results of the PREVENT trial, implementation scientists at IUCAR began work on converting the research model into Eskenazi's first specialty clinic for memory care, the Healthy Aging Brain Center (HABC). The history of the HABC is detailed in our earlier work[3] and is also recounted in more recent work chronicling the evolution of the program.[4] A brief description of the development, structure, and services of the clinic follows.

The HABC was designed to assist the primary care physician in the identification and management of dementia by providing a state-of-the-art diagnostic evaluation and personalized care management for both the patient and the caregiver throughout the course of the disease.[3,4] Minimum specifications for the clinic were determined by an implementation team composed of representatives from each of the disciplines providing dementia care at Eskenazi.[3,4] The fundamental mission of this team was to adapt the model tested in the PREVENT trial to the real-world clinical care environment at Eskenazi while maintaining fidelity to the critical elements of the proven intervention.[3,4] The implementation team completed its work within four months and delivered the seven minimum care delivery requirements of the HABC described in Box 8.2.[3,4] On January 7, 2008, the HABC opened its doors and began serving patients with a multidisciplinary team composed of a physician, two care coordinators [one registered nurse (RN) and one social worker], a medical assistant, and an individual with specialized training in the administration of neuropsychological testing.[3,4]

Care delivery in the HABC takes place in 2 phases—the initial assessment phase and the follow-up

BOX 8.2

MINIMUM CARE DELIVERY REQUIREMENTS OF THE HABC

1. **Use practical, reliable tools such as the Mini Mental Status Exam[5] and the Healthy Aging Brain Center Monitor[6] to periodically assess and monitor cognitive, functional, behavioral, and psychological patient symptoms and the associated caregiver stress, and to evaluate the effectiveness of the care plan.**
2. **Implement psychosocial interventions (e.g., advance care planning, behavioral activation, and peer support groups) aimed at preventing or reducing the patient's symptoms and associated caregiver stress.**
3. **Use self-management tools (e.g., the educational materials tested in the PREVENT study) to enhance the patient's and caregiver's skills in managing symptoms and navigating the health care system.**
4. **Offer medications (e.g., cholinesterase inhibitors and medications to treat depression, diabetes, and hypertension) to improve adherence, treat symptoms, reduce cerebrovascular risk factors, and limit exposure to anticholinergics.**
5. **Prevent and treat conditions superimposed on dementia (e.g., depression, delirium, and pain).**
6. **Use case management and coordinate with community resources.**
7. **Assess the patient's physical home environment and the modifications needed to compensate for disability related to cognitive impairment.**

phase. Each phase includes multiple components.[3,4] Fifty percent of each care coordinator's time is allocated to care coordination activities that typically do not involve face-to-face exchanges with patients.

Initial Patient Assessment Phase

Prior to the patient's first appointment, a care coordinator conducts a structured telephone interview with the patient's caregiver to assess the patient's symptoms, functional status, medical history, and social situation and to determine the caregiver's immediate needs.[3,4] The first clinic visit involves a complete diagnostic evaluation, including a medical assessment, a structured physical and neurological examination, neuropsychological testing that includes a depression assessment, blood work, and brain imaging.[3,4] After all test results are returned, the HABC physician and the care coordinators meet face to face with the patient and family during an extended second clinic visit (referred to as the "family conference visit") to disclose the diagnosis, answer any questions, and initiate the plan of care.[3,4]

Follow-Up Phase

Follow-up care in the HABC may be delivered in person or by telephone.[3,4] The frequency of follow-up appointments is personalized based on the diagnosis and the emergent needs of the patient and caregiver.[3,4] Patients and caregivers are encouraged to contact their care coordinator between visits to ask questions and obtain information and assistance.[3,4] During follow-up contacts, the HABC team assesses the patient's symptoms and the caregiver's stress and may modify the care plan as necessary to address developing needs and concerns.[3,4]

The HABC team serves as the liaison between the patient and caregiver, the primary care physician, specialty care providers, and community resources, all in an effort to facilitate communication and coordinate care for the benefit of the patient and caregivers. The team communicates periodically with primary care providers to discuss patient care issues, share information, and make recommendations. Most communication occurs by telephone or email. Thus, the HABC model would be characterized by Doherty et al as a Level 2 integration within primary care practice, Basic Collaboration at a Distance.[5–7] However, unlike Level 2, the health care providers share the same systems for charting and can see providers' clinical notes.

Within the first year of operation, the model developed in the research laboratory had been successfully converted to a health care delivery program that has positive effects on the quality of dementia care at Eskenazi.[3,4] The reach and impact of the program, however, were constrained by several factors:

1. The clinical setting was limited by the availability of memory care physicians and the limitations of the physical space.[4,8] The clinic was operating three half-day sessions per week with three examination rooms available per session.[3]
2. The clinical setting was limited by the need for two care coordinators [one registered nurse (RN) and one social worker] to come to the clinic.[4,8] Transportation problems, complex social situations, concerns about the stigma related to a diagnosis of dementia, and a general distrust of the health care system all contributed to the failure of patients to show up reliably for visits.[4]
3. The integration of the HABC within primary care was incomplete.[4,8] The physical distance between most primary care clinics and the HABC became a barrier to effective communication and collaboration with primary care physicians.[4]
4. Time and resource constraints posed obstacles to providing comprehensive, evidence-based depression care.[4] As a result, many patients with a primary diagnosis of depression were referred to psychiatry.[4]

THE AGING BRAIN CARE MEDICAL HOME PILOT PROGRAM

In 2009, Eskenazi formed an implementation team to develop a second integrated care program to address the limitations of the HABC and expand the reach and impact of the model beyond the clinical setting. The result was the first prototype of the Aging Brain Care Medical Home (ABC Med Home), a mobile program designed to act as the community outreach arm of the HABC. The mobile design facilitated an increase in the number of face-to-face interactions between the ABC team and the primary care providers at all the clinical sites, thereby upgrading the level of integration within primary care from a Level 2 to a Level 4.[7] The creation and subsequent development of the ABC Med Home was described in detail in our earlier work.[4,8,9] A summary of the history of the current program follows.

The ABC Med Home began as a small pilot program serving older adults with a diagnosis of dementia and/or depression.[4,9] Eligible patients were identified by ICD-9 codes and enrolled following an acute-care event resulting in a hospital stay.[4,9] Given the high rate of unrecognized dementia in primary care,[10,11] a wide range of ICD-9 codes were included, with a preference for sensitivity over specificity. The pilot program began with only one clinical provider, a geriatric nurse practitioner, who was supported by a medical director with specialized training in geriatric care.[4,9] In October 2011, when enrollment reached about 300 patients, a social worker care coordinator was added to the team.[4] The minimum care delivery requirements for the ABC Med Home were the same as those specified for the HABC, but the new program targeted older adults with depression as well as dementia and used several additional tools to support care delivery.[4,9] The ABC Med Home care coordinators were trained in the IMPACT model of care including problem-solving therapy, behavioral activation, relapse prevention, and all other tools of the IMPACT model.[4] In addition, the ABC Med Home used the "mobile office" concept, which allowed the ABC care coordinators to consider the physical and psychosocial comfort of both the patient and caregiver when determining the appointment site.[4] Appointments commonly took place in the patients' and/or caregivers' homes, the primary care or specialty clinics, and other locations within the community selected by the patients and caregivers.[4,9] Finally, the ABC Med Home was supported by a variety of information technology tools, such as laptops with wireless Internet access, cellphones, and the Enhanced Medical Record–Aging Brain Care (eMR-ABC), a web-based care coordination software.[4,9,12]

EXPANSION OF THE ABC MED HOME

Although the pilot program addressed most of the limitations of the HABC, it actually did little to expand the clinic's reach and impact. Like the HABC, the ABC Med Home was limited by the availability of providers and the pilot model was not scalable financially. In the summer of 2012, however, the ABC Med Home was chosen to receive one of the 107 Health Care Innovation Awards from the Centers for Medicare & Medicaid Services (CMS).[4,8] With the support of this funding, the

ABC Med Home solved the scalability problem and expanded services to 1,500 patients across the entire system of community health centers associated with Eskenazi.[4,8] Simultaneously, it altered the platform of its care model from case management to population health management.[4,8] Adopting a population health management approach meant assuming accountability for both the quality and the cost of care provided to enrolled patients. Both outcomes and processes were measured and monitored frequently. Although all patients were actively managed, not all patients received the same "dose" of the intervention. Enrolled patients were continuously stratified by need. Highest-need patients were those not responding to the intervention, as evidenced by poor measured outcomes. If an individual patient was not achieving personal goals, then more resources were allocated to improving his or her health outcomes. In this way, program resources were continuously reallocated where needed most.

Workforce Development of the ABC Med Home

The scalability of the program depended on one critical feature: the development of a brand-new workforce of direct care workers, the care coordinator assistants (CCAs).[4,8] The CCA position is modeled on the concept of "task shifting": tasks requiring less training and experience are delegated to less expensive members of the team who operate under the close supervision of the professional staff, thereby allowing each clinical provider to work at the top of his or her license.[4,8,13,14] CCAs are required to have at least a high school diploma and receive comprehensive training in the knowledge and skills necessary to provide care for older adults with dementia and depression.[4,8,13] The CCAs assist and increase the capacity of the care coordinators by performing visits, administering biopsychosocial needs assessments, delivering psychosocial interventions, educating patients and caregivers, and monitoring medications.[4,8,13]

The CCAs were selected using an innovative process designed by a workforce development team that included experts in medical education, curriculum development and evaluation, dementia care (including caregiver counseling), and team-based care. Eskenazi's human resources department was integrated into the selection process.[4,13] First, the human resources department identified candidates meeting the basic requirements for employment.[4,13] These candidates then participated in preliminary interviews with the department that included questions designed by the workforce team to assess their attitudes and work experience related to the elderly.[4,13] Those who performed best during the interviews were invited to participate in the Multiple Mini Interview (MMI), a process that allowed candidates to demonstrate, rather than simply talk about, their abilities.[4,13] The MMI included six stations, each designed to assess necessary skills that are difficult, if not impossible, to teach, such as the ability to demonstrate compassion, to maintain composure under stress, to educate a caregiver and patient, and to prioritize multiple needs.[4,13] Moving from station to station, candidates interacted with "standardized patients" (trained actors who played the roles of older adults and their caregivers).[4,13] Interviewers simply observed and then assessed the candidates using 1- to 5-point Likert scales developed by the workforce team.[4,13]

When the entire process was complete, the interviewers participated in a group debriefing to discuss and rank the overall performance of each candidate.[4,13] The top candidates were offered employment.[4,13] The new hires received intensive training to prepare for the CCA role. The initial 10-day program included three types of sessions:[4]

1. *Interactive sessions.* Didactic lectures were used to explain the disease process and the common challenges faced by caregivers. We also used (a) video sessions featuring selections from both documentary and modern dramatic films; (b) reflective reading and writing exercises; (c) team-building exercises, including discussions about professionalism, interdisciplinary care, and communication; and (d) a presentation by the local Alzheimer's Association staff detailing available community resources.[4]
2. *Simulation Training.* During two half-day sessions, each CCA conducted a "home visit" with standardized patients while being videotaped. Immediately following the session, the standardized patients provided feedback on the interaction to the CCA. The CCA watched the videotape of the exercise, completed a self-assessment, and then participated in small-group debriefing of the experience. Videotapes of several CCAs were viewed and the group identified

areas of strength and areas in need of improvement focusing on communication skills, active listening, and nonverbal behaviors. Finally, each CCA conducted the exercise a second time, again while being videotaped, attempting to improve his or her performance and comfort with the interaction.[4]

3. *Immersion Training.* Each CCA shadowed the clinical staff of the HABC as well as the ABC Med Home care coordinators. In addition, each CCA received preliminary training on the use of the eMR-ABC care coordination software. Following the immersion sessions, CCAs participated in large-group debriefing sessions with the trainer and the current ABC Med Home staff.[4]

Immediately following the 10-day training, the CCAs were deployed to begin providing care to patients and caregivers. While working in the field, CCAs received additional training in the IMPACT model of depression care as well as specialized training in advanced care planning.[4] Additional professional development and education were provided regularly by local dementia care experts. CCAs also had a number of opportunities to attend educational programs related to dementia and/or depression care that were offered on campus and in the community.[4] In addition, the dementia care trainer met alone with the CCAs once a month over the course of the award; no care coordinators or administrators were present, permitting the CCAs to report any concerns and to provide feedback about the program in a safe environment.

Staffing of the ABC Med Home

Originally, the ABC Med Home comprised three care teams, each serving approximately 500 patients. Each team was led by a 1.0 full-time equivalent (FTE) nurse practitioner (NP) and a 0.5 FTE social worker who served as the care coordinators and jointly supervised five CCAs. Each CCA was responsible for approximately 100 patients. Four members of the teams (one social worker and one CCA from each team) were employed by CICOA Aging & In-Home Solutions, Indiana's largest area agency on aging (See Figure 8.1 for the staffing model.) These team members were trained by CICOA in the art of "options counseling" (i.e., connecting patients and caregivers in need with available community resources).

In late 2013, both NPs left the program and the staffing model was modified based on lessons learned from the first year of operations. NPs were replaced with RNs; few qualified NPs were interested in the care coordinator position, few applied, and many of those interviewed wanted to practice independently rather than as part of a team. In addition, the NPs were expensive and were not working at the top of their skillset. For example, they did not prescribe medications, because the primary care physicians preferred to be consulted before any medication was changed or added. Ultimately we determined that the program would be better served by experienced RNs with team care and management skills.

At the same time, we recognized that the CCAs were not being used to capacity. Because depression is a chronic illness, individuals who have suffered a major depression are at risk for another depressive episode. Therefore, patients who had an ICD-9 code indicating a diagnosis of depression but did not meet the criteria for major depressive disorder, as evidenced by the Patient Health Questionnaire (PHQ-9)[14] administered at the time of enrollment, were still included in the program. At any given time, many of those patients required little attention other than monitoring, allowing the CCAs to expand their panel size from 100 to 150 patients. This permitted the program to continue serving the same population using only two care teams, as illustrated in Figure 8.2.

Enrollment

The enrollment criteria were also modified for the demonstration project; hospitalization no longer served as the trigger for enrollment in the program. To be eligible for enrollment, a patient had to (1) be a Medicare or a Medicaid beneficiary, (2) be 65 years of age or older, (3) have at least one dementia or depression ICD-9 code, and (4) have made at least one visit to one of Eskenazi's primary care practices or the HABC within the previous two years.[4,8]

Eligible patients were identified using Eskenazi's billing records and then grouped together by primary care physician or HABC provider. A list of each physician's eligible patients was then sent to that provider along with a letter explaining the program. Enrollment was an administrative process accomplished by entering the patient in the eMR-ABC.[4,8] Enrolled patients remained active in the eMR-ABC unless (1) the patient, caregiver, primary care physician, or HABC physician requested

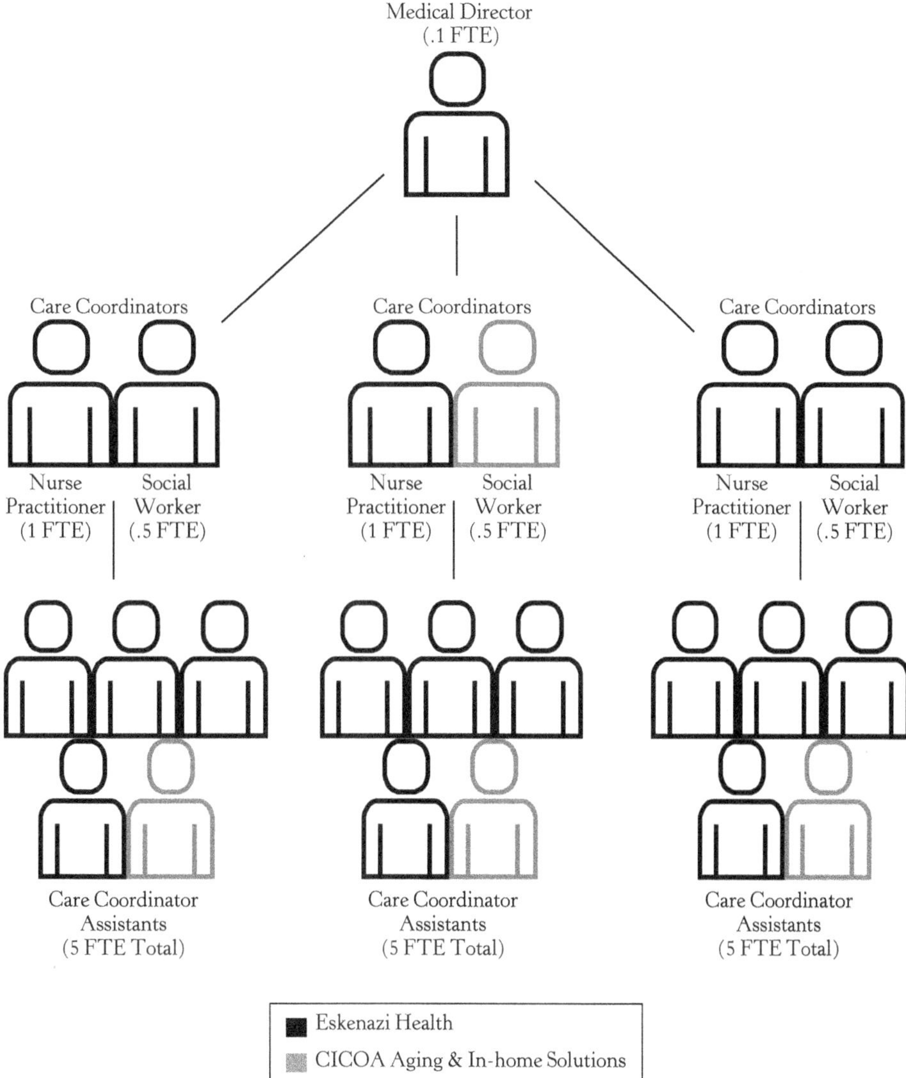

FIGURE 8.1. ABC Medical Home Staffing: Model 1.

no further contact by the program, (2) the patient died, or (3) the patient moved to long-term care or outside of the geographical area served by the program.[4,8] New referrals to the ABC Med Home were also accepted from primary care physicians, HABC physicians, other specialists, informal caregivers, and patients themselves.[4,8]

Care Delivery

The minimum specifications for the day-to-day operations of the ABC Med Home are set forth in the ABC's standard operating procedures (SOPs). The SOPs describe the program structure, the responsibilities associated with each role, and the phases of care delivery. Team members work together to meet the diverse needs of all patients and caregivers; however, individual team members have primary responsibility for certain types of visits. CCAs are primarily responsible for the initial home visit and for completing follow-up home visits at least once a month for the first three months following the initial home visit, and at least once every three months thereafter. RN care coordinators are primarily responsible for home visits to patients recently discharged from the hospital and to patients with urgent medical problems. Social worker care coordinators are primarily responsible for providing home visits to patients living in unsafe

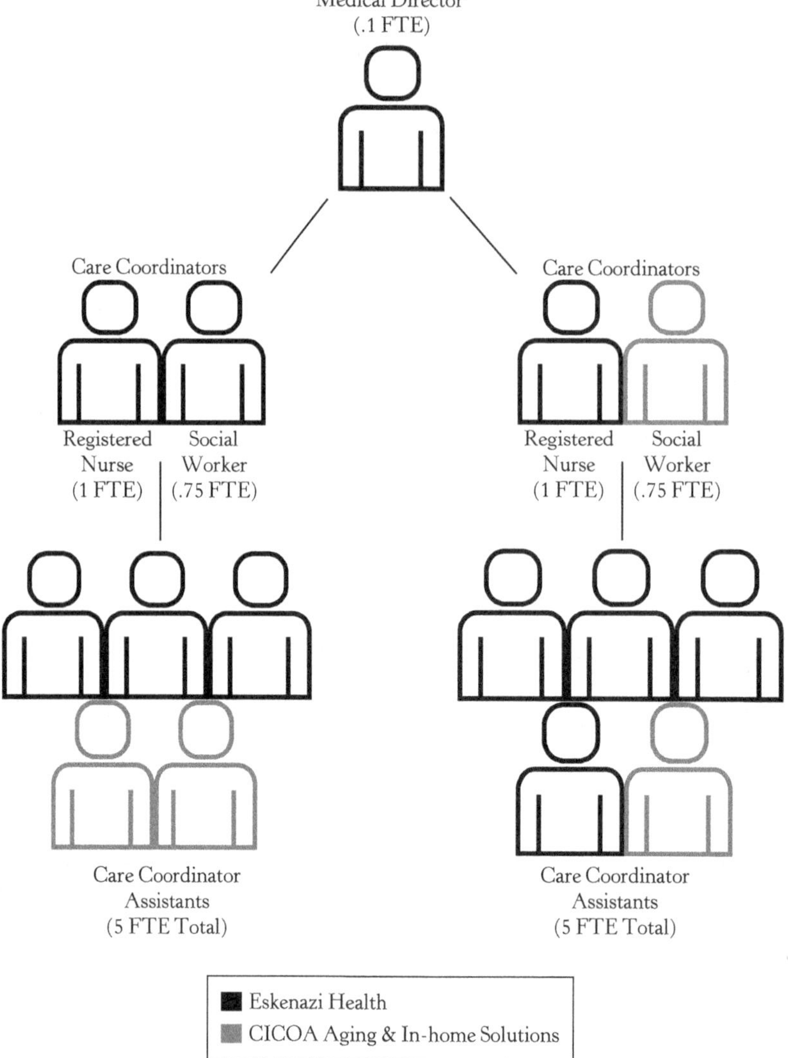

FIGURE 8.2. ABC Medical Home Staffing: Model 2.

conditions or experiencing other serious social situations.

Like the HABC, care is delivered in the ABC Med Home in phases, each one comprising multiple components.

Initial Assessment Phase

Immediately following enrollment, the CCA contacts the patient to explain the ABC program and schedule the first visit.[4,8] The initial visit is ideally conducted in the patient's home but, if requested by the patient or caregiver, may take place in another location.[4,8] During the initial visit, the CCA reviews the hospital's consent form with the patient and/or caregiver and obtains the responsible person's signature. Next, the CCA assesses the symptoms of dementia and depression using the Mini Mental Status Exam,[5] the PHQ-9,[14] and the self-report and caregiver versions of the Healthy Aging Brain Care Monitor (HABC Monitor).[4,8,15–17] The CCA also completes the Physical Self-Maintenance Scale[18] and performs a home safety evaluation. Finally, the CCA provides the patient and/or the caregiver with contact information for all members of the patient's team as well as a number to call for assistance during evening and weekend hours.

Following the initial visit, the CCA meets with the RN and social worker care coordinators to review the results of the initial assessments and determine the severity of the patient's illness and related needs of the patient and caregiver.[4,8] Together, they develop an individualized care plan that may include any of a variety of tools tested in the original clinical trials, including medications (prescribed by the primary care provider at the recommendation of the RN care coordinator), nonpharmacological caregiver interventions, self-management educational materials for both patients and caregivers, behavioral activation, relapse prevention, problem-solving therapy, and coordination with resources in the community.[4,8] The care plan is initiated by the CCA at the next scheduled visit.

Follow-Up Phase

The frequency of follow-up visits is based on the changing needs of the patient and caregiver over time.[4,8] At the request of the patient or caregiver, follow-up visits may occur at any of the mobile office sites or may take place by telephone; however, every patient must receive the minimum number of home visits specified in the SOPs. During all follow-up visits, the RN and social worker care coordinators and the CCAs assess and monitor the cognitive, functional, behavioral, and psychological symptoms of the patient as well as the caregiver's stress using repeat measure of the PHQ-9[14] and the HABC Monitor.[4,6] When symptoms either do not improve or worsen, modifications are made to the plan of care.[4,8] At any time during the follow-up phase the RN care coordinator may determine (after consultation with the medical director) that a patient requires a more extensive evaluation by an HABC physician, psychiatrist, or other medical or mental health specialist.[4,8]

Acute Care Transition Phase

The eMR-ABC receives an alert from the local health information exchange whenever an HABC or ABC Med Home patient is admitted to any hospital or emergency room participating in the Indiana Network for Patient Care.[4,8] Whenever possible, CCAs attempt to visit the patient in the hospital or emergency department to provide information about the patient's medical and social history to the hospital team and to support the patient and family. RN care coordinators are required to visit hospitalized patients within 72 hours of discharge to reconcile the patient's medications and to help coordinate the discharge care plan.[4,8]

Team Meetings

Each of the two clinical teams meets once a week for approximately one hour. Meetings are jointly conducted by the RN and the social worker care coordinators. Prior to the meeting, each CCA provides the care coordinators with a list of all patients who (1) have had a home or clinic visit during the prior week and/or (2) have specific issues and concerns that require input from the interdisciplinary team (e.g., assessment scores are moving in the wrong direction or the patient was hospitalized). The care coordinators review the lists to determine which patients will be discussed during the team meeting. During the meeting each CCA provides a brief overview of the patient, including findings from the last visit, current plan of care, and progress toward implementation of the plan. The team then engages in brainstorming and problem solving to revise the plan of care to meet the needs of the patient and caregiver.

eMR-ABC Population Health Management Software

The first prototype of the eMR-ABC was developed in accordance with Health Insurance Portability and Accountability Act (HIPAA) guidelines and was designed with a goal of creating an intuitive interface for users with little or no knowledge of the system's functionalities.[12] The original design was deployed in 2010 for use in the ABC pilot program and allowed the user to record and update patient demographic data and contact information as well as perform basic case management functions, including recording and monitoring program visits and assessment scores.[12] The system also offered decision support by recommending treatment protocols based on the results of the assessments.[12] These protocols were tested in the foundational PREVENT study and shown to be effective in reducing the behavioral and psychological symptoms of dementia.[2,19] From 2012 to 2015, with the support of CMS funding, the eMR-ABC was expanded to add new population-health management functions to the existing case management tools. New self-monitoring process and outcomes measures were developed to monitor the progress of the ABC Med Home toward achieving the goals of better health, better care, and lower cost through improved quality. The enhanced software calculates each measure (and graphs trends over time), thereby allowing the user to assess the performance of the entire population (or a particular team member's patient panel) and then quickly shift attention to the status of an individual patient. With this information, the team can identify patients with suboptimal outcomes and adjust the plan of care and/or reallocate program resources where needed. New functions were also developed to monitor adherence to the SOPs, identify problems with performance, and provide feedback to the staff electronically. For example, each CCA receives a quarterly alert providing information about his or her performance with respect to number of visits and number of required assessments completed. Administrators can access reports identifying patients who were not visited at home during the past three months (as required by the SOPs). In addition, a dashboard now presents a picture of the entire population at any point in time; pie charts are used to represent the makeup of the population based on a number of different variables, including diagnosis, gender, age, assessment scores, and use of acute care. Finally, a scheduling and optimization algorithm was developed to generate visit schedules for each of the CCAs; the algorithm identifies those patients who may require a visit based on the minimum visit specifications of the SOPs and/or the results of the most recent assessments.[4]

Success Stories and Lessons Learned

The CMS demonstration project offered many opportunities for program leadership to reflect on program successes, challenges, and, most importantly, lessons learned along the way. Similarly, the clinical staff members were asked each quarter to provide "stories from the field" highlighting the value of the intervention, the impact on patients and caregivers, and difficulties overcome in providing care to this population.

Through these reflective exercises, the team has identified four factors critical to the success of the project.

The first is that *the support and engagement of organizational and community stakeholders created the foundation of the project.*[4,8] This support is rooted in a collaboration between Eskenazi, IUCAR, and CICOA that spans multiple projects over several years. These three partners brought a "systems focus" to the project, providing our team with easy access to a much broader range of high-value resources than would otherwise have been possible.

The second factor is that *building trusting relationships with the patient and/or caregiver is fundamental to our intervention.*[4,8] Without trust, patient and caregivers will not seek or accept help; however, building trust takes time. Many staff members have noted that patients and caregivers typically share very little at the initial visit and report few, if any, symptoms. Over the next few weeks and months, however, they begin to open up about their struggles and, during this time, the assessment scores often worsen. Once the trusting relationship is established, the team can begin to engage the patient and caregiver as full partners in their care.

The third factor is that *this work would not be possible without our CCAs.* The time and effort required to select the right people and to provide ongoing support and training has been well worth it. We have had very little turnover in our staff, leading to better continuity of care for our patients. A qualitative analysis of 73 stories submitted by the clinical staff highlights the strengths of our CCAs.[20] CCAs made a mean number of 15.7 (SD = 15.6) visits, with most visits for coordination of care services, followed by home visits and phone visits to over 1,200 patients in 12 months. Six themes were identified, each one describing a skill demonstrated by our staff that leads to the delivery of person-centered care:

1. *Patient familiarity, understanding and communication*: CCAs and the team develop the ability to get to know the patient, customize care, and develop communication based on that patient's individual needs.
2. *Patient interest, autonomy, and engagement*: CCAs encourage patients to engage in activities that promote well-being and autonomy based on the patient's interests as identified by the patient or caregiver.
3. *Flexibility and continuity of care*: CCAs develop a meaningful relationship with patients over time and the ability to adapt to varied and often challenging environments while maintaining continuity of care for the patient and caregiver.
4. *Caregiver support and engagement*: CCAs provide education and support to the patient's primary caregiver and make recommendations important for the overall well-being of both the patient and caregiver.
5. *Effective utilization and integration of training*: CCAs demonstrate an ability to apply the training they received in their daily interactions with patients and caregivers.
6. *Teamwork*: Communication and teamwork result in more comprehensive and better care for all of our patients and caregivers.

Most frequently reported themes were patient familiarity, teamwork, and flexibility and continuity of care: 91.8% of case reports included a reference to patient familiarity, 67.1% included references to teamwork, and 61.6% included the theme of flexibility and continuity of care.[20] Person-centered care has been successfully implemented by our carefully chosen and well-trained CCAs.

The fourth and final factor critical to the success of the project is that *the eMR-ABC provides the real-time feedback required for effective population health management.*[4,8] With the support of CMS funding, we were able to link precisely defined outcomes to an electronic tracking system, allowing for continuous measuring and monitoring of results over time.[4,8]

Despite the many successes of the project, expansion of the ABC Med Home was not without challenges. The first was that *engaging patients can be difficult even with widespread organizational and community support.* Our team has continuously struggled with access to patients since the beginning of the program.[4,8] Staff members have developed innovative strategies to successfully contact patients and caregivers and enroll them in the program, but engagement remains a challenge.[4,8]

Second, *while we have expanded our program from 200 patients in one primary care center to 1,500 patients across all the primary care sites within Eskenazi, the reach of our clinical staff is still limited.* Serving areas where the population density is low presents challenges to providing home visits efficiently.

Third, the ABC Med Home has exceeded HABC by achieving a Level 4 integration within primary care. *However, there is still work to be done to achieve full integration within the primary care team,* including expanding the concept of "team" beyond the ABC clinical staff to include all primary care and specialty providers and staff as well as the agencies serving our patients and caregivers within the community.

Ultimately, the success of the ABC Med Home will be determined by its ability to achieve the triple aims of improving the patient experience, delivering population health, and lowering cost. Independent evaluators have been hired by CMS to identify the relevant measures and conduct the analysis. Our early performance data from the eMR-ABC suggest substantial progress toward improving population health outcomes.[4,8] Furthermore, in recent work we established the financial viability of the HABC based on savings achieved through a reduction in costs associated with the use of acute care.[4,21] The analysis shows promise for the ABC Med Home given that the minimum care delivery requirements are identical for the two programs. However, the current system of reimbursement does not provide incentives for a reduction in acute care costs;[4,21] in fact, current reimbursement processes favor medical procedures and volume-based activities.[4,21] Reform is needed to align reimbursement with the quality of care necessary to effectively serve patients with dementia and depression and keep them out of the hospital.[4,21]

REPLICATION

Although the ABC model was developed in a safety-net hospital system in Indianapolis, we believe the model can be replicated in other settings, although successful replication requires localizing the solution to the unique needs and characteristics of the host environment. The steps set forth in Box 8.3 provide the framework for successful replication, including tips for adapting the intervention for use in communities with limited resources.

In early 2015, the ABC model was licensed to Preferred Population Health Management (PPHM), an Indiana limited liability company engaged in the business of providing aging brain care products to health care providers. PPHM serves as the distribution agent for our program. For more information, contact Jim Vandergrifft, President/CEO, PPHM, at 317-245-7482 or jim@preferredphm.com.

PLANS FOR THE FUTURE

The future is promising for the ABC programs at Eskenazi in Indiana. Eskenazi has committed to continuing the program (after the CMS grant) and recently announced plans to fund a new Center for Brain Care Innovation (CBCI). The ABC Med Home and the HABC are two of the four flagship programs of the new center.

CBCI has adopted a rather daunting mission, that of providing the best brain care services available (both prevention and treatment) to the entire country. Toward that end, the ABC programs have been asked to develop a plan for expanding services to all patients with cognitive impairment across Indiana. New approaches to the existing challenges and limitations facing the program include the following:

1. New strategies for enrolling patients and keeping them engaged
2. New strategies for improving the integration of the current program in anticipation of developing an even broader definition of "team"

BOX 8.3

STEPS TO FOLLOW TO REPLICATE ABC MED HOME

1. *Engage organizational leaders in the development and implementation effort from the beginning.* Support from leadership is essential to help reduce resistance and eliminate barriers to implementation.
2. *Engage primary care leaders in program design.* The program should be integrated in the existing primary care system to help primary care providers in delivering better care without creating additional burden.
3. *Engage community stakeholders in a shared mission to promote and support your program.* "It takes a village" to care for our patients. Support from community agencies will expand the resources available to meet the needs of patients and caregivers. While many communities have limited resources, all communities have access to the services provided by the local Area Agency on Aging (can be found by ZIP code at n4a.org). In addition, all communities have access to the services provided by the local chapter of the Alzheimer's Association, which includes a 24/7 helpline for caregivers of persons with dementia (available in more than 200 languages; visit alz.org). Similarly, the Association for Frontotemporal Degeneration (FTD) (aftd.org) provide online resources and information for people with FTD and their caregivers. Informal support for patients and caregivers is often available from local religious institutions and other community organizations (e.g., voluntary health organizations like the American Diabetes Association, the Heart and Stroke Association, National Alliance on Mental Illness, American Cancer Society, and many others have online resources and local services such as transportation and support groups).
4. *In collaboration with all stakeholders, clearly define what success will look like.* Link precise and measurable processes and outcomes to an electronic tracking system that allows continuous monitoring of progress toward the goals. If a sophisticated electronic system is not available, use a simple electronic or paper database. The format is not important as long as you are measuring and monitoring progress.
5. *Get the right people on the team.* When hiring new staff, invest time and resources up front to select clinical staff most likely to achieve long-term success. First, screen candidates for the skills and qualities that cannot be taught (e.g., compassion, empathy, building rapport); then consider a nontraditional interview process designed to let candidates show you rather than tell you what they can do. If hiring new staff is not feasible, consider reassigning existing employees and training them to manage patients with dementia in a single primary care site. If home visits are not practical or cost effective, consider delivering a combination of a clinic-based and telephone-based intervention.
6. *Provide the training and tools necessary for success.* Take care of your staff and they will take care of your patients. Include teamwork as well as dementia care skills in the curriculum. Provide opportunities to practice new skills in a safe and structured environment before staff begin working with patients and caregivers. Ongoing training, development, and support are necessary to prevent staff burnout.
7. *Engage patients and caregivers as true partners in their own care to ensure everyone is working toward the same mutually agreed-upon goals.*
8. *Define minimum standard specifications for operations, but avoid overprescribing and micromanaging.* Enforce compliance with the standard operating procedures, but remember that following procedures does not ensure positive outcomes. Continuously monitor both process and outcome measures. If assessments are moving in the wrong direction despite adherence to the SOPs, allow your clinicians the freedom to find creative solutions for difficult problems by developing new options for providing needed care.
9. *Don't expect to get it right the first time.* Learn from failures and challenges and adapt your program to incorporate lessons learned. Continuous monitoring will help you identify problems quickly.

3. New strategies for expanding the reach of the current clinical team, including telehealth and video conferencing visits from staff and the development of new technologies that will allow parts of the intervention to be delivered in the space between the patient or caregiver and a mobile device without the need for human intervention

Any future program development or quality improvement must include feedback from our patients and caregivers. To obtain that feedback, CBCI has established a "patient experience working group" to identify outcomes of interest, unmet needs, and other concerns of patients and caregivers. This information will be used to inform decisions regarding changes to the intervention and/or the need for additional staff training.

The CBCI presents us with both a challenge and an opportunity not only to sustain the ABC programs, but also to innovate and re-invent the programs as we continue efforts to meet the needs of the rapidly aging population. Box 8.4 summarizes recommended approaches and relevant evidence for the ABC programs.

ACKNOWLEDGMENTS

Funding/Support: The project described was supported by Grant Number 1C1CMS331000-01-00 from the Department of Health and Human Services, Centers for Medicare & Medicaid Services. The contents of this publication are solely the responsibility of the authors and do not necessarily represent the official views of the U.S. Department of Health and Human Services or any of its agencies. M.G. Austrom is also supported in part by the Indiana Alzheimer's Disease Center funded by NIA P30AG10133.

Additional Contributions: The authors thank Tiffany Campbell, Program Manager for the Indiana University Center for Aging Research, for creating the diagrams representing the evolution of the ABC Med Home staffing model.

BOX 8.4

SUMMARY OF RECOMMENDED TREATMENT APPROACHES AND RELEVANT EVIDENCE

Strength of recommendation taxonomy (SOR A, B, or C)

- **The IMPACT depression care model is a collaborative care model for depression providing personalized, patient-centered care including both antidepressant medications and problem-solving therapy in collaboration with primary care.[1] (SOR A)**
- **The PREVENT dementia care model is a model of care for dementia, based on the success of the IMPACT model and incorporating the same personalized, patient-centered, and collaborative care approach with primary care.[2] (SOR A)**
- **The HABC is a specialty clinic for memory care within Eskenazi Health that represents the successful adaptation and implementation of the PREVENT research model into a real-world clinical care environment.[3,4] (SOR A)**
- **The ABC Med Home, the community outreach arm of the HABC, is a mobile population health management program serving patients primarily in the community. The ABC Med Home successfully expanded the reach and impact of HABC.[4,8,9] (SOR A)**
- **Task shifting to improve workforce efficiency: Tasks requiring less training and experience are delegated to members of the team with less training and professional experience who operate under the close supervision of licensed staff, thereby allowing each clinical provider to work at the top of his or her license.[13,15] (SOR B)**
- **Use of the Multiple Mini Interview (MMI) format to screen and recruit CCAs: These structured mini-interviews are designed to screen for one or more abilities. The MMI has been demonstrated to assess noncognitive traits (with reliability and validity) and to predict performance in school admissions processes.[13,22–26] (SOR A)**

REFERENCES

1. Unützer J, Katon W, Callahan CM, et al. Collaborative care management of late-life depression in the primary care setting. JAMA. 2002;288(22):2836–2845.
2. Callahan CM, Boustani MA, Unverzagt FW, et al. Effectiveness of collaborative care for older adults with Alzheimer disease in primary care: A randomized controlled trial. JAMA. 2006;295(18):2148–2157.
3. Boustani MA, Sachs GA, Alder CA, et al. Implementing innovative models of dementia care: The Healthy Aging Brain Center. Aging & Mental Health. 2011;15(1):13–22.
4. Alder CA, LaMantia MA, Austrom MG, Boustani MA. The Indiana Aging Brain Care Project. In Malone ML, Capezuti EA, Palmer RM, eds., Geriatrics Models of Care. Switzerland: Springer; 2015:231–237.
5. Folstein MF, Folstein SE, McHugh PR. "Mini-Mental State": A practical method for grading the cognitive state of patients for the clinician. J Psychiatr Res. 1975;12(3):189–198.
6. Health Aging Brain Center Monitor. http://www.agingbraincare.org/tools/habc-monitor. Published 2016. Accessed March 15, 2016.
7. Doherty W, McDaniel S, Baird M. Five Levels of Primary Care. Behavioral Healthcare Collaboration; 1996.
8. LaMantia MA, Alder CA, Callahan CM, et al. The Aging Brain Care Medical Home: Preliminary data. J Am Geriatrics Soc. 2015;63(6):1209–1213.
9. Callahan CM, Boustani MA, Weiner M, et al. Implementing dementia care models in primary care settings: The Aging Brain Care Medical Home. Aging & Mental Health. 2011;15(1):5–12.
10. Boustani M, Sachs G, Callahan C. Can primary care meet the biopsychosocial needs of older adults with dementia? J Gen Intern Med. 2007;22(11):1625–1627.
11. Cordell CB, Borson S, Boustani M, et al. Alzheimer's Association recommendations for operationalizing the detection of cognitive impairment during the Medicare Annual Wellness Visit in a primary care setting. Alzheimer's & Dementia. 2013;9(2):141–150.
12. Frame A, LaMantia M, Reddy Bynagari BB, Dexter P, Boustani M. Development and implementation of an electronic decision support to manage the health of a high-risk population: The enhanced Electronic Medical Record Aging Brain Care Software (eMR-ABC). eGEMs (Generating Evidence & Methods to Improve Patient Outcomes). 2013;1(1):8.
13. Cottingham AH, Alder C, Austrom MG, Johnson CS, Boustani MA, Litzelman DK. New workforce development in dementia care: Screening for "Caring": Preliminary data. J Am Geriatrics Soc. 2014;62(7):1364–1368.
14. Spitzer RL, Kroenke K, Williams JB. Validation and utility of a self-report version of PRIME-MD: The PHQ primary care study. JAMA. 1999;282(18):1737–1744.
15. World Health Organization. Task Shifting to Tackle Health Worker Shortages. Geneva: World Health Organization; 2007.
16. Monahan PO, Alder CA, Khan BA, Stump T, Boustani MA. The Healthy Aging Brain Care (HABC) Monitor: Validation of the Patient Self-Report Version of the clinical tool designed to measure and monitor cognitive, functional, and psychological health. Clinical Interventions in Aging. 2014;9:2123–2132.
17. Monahan PO, Boustani MA, Alder C, et al. Practical clinical tool to monitor dementia symptoms: The HABC Monitor. Clinical Interventions in Aging. 2012;7:143–157.
18. Lawton M, Brody E. Physical Self-Maintenance Scale (PSMS): Original observer-related version. Psychopharmacol Bull. 1988;24:793–794.
19. Guerriero Austrom M, Damush TM, Hartwell CW, et al. Development and implementation of non-pharmacologic protocols for the management of patients with Alzheimer's disease and their families in a multiracial primary care setting. Gerontologist. 2004;44(4):548–553.
20. Austrom MG, Carvell CA, Alder CA, Gao S, Boustani M, LaMantia M. Workforce development to provide person-centered care. Aging Ment Health. 2016;20(8):781–792.
21. French DD, LaMantia MA, Livin LR, Herceg D, Alder CA, Boustani MA. Healthy Aging Brain Center improved care coordination and produced net savings. Health Affairs (Project Hope). 2014;33(4):613–618.
22. Lemay J-F, Lockyer JM, Collin VT, Brownell AKW. Assessment of non-cognitive traits through the admissions Multiple Mini-Interview. Medical Education. 2007;41(6):573–579.
23. Cameron AJ, MacKeigan LD. Development and pilot testing of a Multiple Mini-Interview for admission to a pharmacy degree program. Am J Pharmaceutical Educ. 2012;76(1):10.
24. McAndrew R, Ellis J. An evaluation of the Multiple Mini-Interview as a selection tool for dental students. Br Dent J. 2012;212(7):331–335.
25. Hecker K, Violato C. A generalizability analysis of a veterinary school Multiple Mini Interview: Effect of number of interviewers, type of interviewers, and number of stations. Teaching and Learning in Medicine. 2011;23(4):331–336.
26. Eva KW, Reiter HI, Rosenfeld J, Norman GR. The ability of the Multiple Mini-Interview to predict preclerkship performance in medical school. Acad Med. 2004;79(10):S40–S42.

9

Telehealth in an Integrated Care Environment

MARYANN WAUGH, DEBBIE VOYLES, JAMES H. SHORE, L. CHAROLETTE LIPPOLIS, AND COREY LYON

BOX 9.1

KEY POINTS

- **Telehealth, the use of technology to provide care at a distance, is a flexible process adapted to a variety of integrated care applications and models.**
- **Telehealth, which has been in use in various forms since the 1920s, can help maximize limited resources and expand the reach of providers.**
- **There is an extensive and growing body of evidence supporting the use of telehealth for improving care access and outcomes across the integrated care continuum.**
  - **Systems in early levels of coordination may use virtual methods for provider education and training as a "force multiplier" (e.g., teaching primary care physicians basic tools for behavioral health management in primary care settings).**
  - **Systems beginning to coordinate care across systems and sites may use virtual methods for screening and assessment. A variety of structured clinical interview tools and other scales for screening and assessing behavioral health and side effects have been validated for videoconference use.**
  - **There is good evidence for using telehealth to provide co-located care through virtual consultation. University specialists have been able to improve care quality for patients through both distal and in-person consultation with primary care physicians in rural and other under-served areas using flexible models of telebehavioral health delivery. Behavioral health providers have completed direct screening/assessments with patients and submitted written reports/recommendations to provider through both in-person and virtual service delivery.**
- **Collaborative care, the most intensive application of integrated primary care consultation, also has a strong evidence base. Telehealth-supported team-based care, with patient-centered goals and shared care plans, has even surpassed traditional in-person applications in ratings of patient satisfaction. Store-and-forward methods are allowing specialists, like psychiatrists, increasingly flexible ways to maximize their professional impact through time-asynchronous opportunities for team-based participation.**
- **Within the current health care environment, telehealth is likely to forward care integration in new and innovative ways that improve care access, patient care experiences, economic return, and value on investment.**

CURRENT STATE OF HEALTH CARE ENVIRONMENT

The health care industry is rapidly evolving in response to increasing costs, poor health outcomes, and consumer dissatisfaction. Americans spent over $3 trillion on health care in 2014. According to a report from actuaries at the Centers for Medicare & Medicaid Services, projections show health care expenditures will increase an average of 5.8% each year until 2022.[1] Unfortunately, health care spending is expected to grow one full percentage point faster than the expected average annual growth in the Gross Domestic Product. Despite spending far more on health care than any nation on earth, America is ranked last or near last among wealthy countries on measures of health access, efficiency, and equity.[1]

Patients with both physical and mental health issues often have high health care costs and utilization with extremely poor outcomes. Untreated and undertreated behavioral health issues place a particularly large burden on the current health care system, by negatively impacting both physical and behavioral health care outcomes.[2] Access to appropriate and timely behavioral health treatment is challenging and causes disproportionate illness burden for those with behavioral health problems. Minority and rural populations suffer an even greater impact from health care disparities.[3] Most patients with a behavioral health issue present in a primary care setting. The fraction of patients receiving behavioral health treatment, will receive it in a primary care setting rather than at a behavioral health specialty service.[4,5] Primary care providers are overburdened, and often lack specific expertise or the needed resources to properly address behavioral health issues.[2,6] Compounding these challenges are health care professional shortages. According to the Health Resources and Services Administration in September 2015, there were 6,218 Primary Medical Health Professional Shortage Areas, which is up from the reported 5,767 in October 2012.[7] For mental health, there are a reported 4,216 mental health shortage areas, up from 3,712 in October 2012.[7]

Increasing professional shortages, and costs, as well as poor outcomes, and consumer satisfaction ratings, indicate there is a great need to change the way health care services are delivered and received. Integrated care represents a conceptual shift from a disease-specific, biomedical approach to a wellness, whole-person approach. Based on the biopsychosocial-cultural model, integrated care has shown great promise to reduce health care costs, while improving health care outcomes. See Chapter 6: Financing Integrated Health Care Models. The Patient Protection and Affordable Care Act of 2010, commonly called the Affordable Care Act, includes provisions providing support and incentives to adopt the practice of integration of primary care and behavioral health care.[8]

Telehealth, the use of technology to provide care at a distance, is proving to be a key component in the expansion of integrated care. See Box 9.1 for a summary of key points related to Telehealth.

Telehealth, considered a process, as well as a technology, is a way to bridge gaps not only in physical distance, but also in communication between providers. Telehealth can help maximize limited resources and expand the reach of providers. There is increasing evidence that telehealth is an effective way to increase access to care and improve care integration, in particular for those with long-term chronic conditions and often comorbid behavioral health needs.[8] It is likely that in this evolving health care environment, telehealth will not only facilitate. but also help drive new and innovative models of care delivery.

This chapter describes the current state of telehealth technology, practice, use, and telehealth related care integration opportunities. It also provides a summary of current research for the use of telehealth across the integration continuum.

TELEHEALTH DESCRIPTION

The Health Resources and Services Administration defines telehealth as "the use of electronic information and telecommunications technologies to support long distance clinical health care, patient and professional health related education, and public health and health administration."[9] The American Telemedicine Association states, "Videoconferencing, transmission of still images, e-health including patient portals, remote monitoring of vital signs, continuing medical education, and nursing call centers are all considered part of telemedicine and telehealth."[10] There are a variety of web-based resources for practitioners looking for practical guidelines and best practices for telehealth implementation, as shown in Table 9.1.

Within this set of telehealth technologies, one particularly popular application is live, interactive videoconferencing. This application allows a specialist and a patient, two specialists, or another combination of users to have face-to-face, real time

TABLE 9.1. WEB-BASED TELEHEALTH RESOURCES

American Telemedicine Association (ATA) website, including practice guidelines	http://www.americantelemed.org/resources/telemedicine-practice-guidelines/telemedicine-practice-guidelines#.Vhgxg_lViko
Health IT.gov Startup Resources Guide	https://www.healthit.gov/sites/default/files/telehealthguide_final_0.pdf
California Telehealth and eResource, including best practices	http://www.telehealthresourcecenter.org/sites/main/files/file-attachments/best_practices.pdf
Agency for Healthcare Research and Quality (AHRQ) Health Information Technology: Telehealth	https://healthit.ahrq.gov/ahrq-funded-projects/emerging-lessons/telehealth

communication, without having to be in the same location. Providers and patients communicate using secure digital videoconferencing, through which participants' image and audio data are captured by a video camera, then digitized, and transmitted over secure, broadband speed telecommunication lines, for live viewing on the other end.

The concept of telehealth has been around since the early 1900s. In the April 1924 issue of *Radio News Magazine*, an article titled, "The Radio Doctor—Maybe!" offered the first consideration of providing health care services through technology. In 1964, through a grant from the U.S. National Institute for Mental Health, the Nebraska Psychiatric Institute, used a two-way closed-circuit TV link to connect to the Norfolk State Hospital, which was 112 miles way. Through the 1960s and 1970s, well-established organizations, such as Massachusetts General Hospital, the U.S. National Library of Medicine's Lister Hill National Center for Biomedical Communications, the National Aeronautics and Space Administration, and the Health Care Technology Division of the U.S. Department of Health, Education, and Welfare implemented a variety of research and demonstration projects using telehealth technology.[11]

Currently, the U.S. Department of Veterans Affairs (VA), is the world leader in the telehealth space. The VA's telehealth program was designed to make health care more patient-centered, by making it more convenient and accessible to veterans with a variety of physical and behavioral health needs. The VA has implemented telehealth services in 151 VA medical centers. and over 700-community based outpatient clinics. In 2013, the VA conducted more than 1.7 million telehealth consultations to 600,000 patients in 53 sites in 16 Veteran Integrated Services Networks, and in 24 states through its telehealth program.[12] See Chapter 7: Integrating Physical and Mental Health Care in the Veterans Health Administration for additional information.

Most early telemedicine programs focused on providing rural and underserved areas with access to specialty care. Since then, growing indices of success have encouraged expansion into a variety of rural and urban settings. With expanding health insurance coverage and more vendors in the telehealth market, there has been a large increase in telehealth activity over the past several years. As of May 2015, 16 states have telemedicine parity laws that require private payers to reimburse allowable, billable services virtually delivered.[13] A survey of 38 telemedicine providers, conducted by the American Telemedicine Association and a private telemedicine provider (AMD), found that over 100 private payers were reimbursing for telehealth services across the United States, both in states with and without parity laws. Blue Cross Blue Shield, for example, is reimbursing for telehealth in 21 states.[14] Medicare currently has a specific list of telehealth reimbursable services for virtual care in specific areas of the country (i.e., rural or professional shortage areas), with anticipated expansion in coming years.[15] Medicaid, through the Centers for Medicare & Medicaid Services, recognizes telehealth as a cost-effective care delivery option and encourages states to use flexible federal laws to create their own innovative telehealth payment methods.[16]

As of 2015, 48 states offered some level of telehealth reimbursement, including some form of telebehavioral health. Connecticut and Rhode Island are the only remaining states lacking a structure for telehealth reimbursement. The most common telebehavioral health services covered by Medicaid include: assessments, individual therapy, psychiatric diagnostic interview exams, and medication management.[13]

Across payers, the number of U.S. patients participating in telehealth services in 2013 was less than 350,000. A new report estimates that the number of telehealth consultations will rise to nearly 27 million in the U.S. market by 2020.[17] Reports project that by 2020, there will have been growth of nearly 25% per year to reach an anticipated 5.4 million telehealth consultations between primary care providers and their patients.[17] Hospitals, provider groups, and even health plans are looking at telehealth to provide better access to care with limited resources and to provide better care coordination.

Telehealth is a means for patients to get high quality care from a variety of professionals and specialists in one setting, particularly in primary care settings. The opportunity for improved primary care holds promise for reducing emergency room visits, where the cost of health care is highest. Major commercial health insurance plans are rapidly expanding telehealth coverage. As noted, in states with parity laws, any medical and/or behavioral health service that can be virtually conducted must be covered by private payers.[13] Some payers are even giving self-funded plan members access to various virtual provider networks that allow patients direct, real time access to primary care providers, using telehealth technology.[17]

The use of telehealth is associated with reduced health care disparities by increasing access to primary and specialty services.[18] Telehealth is transforming the way that health care is being provided, by increasing a patient's access to routine and specialty care, and increasing providers' access to colleagues in other specialty areas.[19] Telehealth can help with medical workforce shortages, by allowing small or underserved communities to recruit and use nurses linked to higher level providers, which can improve local health care services. This paradigm allows patients to receive care in their communities, and reduces geographical isolation issues for patients and providers. Research is showing that telehealth can improve patient outcomes through earlier interventions, reduced complications, and consistent use of evidence-based medicine.[18,20] According to the Trend Watch article, "Realizing the Promise of Telehealth," telehealth will continue to penetrate the health care arena, and become a natural extension of existing team care models.[8]

TELEHEALTH CAN SUPPORT CARE INTEGRATION

Integrated care, sometimes referred to as *interdisciplinary care*, requires providers from distinct arenas of health care to work collaboratively with one another, patients, and families. An integrated approach to patient care relies upon shared medical, psychological, and social information, and a single care plan developed and implemented by a team of professionals. This medical team can include the primary care provider, specialty medical providers, behavioral health providers, care coordinators/social workers, occupational and physical therapists, and others, depending on the needs of patients and/or their families.[21] Research shows that integrating behavioral health services into the primary care setting can improve access to services, improve quality of care, and in turn, lower overall health care costs.[22] Full integration of behavioral health within primary care requires consideration of the salary and office space needed to add behavioral health professionals, bridging the cultural differences in care practices, billing challenges, and effective resource management, particularly for smaller primary care practices. Telehealth leverages technology to mitigate some of these existing challenges, and supports implementation of a variety of integrated care models across diverse care settings.

There is a continuum of behavioral health care integration with medical services. Telehealth-based care can be used across this continuum. While current fee-for-service models still hamper large-scale implementation and sustainability, VA projects, grant-funded models, and alternative-funded initiatives provide good examples of both effective clinical and payment models.[2,3,6,22] Behavioral health integration into primary care settings is the most prevalent application of the integration model.[23]

Integration Continuum

The Substance Abuse and Mental Health Services Administration (SAMHSA) Center for Integrated Health Solutions, has identified six levels of health care integration, from minimal collaboration to full integration, as detailed in Table 9.2.

SAMHSA based these levels of health care integration on the work of Doherty, McDaniel, and Baird, who proposed the first classification system to encompass both the extent of existing collaboration, and the capacity for collaboration between behavioral and primary care in a given setting.[22] The premise was that as the levels of collaboration

TABLE 9.2. LEVELS OF INTEGRATION AND TELEHEALTH APPLICATION

	Coordinated		Co-located		Integrated	
Levels of Care/ Integration	Minimal Collaboration	Basic Collaboration From a Distance	Basic Collaboration Onsite	Close Collaboration Partly Integrated	Close Collaboration Approaching Integration	Fully Integrated
Systems	Separate systems	Separate systems	Separate systems	Some shared systems	Actively increasing shared systems	Shared systems
Facilities	Separate facilities	Separate facilities	Shared facilities	Shared facilities	Shared facilities	Shared facilities
Communication	Communication is rare.	Periodic focused communication; mostly written	Regular communication, occasionally face-to-face	Face-to-face consultation; coordinated treatment plans	Regular face-to-face consultative and team meetings	Collaborative routines are regular and smooth.
Culture	Little appreciation of each other's culture	View each other as outside resources	Some appreciation of each other's role and general sense of the larger picture	Basic appreciation of each other's role and cultures	In-depth appreciation of roles and culture	Have roles and cultures that blur or blend
Attitude	"Nobody knows my name. Who are you?"	"I help *your* consumers."	"I am *your* consultant."	"*We* are a team in the care of consumers."	"*We* are a team with individual consumers."	"*We* are part of a care system."
Telehealth	Used primarily to distally provide care as usual or refer	Referral with some follow-up; mostly written	Referral and regular follow up, some face-to-face	Education, consultation, and support	Team-based care	Team-based care, shared electronic health record and integrated procedures

Adapted from SAMHSA's Center for Integrated Health Solutions, "A Standard Framework for Levels of Integrated Healthcare."[18]

increased, so too would the adequate handling of complex patients. The levels do not dictate a particular model that would be best for all health care settings, but rather function as a foundation from which to test the strengths and limitations of a variety of solutions.[22]

Telehealth solutions can support practices and systems across a continuum, from completely separate to fully integrated, adding flexibility to the integration construct. Models of integration range from remote infrequent education and consultation, to disease specific care and full integration. The Center for Integrated Health Solutions uses the terms "coordinated," "co-located," and "integrated" to simplify this continuum of collaboration and integration of behavioral health treatment into primary care settings.

Integrated care delivery models across this integration continuum are associated with improved outcomes,[24] but leave unaddressed a myriad of care access, stigma, financial, and other issues. To address the current health care crisis, health care service delivery must be improved. Clinical practices, housed in traditional brick-and-mortar buildings with traditional daytime office hours, do not allow people access to the health care they need, when needed. In rural and underserved communities, access to specialty health care is very limited, and in some cases access to even basic health care is a challenge.[25] Telehealth supports expanded flexibility in integrated care delivery across the integration continuum. Telebehavioral health has been used with promising results for screening and assessment, medication management, case management, psycho-education, direct patient care, psychotherapy, professional supervision and training, and administrative and managerial tasks related to all of these applications.[26]

Separate Health Care Systems

For systems in which physical and behavioral health care are still completely distinct, telehealth can be used to enhance behavioral health awareness/resources, education, and training through "force multiplication," defined by the Robert Wood Johnson Foundation as, "an approach that multiplies impact."[27] These approaches often use a combination of education and consultation to spread the knowledge of an insufficient number of specialists (e.g., psychiatrists) to much larger populations of general practitioners. Expanding access of services can be accomplished by a train-the-trainers model. One psychiatrist can hold only a limited number of patient appointments in one day but can help an infinite number of patients access psychiatric support by training their primary care doctors to better manage and prescribe psychotropic medications.

The Project for the Extension for Community Healthcare Outcomes (Project ECHO) is an example of expansion of services.[28] ECHO initially began in New Mexico, as an initiative to reduce health disparities and curb a viral hepatitis epidemic. ECHO has since been extended to include behavioral health and pain management initiatives. Using televideo technology, the ECHO model links providers in rural and underserved areas, with education, mentoring, and support from university experts. The model supports adherence to best practices to reduce variation in care, using case-based learning and outcomes monitoring. A *New England Journal of Medicine* study found that care delivered by primary care physicians trained via ECHO was of equal quality to care delivered by specialists.[29]

The ECHO pain project adapted the model to accommodate a long waiting list for care at a university pain center, and to provide statewide continuing-education credit opportunities for primary care clinicians. ECHO pain specialists facilitate live weekly half-hour clinics, where they present didactic and case study material. Using international guidelines and curriculum, the material is used to stimulate diagnosis and discussion while addressing the multidimensional nature of pain experience and treatment. Participants demonstrated statistically significant improvements in knowledge, skills, and practice, and reported positive experiences with a more team-based approach to treatment, particularly providers working in rural and other isolated locations.[28]

Coordinated Care: Screening and Assessment

As defined by the Agency for Healthcare Research and Quality, care coordination in primary care settings involves deliberately organizing care activities, and sharing information to achieve safer and more effective care. Care coordination is associated with a set of specific coordination activities, including screening and assessing for patient needs and goals.[30] Screening and assessing for behavioral health disorders via videoconferencing has documented efficacy for a variety of subpopulations, including youth, adult, geriatric, and Spanish-speaking populations.

Tools validated for videoconferencing application, include the Structured Clinical Interview for the Diagnostic and Statistical Manual (DSM-5),[31] the Brief Psychiatric Rating Scale,[32] Scales for the Assessment of Negative and Positive Symptoms,[33,34] the Hamilton Depression Rating Scale,[35] and the Abnormal Involuntary Movement Scale.[36] A variety of additional tools have documented efficacy for distal, videoconference-based screening and assessment for a broad range of cognitive and neuropsychiatric indicators, as well as specific symptoms and disorders.[24] These kind of assessments have also been demonstrated to be equally effective as in-person administration (given appropriate in-person safety procedures and personnel) for evaluating the need for emergency psychiatric hospitalization (e.g., when a patient in a primary care or emergency setting is suicidal, homicidal, gravely disabled, or presenting with symptoms of dementia or acute psychosis).[37]

Coordinated Care: Basic Collaboration from a Distance

For practices at early levels of integration, there is research to support the use of telebehavioral health to enhance distal physicians' ability to provide higher-quality primary care. In a study of youth telepsychiatry feasibility and patient acceptability,[20] psychiatrists at the University of Washington provided evidence-based diagnostic services, medication management, and recommendations via videoconferencing to youth and family members in four rural communities. Youth were referred by their primary care physicians or pediatricians for symptoms of, in order of prevalence, attention-deficit/hyperactivity disorder, disruptive behavior disorder, mood disorder, and developmental disorders, including autism spectrum. Following virtual patient sessions, psychiatrists sent practitioners immediate notes on session outcomes, and followed up with formal reports.[20] In this study, physicians, while invited, did not participate with the child/family and psychiatrist activities. Behavioral and primary care systems remained completely separate, and communication between providers took the form of periodic written reports.

Even at this limited level of integration, indices of improved care quality were strong. Physician/pediatrician endorsements of their improved ability to effectively manage patient care were high, as were doctor and patient endorsements of satisfaction with the care provided and the virtual mode of care delivery.[20] This study gave good evidence for the feasibility of using telebehavioral health to bring evidence-based psychiatry support to medical practices, operating at a very limited level of coordination and collaboration. The same telebehavioral model could also serve to move practices along the integration continuum, if the written reports were replaced with regular face-to-face communication between behavioral health and physical health providers.

Co-located Care: Consultation in Primary Care Settings

Telehealth has been effectively used to provide co-located mental health consultation in primary care settings. At this level of integration, behavioral health and primary care providers still maintain separate systems. In traditional models, the primary care provider looks to a virtually co-located psychiatrist to provide case-specific advice to help the provider manage the diagnostic/medication/referral needs of the patient. Research shows that most often, telepsychiatry consultations result in diagnostic changes (for as many as 91% of patients in one sample) and medication changes. These changes are typically associated with improved outcomes.[38]

The University of California at Davis, has conducted two studies,[39] which are specific examples of practices, using telebehavioral health to support primary care providers with consultative levels of integration. The behavioral and physical care systems remained separate, but the providers from each system had face-to-face consultation. The UC Davis Center for Health and Technology conducted a grant-funded study to provide telepsychiatry and telepsychology to 10 rural primary care sites. Project goals were to increase use of mental health consultation services, improve on-site ability to triage mental health cases, and shift the consultation method to a more efficient model of predominant phone and email use, with videoconferencing, as needed. Preliminary project results were positive, indicating that primary care physicians perceived the consultative service as a benefit to their ability to manage and triage caseloads. Physicians seemed to resist transition to email and phone consultation, indicating a preference for the face-to-face video consultation.[39]

A second UC Davis initiative[39] included culturally informed consultation as part of a rural, primary care, telemedicine collaboration. Again, the primary care and behavioral care systems maintained separate care processes, payment methods, records, and administration. Using videoconferencing, psychiatrists with more diverse cultural backgrounds and experience were able to support primary care physicians with accurate diagnoses and increased medication adherence for a culturally diverse patient population. In some cases, patient cultural interpretation of mental health stigma, and appropriate patient-to-provider communication had previously interfered with treatment adherence, and could be adjusted following culturally appropriate psychiatric consultation.[39]

Co-located Care: Collaborative Care in Primary Care Settings

In 2013, Hilty, et al described collaborative care as the most intensive application of primary care telebehavioral health consultation.[24] As previously noted, this level of integration requires disruptive transformation, discontinuing the use of separate systems, and developing new systems and processes shared by behavioral and physical health providers. The University of Washington's Advancing Integrated Mental Health Solutions (AIMS) Center[40] has identified five key components of collaborative care: (1) a patient-centered care team, (2) population-based care, (3) targeted measurement-based treatment, (4) evidence-based care, and (5) accountable care.[40] These components empower patients and family members to become active participants in their care, support care plan adjustments based on individual progress, systematically track all patients, use resources for population-specific needs, and ensure effective care through team-based accountability.

Practice-based collaborative care (PBCC), is an evidence-based practice based on this model of care. PBCC includes co-located primary and mental health care providers, and care managers providing team-based care in the primary care setting.[41] While well documented in terms of efficacy, PBCC, and collaborative care in general, includes a daunting list of critical components. It is difficult to implement this model of care with fidelity, particularly for smaller, rural, and/or less resourced practices. Telehealth solutions were initially conceptualized as a solution to bring equivalent, if not second tier, services to these smaller and less resourced practices. Emerging research, however, is revealing that these tech-based solutions, once considered second tier, are actually associated with better outcomes and higher ratings of patient satisfaction at all levels of care.[41]

A pragmatic randomized trial compared in-person (called "practice-based," as all team members are physically based in the practice) to telehealth-based collaborative care for depression for rural, uninsured, treatment-resistant primary care patients across five federally qualified health centers.[42] Patients were randomized to on-site care (using the Depression Health Disparities Collaborative), including a primary care physician, and an on-site registered nurse or licensed practical nurse depression care manager, or to telehealth-based care, including a primary care physician and a remote university team, which included a registered nurse depression care manager, pharmacist, psychologist, and psychiatrist.

In both conditions, the depression care manager was an individual without prior mental health training, who completed one day of program-specific training. The practice-based individual had access to online decision support (a web-based system that guides care managers through self-documenting patient encounters, using evidence-based scripts and self-scoring instruments).[42] In contrast, the telehealth-based individual had access to a university mental health team. The remote university team members were employed full time across this and other projects. Compared to patients randomized to practice-based care, those randomized to telehealth-based care had greater treatment response rates, larger reductions in depression severity, and increases in overall mental health status and quality of life, despite no significant difference between number of direct care visits and antidepressant prescription or adherence. These outcomes were statistically associated with greater fidelity to the depression care manager model in the telehealth group, despite equivalent prior experience and training.

The authors theorize that the telehealth-based collaborative care had better outcomes than the in-person collaborative care, because the telehealth-based care manager had (1) more clinical supervision, (2) access to a team that worked together full time (even if not full time for that specific practice site), and, (3) the additional supervision and team-based support, was able to better motivate patients toward engaged care and self-management.[41] This project is an example of telehealth supporting health care evolution, as well as using technology to drive this evolution toward a higher level of fidelity and efficacy. In this project, technology allowed one site to enjoy the benefits of an efficient full-time team, inasmuch as multiple projects financially supported that team. Rarely could the resources of one practice support such a team on-site.

This telehealth collaborative care project is not an isolated example. In a review of telebehavioral health effectiveness, Hilty, et al,[24] describe a variety of collaborative care models that have leveraged telebehavioral health to document positive behavioral and physical outcomes in primary care settings, with an increasing number of studies documenting even better outcomes, with a virtual collaborative care team, than with traditional primary care psychiatry service.[24] Hilty, et al, noted that patients with disorders, such as autism, often prefer virtual, over in-person care, and are more willing to engage in treatment. Patients of varied diagnoses have also reported feeling more comfortable and able to provide full and honest disclosure when they could receive care in their own homes. Increased patient engagement and better-informed providers both drive better health outcomes. Virtual collaborative models that are as effective, or more effective, than usual care include: (1) disease management for depression using telepsychiatry consultation in rural primary care, (2) cultural telebehavioral health consultation to rural primary care, (3) virtual training and mental health consultation for disaster response following bioterrorism attack, and (4) co-provision of medication for depressed primary care patients by the telepsychiatrist and a rural primary care provider.[24]

Some of the leading researchers in the field are finding that videoconference-based assessment accuracy and therapeutic engagement are higher for certain groups of adults and particularly for youth.[43] When the only provider in the room is virtually present, various studies have found the following: (1) young children often exhibit less inhibition, (2) children with behavior issues are more expressive, (3) those with trust, abuse, and dependency issues, feel more comfortable sharing painful details (reporting they feel less "judged"), (4) people with social anxiety and autism spectrum disorders seem better able to engage via telemedicine, and (5) older children, parents, and adult patients have reported a lowered sense of stigma.[43]

The variety in effective collaborative models speaks to the flexibility inherent in telebehavioral health-based solutions. Child and adolescent telepsychiatry programs are now embedded in pediatric practices, schools, and daycare facilities. Adult and youth telepsychiatry programs are in family and general practices, community mental health centers, and correctional and private practice settings.[43] Telehealth-based collaborative models set practices on a path to successful integration by leveraging technology to combine electronic health records and care plans, and support team-based care decisions informed by ongoing and regular review of patient progress. Telepsychiatry can facilitate a stepped-care approach, by starting patients on a low-intensity intervention and increasing the intensity for those who, based on regular review, do not respond to treatment.[24] Telehealth technology can weave stepped practices into the standard course of care by integrating registries, brief electronic communication, and short virtual assessments and reassessments with consultations and team meetings.

Integrated Care: Asynchronous Telepsychiatry

Asynchronous telepsychiatry (ATP), or store-and-forward services, is a great example of how telehealth has helped partial and full integration models move forward in an innovative way. ATP can move systems toward true integration, by addressing the time and operational barriers that make collaborative routines difficult to sustain, even once cultures and attitudes have become team based. ATP records a videoconferencing session with an onsite patient and provider, and forwards the recording, along with electronic patient records, and other relevant documents (i.e., current care plans), to a distal psychiatrist.[24] When shared electronic records and payment options can support this innovative approach, psychiatrists can avoid the challenge of both travel and scheduling. With the freedom to review recordings during even short stretches of available time, including during no-show appointments, psychiatrists can be more productive, increase revenues, and achieve greater personal work flexibility. ATP mitigates both time and operational barriers with one step.

A cost-comparison study of ATP versus synchronous telepsychiatry, in which the psychiatrist conducts a real-time, live session with a patient, identified significant ATP related cost savings. These cost saving were figured using fixed and marginal costs, calculated using equipment costs, time spent by providers and support staff, and hourly salaries. The primary cost-savings driver was the use of low-cost providers over psychiatrists and other specialists for the in-person collection of patient data. The researchers describe ATP as a disruptive health care transformation process. Leveraging telehealth technology within this innovative protocol could create opportunities for greater access, and better care delivery to a larger population of patients at a more affordable cost.[44]

Integrated Care: Clinical Models

As previously noted, part of the true innovation potential of telehealth is the flexibility it offers to individualize clinical practices across all levels of the integration continuum.

Figure 9.1 is an applied example of a virtual integrated specialist clinical workflow. This example is from a virtual care integration pilot, using a child and adolescent psychiatrist to enhance care integration in six accountable care organization pediatric and primary care practices in Colorado.

SUMMARY AND CONCLUSIONS

In response to escalating costs, poor outcomes, and health care provider shortages, the health care system is rapidly developing new and innovative means of integrating health care delivery. Studies demonstrating the efficacy of telehealth are summarized in Box 9.2. Health care now has a focus on the "triple aim" of improved patient experiences, population health, and lower costs. Telehealth is supporting and forwarding the implementation of evidence-based and innovative models of integrated care, with support from agencies, such as the Center for Medicare and Medicaid Innovation, created by Congress to develop and test various payment and service delivery models to reduce program costs, while preserving or improving the quality of care.[45]

The movement toward integrated care is complex, and requires unprecedented collaboration across previously distinct health care systems, training providers to interact in a team-based manner with patients and other providers, addressing system-level cultural differences, developing new health care delivery policies, and creating and enacting new payment methods. Provider ingenuity and telehealth technology are leading to innovative models designed to meet these daunting challenges. The evidence for telehealth as an effective way to implement and forward integrated care is strong and growing. A body of telehealth research finds telehealth delivery on par with in-person care. In a growing number of studies, collaborative models of care leveraging telehealth technology were actually

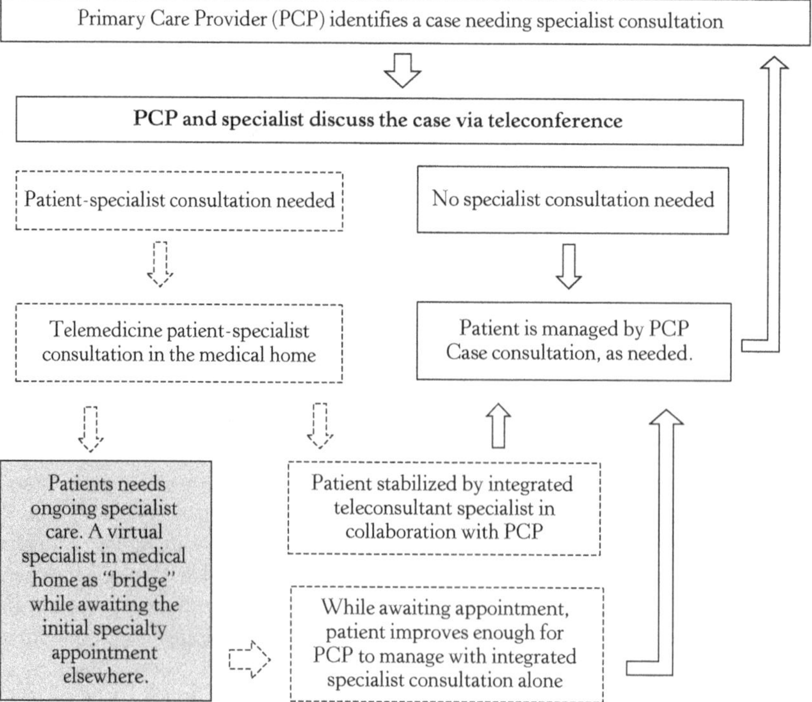

FIGURE 9.1. An Applied Example of a Virtual integrated specialist clinical workflow.

BOX 9.2
SUMMARY OF RECOMMENDED TREATMENT APPROACHES AND RELEVANT EVIDENCE

Strength of recommendation taxonomy (SOR A, B, or C)

- **Extension for Community Healthcare Outcomes (Project ECHO): Specialist education/support to primary care. Telehealth is used to link providers in rural and underserved areas with education, mentoring, and support from university experts. The model supports adherence to best practices in reducing variation in care, using case-based learning, and outcomes monitoring using force multiplication.[27–29] (SOR A)**
- **University of Washington's Advancing Integrated Mental Health Solutions [AIMS] Center: has identified five key components of collaborative care: (1) a patient-centered care team, (2) population-based care, (3) targeted measurement-based treatment, (4) evidence-based care, and (5) accountable care. These components have been shown to empower patients and family members to become active participants in their care, support care plan adjustments based on individual progress, systematically track all patients, use resources for population-specific needs, and ensure effective care through team-based accountability.**
- **Telehealth technology can be used for psychiatric/behavioral health direct screening and assessment of patients. Screening/assessments using televideo include: DSM-IV, GAD, Brief Psychiatric Rating Scale, Hamilton Depression Rating Scale. There is evidence for use of this model for effectively coordinating care (i.e., written specialist report to primary care provider) and increasing levels of integration (e.g. specialist and primary care providers have face-to-face discussion and integrate results into shared care plans).[24,37,46] (SOR A)**
- **Massachusetts Child Psychiatry Access Project, PAC-net, UC Davis project: Primary care consultation. Psychiatrist/BHS provides case-specific consultation and primary care provider retains full responsibility for patient care. This approach has improved outcomes.[20,38,39,43,47] (SOR A)**
- **Practice-based collaborative care (PBCC) has demonstrated efficacy for store-and-forward telepsychiatry.[41,44,48] (SOR A)**
- **Patient in-home direct care via telehealth improves patient satisfaction.[49] (SOR C)**

The citations included here represent only a fraction of studies conducted, and summary articles are cited wherever possible. Patient satisfaction is included as a critical outcome as satisfaction and engagement are critical precursors to effective behavioral health care plans.

associated with better outcomes than in-person care integration.[24]

Telehealth has been able to support care integration in a variety of situations (i.e., rural areas, provider shortage areas, small practices), in which in-person specialist care would not be financially or practically feasible. It has also been associated with increased flexibility and innovation, that has driven integration forward in new ways along the integration continuum. While professional conferences, continuing medical education, and "train-the-trainers" models of professional impact and growth are common across a variety of industries and settings, it is really the videoconferencing technology that has allowed the expertise of limited-supply health care specialists, like psychiatrists, to significantly magnify their professional impact, and has increased patient access to specialty care. Telehealth has allowed providers and practices to substantially improve their ability to manage populations in addition to individuals. Practices across all integration levels can benefit from didactic sessions virtually delivered to an entire practice team, and more integrated practices also improve population health through quick video conference–based primary care consultations. While costly specialist time was once consumed by travel time, constrained by scheduled visits, and wasted by no-show appointments, professional opportunity can now be maximized with these virtual didactic sessions, consultations, drop-in times, as well as store-and-forward assessments unconstrained by tight schedules. As telehealth continues to advance, it offers a platform for innovation and an obvious path toward improved patient-centered, value-based health care delivery options, and helps make the triple aim attainable.

REFERENCES

1. Centers for Medicare & Medicaid Services. National Health Expenditure Projections 2012–2022. https://www.cms.gov/research-statistics-data-and-systems/statistics-trends-and-reports/nationalhealthexpenddata/downloads/proj2012.pdf. Accessed January 18, 2016.
2. McQuaid JR, Stein MB, Laffaye C, McCahill ME. Depression in a primary care clinic: The prevalence and impact of an unrecognized disorder. J Affect Disord. 2010;55(1): 1–10.
3. Funk M, Ivbijaro G. Integrating Mental Health into Primary Care: A Global Perspective. World Health Organization and World Organization of Family Doctors; 2008.
4. Raney LE. Integrating primary care and behavioral health: The role of the psychiatrist in the collaborative care model. Am J Psychiatry. 2015;172(8):721–728.
5. Wang PS, Lane M, Olfson M, Pincus HA, Wells KB, Kessler RC. Twelve-month use of mental health services in the United States: Results from the National Comorbidity Survey Replication. Arch Gen Psychiatry. 2005;62(6):629–640.
6. Collins C, Hewson DL, Munger R, Wade T. Evolving Models of Behavioral Health Integration in Primary Care. New York: Milbank Memorial Fund; 2010.
7. DHS Shortage Areas: HRSA Data Warehouse. http://datawarehouse.hrsa.gov/Topics/ShortageAreas.aspx. Published 2015. Accessed September 17, 2015.
8. American Hospital Association. Realizing the Promise of Telehealth: Understanding the Legal and Regulatory Challenges. American Hospital Association Trend Watch. http://www.aha.org/research/reports/tw/15may-tw-telehealth.pdf. Published May 2015. Accessed January 19, 2016.
9. U.S. Department of Health and Human Services, Health Resources and Services Administration. Telehealth. http://www.hrsa.gov/healthit/toolbox/ruralhealthittoolbox/telehealth/ Accessed January 19, 2016.
10. American Telemedicine Association. What Is Telemedicine? http://www.americantelemed.org/about-telemedicine/what-is-telemedicine#.Vhfql_lVikq. Published 2012. Accessed July 18, 2015.
11. Roger A. A Brief History of Telemedicine. http://electronicdesign.com/components/brief-history-telemedicine. Published 2006. Accessed August 17, 2015.
12. American Hospital Association. The Promise of Telehealth for Hospitals, Health Systems and Their Communities. American Hospital Association, Trend Watch. 2015. http://www.aha.org/research/index.shtml. Accessed August 18, 2015.
13. Thomas L, Capistrant G. State telemedicine gaps analysis: Coverage and reimbursement. http://www.americantelemed.org/docs/default-source/policy/50-state-telemedicine-gaps-analysis---coverage-and-reimbursement.pdf. Accessed May 1, 2015.
14. American Telemedicine. Private Payer Reimbursement Directory, 2015. http://www.amdtelemedicine.com/telemedicine/resources/private_payerabout_survey.html. Accessed November 23, 2015.
15. Centers for Medicare & Medicaid Services. Telehealth Services. https://www.cms.gov/Outreach-and-Education/Medicare-Learning-Network-MLN/MLNProducts/downloads/TelehealthSrvcsfctsht.pdf. Accessed May 10, 2015.
16. Medicaid. Telemedicine. http://www.medicaid.gov/Medicaid-CHIP-Program-Information/By-Topics/Delivery-Systems/Telemedicine.html. Accessed May 10, 2015.
17. Japsen B. Doctors' virtual consults with patients to double by 2020. Forbes. http://www.forbes.com/sites/brucejapsen/2015/08/09/as-telehealth-booms-doctor-video-consults-to-double-by-2020. Accessed August 18, 2015.
18. U.S. Department of Health and Human Services. Understanding the Impact of Health IT in Underserved Communities and Those with Health Disparities. https://www.healthit.gov/sites/default/files/pdf/hit-underserved-communities-health-disparities.pdf. Published 2010. Accessed November 23, 2015.
19. UnitedHealth. Modernizing Rural Health Care: Coverage, Quality and Innovation. Working paper, July 6, 2011. http://www.unitedhealthgroup.com/~/media/UHG/PDF/2011/UNH-Working-Paper-6.ashx. Published July 2011. Accessed July 18, 2015.
20. Myers KM, Valentine JM, Melzer SM. Feasibility, acceptability, and sustainability of telepsychiatry for children and adolescents. Psychiatr Serv. 2007;58(11):1493–1496.
21. American Psychological Association. Health Care Reform: Integrated Health Care. http://www.apa.org/about/gr/issues/health-care/integrated.aspx. Accessed August 12, 2015.
22. Substance Abuse and Mental Health Services Administration. Integrated Care Models. http://www.integration.samhsa.gov/integrated-care-models. Accessed August 18, 2015.
23. Substance Abuse and Mental Health Services Administration. Primary Care in Behavioral Health. http://www.integration.samhsa.gov/

integrated-care-models/primary-care-in-behavioral-health. Accessed October 9, 2015.
24. Hilty DM, Ferrer DC, Parish MB, Johnston B, Callahan EJ, Yellowlees PM. The effectiveness of telemental health: A 2013 review. Telemed J. 2013;19(6):444–454.
25. Moscovice I, Casey M. Challenges for Improving Health Care Access in Rural America. A Compendium of Research and Policy Analysis Studies of Rural Health Research and Policy Analysis Centers 2009–2010. https://www.ruralhealthinfo.org/pdf/research_compendium.pdf. Accessed January 19, 2016.
26. Richardson LK, Frueh C, Grubaugh AL, Egede L, Elhai JD. Current directions in videoconferencing tele-mental health research. Clin Psychol Rev. 2009;16(3):323–338.
27. Robert Wood Johnson Foundation. Force multipliers. http://www.rwjf.org/en/about-rwjf/40th-anniversary/force-multipliers.html. Published 2007. Accessed October 30, 2014.
28. Katzman J, Comerci GJ, Boyle J, et al. Innovative telementoring for pain management: Project ECHO pain. J Cont Ed Hlth Prof. 2014;34(1):68–75.
29. Arora S, Thornton K, Murata G, et al. Outcomes of treatment of hepatitis C virus infection by primary care providers. N Engl J Med. 2011;364(23):2199–2207.
30. Agency for Healthcare Research and Policy. Care Coordination. http://www.ahrq.gov/professionals/prevention-chronic-care/improve/coordination/index.html. Accessed September 23, 2015.
31. American Psychiatric Association. Diagnostic and statistical manual of mental health disorders: DSM-5 (5th ed.). Washington, D.C.: American Psychiatric Publishing; 2013.
32. Overall J, Gorham D. The Brief Psychiatric Rating Scale. Psychol Rep. 1962;10(3):799–812.
33. Andreasen NC. Scale for the Assessment of Positive Symptoms (SAPS). Iowa City: University of Iowa; 1984.
34. Andreasen N. The Scale for the Assessment of Negative Symptoms (SANS). Iowa City: University of Iowa; 1983.
35. Hamilton M. A rating scale for depression. J Neurol Neurosurg Psychiat. 1960;23(1):56–62.
36. Guy W. Assessment manual for psychopharmacology, revised. Rockville, MD: U.S. Department of Health, Education and Welfare, Public Health Service, Alcohol, Drug Abuse and Mental Health Administration, NIMH Psychopharmacology Research Branch, Division of Extramural Research Programs; 1976.
37. Yellowlees PM, Shore J, Roberts L. Practice Guidelines for Videoconferencing-Based Telemental Health, October 2009. http://www.americantelemed.org/docs/default-source/standards/practice-guidelines-for-videoconferencing-based-telemental-health.pdf?sfvrsn=6. Accessed January 19, 2016.
38. Hilty DM, Marks SL, Urness D, Yellowlees PM, Nesbitt TS. Clinical and educational telepsychiatry applications: A review. Can J Psychiatry. 2004;49(1):12–23.
39. Hilty DM, Yellowlees PM, Cobb HC, Bourgeeois JA, Neufeld JD, Nesbitt TS. Models of telepsychiatry consultation–liaison service to rural primary care. Psychosomatics. 2006;47(2):152–157.
40. University of Washington Psychiatry and Behavioral Sciences. Principles of Effective Integrated Health Care, 2013. http://aims.uw.edu/sites/default/files/Five_Principles.pdf. Accessed September 23, 2015.
41. Fortney JC, Pyne JM, Mouden SB, et al. Practice-based versus telemedicine-based collaborative care for depression in rural Federally Qualified Health Centers: A pragmatic randomized comparative effectiveness trial. Am J Psychiatry. 2013;170(4):1–23.
42. Fortney JC, Pyne JM, Steven CA, et al. A web-based clinical decision support system for depression care management. Am J Managed Care. 2010;16(11):849–854.
43. Pakyurek M, Yellowlees PM, Hilty DM. The child and adolescent telepsychiatry consultation: Can it be a more effective clinical process for certain patients than conventional practice? Telemed J. 2010;16(3):289–292.
44. Butler TM, Yellowlees PM. Cost analysis of store-and-forward telepsychiatry as a consultation model for primary care. Telemed J. 2012;18(1):74–77.
45. U.S. Department of Health and Human Services, Agency for Healthcare Research and Quality. 2014 Annual Progress Report to Congress: National Strategy for Quality Improvement in Health Care. http://www.ahrq.gov/workingforquality/reports/annual-reports/nqs2014annlrpt.htm. Published 2014. Accessed August 12, 2015.
46. Neufeld JD, Yellowlees PM, Hilty DM, Cobb H, Bourgeois JA. The e-mental health consultation service: Providing enhanced primary care through telemedicine. Psychosomatics. 2007;48(2):135–141.
47. Holt W. The Massachusetts Child Psychiatry Access Project: Supporting mental health treatment in primary care. Commonwealth Fund, 2010. http://www.commonwealthfund.org/~/media/Files/Publications/Case%20Study/2010/Mar/1378_Holt_MCPAP_case_study_32.pdf. Accessed January 19, 2016.
48. Fortney JC, Jeffrey MP, Kimbrell TA, et al. Telemedicine-based collaborative care for posttraumatic stress disorder: A randomized clinical trial. J Am Med Assoc Psychiat. 2015;72(1):58–67.
49. Egede LE, Frueh CB, Richardson LK, et al. Rational and design: Telepsychology service delivery for depressed elderly veterans. Trials. 2009;109(1):10–22.

10

Automated Mental Health Assessment for Integrated Care

The Quick PsychoDiagnostics Panel Meets Real-World Clinical Needs

JONATHAN SHEDLER

BOX 10.1

KEY POINTS

- **Quality mental health care begins with thorough assessment.**
- **Commonly-used assessment tools do not meet medical providers' clinical needs.**
- **A clinically useful mental health assessment tool must assess the range of conditions commonly seen in medical settings, provide clinically actionable information, and integrate seamlessly into busy practice settings.**
- **The Quick PsychoDiagnostics Panel (QPD Panel) is a fully automated assessment tool that assesses 11 common mental health conditions. It is self-administered by patients, typically on a tablet device in the clinic waiting room.**
- **Providers immediately receive a computer-generated, chart-ready assessment report in a familiar lab report format.**
- **The QPD Panel can be readministered as often as desired for progress monitoring and outcome assessment.**
- **Primary care providers agreed or strongly agreed that the QPD Panel helps provide better patient care, is well accepted by patients, and can be used immediately by any physician without additional training.**
- **The QPD Panel is a revenue generator for health care organizations. QPD Panel administration is billable to third-party payers using Current Procedural Terminology (CPT) code 96103 for computerized psychological testing.**
- **Visit www QPDPanel.com to request a free trial.**

INTRODUCTION

This chapter discusses the challenges of mental health assessment in primary care and general medical settings, and describes the QPD Panel, an automated mental health assessment tool that assesses eleven common mental disorders and meets the real-world clinical needs of medical providers. See Box 10.1 for a summary of Key Points.

At least 20% of primary care patients have mental health conditions, most of which go unrecognized, untreated, or inadequately treated.[1–15] The overwhelming majority of patients with mental health conditions seek care from primary care providers, not mental health providers.[16,17] For better or worse, primary care is the de facto mental health services system for most patients.[18] To make things more difficult, patients with mental health conditions commonly present with somatic rather than mental health complaints, making mental health conditions harder to recognize in general medical practice.

THE CHALLENGE OF ASSESSMENT

As with all areas of health care, good mental health care begins with thorough assessment. Despite frequent assertions to the contrary, medical providers have generally *not* had access to clinically helpful mental health assessment tools. It is not that there is a dearth of assessment tools; on the contrary, the number of such tools can seem overwhelming. The problem, rather, is that the assessment tools commonly given to medical providers do not meet their clinical needs.

Over the past decades, demands on primary care providers have increased relentlessly. Health care organizations and regulatory agencies have expected providers to do more and more in less and less time.[19] Far from easing the burden on providers, the mental health screening tools most often used in primary care add to that burden, hampering rather than facilitating providers' clinical workflow.[20] When medical providers do use mental health screening tools, it is more often because their use is mandated by regulatory and accrediting bodies than because providers perceive compelling clinical benefits.

These comments require explanation. The high prevalence of mental health conditions in primary care and general medical practice is not a recent discovery; it was well documented at least a quarter of a century ago. Then as now, mental health case-finding tools were readily available, but medical providers rarely used them. Beginning in the mid-1990s, screening tools were developed specifically for primary care, and research projects (generally funded by pharmaceutical companies marketing antidepressants) were conducted with the aim of promoting their routine use. The results of these research projects were nearly always the same: Reports in prestigious medical journals documented the validity of the screening tools[2,21] but failed to mention that the medical providers used the screening tools only for the duration of the research projects, while they received external support and incentives.[22,23] When external support and incentives ended, providers stopped using the tools, essentially "voting with their feet" regarding their perceived utility in day-to-day practice.

The health care landscape has since changed. There is now greater awareness of the prevalence of mental disorders, their high societal cost, and the interrelatedness of mental and physical conditions.[3] Use of mental health screening and case-finding instruments has been recommended, for example, by the U.S. Preventive Services Task Force,[24] the Canadian Task Force on Preventive Health Care,[25] and the UK National Institute of Clinical Excellence.[26] Regulatory and accrediting bodies such as the National Center for Quality Assurance (NCQA) now mandate routine depression screening in many medical settings. The nine-question PHQ-9 depression screen[27] and the two-question PHQ-2 depression screen[28] are now commonly integrated into medical office visits and typically administered by medical assistants or nurses along with vital signs.

What has not changed is that providers still do not find these assessment tools especially clinically helpful, nor has their use had a meaningful impact on patient outcomes. A recent rigorous meta-analysis examined the impact of depression screening tools and bluntly concluded, "We found no substantial effect of screening or case-finding instruments on the overall recognition rates of depression, the management of depression by clinicians or on depression outcomes. These findings were true for both primary care and general hospital settings."[29]

A recent study examined physicians' actions following a positive PHQ-2 depression screen in a primary care practice setting where the PHQ-2 was routinely administered to patients at intake per NCQA guidelines.[30] The PHQ-2 comprises the first two questions of the nine-question PHQ-9 depression screen and positive results should be followed by administration of the full PHQ-9.[28] However, 95% of the time, physicians did *not* administer the PHQ-9 after a positive PHQ-2 screen, again "voting with their feet" regarding its perceived utility. In many cases, providers did not even review the PHQ-2 results. Reasons physicians cited included time limitations, other issues taking precedence, and the belief that the patient's depression status was already known.

Such results are commonly explained in terms of need for practice support.[31] Conventional wisdom holds that mental health assessment tools will gain traction in general medical practice when there is enhanced systemic support for behavioral health care, including ready access to behavioral health providers, availability of psychiatric consultation-liaison, availability of care teams and case managers, and so on. These assumptions and principles underlie the integrated care movement. The conventional wisdom obviously has validity, as there is little point in identifying that a need for services exists, if the needed services are not accessible.

However, the conventional wisdom bypasses the question of whether or not the mental health assessment tools typically provided to physicians truly meet their clinical needs. In fact, in the study just described, which showed that physicians rarely administered the PHQ-9 even after a positive initial depression screen,[30] behavioral health support was excellent. The findings indicate that the physicians did not make more use of the depression screening tools, not because of lack of practice support for behavioral health care, but because they did not find the assessment tools sufficiently clinically helpful.

WHAT MEDICAL PROVIDERS DO AND DON'T WANT

One reason these widely distributed screening tools have not gained greater traction in clinical practice is that they were developed and disseminated via a "top down" strategy. Researchers and policymakers made a priori decisions about what kind of mental health assessment tools primary care providers should use, without real input from primary care providers, with the expectation that providers would simply adopt what they were given. An alternative to a "top down" strategy is a "bottom up" strategy, which begins with a thorough investigation into the needs and wants of primary care clinicians. An assessment tool can then be designed in accord with clinicians' specifications, ensuring that it meets a legitimate clinical need "on the ground." This was the strategy used to develop the Quick PsychoDiagnostics Panel (QPD Panel).

In the early 1990s, interviews and focus groups were conducted with primary care physicians, with the aim of discovering (1) why primary care providers did not use existing mental health assessment tools and (2) what the providers would want in a hypothetical, ideal mental health assessment tool that they would want to use.

The answer to the first question was relatively straightforward. In some cases, physicians felt uncomfortable delving into patients' emotional matters or believed, incorrectly, that their patients would be uncomfortable. Some felt their training in psychiatry was inadequate. But the biggest concern, by far, was time. The physicians felt overburdened with responsibilities ("besieged on all sides," as one put it), with barely enough time to address the medical issues that were their primary concern. The last thing they wanted was a mental health assessment tool that required still more of their time or added to their clinical workload.

A PROVIDER WISH LIST

The primary care physicians were asked to describe a hypothetical, ideal mental health assessment tool—one that they would want to use and keep on using.[20] From the interviews and focus groups, the following "wish list" emerged:

(1) The test should require no time from physicians or medical staff. (Note that the desire was not for a test that required little time, but *no* time.)
(2) The test should require no training to use.
(3) The test should diagnose the full spectrum of mental health conditions commonly encountered in general medical settings. *The physicians felt that tools that screened for depression alone did not provide enough information to be truly clinically helpful.* (The general attitude seemed to be, "Give me enough diagnostic information to address the range of mental health issues I'll now have to deal with, or don't bother me.")
(4) The test should provide specific psychiatric diagnoses and symptoms. (Physicians did not just want numeric scores with cutoff points; they wanted actual diagnoses based on the *Diagnostic and Statistical Manual of Mental Disorders* [DSM]).[32]
(5) The test should not require forms or paperwork.
(6) The test should not require change in office routines or interfere with patient flow.
(7) The test should be liked and accepted by patients. (Physicians did not want their patients to feel they were being asked inappropriately personal questions or being treated impersonally.)

These requirements may seem excessive or unreasonable from the perspective of a mental health test developer, but they make sense from the frame of reference of medical providers. That frame of reference is a *medical lab test*. Lab tests do not take up provider time or staff time or create busywork. They do not disrupt office routines or patient flow. They do not add to the burden on providers or staff.

Providers simply *order* lab tests and get back the diagnostic information they need.

COMPREHENSIVE ASSESSMENT IS CRUCIAL

The primary care physicians felt that tools that screened for depression alone had limited utility because they did not provide enough information to guide treatment decisions (item 3 in the "wish list"). The physicians were, in fact, correct. Comorbidity of psychiatric disorders is the norm, and cases of depression alone are relatively rare. Epidemiologically, 78.5% of cases (12-month prevalence) of major depressive disorder (MDD) have additional psychiatric comorbidity, "*with MDD only rarely primary*" (emphasis added).[33] In practice, this means that physicians see depression accompanied by generalized anxiety, substance abuse, trauma, panic disorder, or any number of other configurations of symptoms and disorders, which have different implications for treatment. For a substantial percentage of patients who screen positive for "depression," treating depression per se may not be the correct treatment decision.

From the perspective of primary care providers, screening for depression alone amounts to opening Pandora's box without providing actionable information for treatment decisions. Given a positive depression screen, providers must still conduct a psychiatric examination before making treatment decisions, or even determining whether a behavioral health referral is warranted. Just how primary care providers are supposed to do this on a routine basis, when patients are presenting with medical complaints that require attention, during office appointments that average 15 minutes or less,[19] is anyone's guess.

A truly clinical useful mental health assessment tool *must* provide a comprehensive assessment. It must assess the spectrum of mental health conditions that providers are called upon to address and provide sufficient information to inform sound treatment decisions.

OVERVIEW OF THE QPD PANEL

The QPD Panel is a fully automated mental health assessment test. It was designed from the ground up to meet the specific clinical needs of medical providers, based on the "wish list" compiled from physician interviews and focus groups.[20,34] The test requires no time from providers or medical staff to administer or score. Rather, patients self-administer the test, typically in less than 10 minutes, using a tablet device, smartphone, or computer web browser.

Patients complete the test by responding to a series of true-or-false questions that require only a fifth-grade reading level. The test screens for 11 mental health disorders commonly seen in primary care and general medical settings (Box 10.2). Most often, patients self-administer the test in the clinic waiting room using a tablet device (iOS, Android, Windows, and Kindle tablets are all supported). In some health care organizations, patients have the option of completing the test online prior to their office appointment. The test can be administered in English or Spanish.

When patients complete the QPD Panel, the provider immediately receives a comprehensive, chart-ready assessment report in a familiar lab report format. The computer-generated report is automatically sent to a local office printer or directed to the patient's electronic medical record in electronic format, depending on the needs of the clinic or health

BOX 10.2
QUICK PSYCHODIAGNOSTICS PANEL: DISORDERS SCREENED

- Major depression
- Persistent depressive disorder
- Bipolar disorder
- Generalized anxiety disorder
- Panic disorder
- Obsessive-compulsive disorder
- Posttraumatic stress disorder
- Substance use disorder
- Binge-eating disorder
- Bulimia nervosa
- Somatic symptom disorder
- Psychosis[a]

[a]*Optional module*

care organization. Thus, providers receive real-time diagnostic information. The word *panel* in the name *QPD Panel* reflects the input of physicians in the initial focus groups (see "What Medical Providers Do and Don't Want") and is intended to underscore that the test can function in a medical setting in much the same way as a familiar lab test such as a blood chemistry panel. The QPD Panel software is currently in its 10th major edition. The assessment procedure is fully compliant with the Health Insurance Portability and Accountability Act (HIPAA).

The base version of the QPD Panel screens for the 11 mental disorders listed in Box 10.2, based on diagnostic criteria specified by the DSM-5.[32] The included disorders reflect the input of primary care physicians regarding the conditions they viewed as most important to assess, as well as epidemiological data about the mental health disorders most prevalent in primary care and general medical settings. In addition to these diagnosable mental health conditions, the QPD Panel screens for suicide risk, recent physical or sexual abuse, and (optionally) danger to others.

The QPD Panel software incorporates advanced logic and branching to maximize efficiency and minimize test administration time. Algorithms determine which questions are presented based on responses to previous questions. Thus, patients who do not have a psychiatric disorder are not asked irrelevant questions, and patients who may have disorders are examined in depth. The initial questions focus on physical symptoms, consistent with what patients expect to be asked during a medical office visit (although they are symptoms associated with depression, anxiety, and other mental health conditions). The questions then lead gradually into content that is more obviously related to mental health.

The QPD Panel software capabilities make the test more efficient than a human interviewer. It is unlikely that any clinician could systematically assess 11 mental health disorders in less than 10 minutes, let alone record the specific symptoms associated with each disorder, track changes from previous assessments, and organize the resulting information optimally for presentation. Also, empirical research consistently shows that respondents "are more honest with computers ... than they are with live interviewers."[35]

The QPD Panel assessment results have high reliability and validity.[20,34] The symptom scores show high convergent validity with established psychiatric rating scales (e.g., the QPD Panel depression scale correlates highly with the Hamilton Depression Inventory, Beck Depression Inventory, Center for Epidemiological Studies Depression Scale, and Zung Self-Rating Depression Scale [range, $r = .78$ to $r = .87$]). The QPD Panel diagnoses show high sensitivity and specificity relative to structured psychiatric interviews (e.g., for major depression, sensitivity and specificity were .81 and .96 respectively; for generalized anxiety disorder, sensitivity and specificity were .79 and .90 respectively). For further information on validity, see references 20 and 34.

THE QPD PANEL ASSESSMENT REPORT

The QPD Panel assessment report reflects the extensive input of primary care providers. The report is designed to communicate diagnostic information simply and efficiently, allowing the test to be used by virtually any physician without additional training. By design, the report has a "look and feel" that is familiar to medical providers, resembling a blood chemistry report. Figure 10.1 shows a sample QPD Panel assessment report.

The QPD Panel assessment report has three sections: (1) symptom scores, (2) diagnostic notes, and (3) symptom list. If the QPD Panel is administered more than once, the report also includes a trending graph showing changes in the severity of depression and anxiety symptoms over time (see section on "Outcome Assessment").

Symptom Scores

The first section of the report, "symptom scores," is in lab test format. Numeric scores measure the severity of symptoms in eight areas (see Fig. 10.1). Normal reference ranges are shown on the report. Scores that fall outside the normal reference ranges indicate clinically significant symptoms that warrant clinical attention. In Figure 10.1, the patient's depression and posttraumatic stress disorder (PTSD) scores fall outside the normal reference ranges.

Diagnostic Notes

If one or more symptom scores are out of range, a diagnostic note is displayed in the "diagnostic notes" section, immediately below the symptom score section. Diagnostic notes indicate whether the patient's symptoms meet formal diagnostic criteria for a specific DSM-5/ICD-10 diagnosis. For example, if the depression symptom score is out of range,

QPDPanel v10.1

www.QPDPanel.com 800.559.9885

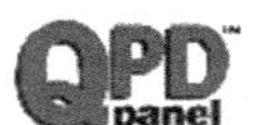

Name: John Doe
ID: 123456789
Date: 2/5/2016 10:25 AM

Sex: M
Age: 44

Symptom Scores

Scale	Results: within range	Results: out of range	Reference Range
Depression*		21	0–10
Manic Episode	0		0–3
Anxiety	9		0–10
Panic Disorder	5		0–8
PTSD		6	0–3
Eating Disorder	0		0–4
Substance Use	1		0–2
Somatization	6		0–11

*11–14 mild/ 15–19 moderate/ >19 severe

DSM-5/ICD-10 Diagnoses:

— Patient appears to meet criteria for Major Depressive Episode
— Patient appears to meet criteria for Posttraumatic Stress Disorder

ID: 123456789
Date: 2/5/2016 10:25 AM

Depression Symptoms

— depressed mood, nearly every day, 2 weeks or longer duration
— diminished interest or pleasure in activities, 2 weeks or longer duration
— weight loss
— insomnia
— fatigue, loss of energy
— feelings of worthlessness or guilt
— impaired concentration
— diminished self-esteem
— hopelessness

PTSD Symptoms

— intrusive recollections of traumatic event
— distressing dreams of traumatic event
— relives or has flashbacks of traumatic event
— distress or physiological reactivity when reminded of traumatic event

Trending: Change in Depression and Anxiety Over Time

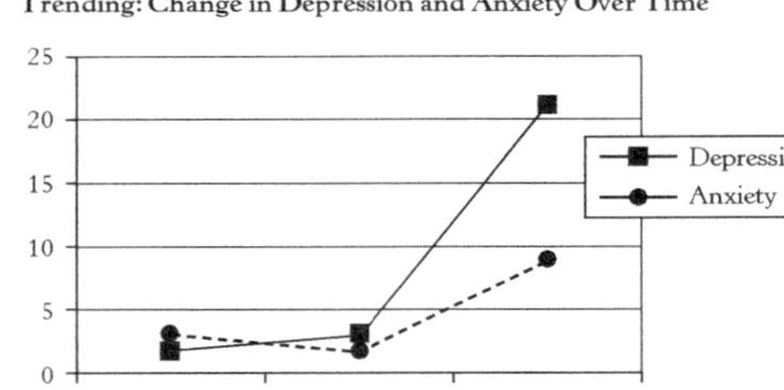

FIGURE 10.1. QPD Panel Sample Report.

the clinician might see one or more of the following diagnostic notes:

- Patient appears to meet criteria for Major Depressive Episode.
- Patient appears to meet criteria for Persistent Depressive Disorder (Dysthymia).
- Clinically significant depression (does not meet formal diagnostic criteria for Major Depressive Episode or Persistent Depressive Disorder).
- Patient appears to meet criteria for Bipolar Mood Disorder.

The notes are generated by pattern-matching algorithms, which match the specific symptoms reported by the patient against applicable DSM-5 diagnostic criteria. The "diagnostic notes" section will also include notes indicating the presence of suicidal ideation, imminent suicide risk, recent sexual or physical abuse, and (optionally) danger to others. In Figure 10.1, the diagnostic notes indicate that the patient has reported symptoms that meet DSM-5 diagnostic criteria for major depressive episode and PTSD.

Symptom List

The second page of the assessment report lists the specific symptoms reported by the patient. The symptom list is valuable for guiding treatment decisions and, if the patient is being referred for behavioral health treatment, for communicating clinically crucial information to the behavioral health provider.

A provider reviewing a QPD Panel report would first review the lab-test format symptom scores. If all scores are within the normal range, the review is done. If one or more out-of-range scores indicate clinically significant symptoms, the provider would then review the diagnostic notes section for applicable DSM-5/ICD-10 diagnoses. Finally, the symptom list provides fine-grained information about the patient's specific symptoms.

Outcome Assessment

Providers can readminister the QPD Panel as often as desired to monitor patient status and for outcome assessment. The QPD Panel software automatically tracks and graphs changes in the depression and anxiety symptom scores over time (see Fig. 10.1), allowing providers to see at-a-glance whether the patient's mental health status is improving or worsening. Both the depression and anxiety symptom scores are sensitive to change.[34] Changes of 5 points or more are clinically meaningful and correspond to approximately one standard deviation of change (for more information, see reference 20).

REVIEWING THE QPD PANEL REPORT WITH PATIENTS

Many providers choose to share the QPD Panel report with patients and find it helpful as a tool for initiating and structuring discussion about mental health problems. The availability of an objective computer-generated report tends to bypass patient resistance and can help providers broach otherwise difficult topics. Providers should review the assessment report findings with patients in a matter-of-fact manner, as they would any other diagnostic findings. For example, the provider might simply say, "Your test results show an elevated level of depression. The normal score range is between 0 and 10, and your score is 16. Let's take a look at the symptoms you're having."

Provider and patient can then review the symptom list section of the report together, which provides an opportunity to educate the patient about the mental health condition and the symptoms associated with it. At this point, provider and patient are already well on the way to a productive discussion about treatment options and a mutually agreed-upon treatment plan. Use of the assessment report in this way, as a tool to structure discussion of mental health issues, helps to keep the discussion focused and productive. The fact that the provider can review a *comprehensive* mental health assessment report, before initiating discussion with the patient, helps ensure that the provider will not be "blindsided" by unexpected mental health problems that he or she did not anticipate having to address (the "Pandora's box" problem described earlier, which is one of the major reasons physicians cite for hesitancy about broaching mental health issues).

The QPD Panel can be readministered on follow-up visits, and provider and patient can review progress together. This way of working facilitates a collaborative working relationship between provider and patient. Regular follow-up assessments allow timely adjustments to be made to the treatment plan, facilitate treatment adherence, and lead to improved outcomes. If the patient is also being seen by a behavioral health provider, follow-up assessments with the QPD Panel enhance collaboration and communication with the behavioral health provider and promote the continuity of care that is a hallmark of quality integrated care.

PHYSICIAN ACCEPTANCE AND PATIENT SATISFACTION

Physician Acceptance

As described in the introduction, the QPD Panel was designed from the ground up to meet the specific clinical needs of primary care medical providers. The extent to which the QPD Panel succeeds in meeting this goal is an empirical question, one appropriately answered by providers. Consequently, we conducted a provider satisfaction study to formally evaluate the utility of the QPD Panel under real-world conditions in busy primary care clinics.[20,34] Table 10.1 presents the results of the provider satisfaction study.

Data were provided by a sample of 26 primary care physicians practicing at one of two outpatient medical facilities in a large group-model health maintenance organization (HMO). Providers in these clinics see approximately 20 to 24 patients per day, with appointments scheduled at 15- to 20-minute intervals. The providers used the QPD Panel on a routine basis for at least one month. Neither the clinics nor the providers received incentives to use the QPD Panel or to participate in the satisfaction study. Providers rated each statement listed in Table 10.1 using a 5-point rating scale (1 = strongly disagree; 5 = strongly agree).

Means for the physician satisfaction items were uniformly high and near the scale maximum of 5.0. As another way of presenting the data, the last column of Table 10.1 lists the percentage of providers who agreed or strongly agreed with each statement. The data demonstrate the high levels of provider acceptance achieved by the QPD Panel, and speak to the soundness of the "bottom up" strategy that guided development of the QPD Panel.

Patient Satisfaction

One item on the provider "wish list" for an ideal mental health assessment tool is that the test should be liked and accepted by patients. To assess patient satisfaction, we asked 77 consecutive primary care patients who completed the QPD Panel to respond to four survey questions, using an agree/disagree response format.[34] The patients completed the QPD Panel using tablet devices during regularly scheduled office appointments, in the primary care clinics in which we collected the provider satisfaction data.

Ninety-seven percent of patients agreed with the statement, "the questionnaire was easy to use"; 99% agreed that "the questions were clear and easy to understand"; 96% agreed that "the questionnaire asks about things that are important for my doctor to know"; and 96% *disagreed* that "the questions were too personal and made me feel uncomfortable." Anecdotally, many patients spontaneously

TABLE 10.1. MEANS FOR PROVIDER SATISFACTION QUESTIONNAIRE (N = 26)

Item	Mean[a] (Standard deviation)	% Agree or Strongly Agree
The QPD Panel is convenient and easy to use.	4.8 (.40)	100
The QPD Panel integrates easily into the primary care clinic.	4.6 (.90)	89
The QPD Panel presents results in a clear, easy-to-understand format.	4.8 (.51)	96
The QPD Panel is well accepted by patients.	4.6 (.50)	100
The QPD Panel helps me provide better patient care.	4.7 (.60)	100
The QPD Panel can be used immediately by any physician, without special training required.	4.6 (.75)	100

[a] On a scale of 1–5, where 1 = strongly disagree, 2 = disagree, 3 = neither agree nor disagree, 4 = agree, and 5 = strongly agree.

commented that the test made them feel good about the quality of care they were receiving, and led them to feel that their doctors cared about them.

INSTITUTIONAL BENEFITS

The QPD Panel offers additional capabilities relevant to health care organizations and systems. Data collected via the QPD Panel are accessible through a HIPAA-compliant database, allowing organizations to conduct statistical analyses of mental health data, for example for population-based needs assessment, outcome assessment, quality metrics, and other statistical and research purposes. From a financial perspective, implementation of the QPD Panel generates positive cash flow. Administration of the QPD Panel and review of QPD Panel test results is a billable procedure. In the United States, physicians and psychologists can bill third-party payers for QPD Panel administration using Current Procedural Terminology (CPT) code 96103 for computerized psychological testing.

IMPROVING PATIENT OUTCOMES: A CASE STUDY IN INTEGRATED CARE

Kaiser Permanente, a group-model HMO that operates in several geographical regions in the United States, developed and implemented a highly successful integrated care program called the Kaiser Permanent Integrated Care Project.[36] The project involved physically locating behavioral health providers (psychologists) in primary care medical clinics, fostering a collaborative team approach to patient care, and systematically tracking outcomes in a sample of patients with mood and anxiety disorders.

The patients self-administered the QPD Panel using tablet devices during regularly scheduled medical appointments, and physicians reviewed the QPD Panel assessment reports during the office visit. One hundred thirteen patients who screened positive on the QPD Panel for depression, generalized anxiety, or panic disorder (which were often comorbid) were enrolled in the project. Exclusion criteria were a positive screen on the QPD Panel for substance abuse, symptoms of psychosis or dementia, or a terminal medical illness. Most patients had medical comorbidities, the most common of which were arthritis or rheumatism, hypertension, sciatica or chronic back pain, asthma, and angina.

Medical providers shared QPD Panel diagnostic findings with the patients, often reviewing

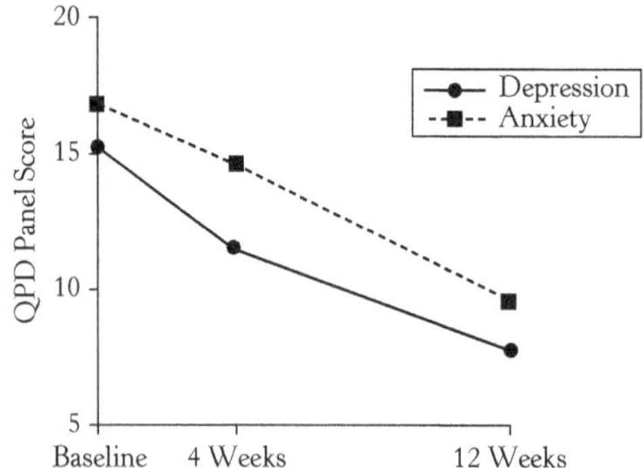

FIGURE 10.2. QPD Panel Depression and Anxiety Scores, Before and After Treatment.

the QPD Panel assessment report together with the patient. The patients were then offered three treatment options, and patients and providers made treatment decisions together. The treatment options included psychotherapy (short-term cognitive-behavioral or interpersonal), antidepressant medication, or a combination of psychotherapy and antidepressants. Most patients chose psychotherapy or combination therapy.

Follow-up assessments were conducted with the QPD Panel at four and 12 weeks after the initial assessment. Figure 10.2 shows QPD Panel depression and anxiety symptom scores at baseline (initial assessment) and at the four-week and 12-week follow-ups. The average depression symptom score at baseline was 15.2, in the moderately severe range. At the 12-week follow-up, the depression score had decreased by approximately 50% (slightly more than a standard deviation) to 7.8, within the normal reference range. The anxiety symptom score showed a comparable decrease, from 16.8 at baseline to 9.7 at the 12-week follow-up. To triangulate on patients' mental health status, patients were also assessed at the same three time points with the Zung depression and anxiety scales and the SF-12 Health Survey; they showed comparable levels of improvement on all measures. The project authors also noted high levels of provider acceptance and patient satisfaction. (For a more complete description of the Kaiser Permanent Integrated Care Project, see reference 36.)

CONCLUSION

Good mental health care begins with thorough assessment. Unfortunately, the mental health screening tools most often given to primary care and general medical providers do not meet providers' clinical needs, and have had little impact on real-world patient outcomes. A mental health assessment tool that is truly clinically useful must provide a *comprehensive* assessment of the range of mental health conditions commonly seen in medical practice (not just a single disorder) and must provide specific, actionable information to guide treatment decisions. Also, it must not hinder clinical workflow or add to the time burden on providers or medical staff.

The QPD Panel is a computerized, fully automated mental health assessment test designed to meet these requirements. Patients self-administer the test, typically in the clinic waiting room using a tablet device, smartphone, or computer web browser. Administration time is generally less than 10 minutes. The test screens for 11 disorders commonly seen in primary care and general medical settings. Physicians immediately receive a chart-ready, comprehensive assessment report, which is printed on a local printer or sent to the patient's electronic medical record. The computer-generated assessment report displays results in lab test format, offering a familiar "look and feel" for medical providers. In addition to initial assessment, the test can be readministered as often as desired for patient monitoring and outcome assessment. The assessment report includes a trending graph that tracks changes in symptom severity, allowing providers to see at a glance whether the patient's mental health status is improving or worsening.

The QPD Panel demonstrated high physician acceptance in a formal provider satisfaction study. In a busy primary care setting, 100% of physicians who used the QPD Panel agreed or strongly agreed that the test is convenient and easy to use, is well accepted by patients, and helps clinicians provide better patient care.

The QPD Panel automates mental health assessment, providing comprehensive and actionable diagnostic information in a user-friendly lab report format. It is a valuable tool for integrated health care. See Box 10.3 for a summary of Relevant Facts. For a demo and free trial of the QPD Panel, visit www.QPDPanel.com.

BOX 10.3

RELEVANT FACTS

1. **Most patients with mental health conditions seek help from primary care providers, not mental health practitioners.[16,17]**
2. **At least 20% of primary care patients have mental health conditions.[1–15]**
3. **Comorbidity of psychiatric disorders is the norm: 78.5% of patients with major depression have additionally psychiatric morbidity, with depression rarely primary.[33]**
4. **The mental health screening and case-finding tools most often used in medical settings do not meet providers' clinical needs,[20] and they have had little impact on patient care or outcomes.[29]**
5. **A clinically useful mental health assessment tool must screen for the range of mental health conditions commonly seen in medical settings (not just one disorder), must provide clinically actionable information, and must not add to the time burden on providers or medical staff.[20]**
6. **The QPD Panel is a computerized, fully automated mental health assessment tool designed to meet the specific clinical needs of medical providers. Patients self-administer the test, typically on a tablet device in the clinic waiting room. Providers immediately receive a computer-generated, chart-ready assessment report in a familiar lab-report format. The test screens for 11 common mental health conditions.[20,34]**
7. **The QPD Panel achieves high provider and patient acceptance. In a provider satisfaction study, primary care providers agreed or strongly agreed that the QPD Panel helps provide better patient care, is convenient to use in busy medical settings, and can be used immediately by any physician without additional training.[20,34]**

REFERENCES

1. Barrett JE, Barrett JA, Oxman TE, Gerber PD. The prevalence of psychiatric disorders in a primary care practice. Arch Gen Psychiatry. 1988;45(12):1100–1106.
2. Spitzer RL, Kroenke K, Williams JB. Validation and utility of a self-report version of PRIME-MD: The PHQ primary care study. JAMA. 1999;282(18):1737–1744.
3. World Health Organization. Integrating Mental Health Into Primary Health Care: A Global Perspective. Geneva: World Health Organization; 2008.
4. Andersen SM, Harthorn BH. The recognition, diagnosis, and treatment of mental disorders by primary care physicians. Med Care. 1989;27(9):869–886.
5. Borus JF, Howes MJ, Devins NP, Rosenberg R, Livingston WW. Primary health care providers' recognition and diagnosis of mental disorders in their patients. Gen Hosp Psychiatry. 1988;10(5):317–321.
6. Katon W. The epidemiology of depression in medical care. Int J Psychiatry Med. 1987;17(1):93–112.
7. Nielsen AC, Williams T. Depression in ambulatory medical patients. Arch Gen Psychiatry. 1980;37:999–1004.
8. Ormel J, Koeter MW, van den Brink W, van de Willige G. Recognition, management, and course of anxiety and depression in general practice. Arch Gen Psychiatry. 1991;48(8):700–706.
9. Rydon P, Redman S, Sanson-Fisher RW, Reid AL. Detection of alcohol-related problems in general practice. J Stud Alcohol. 1992;53(3):197–202.
10. Schulberg HC, Burns BJ. Mental disorders in primary care: Epidemiologic, diagnostic, and treatment research directions. Gen Hosp Psychiatry. 1988;10(2):79–87.
11. Schulberg HC, Saul M, McClelland M, Ganguli M, Christy W, Frank R. Assessing depression in primary medical and psychiatric practices. Arch Gen Psychiatry. 1985;42(12):1164–1170.
12. Kessler LG, Cleary PD, Burke JD, Jr. Psychiatric disorders in primary care. Results of a follow-up study. Arch Gen Psychiatry. 1985;42(6):583–587.
13. Katon W, Ciechanowski P. Impact of major depression on chronic medical illness. J Psychosom Res. 2002;53(4):859–863.
14. Simon GE, VonKorff M. Recognition, management, and outcomes of depression in primary care. Arch Fam Med. 1995;4(2):99–105.
15. Wittchen HU, Muhlig S, Beesdo K. Mental disorders in primary care. Dialogues Clin Neurosci. 2003;5(2):115–128.
16. Bland R. Depression and its management in primary care. Can J Psychiatry. 2007;52(2):75–76.
17. Edlund MJ, Unutzer J, Wells KB. Clinician screening and treatment of alcohol, drug, and mental problems in primary care: Results from healthcare for communities. Med Care. 2004;42(12):1158–1166.
18. Regier DA, Goldberg ID, Taube CA. The de facto US mental health services system: A public health perspective. Arch Gen Psychiatry. 1978;35(6):685–693.
19. Schappert SM. National Ambulatory Medical Care Survey: 1989 summary. Vital Health Statistics 13. 1992(110):1–80.
20. Shedler J. The Shedler QPD Panel (Quick PsychoDiagnostics Panel): A psychiatric "lab test" for primary care. In: Maruish M, ed. Handbook of Psychological Assessment in Primary Care Settings. Mahwah, NJ: Lawrence Erlbaum Associates; 2000.
21. Spitzer RL, Williams JB, Kroenke K, et al. Utility of a new procedure for diagnosing mental disorders in primary care. The PRIME-MD 1000 study. JAMA. 1994;272(22):1749–1756.
22. Gilbody S, Sheldon T, Wessely S. Should we screen for depression? BMJ. 2006;332(7548):1027–1030.
23. Valenstein M, Dalack G, Blow F, Figueroa S, Standiford C, Douglass A. Screening for psychiatric illness with a combined screening and diagnostic instrument. J Gen Intern Med. 1997;12(11):679–685.
24. Agency for Healthcare Research and Quality. Screening for Depression: Systematic Evidence Review Number 6. Rockville, MD; 2002.
25. MacMillan HL, Patterson CJ, Wathen CN, et al. Screening for depression in primary care: Recommendation statement from the Canadian Task Force on Preventive Health Care. CMAJ. 2005;172(1):33–35.
26. National Institute for Clinical Excellence. Depression: Core Interventions in the Management of Depression in Primary and Secondary Care. London, UK; 2004.
27. Kroenke K, Spitzer RL, Williams JB. The PHQ-9: Balidity of a brief depression severity measure. J Gen Intern Med. 2001;16(9):606–613.
28. Kroenke K, Spitzer RL, Williams JB. The Patient Health Questionnaire-2: Validity of a two-item depression screener. Med Care. 2003;41(11):1284–1292.
29. Gilbody S, Sheldon T, House A. Screening and case-finding instruments for depression: A meta-analysis. CMAJ. 2008;178(8):997–1003.
30. Fuchs CH, Haradhvala N, Hubley S, et al. Physician actions following a positive PHQ-2: Implications for the implementation of depression screening in family medicine practice. Fam Syst Health. 2015;33(1):18–27.
31. U.S. Preventive Services Task Force. Screening for depression in adults. Ann Intern Med 2009;151(11):784–792.
32. American Psychiatric Association. Diagnostic and Statistical Manual of Mental Disorders (5th ed.). Washington, D.C.: American Psychiatric Association; 2013.

33. Kessler RC, Berglund P, Demler O, et al. The epidemiology of major depressive disorder: Results from the National Comorbidity Survey Replication (NCS-R). JAMA. 2003;289(23):3095–3105.
34. Shedler J, Beck A, Bensen S. Practical mental health assessment in primary care. Validity and utility of the Quick PsychoDiagnostics Panel. J Fam Pract. 2000;49(7):614–621.
35. Rogers WH, Lerner D, Adler DA. Technological approaches to screening and case finding for depression. In: Mitchell AJ, Coyne JC, ed. Screening for Depression in Clinical Practice: An Evidence-Based Guide. New York: Oxford University Press; 2010.
36. Beck A, Nimmer C. A case study: The Kaiser Permanente integrated care project. In: Maruish M, ed. Handbook of Psychological Assessment in Primary Care Settings. Mahwah, NJ: Lawrence Erlbaum Associates; 2000.

PART II

Integrative Care for Psychiatry and Primary Care

11

Integrated Care for Anxiety Disorders

ROBERT D. DAVIES, ISABELLE GUILLEMET, AND ADAM TROSTERMAN

BOX 11.1

KEY POINTS

- **Anxiety disorders are prevalent in primary care settings but most often go undiagnosed and untreated.**
- **Brief targeted screening of primary care patients can increase the rates of diagnosis of anxiety disorders.**
- **Serotonin specific reuptake inhibitors (SSRIs) are considered first-line treatment for all anxiety disorders. Serotonin norepinephrine reuptake inhibitors (SNRIs) are also considered first-line treatment for all anxiety disorders, excluding obsessive-compulsive disorder (OCD).**
- **Benzodiazepines are commonly used in the treatment of anxiety disorders and have proven efficacy, but they are not considered first-line treatments because of the risk of dependency.**
- **Psychoeducation, exercise, and lifestyle modification can be of particular benefit for individuals with mild forms of anxiety disorders.**
- **Relaxation response training has been shown to be helpful in the treatment of panic attacks, generalized anxiety disorder, and other anxiety disorders.**
- **Mindfulness meditation is beneficial in the reduction of anxiety and stress. Mindfulness-based cognitive therapy goes a step further and incorporates concepts of mindfulness into more traditional cognitive-behavioral therapy (CBT).**
- **CBT has been shown to be as effective as medications in the treatment of anxiety disorders.**
- **Group CBT may be particularly appropriate in an integrated care setting as it is an efficient use of therapist time and practice resources.**
- **Exposure and response prevention therapy is indicated for treatment of OCD.**
- **Treatments for posttraumatic stress disorder include trauma-focused CBT, prolonged exposure therapy, and eye movement desensitization and reprocessing (EMDR).**
- **Multidisciplinary, integrated collaborative models of care have been shown to be effective approaches to treating anxiety disorders in the primary care setting.**

INTRODUCTION

This chapter addresses an integrated care approach for assessing and managing the most common anxiety disorders seen in primary care settings. An overview of the key elements of the integrated care approach is contained in Box 11.1. As a group, anxiety disorders are among the most prevalent disorders seen in primary care, with approximately 19.5% of primary care patients having at least one anxiety disorder.[1] Generalized anxiety disorder (GAD), panic disorder (PD), social phobia (SP), obsessive-compulsive disorder (OCD), and posttraumatic stress disorder (PTSD) are among the most common.[2] Unfortunately, very few individuals with an anxiety disorder realize the need to seek help, and even fewer (14%) actually do seek help.[3] Individuals in the general population are half as likely to seek help for anxiety than for depression, with fewer than one-third ever receiving appropriate treatment.[4] The majority of patients with either mood or anxiety disorders present to primary care with somatic, rather than psychological, complaints.[5] This is particularly true of anxiety disorders, as unexplained, vague, and often frightening physical symptoms are integral components of most anxiety disorders. When patients with anxiety disorders present with somatic complaints, the likelihood of their anxiety disorder being recognized and diagnosed drops dramatically, which in turn results in them not receiving appropriate treatment.[6] Primary care physicians (PCPs) should be aware that 40% to 50% of primary care patients with medically unexplained symptoms have an anxiety disorder,[7] with the number of individual somatic complaints having a positive correlation to the likelihood of either a depressive, anxiety, or somatoform disorder.[8,9] The failure to recognize and diagnose anxiety disorders results not only in the lack of appropriate treatment, but also in a significant time and resource burden for the PCP. Once identified and diagnosed, however, anxiety disorders are responsive to a variety of effective pharmacologic and nonpharmacologic psychotherapeutic interventions.

ANXIETY DISORDERS

Panic Disorder

Epidemiology, Clinical Presentation, and Diagnosis

The lifetime prevalence of PD is 3.5%, with women being twice as likely to be afflicted.[10] The onset of symptoms for PD is typically between the ages of 18 and 45, with the average age of onset being 24.

Patients typically present with unexplained physical symptoms such as palpitations, shortness of breath, chest pain, or abdominal distress. Patients most often present for medical attention complaining of these physical symptoms. Panic attacks are defined by the sudden onset of intense fear or discomfort, accompanied by at least four of the following physical or psychological symptoms: palpitations, sweating, trembling, shortness of breath, choking sensation, chest pain, nausea, dizziness, chills or hot flushes, paresthesias, feelings of unreality (derealization) or being detached from oneself (depersonalization), fear of losing control or "going crazy," and fear of dying. These symptoms typically peak within minutes. PD is diagnosed in individuals when they experience recurrent, unexpected panic attacks, and then worry about future attacks or the consequences of attacks, or modify their behavior in order to avoid future attacks.[11]

Course and Comorbidities

PD tends to be a chronic disorder that waxes and wanes in severity over time. Individuals with PD have high rates of medical and psychiatric comorbidities, including chronic obstructive pulmonary disease, cardiovascular diseases, asthma, irritable bowel syndrome, migraines, fatigue, and major depression,[12–14] that further complicate the accurate diagnosis and treatment. These individuals also have higher risks of alcohol use disorders and suicide than the normal population.[15]

Differential Diagnosis

The psychiatric differential diagnoses include distinguishing panic disorder from GAD, SP, PTSD, OCD, and some personality disorders (e.g., borderline, avoidant, and obsessive-compulsive personality disorders [OCPD]).

The medical differential diagnosis (in particular for PD and GAD) includes conditions that may have similar symptoms or clinical presentations, such as hyperthyroidism, hyperparathyroidism, arrhythmias, valvular disease, obstructive pulmonary diseases, transient ischemic attacks, temporal lobe epilepsy, and substance-induced panic disorders. See Figure 11.1 for differential diagnosis and Table 11.1, which outlines the common medical conditions associated with all anxiety disorders.

It is also important to exclude other medications, substance use or withdrawal, and exposure to environmental or occupational toxins as potential causes of anxiety symptoms.[16] See Table 11.2.

Neurobiology

The neurobiology of PD is believed to involve excessive activity of the amygdala, as well as its efferent and afferent projections. Misinterpretation of somatic inputs results in triggering the fear response involving

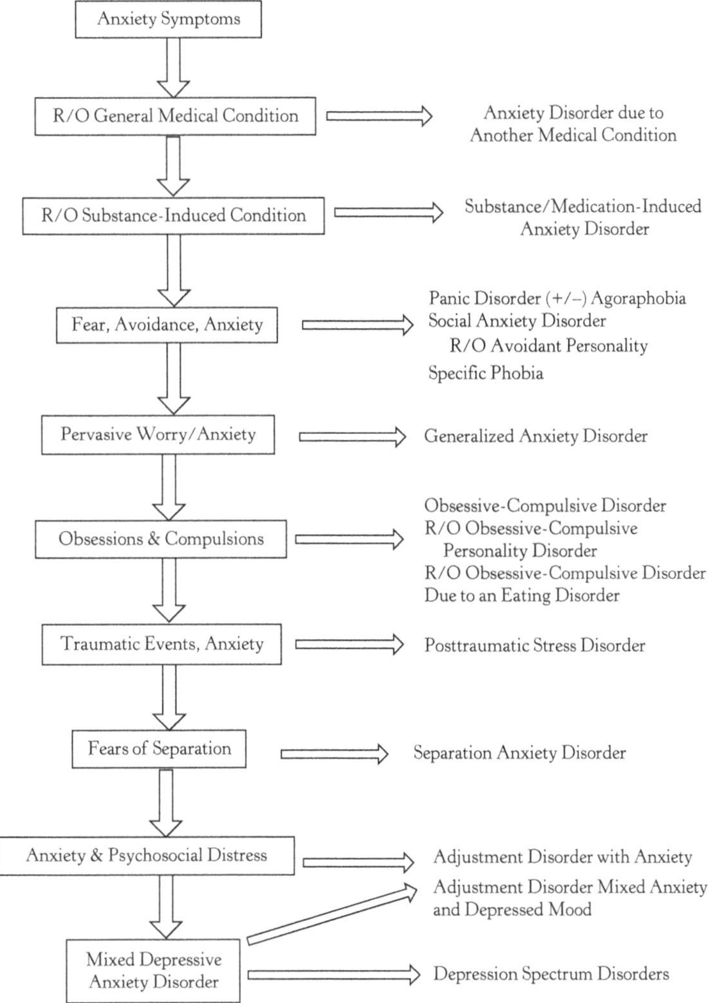

FIGURE 11.1. Differential diagnosis of anxiety disorders.

the autonomic nervous system. Serotonin is thought to modulate the resulting hyper-noradrenergic state.

Generalized Anxiety Disorder

Epidemiology, Clinical Presentation, and Diagnosis

The lifetime prevalence for GAD in the U.S. population is 3.1%; it occurs twice as often in women as in men. The average age of onset is 30 years of age.[10] GAD is diagnosed by the presence for more than six months of excessive anxiety and/or worry about a variety of topics (e.g., finances, work, health, or safety). The anxiety or worry is accompanied by at least three other physical or cognitive symptoms, including edginess or restlessness, fatigue, impaired concentration, irritability, muscle aches or soreness, and trouble sleeping.[11] Patients presenting with GAD may complain of numerous vague health concerns or may report the associated GAD physical symptoms.

Course and Comorbidities

Many patients with GAD have symptoms that have an onset during childhood and adolescence, though many patients also present for the first time in their twenties. GAD has a chronic and often fluctuating course, which is easily exacerbated by stress.

Individuals with GAD have higher rates of psychiatric comorbidity than those with other anxiety disorders, and it is one of the most common comorbid conditions with other disorders. The most common comorbid conditions seen with

TABLE 11.1. MEDICAL CONDITIONS ASSOCIATED WITH ANXIETY DISORDERS

Medical Condition	Associated Anxiety Disorder	Patients with Anxiety Disorder
	Cardiac Conditions	
Atypical chest pain seen in the emergency department	PD	16%
Chest pain and normal coronaries	PD	34%
Negative cardiac workup	PD	55%
Cardiologist office	All anxiety disorders	57%
Intensive care unit patients	PD	33%
Post infarction failure	PD	16%
Cardiomyopathy	PD	83%
Cardiovascular transplantation	PD	16%
	Respiratory Conditions	
Chronic obstructive pulmonary disease	PD	24%
Asthma (children)	All anxiety disorders	43.2%
	Separation disorder	32.4%
	Gastrointestinal	
Primary biliary cirrhosis	Panic and phobia	10%
Irritable bowel	All anxiety disorders	29%
	PD	18%
	Neurological	
Parkinson disease	PD/SP	21–17%
Sydenham chorea	OCD	13%
Tourette syndrome	OCD	35–50%
Tics	OCD	20%
Seizures	Panic/GAD and OCD	Unknown
Postconcussive/transient ischemic attack	Panic/GAD	Unknown
	Endocrine	
Thyroid disease	GAD/PD	62%
Adrenal disease	GAD/PD	Unknown
	Others	
Pheochromocytoma	Panic attacks	Common
Porphyria	Panic attacks	Common
Sjögren syndrome	Phobia	10%
Chronic pain	Panic attacks	16%
Sleep disorders	Panic attacks	Occasional
Toxic gas	PTSD	Unknown
Infections	All anxiety disorders	Rare

GAD are major depressive disorder and dysthymia, although there are also high rates of bipolar disorder, SP, PD, and substance use disorders (particularly alcohol).[17]

Differential Diagnosis

In assessing the differential diagnosis for patient with GAD, review Figure 11.1 and Tables 11.1 and 11.2.

TABLE 11.2. DRUGS OF ABUSE, MEDICATIONS, AND TOXINS INDUCING ANXIETY SYMPTOMS

Drug Intoxications	Drug Withdrawal	Medications Inducing Anxiety	Psychiatric Medications	Environmental Toxins
• Caffeine • Alcohol • Cocaine • Amphetamine • Cannabis • Hallucinogens • Inhalants • Phencyclidine	• Alcohol • Sedatives/ hypnotics • Opiates • Cocaine	• Antihypertensive and cardiovascular medications • Calcium channel blockers and digitalis • Sympathomimetics and bronchodilators • Anesthetics • Analgesics • Anticholinergic and antiparkinsonian agents • Insulin • Thyroid preparations • Oral contraceptives and/ or hormone replacement • Antihistamines • Anticonvulsants	• Lithium • Antidepressants • Antipsychotics	• Gasoline • Paint • Organophosphate • Insecticides • Carbon dioxide • Carbon monoxide • Nerve gas

Neurobiology

GAD is believed to result from hyperactive, dysregulated brain circuits, including the thalamus, basal ganglia, temporal lobe, and fronto/cingulate cortex. Serotonin and norepinephrine play primary roles in these circuits, with individuals with GAD having low levels of serotonin and high levels of norepinephrine in their cerebrospinal fluid. Dysregulated benzodiazepine receptors appear to play a role as well.[18] These hyperactive circuits result in hypervigilance, motor tension, worry, and autonomic response.

Social Phobia

Epidemiology, Clinical Presentation, and Diagnosis

SP is the most common anxiety disorder, and therefore one of the most common psychiatric disorders, with a one-year prevalence of 5% to 8%[19–21] and a lifetime prevalence of 13.3%.[10] The onset of SP is typically between the ages of 11 and 19.[22] Unlike GAD and PD, there is no gender difference in the prevalence of SP.[23]

Patients often present with a childhood history of social inhibition or shyness, but SP is more disabling than just mere shyness, as individuals with SP experience a persistent, intense fear of one or more social or performance situations that impacts their ability to function. Since individuals with SP know specifically what triggers their anxiety, and avoid those situations, they are less likely to seek treatment than those with either PD or GAD, and therefore commonly go undiagnosed.[24] Most patients with SP fear public speaking, may be afraid of speaking to or meeting strangers, and may fear using public restrooms or eating, drinking, or writing in public. Cognitively, these individuals fear that they will humiliate or embarrass themselves.[11]

Course and Comorbidities

SP tends to be a chronic condition that can have a significant deleterious effect on an individual's ability to function effectively in relationships, academics, and work settings.[22,25] Approximately half of patients with SP have comorbid psychiatric conditions, including major depression, dysthymia, OCD, PD, bipolar disorder, or substance use disorders (most commonly alcohol use disorders).[26,27] SP most commonly precedes the onset of these comorbidities, suggesting that untreated SP may play a role in the development of the other disorders.[22,25]

Differential Diagnosis

When assessing the differential diagnosis for patients with SP, also consider avoidant personality disorder in the differential diagnosis. Review Figure 11.1 and Table 11.1 and Table 11.2.

Neurobiology

A clear biological basis for SP has yet to be elucidated, although neuroimaging studies have suggested a primary role of the amygdala and insula, with norepinephrine, dopamine, and serotonin systems likely contributing to the pathophysiology.[24]

Obsessive-Compulsive Disorder

Epidemiology, Clinical Presentation, and Diagnosis

OCD has a lifetime prevalence of 1.6% and an average age of onset of 19.[28] The gender ratio in OCD is 1:1, although males tend to have an earlier onset.[29] OCD patients are likely to present for medical attention not for their anxiety but for the physical sequelae of their compulsive behaviors, such as dermatologic excoriation (from excessive handwashing) or dramatic weight loss (from fears of contamination from food). Most people who have OCD know that their obsessions and compulsions are illogical, yet they feel powerless to stop them. OCD patients can spend hours performing complex rituals involving handwashing, checking, or counting to ward off persistent, troubling thoughts, feelings, or fantasies. Obsessions and compulsions can interfere with the person's normal routine, schoolwork, job, family, or social activities. The focus on obsessive thoughts and performing rituals can make daily functioning difficult. An individual having either obsessions or compulsions defines OCD, although the majority of sufferers experience both. Obsessions are recurrent, intrusive thoughts, images, or urges, while compulsions are recurrent, compulsive physical or mental acts.[11]

Course and Comorbidities

OCD usually follows a chronic waxing and waning course. If untreated, OCD can progress to a severe disability. Symptoms can partially remit for months or years, only to return and worsen. Spontaneous remission is rare. Many patients experience progressive worsening of their symptoms. Stress exacerbates OCD. Most people with OCD feel better if they keep busy, as idleness can increase obsessional thinking. Women with OCD often report an increase in symptoms prior to their menstrual periods.

Individuals with OCD have high rates of comorbid depression, OCPD, other personality disorders, eating disorders (including both anorexia nervosa and bulimia nervosa), attention-deficit/hyperactivity disorder, PD, and GAD.[30,31] Unlike other anxiety disorders, the rate of substance use disorders in OCD is no greater than in the general population.[31]

Differential Diagnosis

OCD was considered an anxiety disorder in the *Diagnostic and Statistical Manual of Mental Disorders, Fourth Edition, Treatment Revision* (DSM-IV-TR)[32] because anxiety symptoms are often severe when a patient is not obsessing or performing compulsions. Because anxiety is prominent in OCD patients, we included it in this chapter despite the fact that the *Diagnostic and Statistical Manual of Mental Disorders, Fifth Edition* (DSM-5) placed OCD in its own category with its related disorders (including body dysmorphic disorder, trichotillomania, and excoriation disorder).[11]

When assessing the differential diagnosis for OCD, review Figure 11.1 and Tables 11.1 and Table 11.2. OCPD must also be considered in the differential. OCPD is often confused with OCD both by physicians and the general public. Individuals with OCPD are preoccupied with control, rules, and orderliness but lack the actual obsessions or compulsions seen in OCD. Chapter 17: Personality Disorders in an Integrated Care Setting provides additional information on differentiating OCD from OCPD.

There is a similarity between OCD and the clinical presentations of obsessions and compulsions that occur as part of an eating disorder. In view of the high rates of co-occurrence, it is essential that a clinical distinction is made between eating disorders and OCD in order to direct appropriate treatment. When they co-occur, the onset of OCD typically precedes the onset of the eating disorder, which suggests that OCD somehow is a vulnerability factor in the development of either anorexia nervosa or bulimia nervosa.[33] The fear of eating in OCD typically relates to contamination obsessions, while in eating disorders the concern is weight gain. See Chapter 15: Integrated Care for Binge Eating Disorder and Other Eating Disorders for a full discussion. OCD is also frequently seen in individuals with temporal lobe epilepsy and stroke and may be associated with streptococcal infection, in children, called pediatric autoimmune neuropsychiatric disorders (PANDAS).

Neurobiology

The neurobiology behind OCD is complex and has yet to be fully elucidated. The growing literature on neuroimaging studies points to involvement of the dorsolateral prefrontal cortex, basal ganglia, thalamus, and limbic system.[34,35] Furthermore, imaging studies have shown decreased serotonin transporter availability in the thalamus and midbrain, as well as decreased dopamine transporter availability in the striatum.[36] This supports the efficacy of pharmacologic interventions targeting these neurotransmitters. Given the suspected role of the basal ganglia, it is not surprising that OCD frequently occurs in individuals with primary basal ganglia dysfunction, such as Tourette syndrome, Sydenham chorea, Huntington disease, and von Economo encephalitis.[37]

Posttraumatic Stress Disorder

Epidemiology, Clinical Presentation, and Diagnosis

The overall lifetime prevalence of PTSD is 6.8%, with the lifetime prevalence in men being 3.6% and in women being 9.7%.[28] Any patient, of any age, who is exposed to a highly traumatic event can develop an acute stress disorder that may or may not lead to PTSD. An acute stress disorder has similar symptoms with duration from two days to four weeks. If symptoms related to a trauma persist beyond four weeks, the disorder is classified as PTSD. The symptoms of PTSD include (1) persistent re-experiencing of the trauma through distressing recollections, dreams, a sense of reliving the event, flashbacks, or psychophysiological reactions when exposed to cues that may represent the event; (2) avoidance of stimuli associated with the trauma; (3) negative alterations in cognitions and mood associated with the trauma, such as a numbing of general responsiveness, the inability to remember important aspects of the trauma, detachment from others, persistent negative beliefs about oneself or others, or persistent negative emotions; and (4) an increase in arousal such as insomnia, startle response, hypervigilance, or reckless, self-destructive behavior. These symptoms can cause significant distress and/or impairment in social or occupational functioning. Traumatic events involve actual or threatened death, serious injury, or sexual violence. Traumas can be experienced directly or may be observed. Hearing about such a trauma involving family or a close friend or repeatedly being exposed to the details of a trauma can also result in symptoms and is called trauma by proxy. Patients often describe survival guilt and avoidance of any situation or people that bring back memories of the traumatic event. Patients with PTSD often develop interpersonal difficulties such as marital conflict, divorce, occupational and social dysfunction, and substance abuse.

Course and Differential Diagnosis

PTSD can occur at any age. Within the first three months after a trauma, symptoms related to the trauma may begin, although at times there may be a long delay in onset (months to years). Initially an acute trauma may meet the criteria for acute stress disorder. The symptoms of PTSD vary over time and duration; many people fully recover from trauma while some individuals have persistent symptoms over their lifetimes. Older isolated patients, with deteriorating health or cognitive functioning, may experience a re-emergence or exacerbation of their PTSD. Children may experience traumas related to neglect, physical or sexual abuse, and/or witnessing intimate partner violence. They typically present with mood, avoidant, or other behavioral disorders. Irritable or aggressive behaviors and symptoms similar to those in adults are common. Some adolescents feel they have been changed by a trauma and no longer fit in with their peer group.

PTSD, like OCD, was considered an anxiety disorder in the DSM-IV-TR because traumatized patients often have prominent anxiety symptoms when reliving or discussing their traumas. For this reason, we included it in this chapter despite the fact that PTSD now appears in its own section, Trauma and Stressor-Related Disorders, in the DSM-5. When assessing the differential diagnosis for PTSD, refer to Figure 11.1 and Tables 11.1 and Table 11.2.

Neurobiology

The neurobiology of PTSD is a complex interplay of brain circuitry, hormonal, and neurochemical changes. The neural circuit involved mediates adaptation to stress and fear conditioning and consists of the hippocampus, amygdala, anterior cingulate gyrus, insula, and orbitofrontal region. In PTSD, this circuit is impacted by abnormal regulation of catecholamine, serotonin, amino acid, peptide, and opioid neurotransmitters, as well as downregulation of pituitary cortisol releasing hormone receptors. This includes an overall dysregulation of the hypothalamic-pituitary axis in response to stressors.[38] Individuals with PTSD have very high rates of psychiatric comorbidity (and often multiple comorbidities), including alcohol and substance use disorders, depressive disorders, psychotic disorders, personality disorders, GAD, and PD, as well as high rates of somatic complaints and disorders. The presence of PTSD also markedly increases the risk for suicide, so individuals with PTSD must be closely monitored.

Mixed Anxiety Depressive Disorder

While anxiety and depressive symptoms often co-occur, there is considerable debate as to whether there is a distinct condition called mixed anxiety depressive disorder. It is estimated that approximately 1% of the population experiences symptoms of both anxiety and depression but do not meet the full criteria for any disorder in either category. Such individuals may be overrepresented in primary care settings. Mixed anxiety depressive disorder was included in the appendix of the DSM-IV-TR as a diagnostic category requiring further research but was not included in the DSM-5. Given the debate, little is known about the epidemiology of this condition. Fortunately, there is considerable overlap between the psychopharmacologic and psychotherapeutic interventions for both depressive disorders and anxiety disorders. Therefore, it is reasonable to expect that these interventions will have efficacy in the combined disorder.

SCREENING FOR ANXIETY DISORDERS IN INTEGRATED CARE SETTINGS

Given the underrecognition and underdiagnosis of anxiety disorders in primary care settings, screening is all the more important. Naturally, it would not be feasible to screen every patient at every visit, but targeted screening could result in a marked improvement in accurate diagnosis and treatment. Four clinical indications increase the likelihood for positive screening of anxiety disorders: (1) patients with a high somatic symptom count, (2) patients with a high severity of somatic symptoms, (3) patients exposed to a recent stressor, or (4) patients with poor self-rated health.[9] Patients presenting with any of these four indicators should be screened for possible anxiety disorders. If screening is positive, they should undergo a more extensive evaluation in order to accurately diagnose their condition. Brief screens with excellent validity include the Overall Anxiety Severity and Impairment Scale (OASIS),[39] the Generalized Anxiety Disorder-7 (GAD-7),[40] and the Generalized Anxiety Disorder-2 (GAD-2).[41] The OASIS is a five-item self-report scale that is good for screening for any single anxiety disorder or multiple co-occurring anxiety disorders.[39] The GAD-2 is a simple two-question general initial screen for anxiety: "Over the past 2 weeks have you (1) been feeling nervous, anxious, or on edge; and (2) not been able to stop or control worrying." If positive, it can be followed up with the GAD-7, which screens more specifically for GAD, PD, and SP,[41] and the Trauma Screening Questionnaire (TSQ)[42] for PTSD. While a good brief initial screening tool for OCD does not exist, patients can be clinically screened using two questions: (1) "Do you ever have a thought or image that keeps coming into your head that you can't dismiss?" and (2) "Do you ever feel the need to repeatedly do certain behaviors that you have a hard time resisting?" If the individual says yes to either of these, then the more extensive Yale-Brown Obsessive Compulsive Scale (Y-BOCS)[43] should be administered.

TREATMENT OF ANXIETY DISORDERS

Pharmacologic Treatment

Serotonin specific reuptake inhibitors (SSRIs), such as fluoxetine, sertraline, paroxetine, citalopram, and escitalopram, are considered first-line treatment for all anxiety disorders.[44–48] Serotonin norepinephrine reuptake inhibitors (SNRIs) such as venlafaxine or duloxetine are also considered first-line treatment for all anxiety disorders, excluding OCD.[44] Both of these medication classes are typically well tolerated, although they may exacerbate anxiety early in treatment. Individuals with anxiety disorders (particularly PD and GAD) may be particularly sensitive to this initial effect, necessitating the starting dose below that typically recommended for the treatment of depression. Although conventional wisdom dictates target doses for GAD, PD, and SP as being typically higher than that for depressive illnesses, the existing literature does not consistently support this, with studies showing individuals responding to a range of dosages.[44] Therefore, it is important to titrate dosages to clinical effect. A positive dose–response relationship does, however, exist for OCD, with higher doses of SSRIs demonstrating greater efficacy.[49]

Benzodiazepines are commonly used in the treatment of anxiety disorders and have proven efficacy.[44,50] However, controversy continues to surround their use owing to risks of dependency as well as other health risks, especially in the elderly.[51] For those reasons, benzodiazepines are not considered first-line treatments and should only be used for brief periods of time, such as during the initiation of SSRI or SNRI treatment.[48] Longer-acting benzodiazepines, such as clonazepam, are preferable to short-acting forms, such as alprazolam and lorazepam. When used, benzodiazepines should be prescribed as a standing dose, with as-needed dosing being reserved for rare anxiety-producing situations such as public speaking or air travel.

Pregabalin, a calcium channel modulator, has been shown to be efficacious in the treatment of GAD[44,52] in doses of 200 to 300 mg/day. One of the benefits of pregabalin over the antidepressants in GAD is that the onset of action can be as early as one to two days.

Gabapentin, at doses of 300 to 400 mg three times a day, does not have the same robust evidence of efficacy as pregabalin, although growing evidence of its benefit as an adjunct treatment in anxiety disorders may make it a safer alternative to benzodiazepines.

The serotonin partial agonist buspirone, in doses of 15 to 30 mg twice a day, was one of the first medications to receive U.S. Food and Drug Administration (FDA) approval for the treatment of GAD and offered a safe alternative to benzodiazepines. Unfortunately, in the intervening years, studies have yielded mixed results, so buspirone is no longer considered a first-line treatment.[53] No evidence supports its use as a primary treatment in the other anxiety disorders.

Atypical antipsychotics have been looked at as potential treatments for anxiety disorders, given their calming effect in psychotic illnesses. Although not considered standalone treatments, quetiapine has been shown to be a beneficial adjunct in the treatment of GAD,[44,54] while risperidone and aripiprazole have shown efficacy as adjuncts in OCD.[55] Studies have evaluated quetiapine, risperidone, and olanzapine as adjunctive medications to SSRIs in the treatment of PTSD with somewhat mixed results.[56]

Anticonvulsants, such as lamotrigine, carbamazepine, valproate, and topiramate, have been used to treat the impulsivity and emotional lability often seen in PTSD, although research findings have been mixed at best.

Prazosin, an alpha-blocker, at doses between 1 and 15 mg at bedtime, is effective in decreasing nightmares and improving sleep in PTSD.

Beta-blockers such as propranolol, at doses of 10 to 80 mg, have been shown to be effective for simple SP (such as performance anxiety) and for decreasing hyperarousal in PTSD.

Table 11.3 outlines medication algorithms for GAD, PD, SP, OCD, and PTSD.

TABLE 11.3. SEQUENCE OF MEDICATION TRIALS FOR ANXIETY DISORDERS

Anxiety Disorder	*Prescribing Sequence*
PD	SSRI or SNRI: Start at very low doses (fluoxetine 5 mg/day or equivalent) and titrate as tolerated to effective dose. If inadequate response, switch SSRI or SNRI, or change to tricyclic antidepressant (TCA). Benzodiazepines may be started concomitantly if anxiety is severe. Long-acting formulations such as clonazepam 0.5–1.0 mg twice daily are preferred. Avoid as-needed scheduling. Benzodiazepines should be discontinued within 4–6 weeks.
GAD	SSRI or SNRI: Start at very low doses (fluoxetine 5 mg/daily or equivalent) and titrate as tolerated to effective dose. Pregabalin 200–300 mg/day may be used as alternative to SSRI or SNRI if those are not tolerated or are ineffective. Buspirone 10–20 mg twice or three times daily may be used as adjunct or alternative to SSRI or SNRI if those are not tolerated.
SP	SSRI or SNRI. Beta-blocker or short-acting benzodiazepine as needed for simple social phobia (i.e., performance anxiety).
OCD	SSRI: Titrate to maximal dosing as tolerated. If unsatisfactory response, switch SSRI or start clomipramine. May use low-dose atypical antipsychotic as adjunct in severe cases (e.g., olanzapine 5 mg).
PTSD	SSRI or SNRI. Prazosin 1–3 mg at bedtime for nightmares and disrupted sleep. Beta-blockers may be added to target hyperarousal symptoms. Atypical antipsychotics may be added as adjunct for associated psychotic symptoms or severe symptomology.

Psychotherapeutic and Other Nonpharmacologic Treatment

Psychoeducation

For individuals with mild forms of anxiety disorders, psychoeducation can be of particular benefit. Many people with anxiety disorders have experienced worrisome symptoms without any understanding of what is going on and may feel that they are going crazy or have some significant medical issues that have yet to be diagnosed. It is not uncommon for patients with anxiety disorders to be dismissed as hypochondriacs, and to be told by medical professionals that there is nothing really wrong, as explained in Chapter 16: Somatic Symptom Disorders and Illness Anxiety in Integrated Care Settings. Clinicians, by merely sharing a clear diagnosis with patients and explaining what is known about the pathophysiology and treatment, may help them experience a significant reduction in their level of anxiety. Recommending that patients read one of the myriad books widely available today on specific anxiety disorders will help them understand they are not unique in their symptomology and may offer self-help interventions. Workbooks such as Bourne's *The Anxiety and Phobia Workbook*,[57] among others, can help patients understand what they are experiencing and guide them through exercises aimed at decreasing their anxiety.

Exercise and Behavioral Activation

Exercise has been shown to be beneficial in the reduction of anxiety, with aerobic exercise showing no more benefit than nonaerobic.[58] The type of exercise may be less important than the acceptability of the exercise program to the individual. Patients with very sedentary lives may not be compliant with an aggressive routine of strenuous exercise; for them, setting a goal of a daily walk may be appropriate. Patients with anxiety and significant cardiovascular symptoms such as palpitations may need to gradually increase their activity in order to become accustomed to a higher heart rate while exercising. Yoga may be of particular benefit in reducing anxiety owing to its impact on both physical relaxation and mental calming.[59] Lack of motivation and poor compliance with regular exercise recommendations are, however, commonly seen and should be addressed with patients. Chapter 22: Wellness: An Integrated Care Approach includes additional discussion.

Behavioral activation is a form of therapy that can help with a lack of motivation and compliance. Behavioral activation focuses on setting goals and scheduling activities in collaboration with patients. It explores their cognitive processes that result in avoidance and helps to facilitate their "buy-in" and improve compliance. Patients should not be overwhelmed by the medical professional's idea of a reasonable exercise routine.

Relaxation Response Training

Relaxation response training (RRT) has been shown to be an effective complementary treatment for many medical conditions and may be particularly helpful in the treatment of panic attacks, GAD, and other anxiety disorders as well. RRT can take many forms, including controlled diaphragmatic breathing, progressive muscle relaxation, and visual imagery. RRT is basically one antidote to the "flight or fight" response. When practiced two or three times per day for 10 to 20 minutes, RRT can lower anxiety levels. RRT is a necessary part of anxiety disorder treatment when used in combination with desensitization therapy.

Mindfulness Meditation

Mindfulness meditation is beneficial in the reduction of anxiety and stress, including among individuals with anxiety disorders. For patients with anxiety disorders in particular, training the mind to let go of ruminative thoughts and focus on the here and now helps interrupt the cognitive aspects of the anxiety cycle. Mindfulness meditation can be done alone, although some form of guided instruction is beneficial. There are numerous smartphone apps for meditation (such as Headspace,[60] Calm,[61] and Stop, Breathe & Think[62]); recorded guided meditations are also available.[63] A more formal approach to mindfulness meditation is the manualized intervention called mindfulness-based stress reduction (MBSR), developed by Kabat-Zinn.[64] MBSR is typically delivered in a group setting and has been shown to be efficacious in the reduction of anxiety symptoms in clinical populations with anxiety disorders, particularly GAD.[65] Mindfulness-based cognitive therapy (MBCT) goes a step further and incorporates concepts of mindfulness into more traditional cognitive-behavioral therapy (CBT).[66] A recent meta-analysis revealed robust clinical responses for patients with anxiety disorders using mindfulness-based interventions (including MBSR and MBCT).[67] Some patients may be wary of these sorts of interventions owing to an erroneous belief that mindfulness meditation is based on religion, so caution should be employed in recommending them.

Cognitive-Behavioral Therapy

CBT has been shown to be as effective as medications in the treatment of anxiety disorders.[68] CBT is actually a group of treatments, all of which have an underlying premise that our thoughts impact our emotions, which then impact our behaviors. CBT typically consists of gradual exposure to and exploration of thoughts about feared situations. Exposure helps patients face feared situations while remaining psychologically engaged. This allows for the normal conditioning processes involved in fear reduction, such as habituation or extinction, to occur. CBT can be delivered through a variety of modalities, including self-guided workbooks (as previously described), individual manualized treatment, clinician-guided computer modules such as CALM,[69,70] and group therapy. Group CBT may be particularly appropriate in an integrated care setting as it is an efficient use of the therapist's time. In addition, research has shown that including patients with different anxiety disorders in the same group is as effective as providing CBT in disorder-specific groups.[71,72] Most courses of CBT last between 12 and 20 weeks. The format for delivering CBT in the primary care setting will depend primarily on the training and preference of the mental health clinician.

A very specific form of CBT called Exposure/Response Prevention is indicated for OCD.[73,74] In this type of therapy, patients are exposed to the stimuli that trigger their anxiety and then are prevented from performing any behaviors (including escape) that decrease their anxiety. Exposure/Response Prevention relies on the phenomenon of extinction of anxiety for its efficacy. This form of therapy requires a specifically trained behavioral health specialist (BHS) who works in an integrated care setting.

Prolonged Exposure Therapy

Prolonged exposure therapy is a form of CBT designed to treat PTSD.[75] It consists of the re-experiencing of traumatic events through remembering and engaging with, rather than avoiding, reminders of the trauma. Through this controlled re-experiencing, the distress from the traumatic events gradually diminishes. A recent meta-analysis of treatments for trauma-related disorders showed prolonged exposure therapy to have the most consistently robust effect.[76] While efficacious, this therapy requires a highly trained mental health professional, and thus may be beyond the scope of what is practical to provide in an integrated care setting.

Eye Movement Desensitization and Reprocessing

Developed in the late 1980s, eye movement desensitization and reprocessing (EMDR)[77] was initially seen as a "fringe" therapy.[78] EMDR involves leading patients in rapidly moving their eyes back and forth while talking about their trauma. While there is no clear evidence to explain how this therapy works, a meta-analysis of treatments for PTSD concluded that, along with trauma-focused CBT, EMDR is a treatment of choice in patients with PTSD.[76] Incorporating EMDR into an integrated care setting, however, is also limited by the availability of BHSs with proper EMDR training and certification.

Choosing a Treatment Modality

The choice of treatment (e.g., pharmacologic, psychotherapeutic, or a combination) depends on many factors, including the severity of the illness, the preference of the patient, and the training of the available mental health clinicians. For adolescents and young adults, the American Academy of Child and Adolescent Psychiatry practice parameters guidelines recommend psychotherapy as the initial treatment for anxiety disorders with a mild severity. Reasons for combining psychotherapy and medication include (1) the need for acute symptom reduction in moderately to severely anxious youth, (2) a comorbid disorder (i.e., depression) that requires concurrent treatment, and (3) partial response to psychotherapy.[79]

SSRIs have emerged as the medication of choice in the treatment of adolescent anxiety disorders. When anxiety disorder symptoms are moderate to severe, or if impairment makes participation in psychotherapy difficult, or if psychotherapy results in a partial response, treatment with medication is recommended.[79] In February 2004, the FDA issued a black-box warning and advised clinicians to carefully monitor pediatric patients and young adults receiving treatment with antidepressants (including SSRIs) for worsening depression, agitation, or suicidality, particularly when initiating medication treatment or during dose changes. This warning was based on a review of studies of adolescents whose primary diagnosis was depression, not studies of youth with anxiety disorders.[79] Benzodiazepines are not recommended in adolescents due to concerns about dependency and side effects.[80]

For mild to moderately severe conditions in adults, the initial plan may be for either patient-directed CBT (via handouts or self-help books), clinician-guided Internet treatment, or clinician-delivered CBT (individual or group). Medications may be added if there is lack of follow-through by the patient or lack of clinical response. Some patients, however, may prefer to take medication in lieu of therapy.

For more severe conditions, a combination of medication and CBT may be indicated. Although it is unclear if the combination of these two modalities improves acute outcomes, there is evidence that CBT added to medications is beneficial in avoiding relapse.[81,82]

INTEGRATED CARE FOR ANXIETY DISORDERS

Integrated care, following the collaborative care model, is particularly suited for patients with anxiety disorders, given its focus on chronic-disease management. A recent meta-analysis of 79 randomized controlled trials of collaborative care for depression and anxiety, compared to treatment as usual, demonstrated significantly greater short-term and long-term improvement in anxiety outcomes for those treated within a collaborative care model. In addition, measures of mental health, quality of life, and patient satisfaction were higher in patients treated in collaborative care settings.[83] Members of such a team should include the front-desk personnel, nurse/medical assistant, PCP, BHS (master's-level therapist, social worker, psychologist), care coordinator, health coach (if available), and consulting psychiatrist (either through referral or, if available, via telemedicine consultation). Table 11.4 shows a clinical pathway for managing patients with anxiety disorders in an integrated care setting.

Initial Team Member Roles

Front Desk Personnel

For new patients, front desk personnel at registration or check-in can conduct preliminary screening using the GAD-2 or OASIS. Targeted screening (diagnostically specific rating scales) for existing patients can also be performed once patients have been identified as having one of the four "high yield" risk factors previously described.

Medical Assistants/Nurses

The medical assistants/nurses should review completed screens. Positive screens should be communicated to the PCP before the patient is seen. If using the GAD-2 for initial screening (rather than the OASIS), the medical assistant can administer the GAD-7. Regardless of the initial screen used, the medical assistant should then administer the TSQ and ask the two OCD screening questions if initial screening is positive. Medical assistants may add their observations and results of screening into patient registries.

Primary Care Physician

Once a patient has screened positive for anxiety, the PCP should conduct a thorough diagnostic evaluation. Such an evaluation should focus not only on the specific diagnostic criteria for the anxiety disorders, but also on physical symptoms that may point to a medical etiology for the symptoms (e.g., hyperthyroidism, anemia), as well as comorbid psychiatric conditions (e.g., somatic symptom disorders) and substance use disorders. Suspicions of an underlying medical etiology should be followed up by the appropriate diagnostic tests and treatments.

Behavioral Health Specialist

Once the PCP has confirmed a diagnosis of an anxiety disorder, the patient should then be seen by the BHS to assess the severity of the condition. Specific tools are available for assessing severity and monitoring response to treatment for each of the anxiety disorders. For individuals with GAD, the GAD-7 should be used for assessing severity. For PD, the Panic Disorder Severity Scale (PDSS)[84] is available in a self-report format. For SP, the Liebowitz Social Anxiety Scale (LSAS)[85] is also available as a self-report scale. Severity of OCD should be assessed using the clinician-administered Yale-Brown Obsessive Compulsive Scale (Y-BOCS).[43] Symptom severity in PTSD should be assessed using the Davidson Trauma Scale (DTS).[86] BHSs, depending on their training, may begin psychoeducation and a discussion of treatment options.

Psychiatrist

Patients with significant comorbid conditions, including significant depression, suicidal ideation, psychosis, or a substance use disorder, should be referred for a live psychiatric consultation/evaluation or may be evaluated via telemedicine. The

TABLE 11.4. CRITICAL PATHWAY: ANXIETY DISORDERS

	Initial Assessment			Week 1–4	1 month–6 months	7 months–1 year
Time	45–60 minutes			30–60 minutes	30–60 minutes	30 minutes
	Screening	Diagnosis	Education, Medications	Education, Medications, Therapy	Education, Medications, Therapy	Coping, Relapse Prevention, Medications, Therapy
	Front Desk • GAD-2[41] or OASIS[39]; if positive, refer to medical assistant (MA). ***MA*** • GAD-7,[40] TSQ,[42] and OCD questions. • Can refer directly to BHS or PCP if patient is suicidal.	*If OASIS or GAD-2 is positive:* ***BHS, PCP*** • If screens are positive, diagnosis to be made by clinical interview. • Rule out medical causes, substance-induced causes. • Look for comorbid psychiatric conditions (depression, substance use disorders, etc.) ***Consult Psychiatrist*** • All cases of suicidal ideation and significant substance use. ***PCP/Psychiatrist*** • As needed: physical exam, complete blood count, Chem 20 panel, drug screen, TSH.	***Nurse, BHS, Health Coach*** • Psycho-education about anxiety disorders and rationale for treatments. • Discuss need to avoid alcohol, drugs, excessive caffeine; need for regular sleep/wake routine. • Discuss use of exercise and/or self-directed mindfulness activities if indicated. ***PCP*** • Initiate medications, SSRIs, SNRIs, others, if indicated. • Consult psychiatrist if questions regarding safety or hospitalization. ***Care Coordinator*** • Assessment of needs (e.g., refer to emergency department, inpatient, community mental health as advised by the team).	***MA*** • Repeat appropriate severity scales based on diagnosis. • Enter patient in registry. ***Nurse, BHS, Health Coach*** • Clinical reassessment. • Assess suicide risk. ***BHS, PCP, Health Coach*** • Psycho-education. • Confirm diagnosis. • Reassess for other psychiatric, substance, medical comorbidities. • Assess symptoms, insight, medication adherence, level of motivation, coping strategies. • Brief therapies: CBT, behavioral activation, exposure, EMDR. • Continued consultation with psychiatrist. • Update registry.	***MA*** • Repeat appropriate severity scales based on diagnosis. ***Nurse, BHS, Health Coach*** • Clinical reassessment. ***BHS, PCP, Health Coach*** • Confirm diagnosis. • Reassess for other psychiatric, substance, medical comorbidities. • Assess symptoms, insight, medication adherence, level of motivation. • Brief therapies: CBT, behavioral activation, exposure, EMDR. • Continued consultation with psychiatrist. • Update registry. ***PCP, Psychiatrist*** • Assess side effects, tolerability, adherence, insight.	***MA*** • Repeat appropriate severity scales based on diagnosis. ***Nurse, BHS, Health Coach*** • Clinical reassessment. ***BHS, PCP Health Coach*** • Reassess for other psychiatric, substance, or medical comorbidities. • Assess for remission. • Discuss need for potential "booster sessions" of brief therapies. • Update registry. ***PCP, Psychiatrist*** • Assess side effects, tolerability, adherence, insight. • Adjust dosing as needed to decrease anxiety symptoms. • Discuss tapering of medications if remission has been achieved.

(continued)

TABLE 11.4. CONTINUED

	Initial Assessment			Week 1–4	1 month–6 months	7 months–1 year
Time	45–60 minutes			30–60 minutes	30–60 minutes	30 minutes
	Screening	Diagnosis	Education, Medications	Education, Medications, Therapy	Education, Medications, Therapy	Coping, Relapse Prevention, Medications, Therapy
				PCP, Psychiatrist • Assess side effects, tolerability, adherence, insight. • Adjust dosing as appropriate to decrease anxiety symptoms. ***Psychiatrist*** • Consult with PCP on medications as needed. • Track patient population in the registry. ***Care Coordinator*** • Coordinate care with other needed medical, psychiatric, substance abuse, or community services as advised by the team.	• Adjust dosing as appropriate to decrease anxiety symptoms. • Begin taper of benzodiazepines, if used. • Need to reassess for adding second agent or changing to alternative primary agent. ***Psychiatrist*** • Consult with PCP on medications, possible switches. • Track patient /population in registry. ***Care Coordinator*** • As needed	***Psychiatrist*** • Consult with PCP on medications, possible switches. • Track patient/population in registry. ***Care Coordinator*** • Coordinate care with other needed medical, psychiatric, substance abuse, or community services as advised by the team.

consulting psychiatrist can then decide whether the integrated care setting or referral to an outside mental health center or other community resource is most appropriate for the management of that patient. Direct communication between the PCP and the consulting psychiatrist, via a "warm hand-off," is important to ensure that the patient does not get lost in the transfer of care.

Other Integrated Team Members

Care coordinators can be used to develop and coordinate the care plan and may begin inputting information in the patient registry. Health coaches may develop a lifestyle- modification plan designed to help reduce anxiety.

Initial Treatment Planning

After the diagnostic evaluation and assessment of severity has been completed, the PCP, BHS, and care coordinator should discuss the initial treatment plan. The consulting psychiatrist should be included in this discussion for patients who have been referred for consultation. The BHS and/or the PCP should meet with the patient for psychoeducation about his or her condition, the rationale behind the treatment options, and the team's recommendations. Patient buy-in to treatment is paramount, so it is important that the patient be involved in all discussions leading to the final decision regarding which treatment modalities are employed.

Some patients may be opposed to either medications or CBT, and this should be taken into consideration by the treatment team. The treatment plan may include a stepped approach, particularly for patients with mild to moderate anxiety. Interventions that require less staff involvement, such as psychoeducation, lifestyle modification (diet, exercise), self-help manuals, or mindfulness meditation, may be suggested first. If the patient has difficulty with motivation and/or compliance, moving to a more structured, clinician-administered intervention such as mindfulness-based therapy or CBT is indicated.

Team Monitoring and Treatment

Front Desk Personnel

The appropriate self-report monitoring tool should be administered at each visit upon check-in and delivered to the BHS or other members of the integrated care team.

Care Coordinator

Based on team recommendations, the care coordinator should facilitate referrals to other medical specialists, community mental health centers, or other community resources. The coordinator, who knows the dates of the initial appointments, must follow up with the patient to make sure appointments are kept. If the patient is not being referred to the community, the coordinator should maintain monthly in-person contact with the patient to assess his or her motivation and adherence to the treatment plan. Frequent check-ins by phone, text, email, or telehealth may be required for patients struggling to follow through with the treatment recommendations.

The care coordinator and/or the BHS should add data to and monitor the patient's progress and treatment plans in the patient registry. The registry should include basic demographic information, initial chief complaints, comorbid medical conditions, initial anxiety severity ratings, treatment approach, and follow-up severity ratings. This registry will aid the PCP and psychiatrist in characterizing a population of patients with anxiety and can assist in developing and instituting evidence-based algorithmic guidelines and tracking of outcomes.

Behavioral Health Specialists

For all of the anxiety disorders, the BHS should review the results of the appropriate monitoring tool with the patient. He or she should administer the Y-BOCS at each visit for patients with OCD, and the DTS for patients with PTSD. Sharing the results of these monitoring tools with patients is important, as it assists in their cognitive perception of improvement and engagement in treatment. Patients who are not demonstrating improvement should be referred back to the PCP or psychiatrist for reassessment of the treatment plan and medications.

For patients who are engaged in self-guided CBT, the BHS should initially meet with the patient monthly to assess progress and symptom improvement. After three months of improvement, the patient should be seen for a follow-up in six months to assess for stability or recurrence of symptoms.

Regardless of the form of CBT preferred by the practice (individual, clinician-guided online treatment, or group), the BHS should meet monthly with the PCP and care coordinator to discuss changes in symptom severity. Worsening of symptoms or lack of improvement over a four-week period should result in a reassessment of the treatment and/or consultation with the psychiatrist. Patients who were initially treated with CBT alone may require re-evaluation for medication.

Health Coaches

Health coaches can work with the patient to develop and implement an exercise program designed to reduce anxiety. In addition, they can offer motivational strategies and recommendation for other lifestyle modifications such as reducing caffeine intake, facilitating smoking cessation, and providing harm-reduction counseling for alcohol or other drug use that may be exacerbating anxiety symptoms. See Chapter 25: Health Coaching in Integrated Care for more information about the scope of practice for these health professionals.

Primary Care Physician

For patients whose treatment plan included medication, the PCP can initiate treatment at low doses, following the guidelines described earlier; review Table 11.3 for medication options. Dosing should be titrated to clinical response and tolerability. After initiating treatment, the PCP should follow up with the patient within two weeks and then monthly thereafter. Once an adequate dose is achieved (or further increase is limited by lack of tolerability), and if there has been no significant clinical response, either an alternative medication should be initiated or an appropriate adjunctive medication should be added. If this results in no significant response, a consultation with the psychiatrist is warranted. For patients initially treated with medications alone,

BOX 11.2

SUMMARY OF RECOMMENDED TREATMENT APPROACHES AND RELEVANT EVIDENCE

Strength of Recommendation Taxonomy (SOR A, B, or C)

- **A meta-analysis of 79 randomized controlled trials of collaborative care for depression and anxiety, compared to treatment as usual, demonstrated significantly greater short-term and long-term improvement in anxiety outcomes for those treated within a collaborative care model. In addition, measures of mental health quality of life and patient satisfaction were higher in patients treated in collaborative care settings.[83] (SOR B)**
- **SSRIs are efficacious and appropriate for first-line medication treatment for all anxiety disorders.[44–48] (SOR A)**
- **SNRIs can be used as a first-line treatment for all anxiety disorders except OCD.[44] (SOR A)**
- **SSRIs are the first-line treatment for OCD. Higher doses of SSRIs are needed for the treatment of OCD compared to other anxiety disorders.[49] (SOR A)**
- **Benzodiazepines are efficacious for short-term use in anxiety disorders.[44,50] (SOR A)**
- **Pregabalin can also be used to treat GAD.[52] (SOR A)**
- **Buspirone may be an effective adjunct in the treatment of GAD and has little addictive risk.[53] (SOR B)**
- **Atypical antipsychotics can be used as adjunctive treatment in GAD, OCD, and PTSD.[54,55] (SOR B)**
- **Increasing regular exercise can be a helpful lifestyle change in the treatment for anxiety disorders.[58] (SOR B)**
- **Mindfulness-based meditation is efficacious as a treatment for anxiety disorders.[67] (SOR A)**
- **CBT has efficacy as a treatment for anxiety disorders.[68] (SOR A)**
- **Group CBT is an effective treatment for anxiety disorders.[71,72] (SOR A)**
- **Exposure/Response Prevention is a first-line treatment for OCD.[73] (SOR A)**
- **Prolonged exposure therapy is an effective treatment as treatment of PTSD.[76] (SOR A)**
- **EMDR is an effective treatment for PTSD.[76] (SOR A)**
- **Combining psychotherapy and medications may be effective when treating anxiety disorders.[81,82] (SOR C)**

poor clinical response may also suggest a need for the addition of CBT.[87] At any point in treatment, the appearance of suicidal ideation, psychosis, manic symptoms, or substance abuse necessitates a referral to the consulting psychiatrist.

Follow-up

Patients who receive pharmacologic treatment from the PCP or psychiatrist should be maintained on the effective dose of medication for at least 12 months after achieving clinical remission.[88] However, since anxiety disorders tend to be chronic conditions, the likelihood of eventual recurrence is high. Patients should be tracked in the registry at every office visit and followed annually for anxiety by a designated member of the integrated care team, rescreened for symptoms, and encouraged to contact the treatment team if they notice a return of their symptoms. Patients who complete a course of CBT should likewise be monitored on an annual basis for signs of recurrence and referred back to the BHS if additional psychotherapy is warranted.

CONCLUSION

The majority of individuals with anxiety disorders choose to seek treatment in a non-psychiatric setting. Unfortunately, many PCPs feel ill equipped to accurately diagnose and treat these individuals. Undiagnosed and untreated anxiety disorders result in significant morbidity for patients. Targeted screening and an organized, collaborative, integrated team-based approach to treatment have been shown to improve time to treatment and to result in a more efficient utilization of resources and improved overall health for this at-risk population. Box 11.2 summarizes the recommended treatment approaches.

REFERENCES

1. Kroenke K, Spitzer RL, Williams JBW, Monohan PO, Lowe B. Anxiety disorders in primary care: Prevalence, impairment, comorbidity and detection. Ann Intern Med. 2007;146(5):317–332.
2. Craske MG, Stein MB, Sullivan G, et al. Disorder-specific impact of coordinated anxiety learning and management treatment for anxiety disorders in primary care. Arch Gen Psychiatry. 2011;68(4):378–388.
3. Mojtabai R, Olfson M, Mechanic D. Perceived need and help-seeking in adults with mood, anxiety, or substance use disorders. Arch Gen Psychiatry. 2002;59(1):77–84.
4. Stein MB, Sherbourne CD, Craske MG, et al. Quality of care for primary care patients with anxiety disorders. Am J Psychiatry. 2004;161(12):2230–2237.
5. Simon GE, Von Korff M, Piccinelli M, Fullerton C, Ormel J. An international study of the relation between somatic symptoms and depression. N Engl J Med. 1999;341(18):1329–1335.
6. Kirmayer LJ, Robbins JM, Dworkind M, Yaffe MJ. Somatization and the recognition of depression and anxiety in primary care. Am J Psychiatry. 1993;150(5):734–741.
7. Kroenke K, Spitzer RL, Williams JBW, et al. Physical symptoms in primary care: Predictors of psychiatric disorders and functional impairment. Arch Fam Med. 1994; 3(9):774–779.
8. Kroenke K, Jackson JL, Chamberlin J. Depressive and anxiety disorders in patients presenting with physical complaints: Clinical predictors and outcome. Am J Med. 1997;103(5):339–347.
9. Kroenke K. Patients presenting with somatic complaints: Epidemiology, psychiatric co-morbidity and management. Int J Method Psych Res. 2003;12(1):34–43.
10. Kessler RC, McGonagle DK, Zhao S, et al. Lifetime and 12-month prevalence of DSM-III-R psychiatric disorders in the United States. Results from the National Comorbidity Survey. Arch Gen Psychiatry. 1994;51(1):8–19.
11. American Psychiatric Association. Diagnostic and Statistical Manual of Mental Disorders. Fifth Edition. Arlington, VA: American Psychiatric Association; 2013.
12. Noyes R Jr, Hoehn-Saric R. Panic disorder and agoraphobia. In: Noyes RJr, Hoehn-Saric R, eds. The Anxiety Disorders. Cambridge, England: Cambridge University Press; 1998:86–157.
13. Hasler G, Gergen PJ, Kleinbaum DG, et al. Asthma and panic in young adults: A 20-year prospective community study. Am J Respir Crit Care Med, 2005;171(11):1224–1230.
14. Beghi E, Allais G, Cortelli P, et al. Headache and anxiety-depressive disorder comorbidity: The HADAS study. Neurol Sci. 2007;28(suppl 2):S217–S219.
15. Fleet RP, Dupuis G, Marchand A, Burelle D, Arsenault A, Beitman BD. Panic disorder in emergency department chest pain patients: prevalence, comorbidity, suicidal ideation, and physician recognition. Am J Med. 1996;101(4):371–380.
16. Locke AB, Kirst N, Schultz CG. Diagnosis and management of generalized anxiety disorder and panic disorder in adults. Am Fam Physician. 2015;91(9):617–662.
17. Simon N. Generalized anxiety disorder and psychiatric comorbidities such as depression, bipolar disorder, and substance abuse. J Clin Psychiatry. 2009;70(suppl 2):10–14.

18. Nutt DJ, Ballenger JC, Sheehan D, Wittchen H-U. Generalized anxiety disorder: Comorbidity, comparative biology and treatment. Int J Neuropsychopharmacol. 2002;5(4):315–325.
19. Simon, N. Generalized anxiety disorder and psychiatric comorbidities such as depression, bipolar disorder, and substance abuse. J Clin Psychiatry. 2009;70(suppl 2):10–14.
20. Magee WJ, Eaton WW, Wittchen HU, McGonagle KA, Kessler RC. Agoraphobia, simple phobia, and social phobia in the National Comorbidity Survey. Arch Gen Psychiatry. 1996;53(2):159–168.
21. Offord DR, Boyle MH, Campbell D, et al. One-year prevalence of psychiatric disorder in Ontarians 15 to 64 years of age. Can J Psychiatry. 1996;41(9):559–563.
22. Stein MB, Kean YM. Disability and quality of life in social phobia: Epidemiologic findings. Am J Psychiatry. 2000;157(10):1606–1613.
23. Schneier FR, Johnson J, Hornig CD, Liebowitz MR, Weissman MM. Social phobia: Comorbidity and morbidity in an epidemiologic sample. Arch Gen Psychiatry. 1992;49(4):282–288.
24. Fink M, Akimova E, Spindelegger C, Hahn A, Lanzenberger R, Kasper S. Social anxiety disorder: epidemiology, biology and treatment. Psychiatr Danub. 2009;21(4):533–542.
25. McLean CP, Asnaani A, Litz BT, Hofmann SG. Gender differences in anxiety disorders: Prevalence, course of illness, comorbidity and burden of illness. J Psychiatr Res. 2011;45(8):1027–1035.
26. Lydiard RB. Social anxiety disorder: comorbidity and its implications. J Clin Psychiatry. 2001;62(suppl 1):17–23.
27. Schneier FR, Martin LY, Liebowitz MR, Gorman JM, Fyer AJ. Alcohol abuse in social phobia. J Anx Disord. 1989;3(1):15–23.
28. Kessler RC, Berglund PA, Demler O, Jin R, Walters EE. Lifetime prevalence and age-of-onset distributions of DSM-IV disorders in the National Comorbidity Survey Replication (NCS-R). Arch Gen Psychiatry. 2005;62(6):593–602.
29. Mathis MA, Alvarenga PD, Funaro G, et al. Gender differences in obsessive-compulsive disorder: A literature review. Rev Bras Psiaquiatr. 2011;33(4):390–399.
30. Weissman MM, Bland RC, Canino GJ, et al. The cross national epidemiology of obsessive-compulsive disorder: The Cross National Collaborative Group. J Clin Psychiatry. 1994;55(suppl 3):5–10.
31. Overbeek T, Schruers K, Vermetten E, Griez E. Comborbidity of obsessive-compulsive disorder and depression: Prevalence, symptom severity, and treatment effect. J Clin Psychiatry. 2002;63(12):1106–1112.
32. American Psychiatric Association. Diagnostic and Statistical Manual of Mental Disorders. Fourth Edition, Text Revision. Washington, D.C.: American Psychiatry Association; 2000.
33. Kaye WH, Bulik CM, Thornton L, Barbarich N, Masters K, Price Foundation Collaborative Group. Comorbidity of anxiety disorders with anorexia and bulimia nervosa. Am J Psychiatry. 2004;161(12):2215–2221.
34. Friedlander L, Desrocher M. Neuroimaging studies of obsessive-compulsive disorder in adults and children. Clin Psychol Dev. 2006;26(1):32–49.
35. Nakao T, Okada K, Kanba S. Neurobiological model of obsessive-compulsive disorder: Evidence from recent neuropsychological and neuroimaging findings. Psychiatry Clin Neurosci. 2014;68(8):587–605.
36. Hesse S, Müller U, Lincke T, et al. Serotonin and dopamine transporter imaging in patients with obsessive-compulsive disorder. Psychiatry Res. 2005;140(1):63–72.
37. Miguel EC, Rauch SL, Jenike MA. Obsessive-compulsive disorder. Psychiatr Clin North Am. 1997;20(4):863–883.
38. Sherin JE, Nemeroff CB. Post-traumatic stress disorder: The neurobiological impact of psychological trauma. Dialogues Clin Neurosci. 2011;13(3):263–278.
39. Campbell-Sills L, Norman SB, Craske MG, et al. Validation of a brief measure of anxiety-related severity and impairment: the Overall Anxiety Severity and Impairment Scale (OASIS). J Affect Disord. 2009;112:92–101.
40. Spitzer RL, Kroenke K, Williams JB, et al. A brief measure for assessing generalized anxiety disorder: The GAD-7. Arch Intern Med. 2007(10);166:1092–1097.
41. Kroenke K, Spitzer RL, Williams JBW, et al. Anxiety disorders in primary care: Prevalence, impairment, comorbidity, and detection. Ann Intern Med. 2007;146(5):317–325.
42. Brewin CR, Rose S, Andrews B, et al. Brief screening instrument for post-traumatic stress disorder. Br J Psychiatry. 2002;181(2):158–162.
43. Goodman WK, Price LH, Rasmussen SA, et al. The Yale-Brown Obsessive Compulsive Scale (Y-BOCS): Part I. Development, use and reliability. Arch Gen Psychiatry. 1989;46(11):1006–1011.
44. Bandelow B, Sher L, Bunevicius R, et al. Guidelines for the pharmacological treatment of anxiety disorders, obsessive-compulsive disorder and posttraumatic stress disorder in primary care. Int J Psychiatry Clin Pract. 2012;16(2):77–84.
45. Baldwin D, Woods R, Lawson R, Taylor D. Efficacy of drug treatments for generalized anxiety disorder: Systematic review and meta-analysis. BMJ. 2011;342:d1199.
46. Kapczinski F, Lima MS, Souza JS, Schmitt R. Antidepressants for generalised anxiety disorder. Cochrane Database Syst Rev. 2003; (2): CD003592. doi:10.1002/14651858.CD003592.
47. Otto MW, Tuby KS, Gould RA, McLean RY, Pollack MH. An effect-size analysis of the relative efficacy and tolerability of serotonin

selective reuptake inhibitors for panic disorder. Am J Psychiatry. 2001;158(12):1989–1992.
48. Zohar J, Westenberg HG. Anxiety disorders: A review of tricyclic antidepressants and selective serotonin reuptake inhibitors. Acta Psychiatr Scand. 2000;101(Suppl S403):39–49.
49. Bloch MH, Maguire J, Landeros-Weisenberger A, Leckman JF, Pittenger C. Meta-analysis of the dose-response of SSRI in obsessive-compulsive disorder. Mol Psychiatr. 2010;15(8):850–855.
50. Starcevic V. The reappraisal of benzodiazepines in the treatment of anxiety and related disorders. Exp Rev Neurotherapeutics. 2014;14(11):1275–1286.
51. Tannenbaum C. Inappropriate benzodiazepine use in elderly patients and its reduction. J Psychiatry Neurosci. 2015;40(3):E27–E28.
52. Frampton JE. Pregabalin: A review of its use in adults with generalized anxiety disorder. CNS Drugs. 2014;28(9):835–854.
53. Mula M, Pini S, Cassano GB. The role of anticonvulsant drugs in the treatment of anxiety disorders: A critical review of the evidence. J Clin Psychopharm. 2007;27(3):263–272.
54. Hershenberg R, Gros DF, Brawman-Mintzer O. Role of atypical antipsychotics in the treatment of generalized anxiety disorder. CNS Drugs. 2014;38(6):519–533.
55. Veale D, Miles S, Smallcombe N, Ghezai H, Goldacre B, Hodsoll J. Atypical antipsychotic augmentation in SSRI treatment refractory obsessive-compulsive disorder: A systematic review and meta-analysis. BMC Psychiatry. 2014;14(1):317.
56. Alexander W. Pharmacotherapy for post-traumatic stress disorder in combat veterans. P&T. 2012;37(1):32–38.
57. Bourne EJ. The Anxiety and Phobia Workbook, 5th ed. Oakland, CA: New Harbinger Publications, Inc.; 2010.
58. Jayakody K, Gunadasa S, Hosker C. Exercise for anxiety disorders: Systematic review. Br J Sports Med. 2013;48(3):187–196.
59. Kirkwood G, Rampes H, Tuffrey V, Richardson J, Pilkington K. Yoga for anxiety: A systematic review of the research evidence. Br J Sports Med. 2005;39(12):884–891.
60. Say Hello to the Headspace meditation app. (n.d.). Accessed April 4, 2016, from https://www.headspace.com/headspace-meditation-app.
61. Calm.com: A free web app for mini-relaxation sessions—Mindful. (2012). Accessed April 4, 2016, from http://www.mindful.org/calm-com-a-free-web-app-for-mini-relaxation-sessions/.
62. Stop, Breathe & Think App. (2014, September 29). Accessed April 4, 2016, from http://stopbreathethink.org/.
63. The Mindfulness Solution: Everyday Practices for Everyday Problems. (2013). Accessed April 4, 2016, from http://mindfulness-solution.com/.
64. Kabat-Zinn J, Massion AO, Kristeller J, et al. Effectiveness of a meditation-based stress reduction program in the treatment of anxiety disorders. Am J Psychiatry. 1992;149(7):936–943.
65. Hoge EA, Bui E, Marques L, et al. Randomized controlled trial of mindfulness meditation for generalized anxiety disorder: Effects on anxiety and stress reactivity. J Clin Psychiatry. 2013;74(8):786–792.
66. Segal ZV, Williams JMG, Teasdale JD. Mindfulness-Based Cognitive Therapy for Depression: A New Approach to Preventing Relapse. New York: Guilford Press; 2002.
67. Hofmann SG, Sawyer AT, Witt AA, Oh D. The effect of mindfulness-based therapy on anxiety and depression: a meta-analytic review. J Consult Clin Psychol. 2010;78(2):169–183.
68. Stewart R, Chambless D. Cognitive-behavioral therapy for adult anxiety disorders in clinical practice: A meta-analysis of effectiveness studies. J Consult Clin Psychol. 2009;77(4):595–606.
69. Titov N, Andrews G, Johnston L, Robinson E, Spence J. Transdiagnostic Internet treatment for anxiety disorders: A randomized controlled trial. Behav Res Ther. 2010;48(9):890–899.
70. Craske MG, Stein MB, Sullivan G, et al. Disorder-specific impact of coordinated anxiety learning and management treatment for anxiety disorders in primary care. Arch Gen Psychiatry. 2011;68(4):378–388.
71. Norton PJ. A randomized clinical trial of transdiagnostic cognitive-behavioral treatments for anxiety disorders by comparison to relaxation training. Behav Ther. 2012;43(3):506–517.
72. Erickson DH, Janeck AS, Tallman K. Transdiagnostic group CBT for anxiety: Clinical experience and practical advice. J Cogn Psychother. 2009;23(1):34–43.
73. Fisher PL, Wells A. How effective are cognitive and behavioral treatments for obsessive-compulsive disorder? A clinical significance analysis. Behav Res Ther. 2005;43(12):1543–1558.
74. Franklin M, Foa E. Cognitive behavioral treatments for obsessive compulsive disorder. In: Nathan PE, Gorman JM, eds., A Guide to Treatments That Work. New York: Oxford University Press; 2002:367–386.
75. Foa EB, Dancu CV, Hembree EA, et al. A comparison of exposure therapy, stress inoculation training, and their combination for reducing posttraumatic stress disorder in female assault victims. J Consult Clin Psychol. 1999;67(2):194–200.
76. Ponniah K, Hollon SD. Empirically supported psychological treatments for adult acute stress disorders and posttraumatic stress disorder: A review. Depress Anxiety. 2009;26(12):1083–1099.
77. Shapiro F. Efficacy of the eye movement desensitization procedure in the treatment of traumatic memories. J Trauma Stress. 1989;2(2):199–223.

78. Davies RD. Wading through the flood of non-traditional therapies. J Nerv Ment Dis. 2013;201(7):636–637.
79. Connolly SD, Bernstein GA. Practice parameter for the assessment and treatment of children and adolescents with anxiety disorders. J Am Acad Child Adolesc Psychiatry. 2007;46(2):267–283.
80. Kendall PC, Peterman JS. CBT for adolescents with anxiety: Mature yet still developing. Am J Psychiatry. 2015;172(6):519–530.
81. Barlow DH, Gorman JM, Shear MK, Woods SW. Cognitive-behavioral therapy, imipramine, or their combination for panic disorder: A randomized controlled trial. JAMA. 2000;283(19):2529–2536.
82. Wetherell JL, Petkus AJ, White KS, et al. Antidepressant medication augmented with cognitive-behavioral therapy for generalized anxiety disorder in older adults. Am J Psychiatry. 2013;170(7):782–789.
83. Archer J, Bower P, Gilbody S, et al. Collaborative care for depression and anxiety problems. Cochrane Database Syst Rev. 2012; 10: CD006525. DOI: 10.1002/14651858.CD006525.pub2.
84. Shear MK, Brown TA, Barlow DH, et al. Multicenter collaborative panic disorder severity scale. Am J Psychiatry. 1997;154(11):1571–1575.
85. Liebowitz MR. Social phobia. Mod Probl Pharmacopsychiatry. 1987;22:141–173.
86. Davidson JRT. Davidson Trauma Scale. Multi-Health Systems, Inc., 1996.
87. Rodrigues H, Figueira I, Concalves R, Mendlowicz M, Macedo T, Ventura P. CBT for pharmacotherapy non-remitters—a systematic review of a next-step strategy. J Affect Disord. 2011;129(1-3):219–228.
88. Rickels K, Etemad B, Khalid-Khan S, Lohoff FW, Rynn MA, Gallop RJ. Time to relapse after 6 and 12 months' treatment of generalized anxiety disorder with venlafaxine extended release. Arch Gen Psychiatry. 2010;67(12):1274–1281.

12

Treating Depression and Bipolar Disorder in Integrated Care Settings

CHRISTOPHER D. SCHNECK

BOX 12.1
KEY POINTS

- **Major depression and bipolar disorder are among the most commonly encountered psychiatric illnesses in primary care settings and can complicate the assessment, treatment, and outcome of comorbid medical diseases.**
- **An established literature supports the use and effectiveness of collaborative models to treat major depression in primary care settings. A growing body of literature supports the effectiveness of collaborative care in treating bipolar patients in primary care settings.**
- **Primary care teams composed of a primary care provider, a behavioral health specialist (psychologist, social worker, or psychiatric nurse practitioner), a care manager, and a consulting psychiatrist can manage the majority of psychiatric patients effectively.**
- **Use of measurement-based care (depression rating scales) is especially important in the diagnosis and management of depression, whether in major depression or bipolar disorder. The Mood Disorder Questionnaire can be helpful in screening for bipolar disorder in those patients in whom bipolar disorder is suspected.**
- **The majority of bipolar patients in primary care settings should have behavioral health consultation early in the course of treatment, given the overall complexity of the illness and the need for rapid assessment and treatment. Bipolar depressed patients should receive psychiatric consultation at the outset of treatment due to the complex nature of their treatment.**
- **Consultation with a psychiatrist should likely occur if a patient has failed to respond to more than one or two antidepressant trials.**
- **Psychotherapy is an important adjunct to treatment of both major depression and bipolar disorder. In major depression, use of cognitive-behavioral therapy and behavioral activation can be extremely helpful to achieve response/remission. In bipolar disorder, illness education, strategies for medication adherence, and relapse-prevention planning are key elements in improving outcome.**

INTRODUCTION

Mood disorders, including major depression and bipolar disorder, are the most common neuropsychiatric causes of disability worldwide.[1] Despite the relative availability of specialty psychiatric care in the United States, most patients with depression or bipolar disorder continue to receive their treatment in primary care settings.[2,3] Patients with medical illness and comorbid mood disorders frequently have poorer outcomes, experience more prolonged and difficult treatment, have higher total health care costs, and have greater morbidity and mortality compared to patients without mood disorders.[4] Conversely, treatment of underlying depressive and bipolar disorders not only improves the emotional well-being of patients, but also improves overall health outcomes and lowers health care costs. Given their frequency, severity, prevalence, morbidity, and mortality, depression and bipolar disorders remain important illnesses for primary care providers (PCPs) to identify and treat. Box 12.1 summarizes key points discussed in this chapter. In addition, an increasing body of evidence demonstrates that better patient outcomes can be achieved using an integrated and collaborative care approach in primary care settings.[3]

DIAGNOSIS OF MOOD DISORDERS

Mood disorders are broadly divided into major depression and bipolar disorder. Within each diagnostic group are subtypes, depending on severity and length of symptoms, types of symptoms present, etiology, and relationship of onset of symptoms to life events (e.g., postpartum depression). Severity of an illness is specified as mild, moderate, or severe, based on the number of criterion symptoms, the severity of the symptoms, and the degree of functional impairment. The *mild* specifier is used when there are few if any symptoms in excess of those required to make the diagnosis, symptoms are manageable, and social and/or occupational functional is minimally disrupted. A *severe* specifier is given, on the other hand, when the number of symptoms is substantially in excess of those required to make the diagnosis, the symptoms are intense and distressing, and they result in marked social and/or occupational functioning. The *moderate* specifier is used when the number and intensity of symptoms fall in between mild and severe. The most recent edition of the *Diagnostic and Statistical Manual of Mental Disorders* (DSM-5)[5] has expanded the number of depressive diagnoses compared to the prior edition (DSM-IV), and now includes major depressive disorder, persistent depressive disorder (formerly dysthymia), substance/medication-induced depressive and related disorder, premenstrual dysphoric disorder, depressive disorder due to a medical condition, disruptive mood dysregulation disorder, other specified depressive disorder, and unspecified depressive disorder. Diagnostic subgroups for bipolar disorder have also expanded in the DSM-5, including bipolar I disorder, bipolar II disorder, cyclothymic disorder, substance/medication-induced and related disorder, other specified bipolar and related disorder, and unspecified bipolar and related disorder. In addition, the DSM-5 allows for a broader number of course and episode specifiers that can be applied to either depression or bipolar disorders, depending on a patient's presentation and illness history. These include anxious distress, peripartum onset, atypical features, psychotic features, mixed features, melancholic features, season pattern, or catatonia. The final course specifier, rapid cycling, can be applied only to bipolar disorder.

A more modern conceptualization of mood disorders is that they exist along a spectrum, with symptoms from the depressed mood pole occasionally co-occurring with symptoms from the manic pole, and vice versa. This mixing of symptoms has been more formally recognized in the DSM-5, which allows for the co-occurrence of subthreshold mood symptoms from opposite poles. Thus, patients with major depression can present with co-occurring subthreshold symptoms of mania or hypomania (e.g., racing thoughts, irritability, pressured speech), classified as major depression with mixed features, while patients with mania or hypomania may have subthreshold depressive symptoms (e.g., depressed mood, anhedonia) and are classified as having bipolar disorder, manic episode with mixed features.[5]

Table 12.1 provides diagnostic criteria and associated features for major depression, persistent depressive disorder, bipolar I disorder, and bipolar II disorder. It also describes differentiating features between bipolar depression and unipolar depression, common medical causes leading to depression or mania, and physical symptoms that may be suggestive of an underlying depressive illness.

EPIDEMIOLOGY

Prevalence estimates of mental disorders in the United States find that mood disorders are second only to anxiety disorders in their frequency. Lifetime prevalence for major depression is estimated to be 14.9% to 16.2%, while approximately 3.9% to 6.2% of Americans have bipolar disorder.[13,14] Rates in primary care clinics for both disorders remain substantially higher than in the general

TABLE 12.1. MOOD DISORDERS DIAGNOSIS AND DIFFERENTIAL DIAGNOSIS

Diagnosis	Symptoms	Associated Features	Notes
Major Depression	• Five or more symptoms (including either depressed mood or anhedonia) • Present during the same 2-week period or longer • Significant change from a patient's previous functioning • Significant symptoms: weight loss or gain; insomnia or hypersomnia; psychomotor agitation or retardation; fatigue or loss of energy; feelings of worthlessness or excessive/inappropriate guilt; diminished ability to think, concentrate, or make decisions; recurrent thoughts of death, suicide, suicidal ideation, plan, or attempt[5]	• Irritable, angry mood may predominate; or explosive, angry outbursts[6] • Severe forms accompanied by psychotic symptoms, e.g., auditory hallucinations, delusional guilt, or certainty of having a disease despite medical evidence to the contrary • Subthreshold manic symptoms can co-occur with major depression.	• Can be superimposed on patients with persistent depressive disorder, often called "double depression" • Bereavement may cause or exacerbate major depression and is no longer an exclusion in making the diagnosis of depression.
Persistent Depressive Disorder (Dysthymia)	• Chronically depressed mood • Occurs most days for at least 2 years • Other symptoms, including feelings of inadequacy, generalized loss of interest or pleasure in activities, social withdrawal, feelings of guilt or brooding about the past, along with decreased activity, productivity, or effectiveness[5]	• Neurovegetative symptoms, e.g., insomnia/hypersomnia, poor appetite or overeating; low energy and poor concentration may be present but are less common than in major depressive episodes	• Major depressive episodes can be superimposed on top of persistent depressive disorder, resulting in "double depression."
Bipolar I Disorder	• Diagnosed with mania (depressive episodes are not necessary for the diagnosis) • *Manic episodes* are distinct periods of persistently elevated, expansive, or irritable mood along with persistently increased goal-directed activity or energy. • Last at least 1 week (or of any duration, if hospitalization is necessary) • Must have at least 3 of the following accompanying symptoms if euphoric or least 4 of these symptoms if irritable: inflated self-esteem or grandiosity, decreased need for sleep, pressured speech, flight of ideas or racing thoughts, distractibility, increased goal-directed activity (either socially, at work, or sexually) or agitation, and/or excessive involvement in pleasurable activities that have a high likelihood of painful consequences (e.g., spending sprees, sexual indiscretions)[5]	• Although manic patients are most often thought to be euphoric, the majority describe a mix of severe irritability, emotional lability, and/or volatility. • Approximately 60% of bipolar I patients experience psychosis, which may involve delusions of grandeur (feeling omnipotent, having special powers or gifts), paranoia, persecutory delusions, or hallucinations (most often auditory, not visual).[7] • Depressive symptoms predominate over manic symptoms by approximately 3:1.[8] • Subthreshold depressive symptoms can occur during manic symptoms, and vice versa.	• Antidepressant treatment can precipitate mania in some vulnerable individuals; when this occurs, bipolar disorder is diagnosed if the mania persists after the physiological effects of the antidepressant are thought to have worn off.

(continued)

TABLE 12.1. CONTINUED

Diagnosis	Symptoms	Associated Features	Notes
Bipolar II Disorder	• Lifetime presence of both hypomanic and major depressive episodes • Hypomanic episodes are similar to full manic episodes. The severity of behaviors is attenuated, and the extreme functional, occupational, and social impairments evident in mania are absent in hypomania. • DSM-5 criteria require that distinct elevations in mood must be present for at least 4 days, must clearly be different from the patient's usual non-depressed mood, and must be accompanied by a change in the patient's usual functioning.[5]	• Depressive episodes predominate over hypomanic episodes during the course of the illness at a ratio of approximately 37:1.[9] • Subthreshold depressive symptoms can occur during hypomanic symptoms, and vice versa.	• Primary care providers are more likely to encounter patients with bipolar II disorder than bipolar I disorder, as patients tend to seek help during their depressive episodes and typically do not report hypomanic episodes as abnormal.[10]
	Differential Diagnosis of Mood Disorders		
Bipolar depression (differentiating from major depression)	• More often associated with: Earlier onset of depression (teens or early 20s) • More severe depressive episodes, especially at a younger age (teens or 20s) • Psychotic depression at a younger age • Severe postpartum depression, or postpartum psychotic depression • Often have shorter depressive episodes (1–3 months) • Sudden onset of depressive episodes (compared to gradually worsening of depression) • Three or more antidepressant failures • Paradoxical reactions to antidepressants (irritability or worsening depression) • Activation/hypomania/mania on antidepressants • Often with seasonal variation of mood (e.g., worse mood in winter, improvement in spring/summer)	• Family history of mood disorders (either bipolar disorder or more commonly, major depression) • Frequent comorbid anxiety disorders • Frequent comorbid substance abuse	• Improper treatment—most often the use of antidepressants unopposed by a mood stabilizer—can lead to worsening mood, rapid cycling, and/or mixed states.

Medical disorders and/or treatments associated with depression	• Endocrine disorders (e.g., Addison disease, hypothyroidism) • Infections (e.g., HIV, influenza, meningitis) • Neurological diseases (e.g., Parkinson disease, stroke, tumors) • Metabolic derangements (e.g., hypercalcemia) • Exogenous steroids (e.g., prednisone bursts)		• Be vigilant for substance abuse, whether open or covert, from intoxication or withdrawal, as it can cause, imitate, or exacerbate an underlying mood disorder. Alcohol abuse often presents as depression.
Medical disorders and/or treatments associated with mania	• Exogenous steroids (e.g., prednisone bursts) • Central nervous system lesions (right side of the brain, multiple sclerosis) • Endocrine disorders (hyperthyroidism) • Other medications (e.g., dopaminergic agents such as amantadine, bromocriptine)		• Be vigilant for substance abuse, whether open or covert, from intoxication or withdrawal, as it can cause, imitate, or exacerbate an underlying mood disorder. Abuse of stimulants and/or cocaine is more likely to produce manic-like symptoms.
Patients with physical complaints suggesting depression	• The majority of patients with such illnesses often present with somatic complaints; only a minority present with purely psychological symptoms and concerns.[11] • May present with multiple physical symptoms (6 or more) • Likely have higher ratings of symptom severity and lower ratings of overall health • More frequently have an encounter that the provider perceives as "difficult"[12]	• Difficulties in diagnosis secondary to patient's inability to articulate psychological problems, reticence to speak of emotional difficulties, short time allowed for patient visits, or PCP's relative lack of training in assessing and treating mental health disorders • Many presenting complaints may be consistent with symptoms of coexisting medical illnesses, further complicating assessment and likely requiring additional etiologic investigation.	

population, with 5% to 12% of patients meeting the criteria for major depression[15] and 9.8% meeting the criteria for bipolar disorder.[16]

Primary care clinics are the de facto treatment settings for patients with mood disorders. Whether this is due to patient difficulties accessing mental health care, greater willingness to talk about mental health issues with PCPs, or stigma associated with going to mental health clinics, the majority of patients seeking psychiatric treatment do so in primary care offices. In a study of 12-month use of mental health services in the United States, nearly 23% of patients were treated by a general medical provider, compared with 12.3% who were treated by a psychiatrist.[17] However, patients with mood disorders seen in general medical settings had far fewer visits (mean 1.5) compared with those seen by psychiatrists (mean 4.5) and less often received care deemed "minimally adequate." Thus, different interventions and strategies for mood disorder patients are needed to improve the quality of care delivered in general medical settings.

COSTS

Depressive and bipolar disorders account for substantial health care costs and thus constitute a major public health and economic concern. The cost of depression in 2000 was estimated to be $83.1 billion, with $26.1 billion (31%) for direct medical costs, $5.4 billion (7%) for suicide-related mortality costs, and $51.5 billion (62%) for work-related costs[18] (e.g., missing days from work, decreased productivity). Bipolar disorder, while less common than major depression, incurs direct and indirect costs nearly three times those of depression, making it the most expensive of the mental illnesses, at $151 billion annually.[3,19] The higher costs are in part from expensive pharmacological treatments and hospitalizations, as well as costs thought to be linked to medical management of these patients, who often have higher rates of obesity, diabetes, smoking, and heart disease.[3]

DISEASE COURSE

Depression and bipolar disorders are, for the most part, chronic illnesses that worsen the longer they remain untreated. While onset of major depression can occur at any age, the median age of onset is 30 years.[14] Depression is a highly recurrent illness; patients experiencing a single episode have a 50% lifetime chance of recurrence, while those with three or more episodes have nearly 100% recurrence of the illness without treatment.[20] In addition, approximately 15% of patients suffering a first episode will go on to have a chronic course. Untreated episodes can last six months or longer and increase the likelihood of relapse and chronicity.[21] Revised and more recent estimates of suicide risk among patients with major depression range from 2.2% to 8.6%, depending on history of hospitalizations for suicidality versus outpatient-only treatment, comorbid conditions, and gender.[22,23]

Bipolar illnesses also are chronic conditions, with more than 90% of patients experiencing a recurrence during their lifetimes.[24] While manias and hypomanias define these illnesses, the majority of mood episodes experienced by bipolar patients are depressions. In a prospective study in which patients were followed for up to 20 years, bipolar I patients were symptomatically ill 47.3% of the time, with depressive symptoms predominating over manic symptoms by a nearly 3:1 ratio.[8] Patients with bipolar II disorder were symptomatic 53.9% of the time during the follow-up period, with depressive symptoms vastly predominating over hypomanic symptoms by a ratio of 37:1.[9] The age of bipolar onset is earlier than in major depression, typically in the 18- to 22-year range. An increasing body of literature also shows that residual, subsyndromal symptoms put bipolar patients at a much higher risk of relapse, and that stable recovery is achieved only when patients become fully asymptomatic.[25] Bipolar disorders carry a substantial risk for death from multiple causes (e.g., suicide, cardiovascular disease, cancers). The standardized mortality ratio—that is, the ratio of those affected by the disease compared to the general population—for patients with a diagnosis of bipolar disorder is 15, compared to a standardized mortality ratio of 20 for patients with unipolar depression and 8.4 for those with schizophrenia.[26]

INTERACTIONS BETWEEN MOOD DISORDERS AND MEDICAL ILLNESS

A complex and reciprocal relationship exists between medical illnesses and mood disorders. Medical illnesses are associated with higher prevalence rates of depression and bipolar disorders, and vice versa. Studies have shown that patients with diabetes, cancer, stroke, myocardial infarction, HIV-related illnesses, Parkinson disease, and epilepsy all have higher rates of depression than patients without such illnesses.[27] Bipolar disorders are commonly associated with increased risks for cardiovascular disease, diabetes, obesity, and thyroid disease. Some of these comorbid diseases may be related to mechanisms intrinsic to the disorder (e.g., bipolar disorder or major depression leading to cognitive dysfunction), some are associated with common comorbid psychiatric illnesses (use of excessive nicotine, alcohol, and other drugs), and still others are the consequences of treatment (e.g., weight gain associated with atypical antipsychotic medications).[28]

Management of these patients is further complicated by the higher rates of unexplained symptoms compared to patients without mood disorders, as well as fragmentation of care across different systems and providers, even after adjusting for the severity of medical illness.[29] An increasing body of literature suggests that patients with medical illness and comorbid depression adapt more poorly to chronic symptoms, such as fatigue or pain, compared to patients without depression. Comorbid patients are more functionally impaired and have more lost workdays, a poorer quality of life, and higher rates of medical utilization.[30] Disease management of these patients is also complicated by higher rates of nonadherence to treatment and self-care regimens, as well as higher rates of risky behaviors (e.g., smoking, overeating, sedentary lifestyle). In addition, patients with bipolar disorder more often have other life stressors, such as homelessness,[31] compared with depressed patients.

OVERVIEW OF SCREENING TOOLS FOR MOOD DISORDERS IN PRIMARY CARE SETTINGS

Self-administered questionnaires that are in the public domain, are well validated in primary care settings, and are sensitive to change over time are the most practical and cost-effective measures to use in a busy practice. Mood disorder screens do not diagnose but rather screen for symptom severity over time, and alert providers that further exploration may be warranted. Positive screens typically indicate that a more in-depth and focused interview is required, as screening will not include many confounding diagnostic variables (e.g., hypothyroidism, substance abuse, bereavement) and provider judgment is required. Patient self-report screening for bipolar disorder is more difficult, since hypomania and mania are typically conditions in which patient insight is clouded or lost. Screening questionnaires, followed by more in-depth interviews, remain the gold standard.

Measurement-based care is a key component of collaborative care models, as it allows for measurable treatment goals and outcomes defined for each patient. Treatments are actively changed and managed until treatment goals are reached. The gold-standard target for both major depression and bipolar disorder is remission of symptoms. Studies have shown that relapse into subsequent mood episodes is higher unless absence of symptoms has been achieved.[32]

Mood questionnaires can be given to patients by front-line staff at the time of check-in, or by medical assistants or nurses who room patients and check vital signs. The questionnaires can be reviewed by the PCP or by the behavioral health specialist (BHS) once the patient's visit begins, and further assessment can take place if warranted.

Screening and Measurement Tool for Depression: Patient Health Questionnaire 9

The Patient Health Questionnaire 9 (PHQ-9) is most often used in primary care settings to screen for depression because of its ease of use, sensitivity to change over time, reliability, and validity.[33] Major depression is diagnosed if five or more of the depressive symptoms have been present at least "more than half the days" in the past two weeks and if one of the symptoms is depressed mood or anhedonia. One of the nine test items ("thought that you would be better off dead or by hurting yourself in some way") counts if present at all, regardless of duration (i.e., the symptom counts toward diagnosis even if present "several days"). Sensitivity ranges from 68% to 95% using cutoff scores from 9 to 15, with specificity from 84% to 95%. Using the cutoff score of 9, sensitivity is 95% and specificity 84%.

Patients scoring at least 10 on the PHQ-9 are considered at high risk for depression and/or dysthymia and require further investigation by the PCP or BHS to confirm a diagnosis of depression and to elicit greater history of depressive episodes. Treatment of the depressive episode should continue until the patient's initial score is reduced by 50% (response) or the patient achieves a PHQ-9 score of less than 5 (remission). The PHQ-9 can also be used in patients with bipolar disorder who are in the midst of a major depressive episode both to screen for a depressive episode and to track its progress.

Screening and Measurement Tool for Bipolar Disorder

The Mood Disorder Questionnaire (MDQ) is a validated tool that combines DSM-IV criteria and clinical experience to screen for bipolar disorder in primary care settings.[34] It is a brief, one-page self-report questionnaire with 13 yes-or-no items and two additional questions regarding functioning and timing of mood symptoms; it typically can be completed in five minutes or less. Seven or more positive responses to questions about manic symptoms plus positive responses to the severity of impairment (moderate or severe) and coincident timing of symptoms yields a positive screen. The specificity and sensitivity of the MDQ vary widely by clinical setting. It works poorly in general community samples (97% specificity but only 28% sensitivity) but much better when given to patients with suspected mood symptoms (93% specificity, 58% sensitivity).[35,36]

Currently, there are no ideal patient self-report measures for tracking hypomanic or manic symptoms. As noted previously, patients in the midst of hypomania or mania often lack insight into the presence or severity of such symptoms. Clinicians may instead need to rely on a clinical interview, family or collateral reports, and assessment of functioning, rather than a measurement-based tool, to determine response to treatment and course of illness.

ASSESSMENT OF MOOD DISORDER PATIENTS IN THE PRIMARY CARE SETTING

Assessment of patients with mood disorders requires establishing a specific diagnosis (or diagnoses), providing a thorough risk assessment (i.e., suicidality, homicidality [see Chapter 18: Violence and Suicide]), judging inability to care for self, assessing the severity of the illness, identifying specific target symptoms to track over time, assessing factors that are likely complicating or exacerbating the illness (e.g., medical illness, substance abuse), and gathering collateral information whenever possible from family, friends, or other providers. Providers should be especially vigilant for the presence of comorbid anxiety disorders (see Chapter 11: Integrated Care for Anxiety Disorders), as these commonly co-occur with both depression and bipolar disorder, and may complicate both psychiatric and medical treatments. For primary care clinics with integrated or co-located behavioral health providers, assessing the complexity of the case and the need for additional collaborative care is best done early in the patient's treatment.

COLLABORATIVE CARE MODELS IN THE TREATMENT OF MOOD DISORDER PATIENTS

Multiple studies have shown that patients with mood disorders have improved outcomes when treated using collaborative care models.[3,15] While treatment of depression using collaborative care models is the best studied, an increasing body of literature also supports the effectiveness of such models in the treatment of bipolar disorder.[3] As described in Chapter 1: Conceptual Framework for Integrated Care: Multiple Models to Achieve Integrated Aims, the central focus of collaborative care models is to reorganize medical care to support an effective partnership between primary care patients and PCPs, BHSs, and other members of the integrated team in order to provide patient-centered care and improved outcomes.[37]

Effective collaborative care involves several key conceptual components and personnel requirements. General conceptual components include the following:

1. A focus on anticipatory patient-centered care, including proactive follow-up visits or telephone contacts
2. Teaching patients self-management skills and providing support so that patients and key family members are equipped with information and skills to effectively manage mood disorders
3. Decision support for PCPs, which may range from provision of practice guidelines to facilitated specialist consultation, typically with a psychiatrist
4. Use of a team, with all members of the team practicing at their highest level of training
5. Information systems that facilitate and support the rapid flow of patient data between all levels of providers and staff, such as widespread use of electronic medical records[15,37]
6. Creation of patient registries that list the patients in the practice who have major depression or bipolar disorder

Key Personnel and Roles for a Collaborative Care Model for Depression

Key personnel in creating a collaborative care model include medical assistants, care managers, BHSs, nurses, consulting psychiatrists, and, of course, the PCP. All members of the team need to work in a fluid and flexible manner with one another, depending on the needs of the patient. Given the frequent complexity of patients presenting in primary care settings, rigid roles and inflexible styles among team members inevitably lead to increased conflict, decreased efficiency, and poorer outcomes. Open communication among team members and a willingness to "do what is necessary at the time for the sake of the patient" is critical for successful management of patients and overall integration into a rapid and changing workflow.

Medical Assistants/Nurses

Medical assistants typically provide the patient with an initial screening measure. Many practices use the PHQ-2,[38] a two-question self-report form that asks about the frequency of depressed mood and anhedonia over the past two weeks. The questionnaire is scored from 0 to 6, with scores of 3 or greater indicating a need for further assessment of mood. If the patient's score exceeds the cut-point score of 3, the medical assistant can then administer a PHQ-9 to more fully assess depressive symptoms. Should the patient score highly on the suicidality question, the medical assistant should alert either a BHS or the patient's PCP. Medical assistants may also add information to the patient's registry.

Nurses can perform mental health screenings and assessments at any time during their routine care of the patient. They also can provide psychoeducation about mood disorders, track outcomes in the registry, and offer ongoing support for patients during treatment. Support may include making outreach calls to patients between appointments to assess medication adherence, side effects, and/or needed dose changes between appointments, or to make referrals to outside mental health resources.

Primary Care Provider

While an entire treatment team shares care of the patient, the PCP directs and oversees the patient's care. PCPs make the initial assessment and diagnosis, may start medications for more straightforward cases, and/or may call for behavioral health consultation either from a BHS or a psychiatrist, depending on the PCP's assessment of patient complexity and need. PCPs are important in introducing the patient to the rest of the treatment team, ideally making a "warm handoff" to the rest of the team to enhance continuity of care and therapeutic alliance. While any member of the treatment team can make assessments of suicidality, PCPs are likely the final arbiters in deciding whether or not a patient requires hospitalization and/or further assessment in an emergency department (ED). PCPs also collaborate with the psychiatrist in complex medical/psychiatric patients to consider interactions between medications and medical illness (e.g., use of atypical antipsychotics in patients with obesity and diabetes). PCPs are likely more comfortable assessing and treating patients with unipolar depression than bipolar disorder, but should seek out consultation on either diagnosis at any point at which a patient's treatment course is not proceeding as expected.

Care Managers

Care managers, who are often case managers, medical assistants, nurses, certified health coaches, psychologists (bachelor's degree in psychology), or social workers, can greatly aid in patient access to services and decrease psychosocial stressors. They can help connect patients with medical specialists and assist the patient with access to housing, transportation, and other community benefits and services, and in so doing greatly support patients and their care. Care managers may also perform mental health assessments and refer patients to BHSs if they appear emotionally distressed or troubled.

Behavioral Health Specialists

BHSs (e.g., psychologists, social workers, psychiatric nurse practitioners, health coaches) will be called on in a variety of ways to help with the management of patients with mood disorders. Often, crisis management or safety assessment skills will be needed (see Chapter 26: Crisis Intervention in Integrated Care and Chapter 18: Violence and Suicide). PCPs or BHSs may encounter patients who score especially high on the PHQ-9, score a 1, 2, or 3 on question 9 ("thoughts you would be better off dead or of hurting yourself in some way"), or are so obviously distressed or upset that the PCP feels that a mental health specialist is needed immediately. In such cases a "warm handoff," whereby the PCP introduces the BHS to the patient during the visit, may be most effective. In situations such as these, a traditional

50-minute therapy visit is impractical. For the treatment of mood disorders in a fast-paced, primary care setting, BHSs need to be skilled in delivering brief psychotherapeutic strategies in pragmatic, abbreviated, but effective ways. BHS skills of particular value in an integrated care environment include crisis intervention, mindfulness skills, behavioral activation, cognitive-behavioral techniques for mood disorders and insomnia, problem-solving therapies, motivational interviewing, and family and group interventions. Information sheets on sleep hygiene and/or sleep restriction therapy, as well as mood disorders diaries, can be especially helpful for this patient population. An example of a patient depression education sheet is shown in Figure 12.1. BHSs may also be called on to help with the management of psychologically complex patients (e.g., patients with histories of trauma, neglect, comorbid substance use) or help sort out "diagnostic dilemma" patients.

BHSs are especially important in managing patients with bipolar disorders in primary care settings, or further assessing patients where bipolar disorder is suspected. Psychoeducation, with a focus on symptom management, problem solving, medication adherence, and tracking patients in registries, is a key element in providing effective collaborative care for bipolar patients. BHSs can further help with the development of relapse-prevention plans (early recognition of signs/symptoms of mania or depression, along with early interventions to deal with worsening symptoms) as well as helping the patient deal with other common topics related to bipolar disorder, such as substance use, anxiety, medication side effects, and relationship management skills.[3] Two excellent resources for patients and the integrated care team are *The Bipolar Disorder Survival Guide*[39] and *Overcoming Bipolar Disorder: A Comprehensive Workbook for Managing Your Symptoms and Achieving Your Life Goals*.[40] Both books are written in workbook style for patients and have assignments, worksheets, and educational sections specifically for patients.

Finally, BHSs are often the providers best suited to manage patient registries. Registry maintenance is typically a shared activity among BHSs and other integrated team members, as all can add to the registry. Registries can help practices track when patient follow-up is needed, inform members of the treatment team which patients are or are not responding to treatment, and help determine patient response to outreach attempts. Registry information often includes the patient's PCP, BHS, visit dates, contact dates, types of contact (in person vs. phone call), PHQ-9 and MDQ scores, and medications.

Psychiatrist

The consulting psychiatrist may offer provider-to-provider consultation or, less frequently, evaluation of the patient on an individual consultation basis. Either interaction can occur in person or via telebehavioral health, depending on a practice's setup. Box 12.2 lists common scenarios for contacting the consulting psychiatrist, including (1) patients failing to respond to two or more antidepressant trials (i.e., treatment-resistant depressions), (2) the presence of psychotic depression, (3) patients becoming activated (manic) on an antidepressant, (4) providing diagnostic clarity for complex mental health patients, (5) helping with the assessment of suicide or violence risk or grave disability, or (6) assisting with the decision to send a patient to an ED or admit a patient for inpatient psychiatric care or substance abuse treatment. On occasion, patients may be sent directly to the psychiatrist for consultation. For example, this may be warranted if the patient has a highly complex, preexisting psychiatric medication list that the PCP feels unable to assess or manage adequately. These decisions are discussed in more detail in the treatment section.

TREATMENT OF MOOD DISORDERS IN PRIMARY CARE SETTINGS

Treatment of Major Depression

Pharmacotherapy and/or psychotherapy are the mainstays for treatment of depression. Pharmacotherapy combined with psychotherapy has been shown to be superior to either modality alone for the management of moderate to severe depression. The goal of treatment for patients with major depression is remission of all symptoms and return to normal functioning. Studies have consistently shown that a lack of remission is associated with higher relapse rates, more severe subsequent depression, shorter durations between episodes, continued impairment in work settings and social relationships, increased risk of all-cause mortality, and increased risk of suicide. BHSs can help in the management of depressed patients by (1) providing education on the temporal course of improvement and on the importance of maintaining (or reestablishing) regular social rhythms (e.g., eating habits, exercise, social

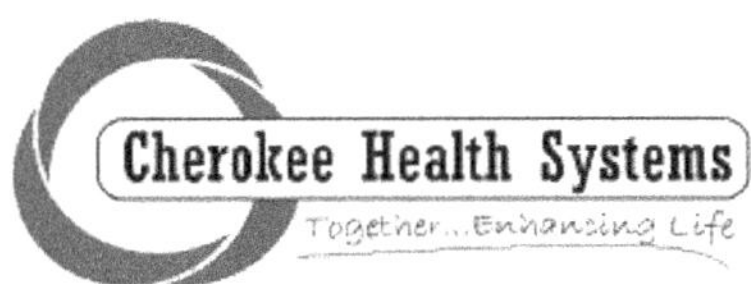

What you can do for Depression:

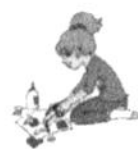

Make time for activities you enjoy. When you are depressed it is easy to leave activities behind that are good for you. Try to do these things again even if you are just "going through the motions" at first.

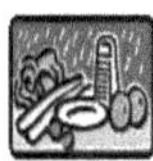

Avoid Junk food. Eat lots of fruit and vegetables. Don't rush. Take your time when you eat. **Get plenty of rest and balance work and play.**

Don't drink alcohol. Limit caffeine to one or two drinks per day. Alcohol may make you feel better 6when you drink it but it has a depressant effect in the long run. Caffeine can make the anxiety and sleep problems that go with depression worse.

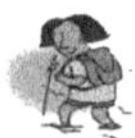

Exercise. 20 minutes or more of brisk exercise per day helps to ease anxiety

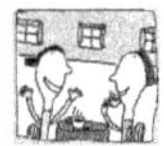

Spend time with people who have a positive effect on you.

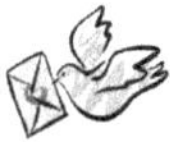

Do something kind for someone else each day.

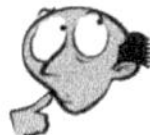

Watch your thoughts. Negative thinking can make depression worse and become a bad habit. Replace realistic, positive thoughts for unreasonable, negative ones.

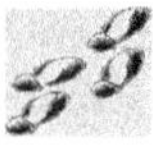

Set simple goals and take small steps. It's easy to feel overwhelmed when you are anxious. Agree with yourself to limit worrying to certain hours each day. Break problems down into small steps and give yourself credit for each step you take.

My Goal Is: ______________________________

Step 1:______________________________

Step 2:______________________________

Step 3:______________________________

FIGURE 12.1. Example of a patient handout for help with depression.

activities, well-regulated sleep); (2) aiding in the development of insight and coping skills (e.g., connecting with family/friends when feeling depressed, scheduling pleasurable activities); and (3) providing a thorough safety assessment and plan. Other key elements at the start of treatment include discussions of medication selection (if indicated) and scheduling of follow-up appointments.

BOX 12.2
CONSULTING WITH BEHAVIORAL HEALTH PROVIDERS

Reasons to consult a behavioral health specialist (e.g., psychologist, social worker, psychiatric nurse practitioner, health coach):

- **Acute suicidality**
- **Presentation complicated by bereavement**
- **Difficulty sorting out medical symptoms from mood symptoms**
- **History of trauma complicating the presentation**
- **Comorbid anxiety**
- **Comorbid substance abuse**
- **Patient diagnosed with bipolar disorder**
- **Diagnostic dilemmas**

Reasons to consult a psychiatrist:

- **Complex polypharmacy, with high likelihood of drug interactions, such as with HIV antiretroviral regimens, blood-thinning agents, anti-epileptic drugs**
- **Concomitant use of medications with likely psychiatric effects, such as steroids, interferons, varenicline**
- **Patient wishes to become pregnant, is currently pregnant, or is breastfeeding and needs psychiatric medications**
- **Patient fails to respond to two or more antidepressant trials**
- **Patient becomes activated (manic) on antidepressant**
- **Presence of psychotic depression**
- **Patient diagnosed with bipolar disorder**

Using BHSs to provide brief therapy, supply handouts, or suggest patient-oriented self-help books, as previously mentioned, on coping and/or behavioral activation, or employing the care coordinator to make referrals into the community for more intensive individual or group therapy can improve the chances of a patient achieving remission. Some patients may choose psychotherapy alone to treat depression. Indeed, psychodynamic therapy, cognitive-behavioral therapy (CBT), interpersonal therapy, and behavioral activation may prove as effective as medication alone for some patients.[41] For patients wanting longer-term therapy, referrals into community resources will likely be necessary as most primary care practices will not be set up for such long-term treatment.

In primary care settings, medications prescribed by the PCP are likely to be considered for the majority of depressed patients, especially those who are suicidal, who are functionally impaired from their depression, who are having recurrent episodes, or whose medical or psychiatric condition is likely to worsen unless their depression is treated (e.g., anxiety, chronic pain, headaches). Mild depression (PHQ-9 score 5–9) may respond to nonpharmacologic interventions alone (e.g., exercise, mindfulness, or brief BHS interventions). Depressive symptoms that persist or respond inadequately to nonpharmacologic interventions warrant more aggressive treatment of the underlying depression. Patients with moderate depression (PHQ-9 score 10–19) or severe depression (PHQ-9 score 20–27) very likely will require medication for adequate treatment. Psychotic depressions require treatment with both an antipsychotic and an antidepressant, and the PCP may need a consultation with a psychiatrist, given the need for complex psychopharmacology and the increased risk for mortality. Patients with severe bipolar mania, psychotic depressions, and co-occurring substance use may be referred by other members of the health care team to the care coordinator to arrange for an ED visit or a referral to an inpatient psychiatry unit, partial hospital program, inpatient addiction unit, or outpatient substance abuse treatment.

Medication Selection for Depression

The effectiveness of antidepressants is generally comparable across classes. Therefore, selection of an antidepressant depends largely on patient preference, side effect profile, drug interactions, previous response to a specific medication, treatment overlap with other psychiatric or medical conditions, and cost. There are few data to suggest that any particular antidepressant has increased efficacy or speed of onset over any other antidepressant. Notable mood changes typically take three to six weeks, although the STAR*D study indicated that patients may require up to 12 to 14 weeks to achieve remission of symptoms.[42]

For most patients, initial treatment with a selective serotonin reuptake inhibitor (SSRI), serotonin-norepinephrine reuptake inhibitor (SNRI), bupropion, or mirtazapine is reasonable. Given the comparable speed and efficacy of antidepressants across classes and within classes, selection of an antidepressant agent may be primarily guided by the side effect profile, possible secondary uses of antidepressants (e.g., treating pain or insomnia), and contraindications to particular agents (e.g., bupropion is to be avoided in patients with a seizure disorder). Table 12.2 lists typical antidepressants, starting and treatment doses, side effects, and characteristics of each antidepressant.

Serotonin Reuptake Inhibitors

SSRIs are safe, effective medications that can be used to treat a variety of psychiatric conditions. All SSRIs operate by the same mechanism of action and are considered equally effective in the treatment of depression. However, failure of one SSRI does not necessarily imply failure of all SSRIs; patients may respond preferentially to one SSRI over another.[43] SSRIs differ substantially in their potential to inhibit particular hepatic cytochrome P-450 metabolic pathways, their half-life, potency, and presence or absence of active metabolites. Clinicians should check for drug interactions in patients receiving complex polypharmacy regimens because drug–drug interactions are constantly being updated and changing. SSRIs have sexual side effects (decreased libido, delayed orgasm, or anorgasmia) and gastrointestinal side effects (nausea, diarrhea). Gastrointestinal side effects likely will remit over time, but sexual effects typically do not attenuate and may require a more detailed sexual assessment (see Chapter 21: Assessing and Treating Sexual Problems in an Integrated Care Environment), treatment with other agents (e.g., a phosphodiesterase inhibitor [e.g., sildenafil], or use of an antidepressant less likely to cause sexual side effects.

Serotonin-Norepinephrine Reuptake Inhibitors

The SNRIs (venlafaxine, desvenlafaxine, duloxetine, and levomilnacipran) are similar in efficacy to SSRIs, although a few studies have suggested a mild advantage of SNRIs over SSRIs.[44] Most clinicians favor use of the venlafaxine XR preparation rather than the immediate-release one given its once-daily dosing and lower likelihood of provoking a withdrawal syndrome on discontinuation of the drug. Desvenlafaxine, the active metabolite of venlafaxine, is more potent than its parent compound, but it is unclear whether it has any advantages over venlafaxine. Unlike venlafaxine, duloxetine provides dual-neurotransmitter reuptake inhibition at any dose, although this does not appear to confer any advantage over other SNRIs in terms of efficacy or the side effect profile. Duloxetine currently is indicated for treatment of chronic pain as well as depression, but this is likely a class effect of SNRIs and not unique to duloxetine. Levomilnacipran is an active enantiomer of the racemic drug milnacipran (U.S. Food and Drug Administration [FDA]-approved for treatment of fibromyalgia). Side effects of SNRIs are similar to those of SSRIs, although because of their increased noradrenergic activity SNRIs also can cause dose-related hypertension, excessive sweating, and dry mouth.

Serotonin-Norepinephrine Modulator

Mirtazapine is a serotonin-norepinephrine modulator that also blocks postsynaptic hydroxytryptamine (HT) receptors, including those in the 5-HT-3 (serotonin) class. Mirtazapine is sedating and can increase appetite, and therefore may be favored when patients have insomnia or decreased appetite and weight loss. Because of a dose-dependent ratio of neurotransmitter blockade involving histamine receptors, mirtazapine is generally more sedating at lower doses than higher. With its 5-HT-3 blockade, mirtazapine may also be helpful when patients complain of GI symptoms, such as nausea, or other side effects from SSRIs. Mirtazapine has fewer sexual side effects than SSRIs or SNRIs and has been tried as an antidote to SSRI-induced sexual side effects. Common side effects from mirtazapine include weight gain and daytime somnolence.

TABLE 12.2. ANTIDEPRESSANTS

Antidepressant	Usual Starting Dose (mg/day)	Usual Dose Range (mg/day)	Side Effects/Specific Comments
SSRIs			All SSRIs can cause sexual side effects, gastrointestinal upset, headache, insomnia or somnolence.
Citalopram	10–20	20–40	Maximum 40 mg in patients < 60 years, 20 mg in patients > 60 years due to cardiac effects
Escitalopram	5–10	10–30	Active enantiomer of citalopram; other indications: generalized anxiety disorder (GAD)
Fluoxetine	10–20	20–80	Active metabolite norfluoxetine T1/2 = 10 days; strong CYP 2D6 inhibitor; other indications: obsessive-compulsive disorder (OCD), panic disorder, bulimia, premenstrual dysphoric disorder (PMDD), pediatric major depression
Paroxetine	10–20	20–60	Immediate-release formulation associated with withdrawal side effects; other indications: OCD, panic disorder, posttraumatic stress disorder (PTSD), GAD, social anxiety
Sertraline	25–50	50–200	Other indications: OCD, panic disorder, PTSD, social anxiety, PMDD
Vilazodone	10–20	20–60	Also a partial agonist of serotonin 5HT1A receptor
SNRIs			All SNRIs can cause sexual dysfunction, hypertension, sweating, nausea, dizziness.
Desvenlafaxine	50	50–100	Active metabolite of venlafaxine
Duloxetine	30	30–120	Inhibits serotonin & norepinephrine at all doses; other indication: chronic pain
Levomilnacipran	20	40–160	Norepinephrine to serotonin reuptake inhibition ratio 2:1, compared to 17:1 for venlafaxine and 27:1 for duloxetine
Venlafaxine	37.5	150–300	Serotonin inhibition at doses <150 mg, SNRI at doses >150; other indications: panic, GAD, social anxiety
TCAs			All TCAs can cause dry mouth, constipation, blurry vision, orthostatic hypotension, weight gain, somnolence, sweating, headache, sexual dysfunction. Can be fatal in overdose.
Amitriptyline	50	100–300	Metabolized to amitriptyline + nortriptyline; therapeutic levels (combined) 120–250 ng/mL, toxic levels >500

Imipramine	50	100–300	Metabolized to imipramine + desipramine
Nortriptyline	25	50–200	Therapeutic levels 50–150 ng/mL
Desipramine	50	100–300	Therapeutic levels 115–250 ng/mL
Norepinephrine-dopamine reuptake inhibitors			Insomnia, dry mouth, tremor, headache, nausea, constipation, anxiety
Bupropion	100–150	300–450	Do not push dose past U.S. Food and Drug Administration maximum of 450 mg due to seizure risk; no sexual side effects; can aid in smoking cessation (marketed as Zyban)
Norepinephrine-serotonin modulators			
Mirtazapine	15–30	30–60	Somnolence, increased appetite, weight gain
Vortioxetine	5–10	20–30	Inhibits serotonin reuptake; 5-HT3 antagonist, 5-HT1A agonist

Note: All antidepressants carry warning for increased risk of suicidality in children, adolescents, and young adults.

Norepinephrine and Dopamine Reuptake Inhibition

Bupropion is pharmacologically unique among antidepressants and is manufactured in immediate-release, slow-release (SR), and extended-release (XL) formulations. Although its primary mechanism of action is unclear, the drug has weak norepinephrine and dopamine reuptake inhibition. Bupropion is an activating drug, making it better suited for patients with poor energy or those who feel they cannot tolerate a sedating medication. It is also virtually free from sexual side effects and has been used with limited success as an antidote for patients with SSRI-induced sexual side effects.[45] Bupropion rarely causes weight gain and is therefore a good choice for patients who are obese or who feel they cannot tolerate weight gain. Unlike SSRIs, SNRIs, and tricyclic antidepressants (TCAs), bupropion does not treat anxiety disorders and may even worsen anxiety in patients because of its activating properties. Bupropion carries a black-box warning against its use in patients with a history of seizures or eating disorders; the latter group was shown to have a higher incidence of seizures in clinical trials. Given its greater propensity for seizures, bupropion dosing should not be pushed above the FDA-recommended dosing limits. Bupropion has also been approved for treatment of smoking cessation and therefore may have particular utility for depressed patients who also want to quit smoking.

A New Antidepressant

Vortioxetine is the drug most recently approved (2013) by the FDA for the treatment of major depression. While it has unique pharmacologic characteristics, acting as an SSRI, a 5HT1A agonist, a partial agonist at 5-HT1B receptors, and an antagonist at 5-HT3, 5-HT1D, and 5-HT7 receptors, it is currently unclear to what extent these characteristics contribute to its antidepressant efficacy or provide any additional advantage over other antidepressants.

Older Antidepressants

TCAs are effective medications for treating depression and pain, although they are more difficult to tolerate and can be fatal in overdose. TCAs offer an advantage over other antidepressants in that blood levels can be checked and dosing individualized. Reasonable evidence suggests TCAs may be more effective in severely depressed patients.[46] Because of cardiac conduction side effects, TCAs must be used with caution in patients who have conduction delays or who are taking class I antiarrhythmic agents. Electrocardiograms should be checked and monitored in patients older than 50 or those with suspected cardiac disease. TCAs also may cause tachycardia and orthostatic hypotension and thus should be used with caution in patients at risk for tachyarrhythmias or falls. The greatest single disadvantage to TCAs is their potential lethality in overdose; a typical 10-day supply can be lethal, and therefore TCAs should be prescribed cautiously in patients at high risk for suicide. TCAs are also used in a variety of headache and pain syndromes and thus may be useful in patients with such comorbidities.

Trazodone is structurally distinct from SSRIs, SNRIs, TCAs, tetracyclics, or monoamine oxidase inhibitors but still inhibits neuronal uptake of serotonin. Although the FDA has approved it as an antidepressant, trazodone is most often used as a sedative-hypnotic. Dosing as an antidepressant is usually 300 to 600 mg, whereas sedative-hypnotic dosing is usually 50 to 150 mg. Risks and side effects of trazodone include sedation, priapism, and myocardial irritability; the latter effect includes the potential of inducing torsades de pointes.

Initiation of Medication Treatment

Once the PCP has initiated the patient's antidepressant, dosing should be optimized to treat depressive symptoms to remission while minimizing side effects. Patients should be monitored for improvement in their mood and their specific array of depressive symptoms. Continued use of measurement-based care tools such as the PHQ-9 can aid in the objective assessment of improvement. Patients should be followed more frequently on initiation of treatment; the time between appointments can be increased as the patient improves. Monitoring for side effects, particularly those that patients may be reluctant to bring up spontaneously, such as sexual side effects, can improve adherence and the therapeutic alliance. Patients should also be monitored for any worsening of mood, increased irritability, impulsivity, insomnia, sudden switches into euphoria, or suicidal ideation. Such symptoms may suggest a bipolar diathesis, in which case discontinuing the antidepressant, consulting the psychiatrist, and changing to mood-stabilizing agents may be indicated. The antidepressant dose should be increased every two to four weeks until the patient shows a response, the maximum dose is reached, or side effects limit further dose changes. Antidepressant doses should continue to be pushed until remission is achieved or the patient has undergone an adequate antidepressant trial (i.e., continuation of a therapeutic dose) for at least four to eight weeks.

Continuation of Medication Treatment

Once symptoms remit, medications should be continued for six to nine months, as the risk of relapse is greater if patients discontinue medications prematurely.[46] Patients who have had multiple episodes of depression should consider long-term pharmacotherapy, as lifetime relapse rates for such patients are 50% to 85%[20] and the risk of recurrence increases by 16% with each successive episode.[47] Ongoing treatment should also be considered for patients who experienced severe functional impairment, severe suicidal ideation, or serious suicide attempts.

Discontinuation of Medication Treatment

For patients who have achieved ongoing remission and want to discontinue their medications, withdrawal of treatment should be gradual and carefully monitored. The decision that a patient has achieved remission should be made after all members of the treatment team, including the patient, agree that the patient is symptom-free. The PCP should gradually withdraw antidepressants to minimize potential withdrawal syndromes and allow for rapid upward titration should depressive symptoms recur. BHSs should discuss early warning signs of relapse (insomnia, early-morning awakening, loss of interest in activities) and instruct patients to contact the practice should such symptoms recur. Nurses, BHSs, or care managers can follow up with the patient at regular intervals to assess the stability of his or her remission. The risk of relapse is greatest in the first few months of discontinuing antidepressants, and thus a scheduled appointment in this period is often needed to monitor for relapse. Patients who relapse after cessation of antidepressants should be restarted on their previous medication and again titrated to remission of symptoms.

Antidepressant Failure

Patients who fail to respond to antidepressants should be carefully reevaluated. The psychiatrist can, on a monthly basis, review the population of patients with mood disorders in the registry with the BHS and/or other members of the integrated care team, tracking progress, medication adherence, adequacy of dosing, treatment duration, diagnosis, comorbid psychiatric illnesses, increased stressors, unaddressed medical or substance comorbidities, and outcomes and adjusting/suggesting medication changes. Initial antidepressant failure may be relatively common; only one-third of patients achieved remission after 12 to 14 weeks of treatment with citalopram in the STAR*D study.[42] If a patient fails to respond to an adequate antidepressant trial, the next possible strategies include (1) switching to a different antidepressant, within the same class or across classes; (2) augmenting the existing antidepressant with a secondary agent; or (3) adding a second antidepressant to the first. The choice of strategy depends on the patient's preference, an assessment of the benefit from the current antidepressant, current side effects, and psychiatric and medical comorbidities.

Switching antidepressants is generally considered when the patient has had little to no response to the first agent or is having intolerable side effects. Across-class switches are most often considered as an initial strategy (e.g., SSRI to SNRI), although within-class switches may also prove useful (e.g., fluoxetine to sertraline). Across-class or within-class switching may yield response rates of 20% to 50%.[48] No clear guidelines exist as to how best to cross-taper medications, although it is generally unwise to stop antidepressants abruptly because withdrawal syndromes may ensue. Medications with a short half-life, such as venlafaxine (immediate release) or paroxetine, have most often been associated with withdrawal syndromes. Typically, patients complain of flu-like symptoms, electric-like shocks in the back of their heads, or dizziness. Consideration of half-life and slow cross-tapers often yield the most tolerable switch.

Augmentation Strategies

Augmentation strategies involve adding a second agent with no intrinsic antidepressant properties to the existing antidepressant. These are often considered when a patient has had a partial response to an antidepressant but has not reached remission; switching to an alternate antidepressant may risk losing the existing response. The two best-studied augmentation strategies for depression are adding lithium and triiodothyronine (T_3). Standard lithium levels of 0.5 to 1.0 mmol/L have most often been used. T_3 augmentation has yielded similar results and is often better tolerated than lithium, usually with doses of 25 to 50 μg/day. Overall remission rates with augmentation in patients unable to achieve remission on antidepressant monotherapy range from 15% to 50%.[49] Atypical antipsychotic drugs have also been used as augmenting agents in nonpsychotic major depression, with beneficial results. Aripiprazole currently has an indication as an augmenting agent, at 2 to 15 mg daily, as does quetiapine XR. Buspirone has also been used as an augmenting agent, as its 5-HT-1A-receptor agonism may enhance SSRI response. In the STAR*D study, 30% of patients who failed to achieve remission on citalopram alone went on to remit with the addition of buspirone, up to 60 mg daily.[50]

Combining two antidepressants to treat refractory depression is based on the theory that targeting a greater number of neurotransmitters will lead to improved antidepressant response. Common strategies include combining mirtazapine and venlafaxine, bupropion and SSRIs, or bupropion and SNRIs. There are few data supporting the practice of combining drugs of a similar class (e.g., SSRI + SSRI or SNRI + SNRI). Venlafaxine combined with mirtazapine and citalopram plus bupropion SR were effective in the STAR*D study when patients failed to achieve remission on their current regimen. Adding bupropion to citalopram achieved a remission rate of approximately 30% in patients whose symptoms failed to remit after 12 weeks of citalopram-alone therapy. The combination of venlafaxine plus mirtazapine was used in a highly treatment-refractory group (failed to respond to three previous medication trials), and approximately 14% of patients achieved remission of symptoms.[51]

Treatment of Bipolar Disorder

Treatment of bipolar disorder is exceptionally complex, and PCPs would likely best be served by obtaining psychiatric consultation early in the course of a patient's illness to optimize care both for the short and long term. The goals of treatment are threefold: (1) acute stabilization, whether the mood episode is manic, hypomanic, mixed, or depressed; (2) establishment of maintenance treatment to prolong euthymia; and (3) relapse prevention, to anticipate and actively manage future episodes. Subthreshold symptoms, most often depressed, are common and have ongoing consequences for interpersonal, social, and occupational functioning. As in the treatment of major depression, remission of all mood symptoms is the goal. Because treatment must control mania and depression and prevent future episodes, and because patients with bipolar disorder commonly have comorbid anxiety, polypharmacy is the norm. Up to 60% of bipolar patients require three or more medications.[52] Patients experiencing fully syndromal manias will almost invariably require hospitalization given their extreme levels of agitation, aggression, impulsivity, and sometimes psychosis. Severely depressed bipolar patients are at substantial risk for suicide, particularly if some symptoms of activation/mixed states are present. In addition, treatment of depressive or manic episodes is complex since the same treatments that alleviate depression may cause mania, hypomania, or rapid cycling, and treatments that alleviate mania may cause depression.[53] Clinical considerations for using antidepressants in bipolar disorders are described in Box 12.3.

BOX 12.3
CLINICAL CONSIDERATIONS IN USING ANTIDEPRESSANTS IN BIPOLAR DISORDER

- **Adjunctive antidepressants may be helpful if the patient has a prior history of response.**
- **Avoid use in patients with two or more concomitant core manic symptoms, in the presence of psychomotor agitation, or in rapid cycling.**
- **Maintenance use of antidepressants may be considered if patient relapses into depression after stopping antidepressant therapy.**
- **Avoid using SNRIs and TCAs as first-line agents, as they may promote more cycling/switches.**
- **There is some evidence that paroxetine may not be effective in bipolar depression.**
- **It is unclear if adjunctive mood stabilizers are protective.**

Pacchiarotti I, Bond DJ, Baldessarini RJ, et al. The International Society for Bipolar Disorders (ISBD) task force report on antidepressant use in bipolar disorders. Am J Psychiatry. 2013;170(11):1249–1262.

It is beyond the scope of this chapter to provide a comprehensive guide to the treatment of bipolar disorder; rather, this section will focus on first steps that PCPs and an integrated team can take in the care of these challenging patients.

Treatment of Mania

A critical pathway for the treatment of bipolar mania is described in Table 12.3.

No fewer than 10 drugs are currently FDA approved for the treatment of mania, though selection can be guided by the differences that exist between agents. While there is evidence of a class effect among antipsychotics in the treatment of mania, a recent meta-analysis revealed that risperidone, olanzapine, and haloperidol appear to have better efficacy-to-tolerability ratios compared to quetiapine, aripiprazole, ziprasidone, or asenapine.[53–55] Lithium also exerts an anti-manic effect, though it does not appear to work as robustly as antipsychotics, and it is further limited by slower dose titration and side effects. However, given its efficacy as a preventive agent, consideration should be given for long-term lithium treatment. Both divalproex and carbamazepine exert anti-manic effect, but they do not have evidence of prophylactic efficacy and have poorer efficacy-to-tolerability ratios compared to atypical antipsychotics. Of note, class effect is *not* seen among anti-epileptic drugs. Other anti-epileptic drugs, such as lamotrigine, topiramate, gabapentin, levitiracetam, and zonisamide, do not have anti-manic effects and therefore should not be used for the treatment of mania.[55] Typical medication treatment options for bipolar mania, bipolar depression, and bipolar maintenance are shown in Table 12.4.

Resolution of Mania

Clinicians should keep in mind that during acute manic episodes, patients can often tolerate very high doses of medications, but as mania resolves, side effects that were initially absent may become evident. Patients can appear increasingly oversedated and have worsening extrapyramidal side effects or poor energy. For patients taking lithium or divalproex, careful monitoring of drug levels in the blood is necessary, as patients can become toxic as mania resolves and blood levels increase. Patients with resolving manias commonly become nonadherent with their medications as side effects increase and insight is still limited. The clinician should carefully taper the dose to control side effects and maintain medication adherence, while remaining cautious and vigilant for any return of mania.

Treatment of Bipolar Depression

Treatment of bipolar depression represents one of the greatest challenges for clinicians, as the majority of episodes experienced by bipolar patients are depressive and few proven treatments exist. Table 12.5 describes a critical pathway for the treatment of bipolar depression by the integrated care team.

Increasing neurobiological, neuroimaging, and clinical evidence demonstrates that major depression and bipolar depression are distinct entities despite the commonality in symptoms. Many medications proven in the treatment of major depression do not work in bipolar depression. Although the practice is widespread, the use of antidepressants in bipolar disorder is controversial, as no large, randomized, adequately powered studies demonstrate efficacy. Furthermore, antidepressants may cause either switches into mania or rapid cycling. In a large bipolar depression trial that included paroxetine or bupropion added to an existing mood stabilizer, no benefit was found with either antidepressant over placebo in achieving durable recovery.[56] However, some evidence has suggested that antidepressants may be of benefit for particular patients, though the clinical characteristics of those patients has yet to be elucidated.[54] Given the complexity of treating bipolar depression, the dearth of FDA-approved treatments, and the risks of inducing cycling and/or mixed states, PCPs should always consult the BHS and/or consulting psychiatrist before initiating treatment in patients with bipolar depression. PCPs may manage patients who gain remission from bipolar depression, but should their mood symptoms reemerge, another consultation with a consulting psychiatrist is advised.

First-Line Treatments for Bipolar Depression

PCPs attempting to treat bipolar depression should consider two of the three FDA-approved treatments for bipolar disorder as first-line treatments for bipolar depression. Quetiapine was FDA approved for the treatment of bipolar depression in 2006 after the agent demonstrated a large effect size in the two pivotal trials submitted to the FDA. Quetiapine was significantly more effective in patients with bipolar I depressive disorder than bipolar II depressive disorder. Common side effects include dry mouth, sedation, somnolence, dizziness, and fatigue;

TABLE 12.3. CRITICAL PATHWAY: BIPOLAR DISORDER; MANIA

	Initial Assessment			Week 1–4	1 month–6 months	7 months –1 year
Time	45–60 minutes			30 minutes	30 minutes	30 Minutes
	Screening	Diagnosis	Education, Medications	Education, Medications, Therapy	Education, Medications, Therapy	Coping, Relapse Prevention, Medications, Therapy
Bipolar I	***Medical Assistant*** MDQ for screening	*If MDQ positive* ***BHS, PCP*** • Diagnosis by clinical interview • Rule out medical causes, substance-induced causes. • Look for comorbid psychiatric conditions (e.g., anxiety, substance use disorders). • Assess severity of manic symptoms, decision-making capacity, and safety. • Enter patient in risk registry. ***PCP*** • As needed: physical exam, complete blood count, Chem 20 panel, drug screen, electrocardiogram, TSH, fasting lipid panel	***Nurse, BHS, Health Coach*** • Psychoeducation about bipolar disorder with patient and family • Discuss need for medication adherence, symptoms of worsening mania, need to access emergency services. • Discuss need to avoid alcohol, drugs, excessive caffeine; need for regular sleep and routine. ***PCP/Psychiatrist*** • Start anti-manic agent according to Box 12.3.	***Nurse, BHS, Health Coach*** • Clinical reassessment ***PCP, BHS, Health Coach*** • Psychoeducation • Confirm diagnosis. • Reassess for other psychiatric, substance, medical comorbidities. • Assess symptoms, insight, need for medication adherence, regular sleep/wake routine. • Assess decision making, impulsivity. • Brief therapy • Follow in registry. ***PCP, Psychiatrist*** • If atypical antipsychotic started, recheck fasting glucose level.	***Nurse, BHS, Health Coach*** • Clinical reassessment (be aware that depression can follow mania) ***PCP, BHS, Health Coach*** • Assessment of symptoms, insight, need for medication adherence, regular sleep/wake schedule • Assess decision making, impulsivity. • Assess for remission. • Create relapse- prevention plan based on prodromal manic symptoms. • Coping strategies • Brief therapies • Relapse-prevention planning • Update registry	***Nurse, BHS, Health Coach*** • Clinical reassessment ***PCP, BHS, Health Coach*** • Reassess other psychiatric, substance, or medical comorbidities. • Assess for remission. • Relapse-prevention plan • Coping strategies • Brief therapies • Relapse-prevention planning • Update registry. ***PCP, Psychiatrist*** • If remission maintained for 6–12 months, continue medications into maintenance phase as in Box 12.3.

	Psychiatrist • PCP, BHS initial consultation with most cases • Consult if questions regarding safety or hospitalization. ***Care Coordinator*** • Assessment of needs (e.g., refer to ED, inpatient, community mental health as advised by team)	• Assess side effects, tolerability, adherence, insight. • Adjust dosing as necessary to decrease manic symptoms. • Consider adding a 2nd agent if inadequate response. ***Care Coordinator*** • Coordinate care with other needed medical, psychiatric, substance abuse, or community services as advised by team.	***PCP, Psychiatrist*** • If atypical antipsychotic started, recheck fasting glucose level, lipid panel. • Assess side effects, tolerability, adherence, insight. • Adjust dosing as necessary to decrease manic symptoms. • If patient has been responding well, may need to consider slowly lowering dose of anti-manic agent(s) as mania resolves ***Care Coordinator*** • As needed	***Care Coordinator*** • Coordinate care with other needed medical, psychiatric, substance abuse, or community services as advised by team.

TABLE 12.4. U.S. FOOD AND DRUG ADMINISTRATION–APPROVED MEDICATIONS FOR TREATMENT OF BIPOLAR MANIA, BIPOLAR DEPRESSION, AND BIPOLAR MAINTENANCE

Medication	Usual Starting Dose (mg/day)	Usual Dose Range (mg/day)	Side Effects/Comments
			Acute bipolar mania
Carbamazepine ER	200 mg bid	600–1,200	Aim for levels of ~8 mcg/mL. Significant hepatic induction will lower levels of other medications metabolized through hepatic CYP systems. Can cause aplastic anemia (rare). Monitor complete blood count (CBC).
Divalproex Divalproex ER	Can load at 20–30 mg/kg	1,000–3,000	Weight gain, sedation, tremor, hair loss, bruising or bleeding. Aim for levels ~80 mcg/mL. Anti-manic, but no evidence of long-term mood stabilization (i.e., prevention of future episodes).
Lithium	300 mg bid	900–1,800	Aim for level ~0.8 mmol/L. Some evidence of anti-suicidal properties. Monitor thyroid, renal function. Approved for maintenance; has some antidepressant effect.
Aripiprazole*	10–20	20–40	Generally nonsedating, minimal weight gain. Approved for use as maintenance drug in bipolar disorder as well. Available in long-acting injectable (Aristada for schizophrenia)
Asenapine*	5–10	20–30	Only available as dissolvable tab
Olanzapine*	10–15	20–40	Very sedating, associated with greater weight gain and changes in lipids/glucose compared to other atypical antipsychotics. Available in dissolvable form (Zydis) and long-acting injectable (Zyprexa Relprevv for schizophrenia). Approved for maintenance treatment in bipolar disorder.
Quetiapine Quetiapine XR	100–300	300–1,200	Very sedating, associated with greater weight gain and changes in lipids/glucose compared to other atypical antipsychotics. Available in extended-release formulation (Seroquel XR). Approved for use in bipolar depression.
Risperidone*	2–3	4–6	Generally nonsedating. Available in dissolvable tab (M-tab) and long-acting injectable (Consta for schizophrenia). Can significantly increase prolactin levels in some patients.
Ziprasidone	60–80	120–240	Available in injectable form. Should be taken with food to increase its absorption. Generally weight-neutral.

			Acute bipolar depression
Lurasidone*	20–40	60–160	Generally weight-neutral. Take with food to increase absorption.
Olanzapine/fluoxetine	3/25	6/50–12/50	Fixed doses of olanzapine/fluoxetine
Quetiapine, XR	50–200	100–800	Very sedating, associated with greater weight gain and changes in lipids/glucose compared to other atypical antipsychotics. Approved for use in mania. Large effect size in treatment of depression.
			Bipolar maintenance
Lithium	600	900–1,800	Aim for level ~0.8 mmol/L. Some evidence of antisuicidal properties. Risk of hypothyroidism and renal concentration defects over long-term treatment.
Lamotrigine	12.5–25	50–400	Must follow recommended titration schedule to minimize risk of Stevens-Johnson syndrome. Some evidence of antidepressant effect, though not FDA-approved for bipolar depression.
Aripiprazole	5–10	10–30	Generally nonsedating, minimal weight gain. Approved for use in acute mania as well.
Olanzapine	5–10	10–20	Very sedating, associated with greater weight gain and changes in lipids/glucose compared to other atypical antipsychotics. Available in dissolvable form (Zydis). Approved for acute mania treatment.

* Approved for monotherapy and adjunctive therapy.
Usual dose range refers to doses that are commonly used in clinical practice, but do not necessarily agree with FDA-recommended dosing.

TABLE 12.5. CRITICAL PATHWAY: BIPOLAR DISORDER DEPRESSION

	Initial Assessment			Week 1–4	1 month–6 months	7 months–1 year
Time	45–60 minutes			30 minutes	30 minutes	30 Minutes
	Screening	Diagnosis	Education, Medications	Education, Medications, Therapy	Education, Medications, Therapy	Coping, Relapse Prevention, Medications, Therapy
	Medical Assistant MDQ PHQ-2 for screening If PHQ-2 positive, do PHQ-9 Can refer directly to BHS or PCP if patient suicidal	*If MDQ positive* ***BHS, PCP*** If MDQ positive, diagnosis made by clinical interview. Be alert for mixed symptoms. Assess need for hospitalization. Rule out medical causes, substance-induced causes. Look for comorbid psychiatric conditions (anxiety, substance use disorders, etc.). ***Consult Psychiatrist*** All cases of bipolar depression ***PCP/Psychiatrist*** As needed: Physical exam Complete blood count, Chem 20 panel, drug screen, electrocardiogram, TSH, fasting lipid panel	***Nurse, BHS, Health Coach*** • Psychoeducation about bipolar disorder with patient/family • Discuss need for medication adherence, symptoms of worsening depression, need to access emergency services. • Discuss need to avoid alcohol, drugs, excessive caffeine, need for regular sleep/wake routine. • Assess for suicide risk. ***PCP*** • Consult with psychiatrist re: FDA-indicated treatment for bipolar depression according to Table 12.5. • Consult if questions re: safety or hospitalization.	***Medical Assistant*** • Repeat PHQ-9. Enter patient in registry. ***Nurse, BHS, Health Coach*** • Clinical reassessment • Assess suicide risk. ***BHS, PCP, Health Coach*** • Psychoeducation • Confirm diagnosis. • Reassess for other psychiatric, substance, medical comorbidities. • Continued reassessment for safety, mixed symptoms, evidence of switching into mania • Assess symptoms, insight, medication adherence, regular sleep/wake routine. • Assess decision making, impulsivity. • Create relapse-prevention plan based on prodromal depressive symptoms. • Coping strategies • Brief therapies: CBT, behavioral activation, problem solving, crisis intervention	***Medical Assistant*** • **Repeat PHQ-9.** ***Nurse, BHS, Health Coach*** • Clinical reassessment • Assess suicide risk. ***BHS, PCP, Health Coach*** • Confirm diagnosis. • Reassess for other psychiatric, substance, medical comorbidities. • Continued reassessment for safety, mixed symptoms, evidence of switch into mania • Assess symptoms, insight, medication adherence, regular sleep/wake routine. • Assess decision making, impulsivity. • Assess for remission. • Discuss relapse-prevention plan. • Coping strategies • Brief therapies: CBT, behavioral activation, problem solving, crisis intervention • Continued consultation with psychiatrist • Update registry.	***Medical Assistant*** • **Repeat PHQ-9.** ***Nurse, BHS, Health Coach*** • Clinical reassessment • Assess suicide risk. ***BHS, PCP, Health Coach*** • Reassess for other psychiatric, substance, or medical comorbidities. • Continued reassessment for safety, mixed symptoms, evidence of switch into mania • Assess for remission. • Discuss relapse-prevention plan. • Coping strategies • Brief therapies: CBT, behavioral activation, problem solving, crisis intervention • Update registry. ***PCP, Psychiatrist*** • Assess side effects, tolerability, adherence, insight. • Adjust dosing as needed to decrease depressive symptoms.

	Psychiatrist • May prescribe instead of the PCP according to Table 12.5 ***Care Coordinator*** • Assessment of needs (e.g., refer to ED, inpatient, community mental health as advised by team)	• Continued consultation with psychiatrist • Update registry. ***PCP, Psychiatrist*** • If atypical antipsychotic started, recheck fasting glucose level. • Assess side effects, tolerability, adherence, insight. • Adjust dosing as needed to decrease depressive symptoms. ***Psychiatrist*** • Consult with PCP on medications. • Track patient/population in registry. ***Care Coordinator*** • Coordinate care with other needed medical, psychiatric, substance abuse, or community services as advised by team.	***PCP, Psychiatrist*** • If atypical antipsychotic started, recheck fasting glucose level, lipid panel. • Assess side effects, tolerability, adherence, insight. • Adjust dosing prn to decrease depressive symptoms. • Need to reassess for addition of second agent or changing to alternative primary agent • If antidepressant used and patient has achieved remission, need to discuss possibility of tapering off antidepressant to minimize risk of switches or cycling as mania resolves. ***Psychiatrist*** • Consult with PCP on medications, possible switches. • Track patient/population in registry. ***Care Coordinator*** • As needed	• Need to reassess for addition of second agent or changing to alternative primary agent • If antidepressant used and patient has achieved remission, need to discuss possibility of tapering off antidepressant to minimize risk of switches or cycling as mania resolves ***Psychiatrist*** • Consult with PCP on medications, possible switches. • Track patient/population in registry. ***Care Coordinator*** • **Coordinate care with other needed medical, psychiatric, substance abuse, or community services as advised by team.**

metabolic disruption (hyperlipidemia, increased glucose levels) is also a limiting side effect for some patients.[57]

Lurasidone was recently approved both for monotherapy treatment of bipolar I depressive disorder in adults and as adjunctive therapy when combined with lithium or divalproex. In the monotherapy trial, lurasidone in both the 20- to 60-mg and 80- to 120-mg groups was significantly superior to placebo in achieving both response and remission of depression (effect size for both, .51). The most common side effects were nausea, headache, akathisia, somnolence, insomnia, and sedation. Importantly, there were no differences between the two active medication groups and the placebo group in terms of weight, body mass index, fasting cholesterol, triglycerides, or glucose. In the adjunctive trial, lurasidone in a dose of 20 to 120 mg was added to either lithium or divalproex. As in the monotherapy study, the lurasidone adjunct treatment was superior to placebo in both response and remission rates, with number needed to treat = 7 (effect size, .34).[57]

The combination of olanzapine and fluoxetine (OFC) was approved for the treatment of bipolar I depression in 2003. OFC comes as a single pill containing different doses of olanzapine/fluoxetine: 3/25, 6/25, 6/50, 12/25, and 12/50 respectively. The effect size for OFC was .68, and the frequency of switches into mania was no different between the dosing groups or the placebo group. Despite its moderate effect size, OFC has not been a treatment used extensively for bipolar disorder, perhaps because of the presence of fixed doses for each medication, the use of the antidepressant fluoxetine, or the side effect profile for olanzapine (weight gain, metabolic derangements).

Second-Line Treatments for Bipolar Depression

Second-line treatments for bipolar depression include lamotrigine and lithium. Lamotrigine is currently FDA approved for maintenance treatment in bipolar I disorder but not for bipolar depression, although it can be used as second-line treatment. This is because lamotrigine failed to show efficacy in its primary outcome measure (the Hamilton Depression Rating Scale), though antidepressant efficacy was shown on its secondary outcome measure (the Montgomery Asberg Rating Scale).[57] A meta-analysis of patient-level data from five trials of lamotrigine in bipolar depression reported a modest treatment effect, though no one trial showed statistically significant benefits of treatment with lamotrigine over placebo.[53] The original lamotrigine trials used doses of 50 mg and 200 mg, and both were significantly more effective than placebo in the seven-week trials on the secondary outcome measure.

Evidence supporting lithium's effectiveness in both acute and long-term treatment of bipolar depression is generally positive, though more recent studies of lithium as a comparator have shown it to be no better than placebo. Earlier studies of lithium in bipolar depression showed its superiority over placebo, and it appears to possess antisuicidal properties. However, the antisuicidal effect of lithium may take weeks, and its narrow therapeutic window, toxicity, and side effect burden may mitigate some of its positives.[58] Because of its proven efficacy in both treatment of mania and prevention of future episodes, and its suicide protective effects, lithium is often a superior choice to other mood-stabilizing agents.

Antidepressants in Bipolar Depression

The use of antidepressants for the treatment of bipolar depression remains controversial, as they can cause switches into mania, mixed states, and/or rapid cycling. While small studies have shown some evidence of their efficacy in bipolar depression, larger, adequately powered studies have not demonstrated their superiority over a mood stabilizer alone.[56] An exceptionally thorough review of all antidepressant trials in bipolar depression reached modest conclusions about their utility in bipolar depression. See Box 12.3.[54] Switch rates from depression to mania may be in the 10% to 20% range, and it is not proven that mood stabilizers protect against mania. That being said, PCPs are advised to use antidepressants very cautiously in patients with bipolar disorder and always consult a BHS and/or psychiatrist.

Maintenance Treatment of Bipolar Disorder

There are currently four medications that have been FDA approved for maintenance treatment of bipolar disorder: lithium, aripiprazole, olanzapine, and lamotrigine. The goals of maintenance therapy include decreasing the number, length, and intensity of mood episodes over time, and in so doing increasing the psychosocial functioning of patients while decreasing the suicide risk.

BOX 12.4

SUMMARY OF RECOMMENDED TREATMENT APPROACHES AND RELEVANT EVIDENCE

Strength of recommendation taxonomy (SOR A, B, or C)

- **Collaborative care models improve treatment outcome for depressed patients in primary care settings.[1] (SOR A)**
- **Collaborative care models improve treatment outcome for bipolar patients in primary care settings.[3,59] (SOR A)**
- **Psychotherapy improves outcomes in both major depression and bipolar disorder.[4] (SOR A)**
- **Antidepressants are effective for the majority of patients with major depression. All classes of antidepressant medications work equally well, though individual patients may respond better to one agent than another.[5,13,46] (SOR A)**
- **Mania is effectively treated with mood stabilizers or atypical antipsychotic medications.[55] (SOR A)**
- **Lithium, lamotrigine, aripiprazole, and olanzapine are effective in preventing future mood episodes in bipolar disorder, though all are more effective in preventing manias than depression.[53,55] (SOR A)**
- **Quetiapine, lurasidone, and olanzapine/fluoxetine are the most effective agents in treating acute bipolar depression.[60–62] (SOR A)**
- **Antidepressants appear beneficial for some patients with bipolar depression, though use of antidepressants includes the risk of switches, rapid cycling, and/or mixed states.[54] (SOR B)**

For patients who are taking stable doses of maintenance medications, management by the PCP is reasonable; growing mood instability would be reasons to have a "curbside consultation" with the psychiatrist or to send the patient back to the psychiatrist for another consultation and management until stable again. Lithium is the best-established medication for long-term treatment. A meta-analysis of five placebo-controlled trials showed that lithium reduced the risk of manic relapse by 38% and depressive relapse by 28%.[53] Aripiprazole, in doses of 15 to 30 mg/day, demonstrated superiority over placebo in preventing manic, but not depressive, relapses. Given its favorable side effect profile compared to olanzapine, aripiprazole is likely the first atypical antipsychotic for PCPs to try if choosing among antipsychotics. Lamotrigine demonstrated a 36% reduction in the risk of relapse over 18 months compared to placebo. There is some evidence that lamotrigine prevents relapses into depression better than relapses into mania. Olanzapine was the first atypical antipsychotic to demonstrate maintenance efficacy in bipolar disorder, and it seemed to show greater efficacy in preventing relapses into mania than depression.

Can Patients with Bipolar Disorder Discontinue Treatment?

Given its extremely high recurrence rates, the substantial morbidity and mortality associated with recurrences, the financial burden imposed from either missed productivity or imprudent financial decisions, and the emotional toll of the illness, patients are best advised to remain on lifelong treatment to prevent recurrences. Recurrent mood episodes also can lessen the effectiveness of previously effective drugs, such as lithium, and negatively alter the course of the illness.[7] Thus, a premium should be put on finding long-term treatments that are both effective and tolerable for patients in order to enhance adherence. Judging the efficacy of a particular treatment often requires several years, given the cyclical and unpredictable nature of mood recurrences. Educating patients about all of these issues is a key component in preventing relapse, enhancing the therapeutic alliance, and practicing collaborative and patient-centered decision making.

CONCLUSION

Given the frequency of mood disorders in primary care settings, the reality that the majority of patients receive their psychiatric care from PCPs, and the growing awareness that treatment of mood disorders improves overall patient outcome while lowering health care costs, an integrated care approach to treating such patients is a necessity. As these treatment strategies become more widespread, further refinements in the models will no doubt take place, driven by expanding health and economic outcomes data and larger studies. This chapter offers initial ideas for providers and practices to transform treatment strategies for these challenging patients, with the full expectation that these models will change in the future. Box 12.4 summarizes the evidence supporting collaborative care of these disorders.

REFERENCES

1. The Global Burden of Disease: 2004 Update. Geneva: World Health Organization; 2008.
2. Spitzer RL, Kroenke K, Williams JB. Validation and utility of a self-report version of PRIME-MD: The PHQ primary care study. JAMA. 1999;282(18):1737–1744.
3. Kilbourne AM, Goodrich DE, O'Donnell AN, Miller CJ. Integrating bipolar disorder management in primary care. Curr Psychiatry Rep. 2012;14(6):687–695.
4. Katon WJ. The Institute of Medicine "Chasm" report: Implications for depression collaborative care models. Gen Hosp Psychiatry. 2003;25(4):222–229.
5. American Psychiatric Association. Diagnostic and Statistical Manual of Mental Disorders (5th ed.). Arlington, VA: American Psychiatric Association; 2013.
6. Fava M, Rosenbaum JF. Anger attacks in patients with depression. J Clin Psychiatry. 1999;60(suppl 15):21–24.
7. Goodwin FK, Jamison KR. Manic Depressive Illness, 2nd ed. New York: Oxford University Press; 2007.
8. Judd LL, Akiskal HS, Schettler PJ, et al. The long-term natural history of the weekly symptomatic status of bipolar I disorder. Arch Gen Psychiatry. 2002;59(6):530–537.
9. Judd LL, Akiskal HS, Schettler PJ, et al. A prospective investigation of the natural history of the long-term weekly symptomatic status of bipolar II disorder. Arch Gen Psychiatry. 2003;60(3):261–269.
10. Manning JS, Haykal RF, Akiskal HS. The role of bipolarity in depression in the family practice setting. Psychiatr Clin North Am. 1999;22(3):689–703.
11. Bridges KW, Goldberg DP. Somatic presentation of DSM III psychiatric disorders in primary care. J Psychosom Res. 1985;29(6):563–569.
12. Kroenke K, Jackson JL, Chamberlin J. Depressive and anxiety disorders in patients presenting with physical complaints: Clinical predictors and outcome. Am J Med. 1997;103(5):339–347.
13. Kessler RC, Wang PS. The descriptive epidemiology of commonly occurring mental disorders in the United States. Annu Rev Public Health. 2008;29:115–129.
14. Kessler RC, Berglund P, Demler O, Jin R, Merikangas KR, Walters EE. Lifetime prevalence and age-of-onset distributions of DSM-IV disorders in the National Comorbidity Survey Replication. Arch Gen Psychiatry. 2005;62(6):593–602.
15. Katon W, Unutzer J, Wells K, Jones L. Collaborative depression care: History, evolution and ways to enhance dissemination and sustainability. Gen Hosp Psychiatry. 2010;32(5):456–464.
16. Das AK, Olfson M, Gameroff MJ, et al. Screening for bipolar disorder in a primary care practice. JAMA. 2005;293(8):956–963.
17. Wang PS, Lane M, Olfson M, Pincus HA, Wells KB, Kessler RC. Twelve-month use of mental health services in the United States: Results from the National Comorbidity Survey Replication. Arch Gen Psychiatry. 2005;62(6):629–640.
18. Greenberg PE, Kessler RC, Birnbaum HG, et al. The economic burden of depression in the US: How did it change 1990–2000? J Clin Psychiatry. 2003;64:1465–1475.
19. Dilsaver SC. An estimate of the minimum economic burden of bipolar I and II disorders in the United States: 2009. J Affect Disord. 2011;129(1–3):79–83.
20. Eaton WW, Shao H, Nestadt G, Lee HB, Bienvenu OJ, Zandi P. Population-based study of first onset and chronicity in major depressive disorder. Arch Gen Psychiatry. 2008;65(5):513–520.
21. Kessler RC, Berglund P, Demler O, et al. The epidemiology of major depressive disorder: Results from the National Comorbidity Survey Replication (NCS-R). JAMA. 2003;289(23):3095–3105.
22. Blair-West GW, Cantor CH, Mellsop GW, Eyeson-Annan ML. Lifetime suicide risk in major depression: Sex and age determinants. J Affect Disord. 1999;55:171–178.
23. Bostwick JM, Pankratz VS. Affective disorders and suicide risk: A reexamination. Am J Psychiatry. 2000;157:1925–1932.
24. Solomon DA, Keitner GI, Miller IW, Shea MT, Keller MB. Course of illness and maintenance treatments for patients with bipolar disorder. J Clin Psychiatry. 1995;56(1):5–13.
25. Judd LL, Schettler PJ, Akiskal HS, et al. Residual symptom recovery from major affective episodes in bipolar disorders and rapid episode relapse/recurrence. Arch Gen Psychiatry. 2008;65(4):386–394.
26. Harris EC, Barraclough B. Suicide as an outcome in mental disorder. A meta-analysis. Br J Psychiatry. 1997;170:205–228.

27. Katon WJ. Clinical and health services relationships between major depression, depressive symptoms, and general medical illness. Biol Psychiatry. 2003;54(3):216–226.
28. Kupfer DJ. The increasing medical burden in bipolar disorder. JAMA. 2005;293(20):2528–2530.
29. Katon WJ, Walker EA. Medically unexplained symptoms in primary care. J Clin Psychiatry. 1998;59:15–21.
30. Simon GE. Social and economic burden of mood disorders. Biol Psychiatry. 2003;54(3):208–215.
31. Cerimele JM, Chan YF, Chwastiak LA, Avery M, Katon W, Unutzer J. Bipolar disorder in primary care: Clinical characteristics of 740 primary care patients with bipolar disorder. Psychiatr Serv. 2014;65(8):1041–1046.
32. Judd LL, Paulus MJ, Schettler PJ, et al. Does incomplete recovery from first lifetime major depressive episode herald a chronic course of illness? Am J Psychiatry. 2000;157(9):1501–1504.
33. Kroenke K, Spitzer RL, Williams JB. The PHQ-9: Validity of a brief depression severity measure. J Gen Intern Med. 2001;16(9):606–613.
34. Hirschfeld RM, Williams JB, Spitzer RL, et al. Development and validation of a screening instrument for bipolar spectrum disorder: The Mood Disorder Questionnaire. Am J Psychiatry. 2000;157(11):1873–1875.
35. Hirschfeld RM, Calabrese JR, Weissman MM, et al. Screening for bipolar disorder in the community. J Clin Psychiatry. 2003;64(1):53–59.
36. Hirschfeld RM, Cass AR, Holt DC, Carlson CA. Screening for bipolar disorder in patients treated for depression in a family medicine clinic. J Am Board Fam Pract. 2005;18(4):233–239.
37. Bauer MS, McBride L, Williford WO, et al. Collaborative care for bipolar disorder: Part I. Intervention and implementation in a randomized effectiveness trial. Psychiatr Serv. 2006;57(7):927–936.
38. Kroenke K, Spitzer RL, Williams JB. The Patient Health Questionnaire-2: Validity of a two-item depression screener. Med Care. 2003;41(11):1284–1292.
39. Miklowitz DJ. The Bipolar Disorder Survival Guide: What You and Your Family Need to Know. New York: Guilford Press; 2011.
40. Bauer MS, Kilbourne AM, Greenwald DE, Ludman EJ. Overcoming Bipolar Disorder: A Comprehensive Workbook for Managing Your Symptoms and Achieving Your Life Goals. Oakland, CA: New Harbinger Publications, Inc.; 2008.
41. DeRubeis RJ, Hollon SD, Amsterdam JD, et al. Cognitive therapy vs medications in the treatment of moderate to severe depression. Arch Gen Psychiatry. 2005;62:409–416.
42. Trivedi MH, Rush AJ, Wisniewski SR, et al. Evaluation of outcomes with citalopram for depression using measurement-based care in STAR*D: Implications for clinical practice. Am J Psychiatry. 2006;163(1):28–40.
43. Rush AJ, Trivedi MH, Wisniewski SR, et al. Bupropion-SR, sertraline, or venlafaxine-XR after failure of SSRIs for depression. N Engl J Med. 2006;354(12):1231–1242.
44. Thase ME, Entsuah AR, Rudolph RL. Remission rates during treatment with venlafaxine or selective serotonin reuptake inhibitors. Br J Psychiatry. 2001;178:234–241.
45. Clayton AH, Warnock JK, Kornstein SG, Pinkerton R, Sheldon-Keller A, McGarvey EL. A placebo-controlled trial of bupropion SR as an antidote for selective serotonin reuptake inhibitor-induced sexual dysfunction. J Clin Psychiatry. 2004;65(1):62–67.
46. American Psychiatric Association. Practice guideline for the treatment of patients with major depressive disorder, 3rd ed. Am J Psychiatry. 2010;167(suppl):1–152.
47. Solomon DA, Keller MB, Leon AC, et al. Multiple recurrences of major depressive disorder. Am J Psychiatry. 2000;157(2):229–233.
48. Thase ME. Are SNRIs more effective than SSRIs? A review of the current state of the controversy. Psychopharm Bull. 2008;41(2):58–85.
49. Nierenberg AA, Fava M, Trivedi MH, et al. A comparison of lithium and T(3) augmentation following two failed medication treatments for depression: A STAR*D report. Am J Psychiatry. 2006;163(9):1519–1530; quiz 1665.
50. TrivediMH,FavaM,WisniewskiSR,etal.Medication augmentation after the failure of SSRIs for depression. N Engl J Med. 2006;354(12):1243–1252.
51. McGrath PJ, Stewart JW, Fava M, et al. Tranylcypromine versus venlafaxine plus mirtazapine following three failed antidepressant medication trials for depression: A STAR*D report. Am J Psychiatry. 2006;163(9):1531–1541; quiz 1666.
52. Goldberg JF, Brooks JO, 3rd, Kurita K, et al. Depressive illness burden associated with complex polypharmacy in patients with bipolar disorder: Findings from the STEP-BD. J Clin Psychiatry. 2009;70(2):155–162.
53. Geddes JR, Miklowitz DJ. Treatment of bipolar disorder. Lancet. 2013;381(9878):1672–1682.
54. Pacchiarotti I, Bond DJ, Baldessarini RJ, et al. The International Society for Bipolar Disorders (ISBD) task force report on antidepressant use in bipolar disorders. Am J Psychiatry. 2013;170(11):1249–1262.
55. Cipriani A, Barbui C, Salanti G, et al. Comparative efficacy and acceptability of antimanic drugs in acute mania: A multiple-treatments meta-analysis. Lancet. 2011;378(9799):1306–1315.
56. Sachs GS, Nierenberg AA, Calabrese JR, et al. Effectiveness of adjunctive antidepressant

treatment for bipolar depression. N Engl J Med. 2007;356(17):1711–1722.

57. McIntyre RS, Cha DS, Kim RD, Mansur RB. A review of FDA-approved treatment options in bipolar depression. CNS Spectr. 2013;18(Suppl 1):4–20; quiz 21.

58. Kasper S, Calabrese JR, Johnson G, et al. International Consensus Group on the evidenced-based pharmacologic treatment of bipolar I and II depression. J Clin Psychiatry. 2008;69(10):1632–1657.

59. Bauer MS, Biswas K, Kilbourne AM. Enhancing multiyear guideline concordance for bipolar disorder through collaborative care. Am J Psychiatry. 2009;166(11):1244–1250.

60. Calabrese JR, Keck PE, Jr., Macfadden W, et al. A randomized, double-blind, placebo-controlled trial of quetiapine in the treatment of bipolar I or II depression. Am J Psychiatry. 2005;162(7):1351–1360.

61. Dube S, Tollefson GD, Thase ME, et al. Onset of antidepressant effect of olanzapine and olanzapine/fluoxetine combination in bipolar depression. Bipolar Disord. 2007;9(6):618–627.

62. Loebel AD, Cucchiaro J, Silva R, et al. Lurasidone monotherapy in the treatment of bipolar I depression: A randomized, double-blind, placebo-controlled study. Am J Psychiatry. 2013;171(2):160–168.

13

The Treatment of Schizophrenia Spectrum and Other Psychotic Disorders in Integrated Primary Care

ELIZABETH LOWDERMILK, NICOLE JOSEPH, AND ROBERT E. FEINSTEIN

BOX 13.1

KEY POINTS

- **Integrated care models have been shown to improve quality and reduce the cost of treatment. While there are the National Institute for Health and Care Excellence practice guidelines for the treatment of schizophrenia spectrum and other psychotic disorders that include portions of care that can be provided in primary care, there are no evidence-based integrated care models that detail the completely successful treatment of these disorders in primary care and no definitive evidence to indicate best practice.**
- **Owing to a growing U.S. population, a decreasing psychiatric workforce, scarcity of resources, socioeconomic factors, and/or patient preference, many patients with psychotic disorders seek treatment in primary care. Primary care, for many patients, may be the only source of mental health treatment available.**
- **Treatment of schizophrenia spectrum and other psychotic disorders in primary care may benefit from a collaborative team approach involving the primary care provider, a behavioral health specialist, and a consulting psychiatrist. The team may also include nurses, social workers, a health coach, a care coordinator, a pharmacist, and clinic navigators.**
- **Targeted screening should be used to identify patients with psychotic symptoms.**
- **A full medical and psychiatric differential diagnosis and assessment should be completed.**
- **Safety concerns, the need for hospitalizations, and medically serious etiologies of psychotic symptoms need immediate assessment and treatment.**
- **When a psychotic disorder is confirmed, treatment should be initiated with a focus on symptom management with medications, psychosocial interventions, and other therapies (e.g., cognitive-behavioral therapy, skill building). Families and/or invested parties should be involved.**
- **Co-occurring medical disorders, including substance use disorders, need to be identified and treated.**
- **Antipsychotic medications require monitoring for effectiveness and management of side effects to avoid medical complications or discontinuation.**

- **Special consideration should be given to psychotic geriatric patients and to women of childbearing age.**
- **Given the large number of patients seen in U.S. primary care practices, registries are key to the management of all patients with psychotic disorders. Special, more frequent monitoring of high-risk psychotic patients (i.e., those who are suicidal or potentially violent, those who have grave disability, or those who are not improving) is warranted.**
- **Practice considerations, including the roles of the team members, day-to-day workflow, and special situations such as the need for hospitalization or specialty referral should be defined before implementing the program.**
- **Team members need to be flexible, using care models that are monitored and adjusted as needed.**
- **A critical pathway outlines the treatment of schizophrenia spectrum and other psychotic disorders in an integrated primary care setting for the first year.**

INTRODUCTION

Traditional paradigms, on which our training programs and current practices are based, would suggest that all schizophrenia spectrum and other psychotic disorders should be treated in a mental health *specialty* practice. So, why consider treating psychotic patients in primary care? The answers are complex and multifactorial:

1. Primary care providers (PCPs) are often the first to identify a patient with a psychotic disorder.
2. Patients often prefer treatment in a primary care practice.
3. An integrated primary care practice may provide better access to mental health care in the current environment of limited availability of specialty psychiatric resources.

Patients with schizophrenia spectrum and other psychotic disorders often present with symptoms or their first psychotic episode in the offices of PCPs, including pediatricians. Schizophrenia typically manifests in the late teens to the mid-30s,[1] at a time in a person's life during which the only existing medical treatment relationship is likely with a PCP. The patient's trust in the PCP may lead him or her to prefer treatment in that practice. The patient may have a strong preference to be treated in primary care because of socioeconomic factors, such as proximity to care, the affordability of a single co-pay, for a primary care appointment rather than the double co-pay required to see both a PCP and a mental health provider, and the fact that "one-stop shopping" in primary care improves mental health access and saves transportation costs that would be required if multiple sites of care were needed.

Multiple systemic factors result in people with psychotic disorders being treated in primary care. Regions vary in the availability of mental health services. In some regions, the PCP may be the only resource for many people with severe and persistent mental illnesses. For systems that care for a large uninsured or publicly insured population, who cannot afford to pay out of pocket for psychiatric care, access to a psychiatrist is often significantly limited: Over half of psychiatrists in private practice do not accept Medicaid and Medicare.[2] Unfortunately, even having private insurance doesn't guarantee access to a psychiatrist, since almost half of currently practicing psychiatrists also do not accept private insurance.[2]

In this chapter, we review the salient clinical features of schizophrenia and psychotic disorders. We briefly describe psychiatric specialty services that integrated care teams should know about so that referrals can be offered as needed. We describe the Denver Health Medical Center (DHMC) model, including lessons learned during its development and implementation. We close by proposing a new integrated care model for the treatment of schizophrenia spectrum and other psychotic disorders in primary care. The proposed model weaves together best practices of specialty mental health care with the fundamentals of integrated care, drawing upon the experience of Integrated Behavioral Health at the DHMC. These key points are summarized in Box 13.1.

ARGUMENTS FOR THE TREATMENT OF SCHIZOPHRENIA SPECTRUM AND OTHER PSYCHOTIC DISORDERS IN PRIMARY CARE

Untreated mental illness increases total health care costs.[3] Currently it is estimated that only 32.2% of those diagnosed with schizophrenia and other nonaffective psychoses are actually receiving treatment.[4] This suggests the potential for significant cost savings by treating psychotic disorders in primary care. A 2001 World Health Report's top recommendation is to address treatment gaps and make mental health treatment accessible in primary care.[5]

In addition to the economic costs of untreated mental illness, there are costs to the patient who is not treated early. A prolonged period of untreated psychotic illness is associated with poorer treatment responses, including lower levels of symptom reduction and poorer functional outcomes.[6] Many psychotic disorders are progressive and, theoretically, the use of antipsychotic medication early in the course of the illness may protect against the progression of the illness and influence the long-term treatment outcomes.[6]

Large numbers of patients with psychotic disorders come to be treated in primary care. A Centers for Disease Control and Prevention (CDC) study noted that 5% of all ambulatory care visits from 2007 to 2008, totaling 47.8 million visits, were made by those with a primary mental health diagnosis.[7] Twenty-three percent of these (11 million visits) occurred for schizophrenia or a primary psychotic disorder. Combine this with the increasing U.S. population and the aging workforce of psychiatrists (55% of the psychiatrists currently practicing are 55 or older),[2] and it is clear that we need to creatively and aggressively develop models within primary care to care for those with serious mental illness.

There is a robust body of literature on the practice of integrated care for depression which demonstrate, evidence-based models that have been shown to improve outcomes[8] and reduce treatment costs.[3] Additionally, there are practice guidelines for the treatment of schizophrenia in *specialty* mental health practices[9,10] and guidelines that allow for portions of treatment to occur in primary care (e.g., maintenance treatment after stabilization).[10] However, these guidelines do not address collaborative treatment of schizophrenia in primary care or best implementation practices, nor do they address barriers to implementation.[11] Robinson and Reiter[12] generally address the application of the Primary Care Behavioral Health Model to patients with serious mental illness. However, there are no evidence-based collaborative care approaches for the treatment of people with schizophrenia, and only low or very low-quality trials in the primary care treatment of the seriously mentally ill.[13]

CARE FOR PATIENTS WITH SCHIZOPHRENIA SPECTRUM AND OTHER PSYCHOTIC DISORDERS

Screening for Schizophrenia and Other Psychotic Disorders

It is not realistic to formally screen every patient for a psychotic disorder. However, initial clinical screening is possible and involves observations of a patient with psychotic symptoms as he or she enters an integrated care practice. Commonly, the patients will present to the front desk, medical assistant, or nurse, who may notice that they appear guarded; withdrawn; suspicious; disorganized in speech, thoughts, or behavior; agitated; or responding to internal stimuli. Patients with mental health conditions who are not adherent to prescribed medical treatment should also be screened for psychosis. In addition to staff observations, the PCP or other team members may have collateral information suggesting psychosis from family members, a review of recent hospitalizations or discharges, emergency department (ED) visits, or a unified electronic medical record.

Patients with a history of mood disorder, anxiety, posttraumatic stress disorder (PTSD), substance abuse, or dementia or with a family history of schizophrenia spectrum and other psychotic disorder may also warrant further investigation. Given the many time constraints inherent in primary care today, the PCP and other team members can focus their detailed screening on patients presenting with (1) an odd affect,[14] strange behaviors, or possible hallucinations, delusions, and/or a thought disorder; (2) a history of schizophrenia, paranoia, or schizotypal/schizoid personality; or (3) a history of mood disorders, substance abuse, or dementia. Once there is a preliminary identification of a psychosis, the PCP or behavioral health specialist (BHS) should routinely review all other psychotic symptoms and, if indicated, complete a full psychiatric assessment.

How to Assess for Psychosis

A clinical interview is required to assess for a psychosis as patient self-report rating scales for psychosis are very unreliable. During the initial interview, when it is important to gain the patient's trust, the PCP may be in the best position for empathic questioning, especially if there has been a previous relationship with the patient.

Clinicians can ask questions to elicit the presence of positive symptoms (e.g., hallucinations, delusions, and/or disorganization), and observe and identify negative symptoms (e.g., withdrawal, paucity of thought, apathy). Typically, one or two questions about each domain are sufficient. A positive diagnostic screen often requires more detailed questioning. The *Diagnostic and Statistical Manual of Mental Disorders, Fifth Edition* (DSM-5)[1] offers an assessment measure, the Clinician-Rated Dimensions of Psychosis Symptom Severity,[1] that can be completed upon initial evaluation and then repeated for ongoing monitoring. It is free and may be reproduced without permission for use with patients.

Questions that are useful for assessing auditory or visual hallucinations include the following:

- "Do you ever hear voices or sounds that others don't seem to hear?"
- "Do you ever hear two people talking about you?"
- "Do you ever hear conversations in your head or hear noises that others don't believe are there?"
- "Do you ever see things that others don't see or don't believe are there?"

Questions about delusions may include the following:

- "Do you ever feel paranoid?"
- "Do you ever think people are watching or following you?"
- "Do you ever think that others can read your mind/insert thoughts into your mind, or control you?"
- "Do you ever believe there are messages meant just for you coming from the TV, newspaper, radio, or Internet?"

The clinician can make important observations about the patient, identifying whether the patient exhibits a coherent, goal-directed, logical thought process or a disorganized thought process, tangential/circumstantial thinking, loose associations (appearing to move from topic to topic with little or no apparent logical connection between thoughts) or has disorganized or incoherent speech. The clinician may observe the patient answering questions in a seemingly irrelevant fashion, or observe disorganized behavior as the patient tries to accomplish basic tasks, such as registration and following instructions. Questions for the patient can include "Do you ever have a hard time making sense of your thoughts?" and "Do you feel your thoughts are confused or do you have difficulty communicating your thoughts to others?"

Negative symptoms, which are often harder to elicit from the patient, may be apparent through the patient's presentation or by obtaining collateral information from family members or friends. Patients may appear withdrawn, have poor eye contact, may give only "yes/no" answers, and may have difficulty initiating conversation. Family members may report that the patient is mostly nonverbal in other settings or may note withdrawal, isolation, and an absence of relationships, activities, or interests.

Direct questions about the patient's history and collateral information from family or friends may also be helpful. A simple, often very informative question to ask the patient is "Have you ever seen a psychiatrist, been hospitalized, or had any previous mental health care?" If yes, ask: "Do you know your diagnosis?" While this question can sometimes result in a list of seemingly discordant diagnoses, the knowledge obtained can help to direct the patient's evaluation and care.

Positive Screens for Psychosis

A positive clinical screen for psychosis leads to identifying and treating emergencies, completing a medical and psychiatric differential diagnosis, and beginning treatment. Clinicians in primary care can work collaboratively, sometimes seeing the patient together or consecutively. The information obtained by one team member often informs the workup by others and drives the considerations for differential diagnosis. For instance, a patient with a reported history of schizophrenia, out of treatment or off medications, presenting with psychotic symptoms, may warrant only a limited medical workup. However, a patient with a new onset of psychosis may require a detailed medical and psychiatric workup. Symptoms of psychosis are not sufficient to determine the specific diagnosis or treatment; a more extensive evaluation is required.

To ensure tight communication and careful monitoring, the PCP and the psychiatrist should develop the initial treatment plan for psychotic patients. New cases should be reviewed at least weekly.

Medical and Psychiatric Emergencies

Emergency situations must be quickly identified. The PCP should assess patients with new-onset psychoses for medical causes that require immediate attention. These include dangerous electrolyte imbalances, metabolic or endocrine abnormalities, infection, space-occupying brain lesions (tumor, bleed), and so forth. In addition, all patients should be assessed for acute intoxication, withdrawal, or drug abuse. A urine drug screen should be routinely obtained as many drugs of abuse (e.g., cocaine, methamphetamine, angel dust) can produce a psychosis that is difficult to differentiate from schizophrenia.[15]

Additionally, the patient should be assessed for psychiatric emergencies. The PCP or psychiatrist should evaluate the risk for suicide and violence (see Chapter 18: Violence and Suicide) and assess for grave disability (the patient is incapacitated and unable to care for himself or herself). These three risks should lead clinicians to consider the need for hospitalization. The team should obtain collateral information and identify the support network and resources available to the patient. The PCP and psychiatrist, focusing on known past medical, mental health, and substance abuse problems, should complete targeted chart reviews. Psychiatric emergencies warrant immediate consultation with the psychiatrist.

Some patients will require psychiatric or substance-related hospitalization. Prior to implementation of an integrated care model, teams should develop a plan for psychiatric hospitalizations with clearly defined staff roles. The team should be familiar with the state regulations regarding involuntary mental health commitment and substance abuse care and treatment. Multiple providers should be trained to initiate the commitment process, and the required forms should be on hand. Clinics with security personnel will need to determine if the security officer may detain a patient in need of an involuntary treatment, and if and when the police will be called. Care should be coordinated with all concerned, including the patient's family, the receiving facility where hospitalization will be arranged, and the receiving inpatient team. It should include helping the family and the health care systems to coordinate discharge plans. Hospitalized patients should remain on the practice registry and their transition plans back to the community should be carefully arranged and tracked.

If there are no emergencies, it may be necessary or helpful for the PCP to start psychiatric antipsychotic medications for the patient's symptomatic relief before completing the full assessment. Inquiring about previous mental health treatment, diagnoses, and medication trials can be invaluable. The consulting psychiatrist can recommend or prescribe medications, and assist the PCP and team to develop and implement the initial treatment and follow-up plan.

Differential Diagnosis

Once emergency conditions have been identified and addressed, and if the patient remains an outpatient, a formal assessment should be completed in one to three weekly visits. The full assessment includes ruling out medical conditions that may be causing the psychosis and completing the psychiatric differential diagnosis.

Medical Assessment and Medical Differential Diagnosis

When a patient presents with a first-break psychosis, or a medical or a substance-induced psychosis is suspected or cannot be ruled out, a comprehensive medical differential diagnosis and workup is warranted. Box 13.2 reviews the medical differential diagnosis for psychosis.

The medical workup includes a collaborative history, a detailed physical examination, a basic laboratory evaluation, and possibly radiologic imaging. At a minimum, the patient should have a complete blood count, electrolyte panel, comprehensive metabolic panel, thyroid function test, vitamin B-12 and folate levels, screening for syphilis and HIV, urinalysis, and urine drug screen. Other laboratory tests to be considered include erythrocyte sedimentation rate, liver function tests, pregnancy test, antinuclear antibody, and ceruloplasm.[14–16] Brain imaging with computed tomography (CT) or magnetic resonance imaging (MRI) should be considered for first-break psychosis, in cases with atypical presentations, when there are abnormalities on neurological examinations, or if there is a poor response to initial treatment.[15,16] Other tests as clinically indicated may

BOX 13.2
DIFFERENTIAL DIAGNOSIS OF PSYCHOTIC SYMPTOMS

PRIMARY PSYCHIATRIC DIAGNOSIS

- **Schizophrenia**
- **Schizoaffective disorder**
- **Delusional disorder (including delusions of parasitosis)**
- **Brief psychotic disorder**
- **Depression or bipolar disorder with psychotic features**
- **Borderline personality disorder**
- **Posttraumatic stress disorder**
- **Schizotypical/schizoid personality disorder**
- **Delirium**

SUBSTANCE OR MEDICATION-INDUCED PSYCHOSIS

- **Alcohol**
- **Cannabinoids (including synthetic)**
- **Sedative/hypnotic/anxiolytics (benzodiazepines, barbiturates)**
- **Stimulants (cocaine, amphetamine, methylphenidate)**
- **Hallucinogens**
- **Antibiotics (floroquinolones, mefloquine, choroquine)**
- **Corticosteroids (prednisone)**
- **Anabolic steroids (testosterone)**
- **Anti-epileptics**
- **Antiparkinsonian agents (levodopa)**
- **Anticholinergics (atropine)**

MEDICAL CONDITIONS CAUSING PSYCHOSIS

- **Endocrine (thyroid, adrenal, insulinoma, pheochromocytoma)**
- **Autoimmune (systemic lupus erythematosus)**
- **Infectious (HIV, neurosyphilis, lyme disease, west nile encephalitis, prion disease)**
- **Metabolic (acute porphyria, Wilson disease)**
- **Electrolyte imbalance (hyponatremia)**
- **Neurological (seizure, stroke, traumatic brain injury, multiple sclerosis, dementia)**
- **Neoplasm: primary or secondary**
- **Central nervous system manifestation of systemic illness (cardiac, respiratory, renal, hepatic)**
- **Nutritional deficiency (vitamin B-12, niacin)**
- **Sleep disturbance (sleep apnea)**

American Psychiatric Association. Diagnostic and Statistical Manual of Mental Disorders, 5th ed. Arlington, VA: American Psychiatric Association; 2013; Carlat DJ. The psychiatric review of symptoms: A screening tool for family physicians. Am Fam Physician. 1998;58(7):1617–1624; Freudenreich O. Differential diagnosis of psychotic symptoms: Medical mimics. Psychiatr Times. 2010;27(12):56–61; and Correll CU, Mendelowitz AJ. First psychotic episode—a window of opportunity: Seize the moment to build a therapeutic alliance. Curr Psychiatr. 2003;2(4):50–67.

include electrocardiogram (ECG), chest x-ray, lumbar puncture/culture, blood and urine culture, arterial blood gas analysis, serum cortisol measurement, toxin screens, drug levels, and genetic testing.[15,16]

If a medically induced psychosis is identified and the PCP has initiated treatment, the psychiatrist can advise, consult, recommend, or deliver additional treatment as needed until the symptoms are controlled or resolved. The BHS and/or the care coordinator should continue monitoring the patient and may be in contact with the patient's family or support network in person, by phone, or via telebehavioral health. Patients should continue to be tracked in the registry.

Psychiatric Assessment and Differential Diagnosis

The PCP and psychiatrist should obtain a psychiatric history and consider the psychiatric differential diagnosis. The PCPs, working within integrated care teams, will increase their knowledge and skills in making psychiatric diagnoses. However, given time restraints, it is rarely realistic for PCPs to routinely complete a full psychiatric evaluation. Complicated cases (e.g., patients with a history of abuse, developmental disorders, or co-occurring substance use disorders) may be referred to a BHS and/or the consulting psychiatrist for further diagnostic evaluation and treatment. The DSM-5[1] is helpful when considering differential diagnosis of psychosis (Table 13.1).

Biopsychosocial-Cultural Evaluation

A mental health professional can take the lead on completing the full biopsychosocial-cultural evaluation. Additional biological and psychiatric history should be obtained, including: (1) a list/review of all current and prior medical conditions; (2) a review of the psychiatric history, including the age of first onset, number of episodes or exacerbations, and severity of episodes, including the need for hospitalization or ED visits; (3) a review of prior psychiatric treatment and any medication taken and the response; and (4) a review of comorbid psychiatric conditions and co-occurring substance use history.

A detailed review of the patient's current life situation and functional status is also essential. Clinicians can ask patients if they (1) are able to independently manage activities of daily living, obtain and prepare food, and pay their bills; (2) can ride the bus or arrange transportation to appointments; (3) can complete applications for Medicaid, Medicare, disability, or medication assistance, as needed; (4) know the medications and the reasons they have been prescribed; (5) take their medications regularly; (6) know how to refill medication; and (7) often miss medications or appointments.

The psychological evaluation should include a history of past traumas, conflicts, coping styles, problem-solving capacity, personality traits, and adaptations to the illness.

The social evaluation should include assessment using Maslow's hierarchy of needs: establishing whether the patient has a place to live, food to eat, financial support, and adequate medical care. Understandably, homelessness, hunger, and poverty may make it nearly impossible for patients to attend appointments, afford medications, or participate in their care. Assessment of the patient's social support network (including family, friends, religious affiliations, and community connections) is essential for treatment planning. Questions to evaluate the social network may include the following:

- "Who is in your life?"
- "Who is important to you and how do they/can they help?"
- "Do your family and/or friends support your need for treatment?"

Some families/friends may not agree with the need for mental health treatment, even advising the patient not to take medications. Others who support the patient can be mobilized to help in a multitude of ways. Obtaining collateral information and working with the patient's supports, as the patient will allow, are keys to understanding the current situation and to implementing a successful treatment plan. Chapter 26: Crisis Intervention in Integrated Care offers information on the development and use of a support network map.

Cultural assessment may also be useful in understanding

> "the cultural identity of the individual; cultural explanations of the individual's illness; cultural factors related to psychosocial environment and levels of functioning; cultural elements of the relationship between the individual and the clinician; and overall cultural assessment for diagnosis and care."[17]

TABLE 13.1. PSYCHIATRIC DIAGNOSIS OF PSYCHOTIC SYMPTOMS	
Schizophrenia Spectrum and Other Psychotic Disorders	
Diagnosis	**Distinguishing Features**
Delusional disorder	Delusions present for a month or longer. No hallucinations; no disorganized, odd, or bizarre behavior.
Brief psychotic disorder	Psychotic symptoms (excluding negative symptoms) are present for more than a day and less than a month. Full return of function after resolution.
Schizophreniform disorder	Psychotic symptoms and signs of illness are present for at least one month but less than six months.
Schizophrenia	Two or more psychotic symptoms (delusions, hallucinations, disorganized speech, grossly disorganized or catatonic behavior and negative symptoms). At least one symptom must include delusions, hallucinations, or disorganized speech. Symptoms present for at least a month (less if treated). Continual signs of the illness for at least six months.
Schizoaffective disorder	Meets criteria for a mood disorder, may have psychotic symptoms during mood episodes, AND psychotic symptoms occur for at least two weeks when mood is stable AND mood episodes are present for the majority of illness duration.
Other Psychiatric Disorders	
Schizotypal personality disorder	May experience magical thinking or odd beliefs that are not as strongly held as delusions. May experience illusions or unusual perceptions. No delusions or hallucinations.
Schizoid personality disorder	Emotionally cold or detached, does not seek or enjoy relationship, prefers solitary activities, takes few pleasures, not interested in sex, and indifferent to praise or criticism.
Mood disorder with psychotic features	Psychotic symptoms occur only during a mood episode.
Substance-induced psychosis	Psychotic symptoms occur only during intoxication or withdrawal.
Borderline personality disorder	May experience transient, stress-related paranoia, psychotic symptoms, or dissociation.[1]
Posttraumatic disorder	Not yet fully understood or formally classified; however, some with complex trauma may have symptoms that appear psychotic.
Delirium	Psychotic symptoms are only present during the course of delirium.
Neurocognitive disorder with behavioral disturbance	Psychotic symptoms are present only after the development of a neurocognitive disorder.
Autistic spectrum disorder	Pronounced deficits in social communication and interaction (may appear similar to negative symptoms like social withdrawal and lack of interest in social interactions) and restricted, repetitive behavior.[1] No delusions or hallucinations.

INTEGRATED CARE AND TREATMENT OF SCHIZOPHRENIA AND OTHER PSYCHOTIC DISORDERS

The NICE guidelines[10] and the American Psychiatric Association's "Practice Guideline for the Treatment of Patients with Schizophrenia,"[9] while focusing on traditional specialty practices, summarize the best treatment practices and are good reference tools for an integrated practice. Treatment begins by developing an alliance with the psychotic patient and offering psychoeducation (with the patient and family) about the illness, developing the management plan, and offering community resources. A complete team-based treatment plan and team member assignments should be developed. A patient registry should be used to monitor the progress, medical care needed community resources used, and will foster regular case review and treatment planning, as needed. See Table 13.2 for a critical pathway summarizing the collaborative care for psychotic patients.

Psychopharmacology for Psychosis

Initiating Medications

Medications are a key aspect of managing patients with psychosis. They should be initiated and monitored with the goals of significant symptom control or remission. Clinicians will need to choose between atypical and typical antipsychotics for the primary treatment of psychotic symptoms. Table 13.3 details medication options and dosing. Both classes of medication are equally efficacious in treating many psychotic symptoms. They vary in scope of side effects and monitoring requirements, but it is important to keep in mind that no medications are curative.

The CATIE study[18] showed no significant differences in the treatment of schizophrenia between numerous atypical antipsychotics (olanzapine, risperidone, quetiapine, and aripiprazole) and a typical antipsychotic (perphenazine). Time to discontinuation was also the same for these atypicals with the exception of olanzapine, which had a longer time to discontinuation because of efficacy but higher discontinuation rates because of side effects.

Negative symptoms (e.g., flat affect, apathy, withdrawal) may be more responsive to atypical antipsychotics, which may also have indications for the treatment of mood episodes/disorders. Atypical antipsychotics also have varying metabolic side effects (e.g., weight gain, diabetes), so current medical conditions should be considered when choosing a medication. Atypicals have lower rates of tardive dyskinesia (TD) and extrapyramidal side effects (EPS) compared with typicals.

The typical antipsychotics (neuroleptics) may have more neurological side effects (including EPS and TD). Table 13.4 reviews common medication side effects. The rates for EPS and TD associated with typicals may be overestimated due to historical uses of higher doses. Also, the lower rates of TD seen with the atypical antipsychotics may be underestimated, as the cumulative effect of lifetime use is not yet known.[19] Table 13.5 outlines medication monitoring requirements.

Clozapine is the most effective medication for schizophrenia. However, it has significant side effects (e.g., possible agranulocytosis, myocarditis, weight gain, drooling); there are specific patient and prescriber requirements (detailed at www.clozapinerems.com), including prescriber and pharmacist certification; and regular laboratory monitoring is needed (weekly for the first six months, less often thereafter, with increased monitoring if signs of agranulocytosis are present). Using clozapine requires the development of a regular practice monitoring process prior to widespread use in integrated care settings. Because of monitoring requirements, clozapine is mostly used for treatment-resistant schizophrenia, defined as two prior failed trials of antipsychotic medication.

Choosing the Initial Antipsychotic Medication

The choice for first-time prescribing is based on provider preference, taking into account efficacy (targeting positive vs. negative symptoms), potential beneficial (e.g., sleep enhancing) versus unwanted (neurological or metabolic) side effects, likely adherence to medication (e.g., administration by mouth or injection), cost, and availability. Patients who are nonadherent to their medications are often good candidates for long-acting injectable medications. See Table 13.3 for treatment options.

Inquiries regarding previous medication trials are helpful. Prior effective doses, duration of treatments and response, and previous side effects all can be used as a guide to the initial medication choice. Titrating to the lowest effective dose may reduce most side effects.[5] A significant number of patients discontinue all medications due to intolerable side

TABLE 13.2. CRITICAL PATHWAY: PSYCHOSIS

	Initial Visit	Week 1–3	Weeks 4–11	Month 3	Month 4–12
Assessment Tools	Clinical Interview Questions at all visits Clinician-Rated Dimensions of Psychosis Severity Scale[1] at all visits				
Main Objectives	• Identification of psychotic symptoms • Identification and treatment of emergent medical, substance use, and psychiatric conditions • Initiation of medications (often before precise diagnosis is known) • Initial plan of care identified and implemented	• Complete assessment, screen for comorbid disorders • Diagnosis • Initial titration of antipsychotic medication • Development of treatment plan • Identification of roles of team members and family • Education of patient and family about illness and system of care • Emergent care? • Needed community resources identified	• Stabilization • Medications monitored for symptom reduction and side effects • Change medication, if needed • Ongoing screening for comorbid disorders • Treatment plan refined • Implementation of strategies to manage symptoms, increase insight and adherence • Focus first on basic needs, linkage to community services, as needed • Identification of health maintenance needs	• Maintenance of stability • Ongoing monitoring of side effects, efficacy, adherence • Ongoing screening for comorbid disorders • Treatment plan refined • When basic needs met, shift focus to strategies to improve daily functioning, management of illness, and quality of life • Drug monitoring • Health maintenance	• Remission/recovery • Ongoing monitoring of side effects, efficacy, adherence • Ongoing screening for comorbid disorders • Treatment plan refined • Illness management, daily functioning and quality-of-life focus • Drug monitoring • Health maintenance
Physical/ Lab/ Diagnostic Tests (Potential)	• Physical exam • Labs: TSH, Chem 7 panel, liver function tests, complete blood count with differential, vitamin B-12, VDRL, HIV, urine toxicology, baseline lipids, HgA1C if starting an atypical antipsychotic • Consider/Optional: ECG, CT/MRI/EEG, pregnancy test		• Urine toxicology	• Physical exam • Labs: urine toxicology, lipids, HgA1C, Ambulatory Involuntary Movement Scale (AIMS) • ECG if indicated	• Labs: urine toxicology, lipids, HgA1C frequency determined by risk factors • AIMS frequency determined by age and type of medication • ECG if indicated
Diagnosis	• Focused on ruling out emergent medical conditions, substance use, psychiatric conditions • Refine diagnosis.	• Diagnosis refined • A Gather collateral information and complete a chart review • Establish timing, duration, course of symptoms, associated mood episodes • Medication workup completed • Medication response: partial response expected; no response leads to reconsideration of diagnosis	• Diagnosis refined • Elicit additional history • Assess for comorbid disorders. • Reconsider diagnoses if no or unexpected response	• Diagnosis including comorbid disorders • Diagnoses revised if additional symptoms arise	

Where	Office	Office or phone	Office and/or phone Community	Office and/or phone Community
Frequency		Every 1 or 2 weeks	Every 1–4 weeks	• Every 1–3 months • More often if specific therapies are being used • More often if medications are being changed
PCP Role	• Screening for psychotic symptoms • Physical exam • Initial lab monitoring • Identification and treatment of urgent medical concerns • Consulting with psychiatrist for initial medication recommendations • Working with BHS and care coordinator to identify initial care plan	• Completion of medical workup • Incorporation of data collected by BHS and/or psychiatrist into assessment • Assess medication adherence, side effects, need for medication changes • Assess need for psychiatrist • Achieve symptom reduction or resolution	• Additional assessment of health status, treatment of medical concerns • Assess medication adherence, side effects, and need for medication changes • Assess need for psychiatrist • Achieve symptom reduction or resolution	• Ongoing monitoring and treatment of psychiatric and medical diagnoses • Assess medication adherence, side effects, need for medication changes • Assess need for psychiatrist • Achieve symptom reduction or resolution • Relapse prevention
BHS Role	• Safety evaluation • Assessment of the need for psychiatric hospitalization • Identification of sources of collateral and support • Education of patient and family re: diagnosis, system of care, how to access urgent/emergent treatment • Implementation of registry monitoring system • Collaboration with psychiatrist for initial medication recommendations and to develop initial treatment plan	• Complete assessment, psychiatric diagnosis • Assess medication adherence, side effects, symptom reduction • Psychosocial assessment, including premorbid functioning social supports, preferences for treatment, goals • Assess ability to do activities of daily living (ADLs), assess skills deficits, need for resources or disability • Need for referral to more intensive treatment • Coordination with psychiatrist • Treatment: psychoeducation with patient and family about illness and system of care • Symptom identification and management	• Refinement of diagnosis • Identification of comorbid disorders • Assess medication adherence, side effects, symptom reduction • Ongoing psychosocial assessment • Assess ability to do ADLs, assess skills deficits, need for resources or disability, patient preferences and goals • Need for referral to intensive treatment • Coordination with psychiatrist • Treatment: ongoing psychoeducation with patient and family about illness and system of care, symptom identification, symptom management, strategies to improve adherence and increase insight	• Refinement of diagnosis • Identification of comorbid disorders • Assess medication adherence, side effects, symptom reduction, progress toward goals • Assess ability to do ADLs, assess skills deficits, need for resources or disability, patient preferences and goals • Assess need for referral to intensive treatment • Coordination with psychiatrist • Treatment: symptom identification, management, life skills, social skills training, strategies to improve adherence • CBT for psychosis • Behavioral activation • Sleep hygiene • Family therapy

(continued)

TABLE 13.2. CONTINUED

	Initial Visit	Week 1–3	Weeks 4–11	Month 3	Month 4–12
		• Strategies to improve adherence • Family involved • Linkage to PCP • Use of registry	• CBT for psychosis • Relaxation techniques • Early skills training • Linkage to PCP • Use of registry	• Health behaviors • Smoking cessation, weight loss, diabetes management • Linkage to PCP • Use of registry	• Follow the same treatment approach as Month 3
Psychiatrist Role	• Provide emergent consultation • Provide initial medication and therapy recommendations	• Review case weekly with BHS; revise diagnosis and treatment plan as needed • Participate in case conferences • Provide medication recommendations and drug monitoring • Recommend needed psycho-social therapy • See patients whose symptoms or dangerousness is not getting better • See severe cases • See patients with unclear diagnoses	• Review case weekly with BHS until symptoms are significantly reduced or resolved • Revise diagnosis and treatment plan as needed • Consider needed referrals • Participate in case conferences • Provide medication recommendations, especially if symptoms are not improving or side effects are intolerable • Recommend needed drug monitoring • See patients whose symptoms or dangerousness is not getting better • See patients with unclear diagnoses	• Review cases weekly with BHS, focusing on those who have severe symptoms, who are dangerous, and/or who are not getting better • Revise diagnosis and treatment plan as needed • Consider needed referrals • Participate in monthly case conferences • Provide medication and drug monitoring recommendations • See patients whose symptoms or dangerousness is not getting better or are worsening • Provide education to the team	
Emergencies	• Assess acute need for hospitalization during all visits. • Assess for risk of suicide, violence, or grave disability during all visits.				
Educational Materials	Education about diagnosis, medication education and tracking sheets Available resources for crisis management, resources for family			Relapse prevention and maintenance	
Consultations	• Psychiatric consult • Medical specialists	• Medical specialist • Psychiatric consultation • Psychiatric referral	• Psychiatric consultation • Psychiatric referral		
Community Resources	National Alliance on Mental Illness (NAMI); vocational rehabilitation services; Department of Human Services; disability lawyers; 12-step programs (Alcoholic/Narcotics Anonymous); community mental health centers; local trauma-specific and substance abuse programs; crisis hotlines; community crisis centers; psychiatric emergency services; nurse advice lines				

TABLE 13.3. ANTIPSYCHOTIC MEDICATIONS

Medications	Doses
Second-Generation Antipsychotics	
Clozapine	• Initial dose 12.5 mg 1 or 2 times/day, target dose 300–450 mg/day (divided doses), maximum 900 mg/day • Requires being a registered provider and specific monitoring; see www.clozapinerems.com
Risperidone	• Oral: Initial dose 1–2 mg/day, target dose 4–6 mg/day, maximum 8 mg/day • Intramuscular: Initial dose 25 mg every 2 weeks, usual dose 37.5–50 mg, maximum 50 mg every 2 weeks
Olanzapine	• Initial dose 5–10 mg/daily, target dose 10–20 mg/day, maximum 20 mg/day
Quetiapine	• Initial dose 50 mg/day, usual dose 150–750 mg, maximum 750 mg/day
Ziprasidone	• Initial dose 40 mg twice daily, usual 40–80 mg twice daily, maximum 160 mg/day (take with food)
Aripiprazole	• Initial dose 5–10 mg/day, maximum 30 mg/day
Lurasidone	• Initial dose 40 mg/day, maximum 160 mg/day
Paliperidone	• Oral: Initial dose 6 mg/day, range 3–12 mg/day, maximum 12 mg/day • Intramuscular: Initial dose 234 mg on day 1, 156 mg in 1 week, then 78–234 mg every month
Asenapine	• Sublingual: 5 mg twice daily, maximum 10 mg twice daily
First-Generation Antipsychotics	
Perphenazine	• Initial dose 4–8 mg three times/day, maximum 24 mg/day
Haloperidol	• Oral: Initial dose 0.5–5 mg 2 or 3 times/day, maximum 30 mg/day • IM: 25–100 mg every 4 weeks

effects.[18] This underlies a common clinical dilemma in which an effective medication is not tolerated and a less effective but more tolerable medication must be substituted.

The current recommendation is to use only one antipsychotic at a time.[5] No evidence exists to support the use of multiple antipsychotics, since polypharmacy just increases the risks of side effects and medication discontinuation. When choosing a medication, clinicians may also need to consider prescribing for affective symptoms, which are part of schizoaffective disorder. See Chapter 12: Treating Depression and Bipolar Disorder in Integrated Care Settings for a review of medications used to target psychotic affective symptoms.

Stabilization Phase

The stabilization phase in the treatment of psychosis (in which symptom reduction is experienced or a remission is occurring) typically happens over months. During this phase, an integrated treatment team can work together, seeing the patient at least monthly. The patient's symptoms and functioning should be tracked in the registry. "Teamlets" (two or three members of a larger integrated care team) can make decisions about the frequency of

TABLE 13.4. COMMON SIDE EFFECTS OF ANTIPSYCHOTIC MEDICATIONS

Side Effect	Description	Caused By	Common Treatments
Extrapyramidal side effects	Parkinsonian symptoms, including muscle stiffness, tremor, cog- wheeling, mask-like faces, drooling	• Any antipsychotic • Variable frequency with atypicals • More common in high-potency typical antipsychotics	• Decrease dose of antipsychotic • Antiparkinsonian drugs: Cogentin (2–6 mg/day) Trehexyphenidyl (4–15 mg/day) Diphenhydramine (25–300 mg/day)
Akathisia	An internal sense of restlessness, may or may not be observable. Often described as anxiety, or feeling unable to sit still	• Common with typicals and some atypical antipsychotics (e.g., risperidone)	• Decrease dose • Antiparkinsonian drugs • Benzodiazepines • Propranolol (30–120 mg/day)
Dystonic reactions	Tonic muscle spasm, typically seen in the tongue, jaw, or neck; oculogyric crisis (eyes forced upward)	• Any antipsychotic	• Antiparkinsonian drugs (IV provides fastest relief) • Benzodiazepines • Once treated, can add scheduled antiparkinsonian drug to prevent recurrence • Patients may prefer change of medication.
Tardive dyskinesia	Abnormal involuntary movements (athetoid or choreiform) often seen in tongue or fingers. Variable onset and course; seen more in the elderly; may be irreversible	• Any antipsychotic • Atypical antipsychotics thought to cause less • Clozapine may not cause tardive dyskinesia, and may treat it	• No evidence-based treatment • Helpful strategies include lowering the dose, changing to clozapine, adding vitamin E (off label), antiparkinsonian drugs, benzodiazepines
Metabolic side effects	Weight gain, increased waist circumference, elevated lipids, elevated blood sugar, hypertension	• Atypicals more than typical antipsychotics • Most with clozapine and olanzapine • Less (or none) with ziprasidone, lurasidone, aripiprazole	• Monitor • Change antipsychotics (especially for weight gain >5%) • Treat the side effect per medical guidelines • Behavioral techniques
Increased prolactin	Lactation, growth of breast tissue (males and females), sexual side effects, change in menstruation and fertility	• Atypical and typical antipsychotics (especially risperidone)	• Decrease dose • Change medication • Rule out medical causes if prolactin level is very elevated or if other symptoms are present

Sedation	Increased hours of sleep, daytime sedation	• Atypical antipsychotics (especially clozapine, olanzapine, quetiapine) • Typical antipsychotics	• Decrease dose • Change medication • Sleep hygiene
Orthostatic hypotension and tachycardia	Dizziness, vital sign abnormalities	• All antipsychotics • Less with high-potency typical antipsychotics, more with low-potency typical antipsychotics • May see more in the elderly	• Decrease dose • Change medication • Behavioral interventions such as rising carefully
QT prolongation	Seen on ECG; syncope	• All antipsychotics • Ziprasidone may cause more than other atypical antipsychotics	• Decrease dose • Change medication • Obtain ECG when symptoms are present, and when patients are on multiple QT-prolonging medications; follow annually if indicated

Goldberg JF, Ernst CL. Managing the Side Effects of Psychotropic Medications. Arlington, VA: American Psychiatric Publishing; 2012 and Schatzberg AF, Cole JO, DeBattista C. Manual of clinical psychopharmacology, 7th ed. Arlington, VA: American Psychiatric Publishing; 2010.

TABLE 13.5. MONITORING ANTIPSYCHOTIC MEDICATIONS

	Atypical Antipsychotics
Baseline	Medical history and family history (obesity, diabetes, dyslipidemia, hypertension, cardiovascular disease). Weight, height, body mass index, waist circumference at umbilicus, blood pressure. Fasting plasma glucose, fasting lipids, urine pregnancy.
Every visit (every 3 months)	Weight, height, body mass index (BMI), waist circumference, blood pressure; consider urine pregnancy.
3 months	Fasting plasma glucose, fasting lipids.
Annually	Fasting plasma glucose (unless frequency otherwise determined by comorbid conditions such as diabetes).
Every 5 years	Fasting lipids (unless frequency otherwise determined by other conditions such as hyperlipidemia or diabetes).
	All Antipsychotics
Abnormal Involuntary Movement Scale (AIMS)	Detects tardive dyskinesia and extrapyramidal symptoms. Check AIMS every 6–12 months, consider increased frequency (every 3–6 months) in geriatrics or if symptoms are present.
Team considerations	Who monitors? Consider having the behavioral health specialist or registered nurse also monitor certain parameters, like weight, BMI, or AIMS. Registries may be used to track data and to help identify the need for intervention; navigators help to ensure appropriate follow-up.

Goldberg JF, Ernst CL. Managing the Side Effects of Psychotropic Medications. Arlington, VA: American Psychiatric Publishing; 2012; Schatzberg AF, Cole JO, DeBattista C. Manual of Clinical Psychopharmacology, 7th ed. Arlington, VA: American Psychiatric Publishing; 2010; and Clark NG. Consensus development conference on antipsychotic drugs and obesity and diabetes. Diabetes Care. 2004;27(2):596–601.

appointments and the provider to be seen (PCP, BHS, health coach, nurse, or psychiatrist). Other team members (e.g., social workers, navigators, health coaches, care coordinators, and pharmacists) may help identify needs and deliver other brief interventions and treatments as recommended in monthly full-team meetings.

During the stabilization phase, specific attention is given to efficacy, adherence to medication regimens, and monitoring and/or treatment of side effects. Medications are changed for lack of efficacy or intolerable side effects. The Clinician-Rated Dimensions of Psychosis Symptom Severity[1] can be used to track symptoms in the registry.

Maintenance Phase

The course of psychotic illnesses varies. Patients with ongoing residual symptoms, or patients with a known recurrent illness, will need to be maintained on lifetime medications. Patients on maintenance medication will need to be followed at least every three months, with the PCP implementing the monitoring guidelines for the medications and side effects while assessing for the return of psychotic symptoms (review Table 13.5). Even with good adherence to medications, 25% to 50% of patients with schizophrenia or schizoaffective disorder will experience a relapse within two years.[20]

During the maintenance phase, a BHS can offer a brief course of psychotherapy, skill training, or referral to the care coordinator for other community resources. The psychiatrist may offer brief visits to treat side effects, suggest changes in the medication regimen, or suggest a referral to a community mental health service as the need for specialty psychiatric care or services arises.

Monitoring the general health and wellness of the patient during the maintenance phase is of utmost importance and will be discussed later in this chapter.

Changing Medications

Medications are often changed because of intolerable side effects or lack of efficacy. When changing medications, the initial medication can be cross-tapered with the increase in the new medication.[5] Cross-medication titrations typically occur over two to four weeks and require weekly contact with the patient. If nonadherence is significant, changing to a long-acting injectable medication should be considered.

Discontinuing Medications

There is no consensus on the length of medication treatment required for patients with a single episode of other psychosis (i.e., not schizophrenia) that has lasted less than six months. For example, a brief psychotic disorder will fully resolve, with return to previous functioning, within a month. In this group, medication can be discontinued. However, one-third of those diagnosed with schizophreniform disorder will recover within the six-month period. Two-thirds of patients diagnosed with schizophreniform disorder will progress to schizophrenia or schizoaffective disorder.[1] For this group of patients, the World Health Organization[5] recommends medications for at least one year following stabilization. However, other experts note that tapering can be considered after symptom resolution for a period of at least three months.[20] In practice, after the first break of schizophrenia or schizoaffective disorder, many practitioners choose to taper medication after a period of six months of complete remission.

For patients who do not require ongoing pharmacotherapy, the medications should be carefully tapered. Medication tapers typically occur over three months. Tapering should be avoided during a period of current or anticipated life stressors.[20] Prior to tapering, the patient and family members or support persons need to be reminded of the early warning signs and symptoms of a relapse. Plans should be in place should symptoms or a relapse recur. During a taper, a patient should be seen every one to two weeks, should be monitored by the care coordinator, and should have ready access to other team members. Once the patient is off medications the BHS should continue to see him or her at least monthly for an additional three months to monitor for relapse.

Symptom Management

Many patients with schizophrenia live their lives with some symptoms, even with optimal treatment. To manage residual symptoms, a BHS can teach the patient relaxation skills, mindfulness techniques, basic coping methods, and problem-solving skills. Patients' insight about their psychotic symptoms and illnesses varies greatly. Those with good insight can learn to identify stressors and can recognize worsening symptoms. Patients may learn problem-solving strategies to manage their symptoms, and can learn to ask for help. For patients who have little insight or who deny their illness, clinicians can assist by correcting reality distortions, using the patient's language for describing his or her symptoms, or by focusing on their need for improved sleep, improved moods, and clear thinking. Patients with little insight or denial of their illness may benefit from family support or referral to specialty psychiatric services.

Substance Use Treatment

There are high rates of co-occurrence of alcohol and substance use disorders among patients with psychotic disorders, so the integrated care team should expect to address these co-occurring disorders. Ideally, the BHS will be comfortable treating mental health and substance abuse disorders. A health coach or substance abuse counselor can facilitate smoking cessation and offer other brief harm-reduction interventions. The care coordinator and other team members should be familiar with other local resources, including 12-step groups and specialty substance abuse programs. The National Institute on Drug Abuse's website (http://www.drugabuse.gov/) includes information for patients, families, and providers. Also see Chapter 14: Integrating the Treatment of Substance Use Disorders into Primary Care Settings.

Health and Wellness

Patients with serious mental illness have a 10- to 25-year reduction in life expectancy.[5] Patients with schizophrenia have a 2 to 2.5 times higher mortality rate because of common problems such as weight gain, diabetes,[21] metabolic syndrome, hypertension, and cardiovascular and pulmonary disease,[5] and because over 50% of patients with schizophrenia smoke.[1] People with serious mental illness report difficulty getting medical care, may have financial issues that delay care, and may not be able to get their prescriptions.[22] While access to care is a factor, patients with serious mental illness have an inherently harder time navigating the system.[22] Patients with psychotic disorders will likely need assistance from team members to navigate the health care system and meet their health needs.

Because of increased health risks, the PCP, health coach, or others on the team may offer a wellness approach to their psychiatric patients focusing on nutrition, weight, exercise, sleep, harm reduction (e.g., smoking cessation or decreasing drug use), and stress management. See Chapter 22: Wellness: An Integrated Care Approach for additional information.

Involving the Family and Community

Family or invested parties need to be involved in the treatment of patients with psychotic disorders. Families of patients with limited insight can help recognize the early warning signs of an exacerbation. They can assist with activities of daily life and skills development in the community and may help the patient meet other health needs by navigating the health care system. Families may benefit from educational and supportive resources such as the National Alliance for the Mentally Ill (https://www.nami.org), support groups, and sometimes their own family treatment. See Chapter 27: Best Practice for Family-Centered Health Care: A Three-Step Model for additional information about working with families.

Patients may also need shelter, food stamps, medical insurance, and transportation resources. Over the course of the illness, many patients may also benefit from social skills training (see below), partial hospitalization programs, and supportive employment, all of which can improve the patient's quality of life. Patients who overuse medical services, driven by severity of illness or poor adherence to treatment, may benefit from assertive community management (home- and/or community-based medication and case management services) and/or linkage to a community mental health center. Emergency community resources include crisis services, mobile services, hotlines, and clinic numbers.

Referral to Specialty Mental Health Services

Referral to a specialty mental health service is often required as part of the care and treatment of psychotic patients. The integrated care practice will need to determine the services it can provide, the services the patient can receive in the community (e.g., addiction treatment, vocational rehabilitation, supportive employment, trauma-specific therapy), and the supports the patient's family may need. The integrated team should try to match the patient's preferences with the resources available. Patients who need long-term involuntary treatment will need to be treated in a specialty mental health setting.

Given the current reality of limited mental health resources, it makes sense for stabilized patients to return to their PCPs, thereby saving mental health resources for more acute or refractory patients. Successful integrated care practices will need relationships with specialty mental health providers, services, and programs and will need to develop processes for regular communication and referrals in both directions. Integrated care practices and mental health services will benefit from using standard communication protocols (e.g., written treatment summaries that include medication trials and reason for discontinuation) and specified protocols for transitioning care between services. Memorandums of understanding for needed levels of care facilitate ready access to the mental health services and/or specialty psychiatric consultation.

SPECIALTY PSYCHIATRIC CARE FOR PATIENTS WITH SCHIZOPHRENIA SPECTRUM AND OTHER PSYCHOTIC DISORDERS

Social Skills Training

Schizophrenia spectrum and other psychotic disorders often appear in teenagers or in young adults, interrupting the acquisition of life skills. In addition, the negative symptoms of the illness often interfere with social skills development. Skills training focusing on social interactions, independent living, and parenting may help improve patient functioning. Psychosocial skills are best taught and used while the patient is functioning within the community and can be taught in groups or individually. The team members should familiarize themselves with local skills-training resources in case these services cannot be provided by the practice.

Vocational Rehabilitation and Supportive Employment

Vocational rehabilitation and supportive employment may be an important part of recovery. Most programs are tailored to patient preferences, assist the patient to seek competitive employment, support individualized placement, and offer ongoing on-the-job vocational support.[23] Such programs can double the rates of patients' competitive employment.[24] Vocational programs offer secondary benefits such as improving quality of life and improving self-esteem.[23]

Cognitive-Behavioral Therapy for Psychosis

Psychotherapies for the management of psychosis may focus on symptom reduction, coping skills, and problem solving and often include supportive therapy, crisis intervention, cognitive-behavioral therapy (CBT), relaxation training, and others. Morrison[25] summarizes the use of CBT as a specialized treatment, offered in a psychiatric specialty environment, for people with schizophrenia. CBT for psychosis may be more effective for the treatment of positive rather than negative psychotic symptoms. For positive symptoms, CBT techniques work best when there is some patient insight into the illness. CBT techniques focus on ameliorating specific delusional beliefs. For instance, CBT focuses on gentle questioning of the logic of delusional beliefs. Patients may also be helped by

1. Offering reality testing of their assumptions about the meanings of various stimuli or situations
2. Introducing doubt regarding their assertions and conclusions
3. Helping patients identify alternative explanations, sometimes by offering them
4. Helping patients control and focus their attention by using switching techniques (shifting attention away from distressing thoughts) or narrowing techniques (restricting the patient's attention to a smaller focus)

Methods for ameliorating negative symptoms include behavioral activation techniques such as (1) monitoring activity levels, (2) developing activity calendars, (3) monitoring responses to activities, and (4) scheduling participation in social activities (e.g., visiting a drop-in center or recreational center). CBT for schizophrenia may improve social functioning and may be helpful when addressing comorbid conditions such as anxiety and depression.

Assertive Community Treatment

Assertive Community Treatment (ACT) psychiatric teams, frequently available through community mental health centers, offer an evidence-based approach to working with a subpopulation of patients with serious and persistent mental illness. ACT services are widely used across the nation. Bond summarizes the ACT model and the supporting research[26] as targeting patients with serious mental illness who (1) cannot effectively use office-based services, (2) regularly miss psychiatric and medical appointments, (3) overuse EDs, or (4) have frequent psychiatric admissions. The ACT team emphasizes delivering care to the patient where he or she lives and works, and regularly involves family members and other invested parties. Treatment focuses on medication adherence and case management services (e.g., offering housing, food, financial management, linkage to financial assistance, medical insurance, and transportation assistance, as needed) and use of other needed community services. Key components include assertive patient outreach by staff and rapid access for the patient to the ACT team members. ACT teams have low staff-to-patient ratios. Research shows that ACT teams facilitate patient engagement, decrease rates of hospitalization, increase housing stability, improve symptoms, and improve patient quality-of-life measures.[26] ACT, with appropriate modifications, can also be applied to medically ill patients.

SPECIAL POPULATIONS WITH SPECIAL CONSIDERATIONS

Women with Psychoses

Given that psychotic patients present in young adulthood and often have lifetime illnesses, integrated care practices will likely be treating psychotic women of childbearing age. The PCP and psychiatrist should always discuss birth control and the patient's future hopes and plans regarding children. Pregnancy testing should be a routine part of the care of these patients. For clinicians prescribing for women with psychotic disorders, women who are pregnant, or postpartum women, a useful review of medication options is provided in Chapter 20: Women's Mental Health Across the Reproductive Lifespan.

Geriatric Patients with Psychoses

Prescribing antipsychotics to geriatric patients with dementias has met with increasing attention and U.S. Food and Drug Administration warnings. For patients with dementias, evidence suggests differences in the mortality risks (mostly cardiovascular) among antipsychotics, with haloperidol having the highest mortality risk and quetiapine having the lowest (though still an increased) mortality risk.[27] However, there is no clear evidence as to how best apply this information to the use of antipsychotics in geriatric patients with schizophrenia spectrum and other psychotic disorders. Antipsychotics may need to be prescribed for elderly patients who are psychotic without dementia. This choice should be considered within the context of the patient's medical and psychiatric needs, considering comorbidities and the efficacy and safety of alternatives. The clinician could reasonably follow the dementia safety literature by preferentially using an atypical antipsychotic (e.g., quetiapine) and avoiding typical agents (e.g., haloperidol).

FUNDAMENTALS OF THE DHMC'S INTEGRATED BEHAVIORAL HEALTH PROGRAM IN THE COMMUNITY HEALTH SERVICES

Many of the approaches discussed above have successfully been implemented at the DHMC. DHMC has developed an integrated behavioral health program in the Community Health Services that spans eight Federally Qualified Health Centers providing services to adults and children, encompassing eight adult and three pediatric clinics. Additionally, there is modified programming in three women's care clinics, in one intensive psychiatric outpatient clinic, and in some medical specialty clinics, including oncology and bariatrics. DHMC serves a large population with a low socioeconomic status and a high burden of mental illness. This population has many barriers to receiving care. Since access to DHMC is not restricted by diagnosis or condition, many patients with schizophrenia spectrum and other psychotic disorders are treated in ambulatory settings. The original program was largely based on the Primary Care Behavioral Health Model.[12] It evolved over time to better meet the needs of the population by adding key components of other integrated care models such as the use of registries[3] and enhanced technology to identify high-risk and high-use patients and populations.

Key staff members of the DHMC model include the PCP, a BHS, the consulting psychiatrist, clinical pharmacists, medical social workers, and care coordinators who are referred to as patient navigators at DHMC. The BHSs are licensed clinical social workers or psychologists who are embedded in the primary care clinics, working side by side with the PCPs.

The BHSs see most of their patients "on the fly," referred in real time by the PCPs. Typical consults include assessments of behavioral health needs (e.g., adjustment to medical conditions, adherence, smoking cessation, weight loss), diagnostic clarification and evaluation of mental health conditions, linkage to the consulting psychiatrist, crisis evaluation, and referral to specialty services. The BHS assessment may lead to a brief course of therapy, typically using evidence-based therapies such as behavioral activation, motivational interviewing, CBT, or crisis intervention.

Care coordinators, in consultation with the BHS, coordinate patient transitions from hospitals and EDs back to community care. Social workers assist with linkage to community resources. Pharmacists provide education and monitor for drug interactions, side effects, and medication adherence.

DHMC psychiatrists serves as consultants, team members, team leader, and educators. The psychiatrist confers regularly with the BHS, is available for urgent consults via pager, and is routinely available by email for consultation. The PCP, who follows the patient with the BHS, can initiate the treatment recommendations. In severe or difficult cases in which the recommendations and interventions do not lead to symptomatic improvement or reduction in dangerousness, the psychiatrist will see the patient (typically for one to three visits, which may be interspersed with PCP and/or BHS visits). In cases of severe illness, it is common for the PCP to simultaneously start medications based on the recommendations of the psychiatrist and to schedule the patient with the psychiatrist. The DHMC psychiatrist has available appointment times at the clinic site, including time for urgent visits. The psychiatrist at two of the DHMC sites also is available for walk-in appointments.

DHMC multidisciplinary primary care team, with the help of the integrated behavioral health team (involved for brief periods and/or intermittently over time), can address the majority of patient care needs. Due to variable access to care, limited resources, and patient preference, a few psychiatric patients are followed over time in a manner consistent with *specialty* mental health practice. Additionally, patients can and do move between primary care and mental health visits in one location depending on their needs.

At DHMC, the BHS sees a large number of patients. Most patients are seen for only one or two visits because of the large population that is served, the fundamental practice of accepting all consultations, and the variety of consultation types needed. As the patient population becomes better understood, specific subpopulations who need intense intervention continue to be identified. These populations include patients with severe illness, those at risk for dangerousness (see Chapter 18: Violence and Suicide), patients with high or unnecessary use of medical resources, and patients transitioning from the hospital/psychiatric ED back to primary care. Standardized reports are generated that identify hospital/psychiatric ED discharges and patients who are high users of medical resources.

The DHMC integrated behavioral health team enters relevant patient information into a limited registry to track the assessments of severely ill and high-risk patients. The registry includes a subjective risk score and can track standardized measures such as the Patient Health Questionnaire-9 (PHQ-9: depression rating scale)[28] and the Generalized Anxiety Scale-7 (GAD-7).[29]

Standardized reports identify hospital/psychiatric ED discharges and patients who are high users of medical services. Clinic-based care coordinators manage the discharge/transition plan using a scripted phone call (see Chapter 18: Violence and Suicide for an example of a safety discharge checklist). Care coordinators ensure follow-up appointments are in place, review discharge instructions (highlighting medication changes), and address barriers to follow-up care (e.g., financial problems, transportation). The care coordinator at DHMC is typically a layperson, so medical backup is provided from nursing, BHS, PCP, or a pharmacist when more skilled needs arise during this scripted phone call.

The BHS reviews the registry and the discharge reports daily to weekly, using them to guide between-visit work and to monitor patient progress. The BHS works with the PCP to coordinate the team's care. The BHS and the psychiatrist review registry cases weekly, focusing on patients who are severely ill, are at high risk, or are not improving. The psychiatrist may provide medication recommendations that are implemented by the PCP and helps to develop the initial treatment plan.

Lessons Learned at DHMC and Other Practice Considerations

Over time the team at DHMC grew to work well together. Initially, however, some of the PCPs felt that they were practicing out of their scope of practice or with limited knowledge when treating serious mental illness. To ameliorate the PCPs' concerns, the psychiatrist and BHS offered formal monthly educational sessions focusing on psychiatric diagnosis, medication use (including monitoring), and related psychological treatments. This helped to increase the PCPs' psychiatric knowledge and comfort. The PCPs also felt reassured when treating patients with mental illness because of the immediate availability of the BHS and consulting psychiatrist. Over time, the clinicians working together gained understanding of each other's approaches, strengths, and styles. The PCPs gradually incorporated psychiatric recommendations into their usual practice.

Initially, the DHMC consulting psychiatrist also felt some anxiety while making recommendations based solely on information provided by the BHS and the PCP. Early conversations with the multidisciplinary team helped to identify the information that the psychiatrist needed in order to provide safe and appropriate consultation. The ongoing collaborative review of cases identified knowledge gaps, afforded opportunity for real-time education, and provided a natural way to monitor the acquisition of knowledge. Ultimately, this process led to increasing trust and cohesion among the team members.

The team-based care at DHMC required adaptation by the PCP when mental health professionals were added to the team. Early on, the primary care team saw the new team members (BHS, social worker, and the psychiatrist) as co-located practitioners. The primary care group had an initial desire to refer all severely mentally ill patients to mental health professionals rather than allowing all members of the fully integrated team to provide some essential mental health care.

Nationwide, BHSs have many different kinds of mental health degrees and expertise (e.g., health coach certification, bachelor's degree in psychology, nursing, social work, psychology). At DHMC, BHSs with social work and psychology degrees are used. As many mental health clinicians did not have training or experience in integrated care, clinicians were hired who had broad mental health experience and psychiatric diagnosis and crisis intervention skills and who were flexible, adaptable, and excited to work in a new and evolving model of care.

The schedule of the BHS is based on his or her expertise and roles, balancing the services delivered with the time needed for integrated visits (on-the-fly visits) and the longer sessions needed for brief individual therapy. Staffing ratios vary based on the complexity of the patient population and the ambitions of each of the particular practices. Specified time is allocated for work between patient visits. In other settings, the optimal patient-to-BHS staffing ratios and practices will need to be determined. Questions to be considered include the following:

How many PCP providers and patients can a single BHS support?

What is the best way to do "warm handoffs" to effectively convey information (e.g., in person, on the phone, via the medical assistant)?

Can the PCPs interrupt the BHSs when they are with patients?

How should the practice manage acute crisis walk-ins?

There should be open communication between the BHS, PCP, psychiatrist, practice leadership, other team members, and patients, as well as a willingness to change processes as needed. Practices in other settings will have to discover their local optimal workflows and best processes for a variety of situations.

Proposed Enhancements to the DHMC Integrated Behavioral Health Model

While the DHMC integrated behavioral health model is based on fundamental integrated care practices, several enhancements to the model may be desirable in order to move toward an expanded or ideal model of care. Proposed enhancements include adding team members, broadening team member functions, expanding the use of the registry, and developing routine case conferences aimed at improved individual and population management. Proposed changes to the team include the addition of health coaches and the expansion of the roles of the care coordinators and the psychiatrist. Health coaches on the team can focus on health and wellness, working with patients on identified needs, such as smoking cessation, harm reduction, and brief interventions related to substance use, nutrition and weight loss, exercise, stress management, sleep, and assistance in the management of other chronic illnesses. See Chapter 25: Health Coaching in Integrated Care. In addition to the care coordinator's primary role in transitions of care, this role could be expanded to use the registry to track patients' psychiatric and medical needs, ensuring that needed appointments are set, tracking laboratory results and referrals for other studies, and reaching out to patients who have missed appointments. The psychiatrist's role could also be expanded to include telebehavioral health consultation and the development of population management algorithms that include screening, assessment, monitoring, and treatment planning for the severely and persistently mentally ill. With additional staff, the registry could be expanded and used by the entire team for population management of all psychotic patients, not just patients with severe illness, those at high risk, or those with symptoms/risk levels that are not improving. The expanded registry could include tracking of the Psychotic Symptom Rating Scale,[1] patient functioning, substance use, wellness variables, and other chronic illnesses, as well as monitoring of lab results, appointments, referrals, and use of community resources.

In an expanded model, monthly case conferences could be added and attended by all the integrated care team members, including the PCP, BHS, psychiatrist, care coordinator, health coach, front desk staff, nurses, medical assistants, social workers, and clinical pharmacists. The team can review cases prioritized by the registry, develop and refine the treatment plans, and assign tasks to multidisciplinary team members. Patients can be reviewed monthly, until stable, and newly prioritized cases can be added as they are identified. Case conferences are an ideal setting to provide education. The psychiatrist can help develop and teach about population management approaches for the severe and persistently mentally ill.

CONCLUSION

Many patients with schizophrenia spectrum and other psychotic disorders are being treated in primary care for systemic and personal reasons. These psychiatric populations and the decreasing number of psychiatrists suggest that, in the future, more psychiatric care will be offered in primary care environments. The lack of evidence-based models for successfully integrating the care and treatment of psychotic patients, and the

BOX 13.3
SUMMARY OF RECOMMENDED TREATMENT APPROACHES AND RELEVANT EVIDENCE

Strength of recommendation taxonomy (SOR A, B, or C)

- **No integrated care models have been shown to be effective in the treatment of schizophrenia and other psychotic disorders. More research is needed.[13] (SOR A)**
- **The Primary Care Behavioral Health Model (SOR C)[12] and the IMPACT model (SOR A)[8] are major models of integrated care, the fundamental principles of which may be applied to the integrated treatment of schizophrenia spectrum and other psychotic disorders in primary care.**
- **Screening for psychosis in primary care is recommended.[14,16] (SOR C)**
- **When psychosis is detected, a workup should be completed to rule out medical/substance-induced causes, especially in first-break psychosis. Some elements of the work up will depend on clinical presentation.[14–16] (SOR C)**
- **A shorter duration of untreated psychosis is associated with an improved response to treatment.[6] (SOR A)**
- **Little difference has been found in the efficacy of antipsychotics, with the exception of olanzapine, but many stop this treatment due to intolerable side effects.[18] (SOR B)**
- **Monitoring of metabolic side effects is recommended for those taking antipsychotics.[20,21] (SOR C)**
- **Patients with one episode of psychosis, lasting less than six months, and now in full remission, should be tapered off medications after a period of stability.[5,20] (SOR C)**
- **Patients with psychotic symptoms persisting longer than six months or with recurrent episodes of psychosis should be maintained on medications.[5,20] (SOR C)**
- **CBT is effective in the treatment of positive symptoms and may reduce negative symptoms.[25] (SOR A)**
- **The Assertiveness Community Treatment (ACT) model is effective in treating a subgroup of the psychotically mentally ill population with high use of hospitals and poor use of traditional clinic services.[26] (SOR A)**

variable readiness of practices and PCPs, can make care of this population a daunting proposition. However, the patient-centered integrated care model described in this chapter offers hope and a method to provide care to psychotic patients living in the community. Further research will be needed to define best practices for the integrated care and treatment of patients with psychotic disorders. Research will be needed to determine (1) the feasibility of delivering population-based care for psychotic patients in an integrated care environment, (2) the quality of care that can be delivered, (3) the efficiency and effectiveness of that care, and (4) cost. Box 13.3 summarizes the recommended treatment approaches and relevant evidence for the integrated care of patients with psychotic symptoms.

REFERENCES

1. American Psychiatric Association. Diagnostic and Statistical Manual of Mental Disorders, Fifth Edition, DSM-5. Arlington, VA: American Psychiatric Association; 2013.
2. Bishop TF, Press MJ, Keyhani S, Pincus HA. Acceptance of insurance by psychiatrists and the implication for access to mental health care. JAMA Psychiatry. 2014;71(2):176–181. doi:10.1001/jamapsychiatry.2013.2862.
3. Raney LE. Integrated Care Working at the Interface of Primary Care and Behavioral Health. Arlington, VA: American Psychiatric Association; 2015.
4. Kohn R, Saxena S, Itzhak L, Saraceno B. The treatment gap in mental health care. Bull World Health Organ. 2004;82(11):858–866.
5. World Health Organization. Pharmacological Treatments of Mental Disorders in Primary Health Care. Geneva, Switzerland: WHO Press; 2009.

6. Perkins DO, Gu H, Boteva K, Lieberman JA. Relationship between duration of untreated psychosis and outcome in first-episode schizophrenia: A critical review and meta-analysis. Am J Psychiatry. 2005;162(10):1785–1804.
7. Reeves WC, Strine TW, Pratt LA, et al. Mental illness surveillance among adults in the United States. MMWR Surveill Summ. 2011;60(Suppl 3):1–29.
8. Unutzer J, Katon W, Callahan CM, et al. Collaborative care management of late-life depression in the primary care setting—A randomized controlled trial. JAMA. 2002;288(22):2836–2845. doi:10.1001/jama.288.22.2836.
9. Lehman AF, Lieberman JA, Dixon LB, et al. Practice Guideline for the Treatment of Patients with Schizophrenia, 2nd ed. American Psychiatric Association; 2010.
10. National Collaborating Centre for Mental Health (UK.) Psychosis and Schizophrenia in Adults: Treatment and Management. (2014).
11. Berry K, Haddock G. The implementation of the NICE guidelines for schizophrenia: Barriers to the implementation of psychological interventions and recommendations for the future. Psychol Psychother. 2008;81:419–436.
12. Robinson PJ, Reiter JT. Behavioral Consultation and Primary Care: A Guide to Integrating Services. New York: Springer Science+Business Media, LLC; 2007.
13. Reilly S, Planner C, Gask L, Hann M, et al. Collaborative care approaches for people with severe mental illness. Cochrane Database Syst Rev. 2013;10(11):1–58.
14. Carlat DJ. The psychiatric review of symptoms: A screening tool for family physicians. Am Fam Physician. 1998;58(7):1617–1624.
15. Freudenreich O. Differential diagnosis of psychotic symptoms: Medical mimics. Psychiatr Times. 2010;27(12):56–61.
16. Correll CU, Mendelowitz AJ. First psychotic episode—a window of opportunity: Seize the moment to build a therapeutic alliance. Curr Psychiatr. 2003;2(4):50–67.
17. Mezzich JE, Caracci G, Fabrega H, Kirmayer LJ. Cultural formulation guidelines. Transcult Psychiatry. 2009;46(3):383–405.
18. Lieberman JA, Stroup TS, McEvoy JP, et al. Effectiveness of antipsychotic drugs in patients with chronic schizophrenia. N Engl J Med. 2005;353(12):1209–1223.
19. Goldberg JF, Ernst CL. Managing the Side Effects of Psychotropic Medications. Arlington, VA: American Psychiatric Publishing; 2012.
20. Schatzberg AF, Cole JO, DeBattista C. Manual of Clinical Psychopharmacology, 7th edition. Arlington, VA: American Psychiatric Publishing; 2010.
21. Clark NG. Consensus development conference on antipsychotic drugs and obesity and diabetes. Diabetes Care. 2004;27(2):596–601.
22. Bradford DW, Kim MM, Braxton LE, Marx, CE, Butterfield M, Elbogen EB. Access to medical care among persons with psychotic and major affective disorders. Psychiatr Serv. 2008;59(8):847–852.
23. Bustillo JR, Lauriello J, Horan WP, Keith SJ. The psychosocial treatment of schizophrenia: An update. Am J Psychiatry. 2001;158(2):163–175.
24. Burns T, Catty J, White S, et al. The impact of supported employment and working on clinical and social functioning: Results of an international study of individual placement and support. Schizophr Bull. 2009;35(5):949–958. doi:10.1093/schbul/sbn024
25. Morrison AK. Cognitive behavioral therapy for people with schizophrenia. Psychiatry (Edgmont). 2009;6(12):32–39.
26. Bond GR, Drake RE, Mueser KT, Latimer E. Assertive community treatment for people with severe mental illness. Dis Manag Health Out. 2001;9(3):141–159.
27. Kales HC, Kim HM, Zivin K, et al. Risk of mortality among individuals antipsychotics in patients with dementia. Am J Psychiatry. 2012;169(1):71–79.
28. Kroenke K, Spitzer RL, Williams JBW. The PHQ-9: Validity of a brief depression severity measure. J Gen Intern Med. 2001;16(9):606–613.
29. Spitzer RL, Kroenke K, Williams JB, Lowe B. A brief measure for assessing generalized anxiety disorder: The GAD-7. Arch Intern Med. 2006;166(10):1092–1097.

14

Treating Substance Use Disorders in Integrated Care Settings

PATRICIA PADE, LAURA MARTIN, AND SOPHIE COLLINS

BOX 14.1

KEY POINTS

- **Substance use disorders (SUDs) and at-risk use of substances, which are often unrecognized by medical providers, contribute to an array of medical, emotional, economic, and societal problems.**
- **Barriers to care exist from provider, patient, and system perspectives.**
- **Primary care providers can contribute significantly to the recognition, intervention, and treatment of SUDs.**
- **For a variety of SUDs, pharmacotherapy and nonpharmacologic treatments can be effectively provided and managed in an integrated care setting.**
- **The integrated team can often provide the necessary monitoring, continuity of care, and support to assist patients in their recovery from SUDs.**

INTRODUCTION

The abuse of substances, including tobacco, alcohol, and illegal and prescription drugs, is among the leading causes of death, disability, and disease in the United States today.[1] Substance use also contributes to suicide, homicide, and unintentional injury and is among the leading causes of injury and death in adolescents. Over the course of a lifetime, one in four Americans will develop a nontobacco substance use disorder (SUD).[2] In 2014, an estimated 21.5 million Americans had a SUD in the past year, including 17 million with alcohol use disorder, 7.1 million with illicit substance use disorder, and 2.6 million with both disorders.[3] The misuse of prescription medications, particularly opioids, has increased since the 1990s, with a corresponding tripling in deaths related to opioid overdose from 1999 to 2012, followed by a rise in heroin deaths from 2002 to 2013.[4,5] The financial burden to society due to the abuse of tobacco, alcohol, and illicit drugs is a staggering $700 billion annually related to crime, lost work productivity, and health care costs.[6] Addiction contributes to societal problems such as homelessness, crime, domestic violence, teen pregnancy, motor vehicle accidents, shattered families, and lost productivity. In addition, substance abuse has been associated with an array of psychiatric and medical conditions that are commonly seen in primary care practice, including depression, anxiety, posttraumatic stress disorder (PTSD), bipolar disorder, respiratory illnesses, heart disease, hypertension, gastrointestinal and liver disorders, stroke, cancer, and a number of infectious diseases such as human immunodeficiency virus (HIV), hepatitis C, hepatitis B, tuberculosis, and sexually transmitted illnesses.

Alcohol and drug use disorders, despite their high prevalence, continue to be undertreated, with only 20% of those with a substance disorder receiving treatment.[7] Furthermore, despite the marked prevalence of medical and psychiatric problems in patients with SUDs, historically, treatment for SUDs and traditional medical care are provided separately. Often, medical care (onsite or offsite) is not offered during SUD treatment despite improvements in clinical outcomes and reduced costs for those receiving primary health care integrated into SUD treatment.[8] On the other hand, in the most comprehensive and largest survey of how primary care providers (PCPs) diagnose, intervene, and treat patients with SUDs, less than 20% had confidence in identifying alcoholism or illicit SUDs and only 30% felt prepared to detect prescription drug abuse.[1] The survey also found that more than 50% of patients stated their PCP did nothing about their SUD and a substantial number continued to prescribe drugs potentially dangerous to addicted individuals. Three out of four patients said their PCP was not involved in their decision to seek treatment for their SUD.[1] Provider, patient, and systems issues can present obstacles to treatment.

Providers may not possess the skills to adequately make the diagnoses or understand the nature of addiction. There traditionally has been a lack of training in medical schools and residency programs about the recognition or the nature of addiction. In the Center on Addiction and Substance Abuse survey in 2000,[1] only 3.6% of physicians believed substance abuse treatment was effective, compared to 85.7% who thought treatment for hypertension was highly effective. A majority (57.7%) said that they did not discuss substance abuse with patients because they believed patients would lie to them. Forty percent of providers found discussion of alcohol abuse difficult, while 47% had difficulty discussing prescription drug abuse. In contrast, only 17.9% found depression difficult to address. One-third of physicians believed that time constraints limited their discussion of SUDs and 11% were concerned that their time would not be compensated. Twenty-five percent of providers were concerned that the discussion would anger their patients and would result in the patient seeking care elsewhere.[1]

From the patient's perspective, the stigma of the disease was identified as a major barrier to receiving treatment.[9] Many patients, despite overwhelming evidence to the contrary, do not believe they have a significant problem, do not believe treatment to be effective, or do not wish to give up their use. Some patients will readily obtain mental health treatment, believing that their use of alcohol or other substances arises from the need to self-medicate their mental health symptoms.[10] Evidence suggests that women with SUDs are less likely to enter treatment over their lifetimes. Economic disparities and fewer social supports among women may influence their treatment entry. When women do enter treatment, they tend to have more medical, psychiatric, and adverse social consequences of their substance use than their male cohorts.[11]

From a system perspective, major barriers have slowed the adoption of a chronic disease model for treatment of SUDs. Most clinics, provider offices, and staff are not adequately educated and skilled at caring for patients with SUDs. Training regarding the use of pharmacotherapy in these disorders is lacking in medical education systems. The enactment of the Parity Act (2008) and the Affordable Care Act (2010) heralded an end to separate and unequal resources for SUD treatment; however, the full realization of this goal is still in progress.[12] Further barriers persist that include the complexities of billing mental health codes, specification of mental health and substance abuse treatment as "carved-out services" by insurance companies, and lack of organizational support for collaborative services. In addition, the confidentiality and privacy regulations are more complex than for typical Health Insurance Portability and Accountability Act (HIPAA) cases, including federal law (42 USC), regulations (42 CFR Part 2), and state-based policies that pose obstacles to communication among various providers and stakeholders.[14]

Despite the historical barriers to the integration of behavioral health care and SUD treatment, an increasing number of studies of systems demonstrate improved outcomes in both adults and children/adolescents when SUD treatment is integrated into primary care sites through integrated, collaborative, or co-located care models.[15] These models offer new and unique opportunities to integrate behavioral health, addiction, and primary care, all three of which were formerly disparate care practices, into a single integrated care practice that can improve patient outcomes. An overview of the key elements of treatment of SUDs in the integrated settings is found in Box 14.1.

ADDICTION IS A BRAIN DISEASE

Over the past two decades, research has increasingly supported the view that addiction is a brain disease. Many neurotransmitters, including γ-aminobutyric acid (GABA), glutamate, acetylcholine, serotonin, endorphins, and cannabinoids, are implicated in producing central nervous system effects by various drugs of abuse. All known addictive drugs activate the reward regions in the midbrain by increasing dopamine, thus mimicking the brain's natural chemicals that respond to natural rewards such as food and water. Over time, repeated drug use desensitizes the reward circuits, diminishing the frequent user's ability to feel pleasure and motivation to perform everyday activities. The brain's reward system becomes less sensitive to stimulation by both drug-related and nondrug-related rewards, changes that are deeply ingrained and not easily reversed after detoxification. In addition, after prolonged drug use changes in the circuitry of the extended amygdala result in an increased vulnerability to stress and the emergence of negative emotions. In the addicted brain, this anti-reward system, which is fueled by stress neurotransmitters such as corticotrophin-releasing factor and dynorphin, becomes overactive, particularly when the drug is withdrawn, creating extreme discomfort and an intense drive for relief of the dysphoria. The desensitization of the dopamine signaling in the reward pathway simultaneously occurs in the prefrontal brain regions. This causes impairment in executive functioning and diminishes the capacity for self-regulation, decision making, watching for and correcting mistakes, as well as assigning appropriate value to a given activity (e.g., becoming upset after hearing some sad news, becoming intoxicated to "feel better" rather than feeding one's child, and then, when the child cries, not asking for help). Thus, the ability to resist strong urges or to follow through on one's resolve to not use the drug is grossly impaired. The combination of the alterations in reward sensitization, negative emotional responses, and impaired prefrontal lobe function creates the development of an addicted disease state whereby the individual has reduced ability to voluntarily stop his or her drug-taking behavior.[6]

DIAGNOSIS OF SUD

The brain changes that occur with addiction ultimately lead to the behaviors that are described as diagnostic criteria for SUD by the *Diagnostic and Statistical Manual of Mental Disorders*, Fifth Edition (DSM-5).[23] The 11 criteria are similar regardless of class of substance, and the clinician should apply the specific substance to the code rather than just the class (e.g., methamphetamine use disorder rather than stimulant use disorder). The 11 criteria are as follows:

1. The substance is used in larger amounts and longer than intended.
2. Efforts to control or cut down use are unsuccessful.
3. A great deal of time is spent either obtaining, using, or recovering from the effects of the substance.
4. Craving for the substance.
5. Failure to fulfill work, school, or home obligations related to use of the substance.
6. Continued use despite social and interpersonal problems caused by the substance.
7. Social, occupational, or recreational activities are curtailed because of use.
8. Recurrent use in situations that are physically dangerous.
9. Continued use despite knowing the substance is harmful physically or psychologically.
10. Tolerance to the substance.
11. Characteristic withdrawal symptoms are present when there is reduced use or discontinuation of the substance.

The DSM-5 SUD diagnosis requires that symptoms lead to clinically-significant impairment and be present within a 12-month period. Severity of SUD is estimated by the number of DSM-5 criteria that are met, with two or three representing a mild disorder, four or five a moderate disorder, and six or more a severe disorder. If criteria for a moderate to severe disorder are met, then that is consistent with what was formerly called substance dependence. Symptoms of tolerance and withdrawal from a prescription medication, taken as directed, do not meet the criteria for a DSM-5 SUD diagnosis.

The involvement of multiple brain circuits and associated behavioral disruptions require a multimodal approach to the treatment of the addicted individual that includes pharmacological and behavioral interventions that inhibit the rewarding effects of the drug, enhance the responsiveness to natural rewards, decrease conditioned responses, and strengthen executive functioning and capacity for self-regulation.

SUDs are chronic illnesses, and the adaptations in the brain resulting from prolonged substance abuse are long-lasting. Once a patient is diagnosed with an SUD, it can go into remission, but the patient will always be vulnerable to relapse. In describing the current symptomatic state of these illnesses, it is helpful to keep in mind that the SUD is considered in remission between one and 12 months after no symptoms of the SUD are present. Emergence of any symptom prior to the 12 months is considered a relapse. An individual who has had more than 12 months without symptoms is considered to be in recovery. Emergence of any symptom during recovery is considered a recurrence.

Only a minority of individuals who use or even misuse drugs or alcohol will ultimately develop an SUD. Many genetic, environmental, developmental, and social factors contribute to a person's susceptibility to developing the brain disease of addiction.[24] Family history of SUD, early exposure to drug use, exposure to high-risk environments with poor familial and social supports, easy access to drugs, and certain mental illnesses such as mood disorders, attention-deficit disorders, psychoses, and anxiety disorders all increase the vulnerability to development of addiction.

INTEGRATED CARE FOR SUDS

Addiction treatment traditionally has occurred outside of mainstream health care and has been delivered in an acute and episodic manner, despite the recognition of addiction as a chronic, relapsing condition. Current models approach SUD like other chronic illnesses such as diabetes, hypertension, and asthma, where the effects of treatment are maximized with ongoing care, medication, and monitoring.[27] The first step in supporting a patient in recovery is to understand the goals for treatment and the meaning of recovery itself.

Whether a patient has problematic substance use or a severe SUD, the ultimate goal is control of substance use. For some less severely-affected individuals or those who have problematic drinking or drug use, the goal may be harm reduction toward moderation. However, for those with more protracted use and severe medical, psychiatric, and social consequences, abstinence may be required. Provider and patient should arrive at similar realistic goals, including (1) reduction of alcohol and drug use (or elimination of use); (2) increase in personal health and decrease in inappropriate use of the health care system; (3) improvement in social functioning such as employment and family and social relationships; and (4) reduction of threat to public health and safety (decrease crime, spread of infectious disease, risk of accidents).

Regardless of the patient's readiness for change, or the treatment intensity and setting, PCPs and integrated care teams may assume a vital role in the ongoing follow-up for patients with SUDs. Whether a patient has undergone treatment in a residential program or has received care in an outpatient setting, health professionals provide the necessary support, disease monitoring, treatments, and resources necessary for recovery.

Integrated care offers the opportunity to use PCPs in a primary care environment that is staffed with behavioral health specialists (BHSs), addiction specialists, care coordinators, and other team members, to deliver coordinated integrated care that is accessible, efficient, and cost saving, to the millions of patients with addictions. Integration of care increases access to care by using a more cost-effective, efficient, and reliable method of screening through the use of medical assistants, followed by the use of health educators, nurses, and other behavioral workers for brief interventions and referral to treatment. An effective method of integration is the incorporation of screening, brief intervention, and referral to treatment (SBIRT) for unhealthy alcohol use into the primary care clinic.[18,19] Another model of integration increases the frequency and effectiveness of PCP-driven pharmacotherapy interventions for alcohol and drug use disorders, and in particular buprenorphine.[20–23] This is especially important in the very high-risk population of individuals with chronic pain who are taking high doses of opioids. Moving forward, implementation research is directed toward five key areas: SBIRT for alcohol use; screening, brief intervention, and treatment for tobacco use; pharmacotherapy prescription and adherence; appropriate opioid prescribing; and disease management.

The Integrated Team

As would be expected, appropriate funding and leadership are associated with the successful integration of SUD treatment into integrated care settings. Technical assistance in the form of leadership support, staff education about the process, and ongoing monitoring of both successes and barriers, using integration checklists, can be used to support successful integration of the integrated team.[28]

The majority of evidence to date supports the provision of some sort of care manager within the primary care clinic.[28] The care manager (a specially trained nurse or health coach, or BHS) screens for appropriate patients, provides brief consultation to the patient to engage and educate, creates a patient outcome tracking mechanism to proactively address less-than-optimal treatment outcomes, and provides effective therapeutic interventions such as motivational enhancement, behavioral activation, and problem-solving strategies. Care managers are also responsible for facilitating collaboration between physicians and coordinating specialty care. Typical caseloads range from 50 to 100 patients. When considering the integration of such an individual within the primary care setting, Miller et al[29] created a helpful resource to outline the necessary core competencies as well as specific examples for each competency. Care managers must be able to (1) identify and activate patients in their care; (2) work as a primary care team member to create and implement care plans that address behavioral health factors (e.g., mental illness, SUDs, physical health problems that benefit from psychosocial interventions); (3) help observe and improve care team function and relationships; (4) communicate effectively with other providers, staff, and patients; (5) provide efficient and effective care delivery that meets the needs of the populations of the primary care setting; (6) provide culturally responsive, whole-person and family-oriented care; and (7) understand, value, and adapt to the diverse professional cultures of an integrated care team.

The training of care managers, BHSs, or addiction counselors in motivational interviewing and brief interventions along with the creation of toolkits (combining SBIRT, motivational enhancement, relapse prevention, and 12-step facilitation techniques) that help tailor behavioral interventions toward medical care settings can enhance a counselor's effectiveness.[16,17]

An addiction medicine or addiction psychiatry specialist is a crucial member of the integrated team. This individual can provide supervision for the care manager and other team members regarding their screening practices, behavioral interventions, recommendations for level of substance use treatment required, and education of primary care providers. Addiction physician specialists also provide direct support to the PCP regarding pharmacologic management via general educational endeavors as well as ongoing case consultation in real time. They can also participate in weekly reviews of the patient caseload or registry along with the care manager to identify patients who are not improving and to make appropriate recommendations to the clinical team, as well as being available for direct consultations with the PCP in real time. A typical caseload for a physician addiction specialist is one hour per 15 to 30 patients managed by a care manager.[30]

Excellent resources for physicians interested in integrating substance use treatment into their practices include the Agency for Healthcare Research and Quality's Academy for Integrating Behavioral health and Primary Care,[31] and the Substance Abuse and Mental Health Services Administration (SAMHSA) website.[32] One caveat is that the majority of this work to date has focused on the integration of primary care into community mental health centers that do not include individuals with primary SUDs, or the integration of depression and anxiety-related treatments into primary care clinics. For instance, of the five collaborative care models highlighted by the American Psychiatric Association and Academy of Psychosomatic Medicine, only two tracked whether SUDs were present.[28] Similarly, in an evaluation of SAMHSA-sponsored integration grant programs, enrollees were less likely to have used substance use–related services than other mental health–related services. Their summary called for increasing adherence to evidence-based practices, ongoing quality improvement processes, and improving processes to engage patients in care.[33] Although the bulk of research on collaborative care models has focused on depression and anxiety, it is our opinion, in the absence of other evidence, that the collaborative care models are likely generalizable to the treatment of SUDs.

Integrated Team Functioning

Systematic identification of patients with SUDs as well as ongoing monitoring of their progress in treatment is an important role for the addiction specialist care manager and physician. An integral tool to accomplish these goals is the patient registry. Our recommended use of a registry is to coordinate and implement screening, tracking of interventions, referrals, and outcomes based on available quality measures for individuals in outpatient settings.

Screening: (1) every patient should be screened at every visit for tobacco use, (2) every patient should be screened on an annual basis for alcohol use, and (3) every chronic-pain patient should be screened for SUDs prior to the prescription of opioid pain medication. We believe this recommendation can be generalized to the prescription of any controlled substance. See Chapter 23: Integrated Chronic Pain and Psychiatric Management for additional information on this topic.

If high-risk alcohol use is present: (1) alcohol-related education and counseling is initiated, and (2) the patient is screened for an alcohol or other drug use disorders.

If a substance use disorder is identified: (1) follow-up treatment is arranged within 14 days, (2) the family is involved in treatment, (3) counseling regarding psychosocial and pharmacotherapy options for alcohol and opioid use disorders (OUDs) is provided. If a patient receives treatment for his or her SUD, follow-up with the PCP should occur within 30 days.

If tobacco use is present: Patients are (1) advised to cut down or quit, (2) referred to a quit line, (3) provided nicotine replacement or other pharmacotherapy, and (4) given behavioral counseling.

Screen for PTSD, anxiety and depression: See Chapter 11: Integrated Care for Anxiety Disorders and Chapter 12: Treating Depression and Bipolar Disorder in Integrated Care Settings for relevant screening instruments.

ALCOHOL USE AND ALCOHOL USE DISORDERS

Alcohol use in the general population is quite common, with a lifetime prevalence of 87%.[34] Twenty-one percent of the general population are "at-risk drinkers" or those exceeding the recommendations but not meeting diagnostic criteria for an alcohol use disorder (AUD). Medically, psychiatrically, and socially, at-risk drinking is considered to be a precursor to more serious alcohol-related problems. More recent studies show that the past-year prevalence and lifetime prevalence of AUD is 13.9% and 29.1%, respectively.[34] Of note, significant associations are found between 12-month and lifetime AUD and other SUDs, major depressive and bipolar I disorders, as well as antisocial and borderline personality disorders across all levels of AUD severity.[34]

Despite the prevalence of AUD in primary care, the presentation of patients can be extremely varied. Not only can signs of these disorders be subtle and often attributed to other problems, but patients are often reluctant to disclose the true nature of their substance use for fear of real or perceived consequences. A nonjudgmental, empathic, and compassionate approach to screening, evaluating, and treating patients with SUDs is essential to provide effective communication and to support a patient's readiness to change.[35]

Screening and Assessment for Alcohol Misuse and AUD

In 2013, the U.S. Preventive Services Task Force (USPSTF) published a recommendation statement endorsing that clinicians use screening and brief intervention (SBI) in adults aged 18 years or older for alcohol misuse.[36] The USPSTF defines "alcohol misuse" as a spectrum of behaviors ranging from drinking more than the recommended daily, weekly, or per-occasion amounts (risky/hazardous drinking) to meeting criteria for DSM-5 AUD. There is limited evidence that brief intervention is actually effective with patients with an AUD. Therefore, the statement specifically applies and targets asymptomatic, at-risk levels of alcohol use in adults, including pregnant women. It does not apply to persons actively seeking evaluation or treatment for alcohol misuse. As very little literature supported SBI in adolescents at the time of the USPSTF review (publications up to 2011), patients age 12 to 17 are subject to an "I" recommendation (current insufficient evidence).[36]

Three screening tools are endorsed through the USPSTF statement: the ten-question Alcohol Use Disorders Identification Test (AUDIT),[37] the three-question AUDIT-Consumption (AUDIT-C),[37] and the single-question National Institute on Alcohol Abuse and Alcoholism (NIAAA) screen.[38] Per the USPSTF, a score of 4 or above on the AUDIT represents the optimal balance between sensitivity (84–85%) and specificity (77–84%) for all forms of alcohol misuse, including AUD. The latter is based on the NIAAA definition of at-risk drinking: more than three drinks per day or seven drinks per week for women, and for men 65 years of age and older, and more than four drinks per day or 14 drinks per week for men under age 65; it has validity when used in primary care settings.[36,38,39] The development of self-administered, single-item screening question is also being investigated to overcome routine practice barriers.[40] See Box 14.2 for single-line screeners for alcohol and drug use.

Other professional societies, including the American Society of Addiction Medicine (ASAM), recommend that PCPs routinely screen for problematic alcohol use. The American Academy of Family Physicians' (AAFP) recommendations are similar to those of the USPSTF. The American College of Obstetricians and Gynecologists (ACOG) encourages clinicians to question all patients directly about their use of drugs (in addition to tobacco and alcohol) as part of periodic assessments.[41] The T-ACE variation (Tolerance, Annoyed, Cut-down, Eye opener) is

BOX 14.2
SINGLE-ITEM SCREENERS

Single-Item Alcohol Screener:[38]

"How many times in the past year have you had five (four in women) or more drinks in a day?"

- **If > 0, it is a positive response.**
- **Sensitivity 82%**
- **Specificity 79%**

Single-Item Drug Use Screener:[39]

"How many times in the past year have you used an illegal drug or used prescription medications for nonmedical reasons?"

- **If > 0, it is a positive response.**
- **Sensitivity 100%**
- **Specificity 74%**

recommended by ACOG, and the 4P-Plus (Parents, Partner, Past, Pregnancy) has also been designed specifically for all perinatal substance use in women of childbearing age.[42,43] Of note, although the effectiveness and specific modalities of brief intervention in adolescents are still being elucidated, the use of a screening tool (Car, Relax, Alone, Forget, Friends, Trouble [CRAFFT]) is still recommended by the American Academy of Pediatrics (AAP) at every preventive visit and appropriate acute care visits.[44]

Following the identification of at-risk drinking, further history should be obtained to determine whether an AUD is present. A medical history and physical examination may detect significant underlying problems, as virtually every system of the body can suffer the consequences of alcohol use. Many of the routine problems seen in primary care are secondary to or complicated by the use of alcohol. See Table 14.1 for a review of medical complications related to alcohol.

Even though the stigma surrounding substance use is somewhat relenting, it still represents a major obstacle preventing individuals who have risky or downright harmful use to admit to high-risk drinking, to acknowledge the existence of a problem, or to reach out for help. In view of this, it should not come as a surprise to the clinician that denial and minimizing are hallmarks of alcohol misuse. When an AUD is identified or there is significant concern for an AUD following a negative screen, other collateral sources of data are important. This is especially the case in the elderly, who may be more likely to hide their substance-related problems, may be socially isolated from individuals who might recognize problematic use, or may be misdiagnosed with dementia or a depressive disorder.[45] These sources of data are also important to confirm the reported severity of an AUD in a patient who is seeking treatment. If the patient formally consents to a release of information to a significant other or family member, an open and honest conversation may ensue, often revealing essential information pertaining to the patient's actual health risk.

Since AUDs have a strong correlation with mental health disorders, it is also important to screen and treat underlying psychiatric conditions, particularly mood disorders such as major depression and bipolar disorders, as well as other SUDs.[46] There is a ten-fold increased risk for suicidal symptoms in AUD, so a safety assessment should be conducted as well.[47] (See Chapter 18: Violence and Suicide for relevant safety assessments.) Conversely, the presence of any of these psychiatric symptoms or disorders in the context of a non–alcohol-related visit should trigger a screen or assessment for an AUD.

Laboratory tests may provide indirect evidence of organ damage attributable to ethanol such as elevated liver transaminases and gamma-glutamyltransferase (GGT), increased mean corpuscular volume (MCV), anemia, and thrombocytopenia secondary to bone marrow suppression. Transaminases and GGT may remain elevated for two to four weeks following abstinence and MCV may require two to three months to return to normal.[48] As for specific detection of alcohol, measurement of blood or breath alcohol level can correlate with levels of impairment. Significant tolerance can be inferred in those persons who do not demonstrate impairment such as ataxia, incoordination, and delayed reaction time at blood levels between 100 and 199 mg%. Elimination of alcohol occurs at a fixed rate of 15 to 20 mg/dL/hr.[49] Generally, alcohol can be detected in the urine for 12 hours after drinking has stopped (depending on the blood alcohol level) and lags behind the blood level due to the collection in the bladder. Two metabolites of alcohol, ethyl glucuronide (EtG) and ethyl sulfate (EtS), can be detected up to five days after the last alcohol ingestion. These tests are extremely sensitive and can be positive after incidental use of alcohol-containing mouthwash and alcohol-containing hand sanitizer; interpretation

TABLE 14.1. MEDICAL COMPLICATIONS RELATED TO ALCOHOL

System	Disorders	System	Disorders
Cardiovascular	Cardiomyopathy Hypertension Myocardial infarction Arrhythmias Sudden death	*Renal*	Hepato-renal syndrome Acute renal failure Volume depletion
Pulmonary	Aspiration pneumonia Sleep apnea Respiratory depression	*Metabolic*	Dehydration Hypophosphatemia Alcoholic ketoacidosis Hypomagnesemia Hypokalemia
Gastrointestinal	Gastritis Esophagitis Pancreatitis GI bleed Esophageal varices Malabsorption (chronic pancreatitis) Parotid gland enlargement Malignancies	*Neurologic*	Peripheral neuropathies Seizures Hepatic encephalopathy Subdural hematomas Traumatic brain injuries Wernicke/Korsakoff syndrome Central pontine myolysis Cerebellar dysfunction Myopathies
Hepatic	Alcoholic hepatitis Cirrhosis Fatty liver Portal hypertension Spontaneous bacterial peritonitis	*Hematologic*	Pancytopenia Leukopenia Thrombocytopenia Macrocytic anemia Coagulopathy Folate deficiency
Infectious Disease	Pneumonia Tuberculosis Sexually transmitted disease Peritonitis Meningitis Hepatitis C	*Endocrine*	Gynecomastia Hypogonadism Hyperadrenalism Osteoporosis Hyperglycemia Hypoglycemia Hyperlipidemia
Perinatal	Fetal alcohol effects and syndrome	*Musculoskeletal*	Rhabdomyolysis Compartment syndromes Gout Fractures Osteonecrosis
Trauma	Motor vehicle accidents Physical abuse Sexual abuse	*Nutritional*	Vitamin B deficiencies Magnesium and calcium deficiencies Vitamin D deficiencies

of the results therefore requires clinical judgment. More sensitive and costly tests such as carbohydrate deficient transferrin (CDT) and phosphatidylethanol (PEth) can be used to detect binge drinking and in conjunction with other clinical data. Drinking four to seven standard drinks per day for one week may raise CDT levels for about two to three weeks. CDT testing is reported as % CDT/total transferrin level to adjust for variations in transferrin, and it has a greater specificity than GGT. PEth is an abnormal phospholipid generated by the presence of alcohol and can be detected up to three weeks following a period of moderate to heavy drinking and is used as a biomarker for binge drinking.[48,50]

Interventions for Alcohol Use and AUD

At-risk drinkers or those above the NIAAA recommended daily or weekly limits respond well to brief interventions. Treatment interventions for individuals with AUD include brief interventions, medical detoxification, psychotherapeutic interventions, medication-assisted treatment, and mutual support groups.

Brief Interventions

SBIRT is a highly effective approach to brief interventions for AUD in the primary care setting.[36,51] SAMHSA defines SBIRT as

> a comprehensive, integrated public health approach to the delivery of early intervention and treatment services for people with SUDs, as well as those who are at risk for developing these disorders. Primary care centers, office-based practices, and other community settings provide opportunities for early intervention with at-risk substance users before more serious consequences occur.[52]

Primary care clinicians are typically well positioned to use SBIRT as prevention of substance use. SBIRT is an ongoing process that leads to raising an inherently difficult topic in the context of a wellness visit, annual discussion of substance use, or whenever changes in behavior, physical health, or major life events occur.[51]

The brief interventions for abstainers and low-risk drinkers include verbal positive reinforcement for limited drinking, health promotion, and ongoing education regarding recommendations for maximum limits of alcohol use. Prevention efforts through education are particularly important for adolescents and women who are pregnant or are planning a pregnancy.

A positive screen for high-risk drinking in the absence of an AUD should trigger a brief intervention based on the transtheoretical stages of change model and motivational interviewing techniques. See Chapter 25: Health Coaching in Integrated Care for a review of these approaches. Together, these interview modalities identify a patient's readiness to change and assist in the continuing movement toward healthy, adaptive responses related to substance use. Brief intervention is recommended, ideally in a six- to 15-minute multicontact format, as very brief (five minutes or less) counseling shows limited effectiveness. The number of brief intervention sessions may vary according to the patient's level of risk, severity of psychosocial consequences related to substance use, and severity of co-occurring medical or psychiatric consequences, as well as individual response to brief intervention.[51] These sessions are aimed at helping the patient move in the right direction along a continuum of health-related behaviors, which is considered the cornerstone of SBIRT. The brief intervention provider must recognize and acknowledge with the patient that progress is rarely linear, thus allowing for setbacks, without compromising the integrity of the clinician–patient relationship. The goal pursued by the patient may be a moving target, oscillating between reduction, status quo, and cessation of substance use.

The acronym FRAMES summarizes six elements that should typically be part of a brief intervention, based on Miller's motivational interviewing principles:[51]

1. **F**eedback to the individual about personal risk or consequences
2. **R**esponsibility for change, placed on the patient
3. **A**dvice to change, given by the provider
4. **M**enu of options for behavioral change, support, and/or treatment
5. **E**mpathic style of counseling
6. **S**elf-efficacy encouraged in the patient

Another approach to brief intervention, the "5 A's," has been put forward by the U.S. Department of Health and Human Services[53] for PCPs and is summarized in Table 14.2.

Positive outcomes from brief interventions range from a 9% to 12% increase in proportion of adults who report adhering to consumption

TABLE 14.2. THE "5 A'S" OF BEHAVIORAL COUNSELING

Assess	Assess behavioral health risks and factors influencing choices.
Advise	Advise about personal health harms and benefits.
Agree	Agree to select goals based on patient's willingness to change behavior.
Assist	Assist the patient in acquiring skills, confidence, and social supports for behavior change, supplemented with adjunctive medical treatments when appropriate.
Arrange	Arrange for follow-up contact for ongoing assistance and adjust the treatment plan as needed including referral to specialized treatment.

From Centers for Medicare & Medicaid Services (CMS), Department of Health and Human Services (DHHS). Screening and behavioral counseling interventions in primary care to reduce alcohol misuse. Publication ICN 907798. CMS; 2013. http://www.integration.samhsa.gov/Screening_and_Behavioral_Counseling_Interventions_in_Primary_Care_to_Reduce_Alcohol_Misuse,_CMS,_Aug_2013.pdf. Accessed July 24, 2016.

guidelines, abstaining from binge drinking (drinking more than four drinks for women or five drinks for men in a two-hour period), and/or using health care within 12 months after the brief intervention.[54,55] Little direct evidence exists as to the long-term effect of SBI on morbidity, mortality, or quality of life. However, one possible outcome, the potential immediate reduction in trauma-related morbidity that is largely associated with heavy drinking patterns in observational studies,[36] makes it possible that SBI may eventually be demonstrated to have a direct effect on burden of disease. Potential harm (e.g., patient anxiety, stigma, interference with clinician–patient relationship, increasing use of other substances following reduction of alcohol) has never been demonstrated to follow implementation of SBI. The USPSTF currently endorses its widespread use.[36]

For individuals with AUD, treatment goals should depend on their stage of change, as well as the extent and severity of the alcohol use. For patients who are not ready to stop alcohol use, harm-reduction strategies can be used to reduce the risk for acute adverse events and injuries, as well as motivational interventions toward abstinence. For patients who have mild or moderate AUD without physical dependence and who are ready to abstain, stopping all alcohol use and treatment with relapse-prevention pharmacotherapy such as naltrexone or acamprosate with ongoing motivational interviewing and brief interventions may be effective.[56] For patients with an AUD that includes physical dependence, medical detoxification may be required. All individuals with an AUD should be prescribed thiamine 100 mg/day to prevent Wernicke encephalopathy. Multivitamins and folic acid 1 mg should be given to correct any underlying nutritional deficiencies, in addition to the follow strategies.

Medical Detoxification

For individuals with an AUD who have physical dependence and are ready to abstain, medical detoxification to mitigate the risk of withdrawal symptoms may be needed prior to the initiation of relapse-prevention medications or relapse-prevention therapies. Withdrawal can occur within several hours after the patient's last drink and may be severe or fatal. Thus, the first step in treatment is determining the likelihood and severity of alcohol withdrawal, which guides the appropriateness of stopping alcohol use in an outpatient or inpatient setting. The severity of alcohol withdrawal symptoms can be measured using scales such as the Clinical Institute Withdrawal Assessment for Alcohol, Revised (CIWA-Ar), which ranks the following symptoms: nausea/vomiting, tactile/auditory/visual disturbance, tremor, sweats, anxiety, headache, agitation, and orientation.[57] Scores range from 0 to 7, except for orientation (0–4), and are added together. Patients eligible for ambulatory detoxification are those with a relatively low risk of complications.[57] Patients presenting with a CIWA-Ar score in the presence of current intoxication or a CIWA-Ar score greater than 15 would be better managed in an inpatient setting. Appropriate candidates for outpatient detoxification are patients who do not have a prior history of seizures or delirium tremens, do not have comorbid benzodiazepine dependence, do not have traumatic brain injury, are not pregnant, are stable medically and psychiatrically, are able to follow instructions, are willing to commit to daily visits, and have family or social support to monitor the patient carefully.[58] Symptoms generally occur for up to seven days, and patients should be monitored daily until their symptoms have resolved. Benzodiazepines remain the standard of care for alcohol withdrawal. All benzodiazepines are effective in reducing symptoms and preventing withdrawal seizures. Particularly good choices are those that are relatively long acting and less reinforcing, such as chlordiazepoxide, chlorazepate, or oxazepam.[59] A fixed schedule for an outpatient detoxification may be more feasible than a symptom-triggered schedule, and medication should be initiated quickly as withdrawal symptoms begin within six hours following the last drink and seizures can occur six to 48 hours after the last drink as well.[60] Anticonvulsants have been shown to reduce cravings and produce less sedation than benzodiazepines, but the data still do not support their use over benzodiazepines at this time.[61,62] It is not recommended to continue long-term use of benzodiazepines following the acute detoxification, and these medications are rarely used longer than ten days.

Psychotherapeutic Treatments

Other psychosocial interventions that can be provided by BHSs, addiction counselors, or trained health coaches include cognitive-behavioral therapy (CBT), motivational enhancement therapy, and 12-step facilitation. The focus of CBT is to change thinking and behavior not only toward the alcohol use but also to other areas of life functionally related to alcohol use, as well as to strengthen coping skills.[63] Motivational enhancement therapy is a less intensive intervention than standard motivational interviewing and utilizes a more structured approach providing systematic assessment and personalized feedback.[64] The goal of 12-step facilitation is to increase patient involvement in Alcoholics Anonymous (AA) or other 12-step groups by following a manualized approach outlined by the NIAAA.[65]

Mutual Support Groups

AA is a mutual support organization of individuals who wish to stop drinking. Not only can patients attend at no cost, but meetings are widely available and diverse in their membership. Studies have shown higher rates of abstinence than CBT among veterans, and the more meetings attended the higher the rate of abstinence.[66,67] Participation in 12-step programs does not conflict with other interventions medically or psychiatrically, and most objections by patients can be overcome with encouragement and support and by finding a compatible meeting or group. In addition to becoming familiar with standard 12-step meetings in the area, clinicians should also be aware of specialty groups and other mutual support groups (e.g., lesbian, bisexual, gay, transgender, queer [LGBTQ],[68] Celebrate Recovery,[69] Smart Recovery,[70] and Life Ring[71]). Professionals with SUDs may have greater concerns about anonymity, may have greater shame related to their illness, and may have more difficulty discussing the consequences of their SUD due to public health concerns. All members of the integrated care team should be aware of the concerns of these patients during their primary care visits, as well as being aware of potential referral to professional treatment programs and mutual support groups (e.g., Birds of a Feather for pilots,[72] International Doctors in AA for physicians or PhDs,[73] The Other Bar for attorneys[74]).

Medication-Assisted Treatment

PCPs and psychiatrists in integrated care settings remain well positioned to prescribe medications approved by the U.S. Food and Drug Administration (FDA) for the treatment of moderate to severe AUD. Whether patients are receiving care for their AUD in a primary care setting/integrated practice or an SUD treatment program, PCPs and psychiatrists should be aware of medications that help prevent relapses and promote recovery and assist with monitoring for side effects and signs of relapse. Naltrexone, acamprosate, disulfiram, and topiramate are recommended based on randomized controlled trials and meta-analyses.[75–78] Naltrexone, acamprosate, and disulfiram are currently FDA approved.

Naltrexone

Naltrexone is an opioid antagonist that reduces cravings, has been shown to prevent relapse to heavy drinking,[79] and has been FDA approved to treat both AUD and OUD. The recommended dosage of 25 mg/day minimizes side effects and the dose can be increased to 50 mg in three to seven days; no clear evidence exists that doses beyond 50 mg/day provide additional therapeutic benefit. Common side effects are transient and include nausea, headache, and dizziness. Long-acting naltrexone is available as a 380-mg dose and administered as a deep intramuscular injection in the gluteal muscle every four weeks.

Injection site reactions can occur and are treatable with local warm compresses and nonsteroidal anti-inflammatory medication. Intramuscular medication increases adherence over the oral formulation. Naltrexone should not be prescribed to patients with severe liver disease due to its potentially hepatotoxic effects and in those on opioid therapy because it precipitates opioid withdrawal with its antagonist action. Initial liver function testing is warranted with periodic follow-up every 3 to 6 months. The benefits for the liver due to the medication's related reduction in alcohol intake may outweigh the rare but serious risk of hepatotoxicity.

Acamprosate

Acamprosate, an alternative to naltrexone, is believed to act on the glutamate and GABA systems to relieve symptoms of post-acute withdrawal.[80] Acamprosate has beneficial effects in reducing drinking days, lengthening the time to relapse, and increasing complete abstinence. Acamprosate may be a particularly good option for patients requiring co-occurring opioid treatment and in those with severe liver disease. However, its three-times-a-day dosing and large tablet size make adherence an issue. Its excretion is renal, not hepatic, so it should be used in caution with patients with reduced creatinine clearance. The starting and maintenance dose is 666 mg three times a day.

Disulfiram

Disulfiram is an alcohol-sensitizing agent that inhibits the enzyme aldehyde dehydrogenase. When alcohol is ingested in the presence of the inhibition of this enzyme, the result is the elevation of acetaldehyde and a disulfiram–ethanol reaction. The intensity of the reaction (warmth, flushing, nausea, vomiting, tachycardia, palpitations, diaphoresis, blurred vision, dizziness, and confusion) relates to both the dose of disulfiram and the volume of alcohol ingested. Occasionally, these reactions can be severe enough to cause cardiovascular collapse or seizures. Only patients who are committed to abstinence and who are in generally good health and have solid social support should take these medications. Due to hepatic side effects, liver function should be monitored regularly, and this medication should not be prescribed to patients with severe cardiac disease or psychosis or those who are incapable of understanding the nature of the reaction. To avoid incidental reactions the clinician should carefully review with the patient the use of substances that contain alcohol, such as cologne, mouthwash, and cough medications. Disulfiram has multiple drug interactions, and the patient must be abstinent for greater than 12 hours before starting this medication. Patients should understand that they may have a reaction up to several weeks after discontinuation of the medication. The usual dose is 250 mg/day with a range between 125 and 500 mg/day.

Other Medications

While topiramate is not approved by the FDA for AUD, it has been shown in studies to reduce days of heavy drinking and to promote abstinence. It is believed to serve as a glutamate antagonist and inhibit dopamine release. It does have well-documented side effects, which include paresthesia/numbness, anorexia, taste abnormalities, weight loss, cognitive impairment, and rash. Some common side effects can usually be managed by lowering the dose. The starting dose is usually 50 mg/day (in two divided doses), and it is titrated over several weeks to 100 mg twice a day.

Gabapentin is also not FDA approved to treat AUD but may be an option for patients with AUD for whom first-line pharmacotherapy is contraindicated or ineffective. The effects of gabapentin likely occur through modulation of GABA activity in the amygdala associated with AUD. In one clinical trial, the addition of gabapentin to oral naltrexone improved drinking outcomes over those obtained with naltrexone alone.[81] There are concerns for abuse of gabapentin and pregabalin, particularly in patients with substance abuse.[82] However, when taken as directed, gabapentin has a high margin of safety, and many PCPs have experience prescribing the drug for non-AUD indications. The starting dose is usually 300 mg with an increase by 300 mg/day to 1,800 mg in three divided doses. Similar to the previous medications discussed, gabapentin is a pregnancy category C drug.

Follow-up Visits

Once the PCP has initiated treatment, follow-up visits should include assessment of drinking amounts, functional status, therapeutic adherence, medication adherence, and medication side effects. An inquiry about other substances used is also important. Asking the patient about support group attendance, use of a sponsor and/or support network, and other aspects of recovery should also be a part of follow-up visits.[38] Patients prescribed pharmacotherapy should continue taking the medications until their recovery is stable and the provider and patient mutually agree that the medication is no longer needed, or side effects emerge precluding their safe use. If side effects to one medication emerge, patients should be offered an alternative medication. The intensity of therapeutic interventions can also be increased.

TOBACCO USE AND TOBACCO USE DISORDERS

Tobacco use disorders (TUDs) account for the deaths of over 435,000 people each year and are associated with both the development and worsened prognosis of a multitude of medical and emotional disorders, as well as damage and injuries related to fire and trauma.[83] Although the neurobiological underpinnings of tobacco dependence parallel those of other SUDs, the relatively increased acceptability, increased availability, and strongly conditioned behavior associated with tobacco use lead to high rates for the development of dependence.[83] PCPs and integrated practices are in an excellent position to intervene on this disorder as a majority of smokers have been seen by a primary care provider in the past year.

Screening and Assessment for Tobacco Use and TUD

It is a Class A recommendation of the USPTF that all patients be screened for TUD. The DHS's "Guide to Treating Tobacco Use and Dependence" (2008 update)[84] advises that clinicians and health care delivery systems consistently identify and document tobacco use status and treat every tobacco user seen in a health care setting. This act alone can increase future quit rates.

Interventions for Tobacco Use and TUD

It is a Class A recommendation of the USPTF that all nonpregnant adults be offered both behavioral therapy and pharmacotherapy. There is currently insufficient evidence to guide the use of pharmacotherapy in pregnant women, so only behavioral interventions are officially recommended. Similar to the treatment of alcohol use, interventions should occur for tobacco users in all stages of change. Treatment interventions for individuals with TUD include brief interventions, psychotherapeutic interventions, medication-assisted treatment, and mutual support groups.[85] Additionally, the DHS's "Guide to Treating Tobacco Use and Dependence" (2008 update)[84] advises the following:

1. Tobacco dependence is a chronic disease that often requires repeated intervention and multiple attempts to quit. Effective treatments exist, however, that can significantly increase rates of long-term abstinence.
2. Tobacco-dependence treatments are effective across a broad range of populations. Clinicians should encourage every patient willing to make a quit attempt to use the counseling treatments and medications recommended in this Guideline.
3. Tobacco-dependence treatments are both clinically effective and highly cost-effective relative to interventions for other clinical disorders. Providing benefits/cost coverage for these treatments increases quit rates. Insurers and purchasers should ensure that all insurance plans include the counseling and medication identified as effective in this guideline as covered benefits.

Despite public awareness campaigns and the presence of numerous recommendations and guidelines for tobacco-related interventions, the number of individuals who seek medical care for tobacco cessation assistance, the number of providers who discuss tobacco cessation with their patients, and the number of patients who abstain following brief interventions by care providers are very limited. Efforts to combat these low success rates include the development of chronic care models and appropriate electronic health care infrastructure to support improved efforts at treating this addiction. Specific interventions include screening by a medical assistant during each visit for tobacco use; an invitation to participate in either harm-reduction or cessation interventions; the use of a smoking-specialist case manager for tracking outcomes and providing counseling; and the modification of the electronic health record to prompt screening, referral, and identification. Effective clinic managers are able to motivate medical assistants who do not adhere to the screening protocol due to their own tobacco use behaviors and beliefs, or inefficiency. Effort-based and non–effort-based rewards as well as a weekly review of goals and sharing of patient testimonials regarding positive aspects of the intervention can improve motivation in clinic staff.[86]

Brief Interventions

The DHS's "Guide to Treating Tobacco Use and Dependence"[84] advises that brief tobacco dependence treatment is effective. This guideline reviews a behavior change model framework for smoking cessation brief interventions called the "5 A's" (see Table 14.2). Greater detail is provided in the guideline itself, as well as various toolkits such as the DIMENSIONS: Tobacco Free Toolkit for Healthcare Providers that have been created to address tobacco cessation in varied populations.[87]

Psychotherapeutic Treatments and Mutual Support

The DHS's "Guide to Treating Tobacco Use and Dependence"[84] advises that "Individual, group, and telephone counseling are effective, and their effectiveness increases with treatment intensity." Two components of this counseling are especially effective, and clinicians should use these when counseling patients making a quit attempt: (1) practical counseling (problem solving and skills training) and social support can be delivered as part of treatment, and (2) patients can be referred to Nicotine Anonymous groups[88] as well as online supports such as the American Lung Association's Freedom From Smoking.[89]

Medication-Assisted Treatment

Three types of medications are currently approved by the FDA for the treatment of TUD.

Bupropion

The mechanism of action for bupropion is unknown, although it appears to be independent of its antidepressant efficacy. Bupropion SR (Zyban) is ideally initiated one to two weeks prior to the quit attempt and should be started at 150 mg for three days and then increased to twice-a-day dosing. This medication may be a good choice in individuals who have co-occurring depression (FDA approved), who are particularly concerned about weight gain with tobacco cessation, who are experiencing sexual dysfunction related to other medications, who have attentional dysfunction (not an FDA-approved use), or who do not have access to behavioral interventions. Side effects include an increased risk for seizures, particularly in individuals with a history of eating disorders, alcohol and sedative use disorders, traumatic brain injury, and co-occurring prescription of other medications that reduce the seizure threshold. Theoretically, a risk of illness exacerbation with the medication may occur in individuals with anxiety, bipolar, or psychotic disorders (neuropsychiatric side effects). The length of treatment is typically three months, with maintenance up to six months, although there is emerging evidence and our anecdotal experience is that some individuals will require longer pharmacotherapeutic support to achieve and sustain abstinence.

Nicotine Replacement

Nicotine replacement currently includes three over-the-counter varieties (gum, patch, and lozenge) and two prescription products (nasal spray and inhaler). Their mechanism of action is as nicotinic agonists to reduce the experience of withdrawal and craving, as well as to prevent the positive reinforcement of other tobacco use. These products can be used on their own or in combinations of short- and long-acting nicotine replacement, or nicotine replacement with bupropion or varenicline. These medications may be better choices in individuals who cannot tolerate or are reluctant to use prescription medications, or who do not have access to other smoking-cessation medications or therapies. Caution should be used in individuals who are at high risk for developing a higher level of dependence on these products. Although each product gives dosing instructions, providers should monitor adherence to recommended dosing techniques and dose levels and also should evaluate whether patients are suboptimally replacing nicotine. Evidence is emerging that nicotine replacement can be used in a harm-reduction approach to not only reduce the number of cigarettes smoked but also to increase the likelihood that unmotivated smokers will make a quit attempt in the future.

Varenicline

Varenicline is the most recently FDA-approved medication for tobacco cessation. As a partial nicotinic agonist, it also reduces the experiences of withdrawal and craving and reduces positive reinforcement of tobacco-use behavior. This medication is typically initiated at a dose of 0.5 mg for three days, then 0.5 mg twice per day for four days, then 1 mg twice a day for 12 weeks to reduce the risk of side effects. Common side effects include nausea and changes in dreams. More serious, albeit rarer, side effects include psychosis and other neuropsychiatric symptoms. All patients should discuss significant changes with their physicians.

Special Considerations in the Treatment of TUDs

Given the increasing use of electronic delivery devices for nicotine (e-cigarettes) by individuals who have never used tobacco, who want to continue to use tobacco, and who are attempting to stop using tobacco, it is important for the integrated care team or PCP to be able to screen for and discuss the use of these nicotine products. Although patients should be advised using clearly evidence-based approaches such as those discussed above (nonpharmacologic and pharmacologic), these approaches may be ineffective or contraindicated for use in some patients who are hoping to stop or reduce their tobacco use. In such cases, the patient should be educated about the conflicting evidence base for the efficacy of e-cigarettes, as a replacement for tobacco in controlled settings, as well as the risks of worsening nicotine dependence, the lack of regulation of nicotine content, and public safety concerns (nicotine poisoning, use of other legal and illegal drugs in the devices, device explosions, risk of addiction, and risk of underage use, as it is harder to detect by smell by authority figures). Additional discussion should include the need to use other smoking cessation behavioral interventions (e.g., setting a quit date) to improve chances for e-cigarette use cessation.[90]

Another special consideration is the large number of individuals with TUDs who also have other co-occurring behavioral health disorders. Historically, both behavioral health providers and medical providers have been less likely to address tobacco use in these individuals. None of the frequently cited reasons for this failure (e.g., self-medication, lack of interest in quitting, inability to quit, worsening of the other behavioral health condition, a low priority for behavioral health patients) have been supported by a multitude of studies. Unfortunately, lack of penetration of these findings to providers in primary care and behavioral health settings, other sources of provider reluctance (e.g., being a smoker, lack of training), and lack of appropriate clinic infrastructure (e.g., outreach to patients who are not regularly making appointments, funding, space, providers) continue to limit the number of individuals with behavioral health disorders who receive smoking cessation treatment. In addition to the guiding principles listed above, considerations for tobacco cessation interventions in individuals with behavioral health disorders include appropriate education regarding the symptoms of nicotine withdrawal and length of time that withdrawal symptoms can persist (up to four weeks, although the worst of the symptoms will resolve within 72 hours). This will increase the likelihood that the patient and provider do not misattribute symptoms to an exacerbation of the underlying condition, as well as guide the need for potentially higher doses of nicotine replacement if that intervention is being used.

Providers should also be aware that transitions from smoking to nicotine use (and the reverse) are associated with CYP-450 interactions and can result in significant and serious medication metabolism interactions with classical behavioral health–related medications such as (1) antipsychotic medications such as clozapine and olanzapine, (2) antihypertensives, anticoagulants, chemotherapeutic medications, and opioid medications used for acute or chronic disease management, or (3) birth control pills. Patients should also be educated regarding the increase in caffeine levels during smoking cessation so that potential symptoms of caffeine intoxication are not misattributed to tobacco cessation or another behavioral health disorder.[91] An additional helpful resource for clinicians is the Smoking Cessation Leadership Center.[92]

OPIOID USE AND OUDS

One of the most complicated and vexing issues in primary care over the past 20 years is chronic pain management involving increasing opioid prescriptions. See Chapter 23: Integrated Chronic Pain and Psychiatric Management for additional information on this topic. Until recently, PCPs were encouraged to treat chronic pain aggressively, often using opioids, despite very little evidence of their long-term efficacy, benefit, and risks, particularly in the management of chronic non-cancer pain. Corresponding to the increase in opioid prescribing rates is an increase in overdose deaths related to opioid pain medication in the United States. In the primary care setting, studies have shown that the prevalence of opioid dependence among chronic pain patients on chronic opioid therapy is 3% to 26%.[93] From 1999 to 2014, more than 165,000 persons died from opioid overdoses.[94] In addition to the rise of prescription opioid misuse and dependence, heroin use has increased over the past six years. A SAMHSA report found that 80% of new heroin users reported nonmedical prescription opioid use, even though less than 4% of nonmedical prescription opioid users transitioned to heroin use.[95]

Screening and Assessment for Opioid Use and OUDs

Several tools have been developed to guide the prescriber, prior to prescribing a course of opioids for pain management, in weighing the risk of whether the patient might develop an OUD. These include the Opioid Risk Tool (ORT), Screener and Opioid Assessment for Patients with Pain–Revised (SOAPP–R), and Brief Risk Interview (BRI).[94] The evidence for their accuracy of risk assessment has been found to be insufficient.[94] The Centers for Disease Control and Prevention (CDC) has issued guidelines and recommendations that are grouped into three areas: (1) determining when to initiate or continue opioids for chronic pain; (2) opioid selection, dosage, duration, follow-up, and discontinuation; and (3) assessing risks and addressing harms of opioid use. The recommendations for PCPs, who account for nearly half of all prescribed opioids, are outlined in Box 14.3.[94]

A history of SUD, young age, older age, major depression, and the use of benzodiazepines and other psychotropic medications are important risk factors that must be assessed.[96] A detailed pain history and physical examination may also reveal signs of opioid use, withdrawal, or intoxication. Complications of opioid use are often related to the route of administration of the drug and include intravenous drug use–related track marks, skin-popping disfiguration, skin abscesses, cellulitis, septic arthritis, brain abscess, osteomyelitis, pulmonary talc granulomatosis, and endocarditis, as well as hepatitis B and C and HIV. Opioid use is also associated with chronic constipation. Endocrinologic problems such as hypogonadism and osteopenia are common with chronic opioid use.

Interventions for Opioid Use and OUDs

Interventions for opioid use and OUDs in individuals with illicit use and individuals with co-occurring pain are similar in that brief interventions are not effective. The best outcomes are seen with the use of medication-assisted therapies, in addition to other psychotherapeutic interventions. Patients with iatrogenic opioid use who develop OUD have the additional complications of pain, which complicates their evaluation and often limits the medication-assisted treatments that are available. Therefore, we first address this difficult population.

Approaches to Iatrogenic Opioid Use and OUDs

The best approach to avoid development of an OUD is to use opioid therapy for chronic pain judiciously and as a last resort. Patient- and disease-specific treatment customized to the cause of pain should be tried first. Nonpharmacologic approaches such as physical therapy, CBT, exercise therapy, and weight loss, if indicated, as well as nonopioid pharmacotherapy are recommended prior to starting opioid therapy.[94] For additional discussion and approaches see Chapter 23: Integrated Chronic Pain and Psychiatric Management.

After adequate trials of nonopioid treatment, if opioid therapy is initiated, universal precautions should be taken. First, the provider must discuss the goals of therapy with the patient, which include both pain relief and improved functioning, and agree to an exit strategy if goals are not met. Goals should be reviewed at each visit. Other components of universal precautions are a written controlled-substance agreement or informed consent, routine monitoring of prescriptions, and urine toxicology testing.[97] All patients should understand the need for monitoring and agree to participate in the appropriate recommendations prior to initiating opioid therapy.

Most states now feature a prescription drug monitoring program (PDMP), which may reveal collateral factual data about controlled substances dispensed by the provider and received by the patient. The PDMP is a useful tool that should be accessed prior to initiating opioid therapy and subsequently at least every 3 months. PDMPs are not systematically integrated across state lines and they typically do not trace prescriptions before the last decade. A formal release of information is necessary to obtain older/out-of-state medical records that could prove useful. Providers should discuss the results of the PDMP query with patients if multiple prescribers or multiple prescriptions for controlled substances are found. In the case of multiple prescribers, clinicians should discuss safety concerns with both the patient and prescriber to coordinate care. The PDMP should be used as a clinical tool, not in a punitive manner. If multiple medications are being prescribed, interventions such as education about overdose, safer prescribing to lower doses of medication, and naloxone opioid overdose prevention should be instituted. This may also be an opportunity to provide effective treatment for an SUD.

Urine drug toxicology is a screening and diagnostic tool that can provide information about drug use not reported by the patient as well as identifying when patients are not taking the opioids prescribed for them. The latter may indicate diversion or overuse of medication, leading the patient to run out of medications. Drug toxicology screening is an integral part of the universal precautions of chronic opioid therapy and is best conducted with the patient's consent and knowledge.

BOX 14.3

CENTERS FOR DISEASE CONTROL GUIDELINES FOR PRESCRIBING OPIOIDS FOR CHRONIC PAIN

DETERMINING WHEN TO INITIATE OR CONTINUE OPIOIDS

1. **Nonpharmacologic therapy or nonopioid pharmacologic therapy is preferred.**
2. **Before starting opioid therapy for chronic pain, clinicians should establish treatment goals for pain and function and consider how opioid therapy will be discontinued if benefits do not outweigh the risk.**
3. **Before starting and periodically during opioid therapy, clinicians should discuss known risks and realistic benefits of opioid therapy with patients.**

OPIOID SELECTION, DOSAGE, DURATION, FOLLOW-UP, AND DISCONTINUATION

4. **When starting opioid therapy for chronic pain, clinicians should prescribe immediate-release opioids instead of extended-release or long-acting opioids.**
5. **When opioids are started, clinicians should prescribe the lowest effective dosage. Dosages ≥ 90 MME per day should be avoided.**
6. **Long-term opioid use often begins with treatment of acute pain. Three days or less of prescription opioids is often sufficient and more than 7 days is rarely needed.**
7. **Clinicians should evaluate benefits and harms with patients within 1 to 4 weeks of starting opioid therapy. Subsequently, the risks and benefits should be evaluated every 3 months or more frequently. Clinicians should work with patients to taper to the lowest dose possible or discontinue opioid therapy if benefits do not outweigh the harms.**

ASSESSING RISKS AND ADDRESSING HARMS OF OPIOID USE

8. **Clinicians should continually assess for opioid-related harms. Overdose prevention and naloxone should be offered when high risk for opioid overdose factors such as history of overdose, history of substance use disorder, higher opioid dosages (≥ 50 MME/day), or concurrent benzodiazepine use are present.**
9. **Clinicians should review the patient's history of controlled-substance prescriptions by accessing the state's prescription drug monitoring program periodically but at a minimum of every three months.**
10. **When prescribing opioids for chronic pain, clinicians should use urine drug testing before starting therapy and consider testing at least annually.**
11. **Clinicians should avoid prescribing opioid pain medication and benzodiazepines concurrently.**
12. **Clinicians should offer or arrange evidence-based treatment with buprenorphine or methadone in combination with behavioral therapies for patients with opioid use disorders.**

Adapted from Dowell D, Haegerich T, Chou R. CDC guideline for prescribing opioids for chronic pain—United States, 2016. MMWR. 2016;65(1):1–49.

The frequency of testing should be determined by the provider's concern for SUD. Most initial screening is done by immunoassays, which are relatively inexpensive but often limited in their ability to detect semi-synthetics such as oxycodone and synthetic opioids such as fentanyl or methadone. The use of confirmatory tests (e.g., gas or liquid chromatography/mass spectrometry) can be costly but may be necessary to detect the presence of specific opioids, or confirm the presence of an unexpected positive immunoassay test result.[98] Consultation with the laboratory scientist or toxicologist may be indicated if results are truly unexpected and the patient cannot provide an adequate and plausible explanation. Clinicians must be familiar with the drugs included in the urine drug test panels in their practice. Urine drug screening tests results can often be subject to misinterpretation, resulting in practices that actually harm patients. Urine toxicology testing should always be performed to properly guide and inform patient care. Table 14.3 is a review of the common categories of drugs tested with the usual cutoff values, length of detection, and major concerns with each class of drug.[99,100]

When starting opioid therapy, the CDC guidelines[94] suggest that immediate-release opioids be used instead of long-acting opioid formulations. Long-acting opioids are appropriate only for those who have received 60 mg of morphine or its equivalent for at least a week. Additionally, the lowest dosage that is effective should be prescribed and escalation should be avoided. Extreme caution is now recommended for doses greater than 50 morphine milligram equivalents (MME) per day, and dosages above 90 MME should be avoided. Opioid medications should not be prescribed with benzodiazepines due to respiratory suppression and heightened risk for overdose when they are taken concurrently.[94]

Differential of Aberrant Opioid Medication Behavior

Problems that arise during treatment may include requests for early refills of medications, unexpected urine toxicology or PDMP results, lost prescriptions, behavioral problems, or reports of ineffective analgesia. Providers often struggle in their conversations with patients regarding their aberrant medication-taking behavior and patients often feel excessively stigmatized, shameful, and scrutinized. Often the physician–patient interaction is uncomfortable for both parties, and this can threaten the primary care relationship. A differential diagnosis of aberrant behaviors arising during opioid therapy with management suggestions is as follows:

1. *Disease Progression:* A patient's flare-up of pain and increased use of medication may be related to progression or changes in the underlying medical problem causing the pain disorder. This would be suggested by new symptoms or changes in the location, character, and quality of pain. The intervention is further diagnostic workup.
2. *Withdrawal Pain:* Short-acting opioids have a half-life of three to four hours. Withdrawal pain commonly occurs in the morning hours, particularly if the patient has not taken medication throughout the night. Patients will experience aching pain in the back and other myalgias. The intervention is to provide more evenly distributed medication administration times or possibly the use of longer-acting opioids.
3. *Analgesia Tolerance:* Tolerance to the effects of short-acting opioids occurs after one to two weeks. Many chronic pain patients have been taking opioids for years. Possible interventions are to use the lowest possible dose of medication, provide opioid rotations and opioid drug-free times, and maximize nonopioid interventions.
4. *Hyperalgesia*: It is theorized that hyperalgesia is related to increased sensitization to pain caused by the opioid. The patient's baseline pain threshold is diminished. Hyperalgesia symptoms include pain that becomes increasingly diffuse and less defined. The patient's pain may actually increase despite increasing opioid doses. Possible interventions include decreasing the dose of opioid, using alpha-2 receptor agonists or COX-2 inhibitors, or trying buprenorphine.[101]
5. *Medicating Symptoms Other than Pain:* Clinicians should avoid using opioids to treat insomnia, anxiety, depression, somatoform disorders, or social anxiety. The best intervention is to taper off opioids and appropriately treat the underlying psychiatric condition.
6. *Diversion:* The patient may or may not be aware of diversion, particularly the elderly patient who often has family members or care providers who are diverting the medications. Patients should be instructed that all medications, especially controlled substances, should be kept in a safe location. If urine results are repeatedly negative for prescribed substances, providers should discontinue prescribing without tapering.
7. *Addiction:* If diagnostic criteria for an OUD are met, such that the patient has loss of control of use of opioids or compulsive use of opioids, or continues to use despite consequences, and describes craving, then treatment for an OUD is indicated and advised.

TABLE 14.3. URINE TOXICOLOGY

Drug Class	Length of Detection	Usual Cutoffs	Issues
Alcohol			Urine alcohol cannot be correlated with blood levels. False positive can exists with urine alcohol testing. EtG and EtS will detect alcohol ingestion longer; however, these tests are highly sensitive and can detect alcohol from mouthwash, hand sanitizers, and other "incidental" alcohol use.
Ethanol	7–12 hrs	0.04 g/dL	
EtG	Up to 5 days	100–500 ng/mL	
EtS	Up to 5 days	75–100 ng/mL	
Cannabis			Detection length determined by level of use. Studies have shown that passive ingestion is highly unlikely to produce a positive result.
Single use	3 days	50 ng/mL (immunoassay)	
Moderate use (2–4 times weekly)	5–7 days		
Heavy use (daily)	10–15 days	15 ng/mL (confirmation)	
Chronic heavy use	>30 days		
Cocaine			Rare to have false-positive results. Consumption of tea and products from coca plant can produce positive result.
Benzoylecgonine	2–4 days	300 ng/mL (immunoassay) 150 ng/mL (confirmation)	
Stimulants			
Amphetamine	48 hrs	1,000 ng/mL (immunoassay) 500 ng/mL (confirmation) Note: Positive methamphetamine must contain >200 ng/mL of amphetamine	Many false positives with immunoassay. Bupropion, pseudoephedrine, trazodone, and a number of other compounds cross-react with the immunoassay tests. Note: Methylphenidate (MDMA) will not react with this test. It has a very low sensitivity for the detection of MDMA, and specific testing for MDMA is required if suspected.
Methamphetamine	48 hrs		
Benzodiazepines			Metabolites are detected in urine. Lorazepam and clonazepam often have limited cross-reactivity with most immunoassays, which can lead to false-negative results. Sertraline can cause false-positive results.
Short acting (lorazepam)	3 days	200–300 ng/mL (immunoassay)	
Long acting (diazepam)	30 days	50–300 ng/mL (confirmation) Depends on lab	
Barbiturates			Abuse potential is generally lower than other substances.
Short acting (pentobarbital)	24 hrs	200–300 ng/mL for both immunoassay and confirmation	
Intermediate (butalbital)	3–8 days		
Long acting (phenobarbital)	21 days		
Opioids		300 ng/mL (immunoassay) 2,000 ng/mL for federal workplace	Immunoassays for opiates will detect codeine, morphine, 6-MAM, and hydromorphone. Oxycodone will not be routinely detected unless urine levels are extremely high. Methadone, oxycodone, fentanyl require specific assays.
Codeine	48 hrs		
Heroin (6-MAM)	48 hours		
Hydromorphone	2–4 days		
Methadone	3 days		
Morphine	48–72 hrs		
Oxycodone	2–4 days		
Fentanyl	Difficult to detect		

Substance Abuse and Mental Health Services Administration. Clinical Drug Testing in Primary Care. Technical Assistance Publication (TAP) 32. HHS Publication No. (SMA) 12-4668. Rockville, MD: Substance Abuse and Mental Health Services Administration; 2012. https://store.samhsa.gov/shin/content/SMA12-4668/SMA12-4668.pdf. Accessed July 24, 2016.
Moeller KE, Lee KC, Kissack JC. Urine drug screening: practical guide for clinicians. Mayo Clin Proc. 2008;83(1):66–76.

Medical Opioid Detoxification

Patients receiving opioid therapy should receive close follow-up, at least every 3 months, especially for patients with opioid doses of more than 50 MME, history of substance abuse, history of overdose, or comorbid psychiatric illness. Patients should be seen more frequently if they are not benefitting in terms of either pain control or functioning, are experiencing untoward side effects, are exhibiting aberrant behavior, or are manifesting any signs of an OUD. In these circumstances, the medication should be tapered or discontinued. The rapidity of the taper should depend on the circumstances, with overdose or other severe adverse events requiring a rapid taper by weekly reductions of 10% to 50%.[102] Patients who consistently have negative urine screens and are diverting medications do not require tapers and the medication can be discontinued. However, a taper that is slower, to minimize withdrawal symptoms, is generally tolerated much better. A decrease in opioid dosage of 10% per week or per month is preferable, particularly if the patient has been taking opioids for a number of years.[94]

Approaches to Non-Iatrogenic Opioid Use and OUD

For patients who are using heroin, who are using their prescribed opioids via the intravenous route, smoking, or snorting, who cannot be safely weaned from their prescriptions, or who cannot safely manage their medications, OUD treatment should be considered and treatment should be initiated. Detoxification alone is unlikely to result in sustained abstinence and is rarely successful.[103,104] Rapid and ultra-rapid detoxification under anesthesia is not only ineffective but potentially fatal and not recommended.[105]

For patients with OUD who have not been abstinent for an extended period of time, and who have not received formal structured treatment for their disorder, maintenance treatment with methadone or buprenorphine is generally preferable to short tapers and detoxification.[103,104] If detoxification is required (e.g., the patient prefers treatment with naltrexone, impending incarceration, or occupational requirement not permitting medication-assisted therapy), then a medically supervised opioid withdrawal employing methadone or buprenorphine followed by a taper is preferred. The choice would depend on availability of an opioid treatment program (OTP) for methadone or buprenorphine from a provider with the appropriate U.S. Drug Enforcement Administration (DEA) authorization. During detoxification, adjunctive medications can be administered. Clonidine (an alpha-2 adrenergic agent that blocks the activation the noradrenergic activity of the locus coeruleus during opioid withdrawal) is reported to reduce lacrimation, rhinorrhea, restlessness, muscle pain, and some gastrointestinal symptoms that commonly occur with opioid withdrawal. Its chief side effect is orthostatic hypotension, which can result in sedation and dizziness.[106] Other adjuvant medications for nausea, diarrhea, abdominal cramps, muscle aches, anxiety, and insomnia can be prescribed as well.

Mutual Support Groups

There are a multitude of 12-step groups for individuals with OUDs to consider. Narcotics Anonymous (NA) is the second-largest 12-step organization and is based on the same 12-step principles as AA but substitutes "addiction" for alcohol. It is open to all drug addicts regardless of the type of drug or combination of drugs used.[106] Individuals with co-occurring pain may wish to consider participating in mutual support groups such as Chronic Pain Anonymous, a 12-step fellowship program for individuals with chronic pain or any chronic illness.[107] The only requirement for membership is the desire to recover from the emotional and spiritual debilitation of chronic pain and chronic illness.

Medication-Assisted Treatment for OUDs

OUDs, more than any other SUDs, have pharmacotherapy alternatives that are highly effective for treatment. Due to the chronic relapsing nature of the disorder, long-term treatment may be necessary as studies have shown frequent relapses after withdrawal from medication-assisted treatment.[108] The following is a review of the OUD pharmacotherapies.

Methadone

Methadone is a full opioid agonist that may be prescribed for pain by a provider with a valid DEA license. However, it is only available for use in the treatment for OUD in a specialized and licensed OTP. There is extensive experience with methadone, which has been shown to effectively reduce drug use, criminal behavior, infectious disease transmission, overdose, and death.[109] Despite these positive outcomes, methadone has some drawbacks. There continues to be significant stigmatization. Clinics are often outside mainstream medical care, limiting the experience most providers have with methadone and hindering continuity of care. Access to OTPs is often limited as well, and most clinics do not have integrated mental health or medical services. Although the structure of OTPs and necessary accountability can support recovery, many patients find the requirement for daily visits (so taking the medication can be observed) to be overwhelming. Patients in methadone clinics are, at first, required to attend six days per week of treatment. Those who are compliant for at least three months can earn take-home doses of medication. PCPs or members of an integrated team can assess a patient's progress by inquiring about take-home medications.

The long half-life of methadone allows for once-a-day dosing for the treatment of opioid dependence. Maintenance doses used for opioid dependence are generally between 80 and 120 mg/day, far higher than those used to treat pain. Common problems associated with methadone are prolongation of the QTc, constipation, and drug interactions (related to concomitantly administered drugs on the CYP-450 system), which can raise or lower methadone levels. Methadone has been associated with overdose deaths involving diverted methadone (mostly diverted from pain treatment settings, not from patients treated at OTPs).[110] There is no fixed time limit to methadone treatment, and patients should continue treatment until they are abstinent from illicit substances and have achieved stability in regard to their medical, psychiatric, social, and legal problems. OTPs do not provide pain management, nor do they provide methadone for pain control. However, OTPs will provide treatment for the OUD arising from the use of prescription opioid medications.

Buprenorphine

Prior to the passage of the Drug Addiction Treatment Act of 2000 (DATA 2000),[111] it was illegal to prescribe certain narcotic drugs for maintenance treatment or detoxification treatment of opioid-dependent patients other than in a federally regulated OTP. DATA 2000 allowed physicians who met the appropriate qualifications to prescribe federally approved Schedule III medications to treat OUDs in an office-based setting. Completion of an approved eight-hour training course is one route for providers who wish to obtain the necessary DEA waiver. Buprenorphine, a high-affinity mu-opioid partial agonist and kappa antagonist, was approved by the FDA for pharmacotherapy of OUDs. This medication has a number of properties that make it ideal to treat OUDs, including a lower ceiling effect so that past a certain dose, there is no further activation of the opioid receptor; this makes an overdose less likely. It has a higher affinity for the opioid receptor than full agonists, therefore blocking their binding and rendering agonists ineffective. Buprenorphine has a long half-life, allowing for once-a-day dosing. Because of the low ceiling effect and higher affinity for the receptor, patients must be in mild to moderate withdrawal to initiate treatment or risk a precipitated withdrawal. Buprenorphine is taken sublingually because it is not absorbed orally. It has two formulations, one with naloxone included and the other without. Naloxone is neither absorbed orally nor sublingually and its presence serves as a deterrent to reduce intravenous abuse of the medication. The usual buprenorphine dose range is between 8 and 24 mg/day. Major side effects are nausea, headache, and constipation.[112]

Multiple studies have compared buprenorphine to methadone and found comparable rates of drug use during treatment, particularly between buprenorphine and methadone. However, methadone is associated with slightly better rates of treatment retention.[113] Since treatment in an office-based setting may be preferable to most patients, it is reasonable to recommend buprenorphine first and then, if more structure is needed, to refer the patient to an OTP for methadone treatment.

The waiver for office-based prescribing of buprenorphine also requires the practitioner to have the ability to refer patients for psychosocial therapy. Psychosocial services for patients can consist of medication management services, monitoring, and support. Higher levels of psychosocial interventions, including CBT, were not more effective than medication management alone.[114,115] Buprenorphine can also be used in the primary care or integrated setting to effectively treat patients with comorbid chronic pain and OUDs.[23] Physicians who wish to prescribe buprenorphine and obtain the waiver can find complete information on SAMHSA's website.[116]

Oral Naltrexone

Naltrexone is a long-acting, oral mu-opioid receptor antagonist that provides complete blockade of opioid effect at the mu-opioid receptor. The usual dose is 50 mg/day. Theoretically, it should be an ideal pharmacotherapeutic agent; however, it has not been particularly effective for treatment of OUD. It lacks the reinforcement effects of methadone or buprenorphine, and cravings may continue. The treatment retention rates with naltrexone alone are only 20% to 30% over 6 months.[117] Naltrexone, if used, should not be started until abstinence from opioids is established for five to seven days for short-acting opioids and seven to ten days for long-acting opioids to avoid precipitating withdrawal.

Injectable Naltrexone

In 2010, the FDA approved the use of extended-release injectable naltrexone for the treatment of opioid dependence based on clinical trials in Russia that showed a 90% abstinence rate, confirmed by urine testing (the placebo group had a 35% abstinence rate).[118] The naltrexone group had greater retention in treatment and reduced cravings compared to the placebo group.[119] The dose is 380 mg every four weeks and the major side effects for both the oral and injectable forms are nausea and fatigue. Injection site reactions are frequent. Studies are ongoing comparing the injectable form of naltrexone to methadone and buprenorphine.

OUD in Pregnancy

Corresponding to the increased use of opioids in the general population, concern for opioid misuse, abuse, and dependence during pregnancy is growing. Since 2012 there has been a four-fold rise in the identification of maternal opioid use at delivery and a three-fold rise in the incidence of neonatal opioid withdrawal. Stillbirth, prematurity, poor fetal growth, and neonatal abstinence syndrome have been associated with maternal opioid use.[119,120] Methadone maintenance for the treatment of opioid dependence in pregnancy has been extensively studied. Prescribing methadone is the standard of care, recommended over opioid withdrawal, as it has been associated with good maternal and neonatal outcomes.[121] Recently studies have shown that buprenorphine can also be used successfully in pregnancy. In a study comparing methadone- versus buprenorphine-treated mothers, Jones et al.[122] found that infants with mothers treated with buprenorphine required significantly lower amounts of morphine to treat neonatal abstinence and had shorter hospital stays. Methadone, however, was associated with greater maternal retention in treatment versus buprenorphine.[123]

The choice of pharmacotherapy depends on treatment availability, patient preference, and primary goals (i.e., treatment retention vs. shorter neonatal abstinence). In addition, to minimize any risks to the fetus, the mono-product of buprenorphine was used versus the formulation with naloxone. However, no clear evidence exists that the naloxone has any effect on fetal health. Providers should weigh the risk of exposure of the fetus to small quantities of naloxone versus the possible risk of misuse and diversion if the mono-product is used.[124]

Opioid Overdose Education and Naloxone Distribution

Patients, family members, and significant others should be provided opioid overdose prevention and naloxone administration training if they are prescribed opioids, if they demonstrate aberrant behaviors, or if they have risk factors for overdose such as a prior overdose history, taking more than 50 mg of morphine or equivalent doses of other opioids, have a history of SUD, are taking benzodiazepines with opioids, have recently lost tolerance to opioids, and/or are at risk for returning to high doses.[94]

SEDATIVE USE AND SEDATIVE USE DISORDERS

Sedative-hypnotic medications are a group of drugs that suppress the central nervous system. Substances in this category include benzodiazepines, "non-benzodiazepine hypnotics," barbiturates, carisoprodol, and related compounds. Typically, these drugs are prescribed as anxiolytics, hypnotics, anticonvulsants, muscle relaxants, and anesthesia induction agents.[125] These medications have abuse potential and their misuse or abuse is problematic because of the risk of addiction and their contribution to overdose deaths. One case-cohort study found concurrent benzodiazepine and opioid prescription to be associated with a four-fold risk of overdose deaths compared to opioid prescription alone.[126] This risk has led the CDC to recommend that opioids and benzodiazepines not be prescribed together except in special circumstances such as severe acute pain in a patient taking a stable low dose of benzodiazepines in the long term.[94]

Benzodiazepines are often used to treat anxiety-related disorders. However, given the risk of overdose, diversion, and addiction, these medications should not be used as a first-line pharmacologic treatment for anxiety. Serotonin reuptake inhibitors and serotonin-noradrenalin reuptake inhibitors are the first-line choice for generalized anxiety disorders. See Chapter 11: Integrated Care for Anxiety Disorder for a full discussion of the treatment of anxiety disorders. Possible short-term side effects of benzodiazepines are subjective sedation, impaired psychomotor effects, impaired cognition, delirium, accidents and injuries, impaired driving skills, and possible disinhibition, especially in the elderly. Although tolerance can occur to some of the short-term effects, long-term use is associated with even more profound cognitive, psychomotor, and practical impairments.[127] Certainly these effects are even more pronounced in combination with alcohol and in the elderly.[128]

Screening and Assessment for Sedative Use and Sedative Use Disorders

Similarly to opioid prescription, screening for the risk of the development of a sedative use disorder should occur prior to prescribing sedatives. The PDMP should also be reviewed, at least on an annual basis, and in all patients prior to prescribing a sedative-hypnotic. If the adverse effects are found to outweigh the continued benefit of prescription, or if there is evidence of diversion, other evidence of misuse, or increasing evidence of addiction, discontinuation of the benzodiazepine should be considered.

Interventions for Sedative Use and Sedative Use Disorders

Brief interventions are ineffective for the treatment of sedative use disorders. Detoxification is often necessary due to the development of tolerance in individuals who regularly take benzodiazepines. Patients should be prescribed behaviorally based treatments. There are no FDA-approved medications for the treatment of benzodiazepine use disorders. Patients may find 12-step program participation or other mutual support groups helpful.

Benzodiazepine discontinuation can be challenging. Symptoms can include reemergence of the symptoms of the original illness (rebound symptoms that are more intensely experienced than the original symptoms) and withdrawal similar to alcohol withdrawal. Symptoms may include seizures, tremors, paresthesia, perceptual symptoms, hallucinations, and delirium tremens. Benzodiazepine withdrawal can be associated with life-threatening symptoms.[127] Providers should taper benzodiazepines gradually to prevent severe withdrawal. A commonly used tapering schedule that has been safely used with moderate success is a reduction of the benzodiazepine dose by 25% every one to two weeks.[128] Individuals who are unsuccessful with attempts at outpatient detoxification or who present at high risk for complicated withdrawal should pursue inpatient detoxification. If both opioids and benzodiazepines are prescribed and require tapering, the opioids should be tapered before the benzodiazepines. If benzodiazepines prescribed for anxiety are tapered or discontinued, or if patients receiving opioids require treatment for anxiety, evidence-based psychotherapies (e.g., CBT) and/or specific antidepressants or other non-benzodiazepine medications approved for anxiety should be offered.[94]

CANNABIS USE AND CANNABIS USE DISORDERS

One in 10 adults and one in six adolescents who use cannabis will develop a cannabis use disorder (CUD). The lifetime prevalence of CUDs is 6% to 19% and the average age of onset is 18.6 years. Of individuals with CUD, 82% will achieve recovery within three years of onset, but up to 30% of these recovered individuals will have a recurrence by the time they are age 30.[129] Only 13% of individuals with CUD will seek mutual support groups or professional treatment.[130] This is especially concerning given evidence that regular cannabis use, as well as cannabis dependence, is associated with being less educated, downward socioeconomic movement, worse financial difficulties, increased relationship conflict (including violence), unprofessional behavior in the workplace, and traffic convictions.[131] For the majority of these realms, there was no difference in decline when compared to individuals with alcohol dependence, with the exception of seeing more financial decline in cannabis-dependent individuals. These findings in cannabis users were not confounded by age of onset, history of convictions, or co-occurring alcohol and other drug use disorders.[131] CUDs are also associated with the presence of other psychiatric illness (e.g., other drug use disorders, mood disorders, anxiety disorders, and personality disorders).[132]

With the widespread national adoption of medical marijuana policy (currently adopted in 25 states, plus Washington, DC) and legalization in four states, the PCP and integrated care team should remain up to date regarding emerging and purported medical indications for cannabis products. To date, there are no FDA indications for any marijuana product. Both dronabinol (synthetic delta-9-tetrahydrocannabinol [THC], Marinol) and nabilone (synthetic delta-9-THC congener, Cesamet) have FDA indications for chemotherapy-induced nausea and vomiting. In a recent meta-analysis of 79 randomized controlled trials (6,462 participants), moderate-quality evidence supported the use of cannabis products for the treatment of chronic pain (nabiximols and smoked THC) and spasticity (nabiximols, THC/CBD capsules, dronabinol, and nabilone).[133] Less clear evidence exists for the treatment of nausea and emesis due to chemotherapy (nabiximols and nabilone), for the promotion of weight gain in individuals with HIV (dronabinol), for insomnia (nabilone and nabiximols), and for motor tics (THC capsules).[133] No evidence supports the use of cannabis for depression, anxiety disorders, psychosis, and glaucoma. Many of the studies included in this meta-analysis were of small size and were at high risk of bias. Meta-analysis data indicate that the regulated products delivered in nonsmokable forms still carry the risk of acute adverse effects, including disorientation (odds ratio [OR] 5.4), dizziness (OR 5.09), euphoria (OR 4.08), confusion (OR 4.03), drowsiness (OR 3.68), and dry mouth (OR 3.5). Acute adverse events with an OR between 2 and 3 include nausea, fatigue, somnolence, asthenia, balance, hallucinations, and paranoia. Furthermore, cannabis increases the risk for depression, emesis, diarrhea, anxiety, and other psychosis. No studies in this meta-analysis addressed the long-term adverse events associated with medical cannabanoids.[133]

In addition to the limited indications for marijuana use, the PCP and members of the integrated care team should keep in mind other potential adverse events associated with marijuana use. Cannabis potency has changed immensely, with a national upward trend in the mean delta-9-THC content of all confiscated cannabis preparations. For example, it increased from 3.4% in 1993 to 8.8% in 2008.[134] Furthermore, the use of vaporizing techniques can increase the intensity of physical and emotional reactions. Thus, much of the literature today may underestimate the rate and severity of adverse events. Additional adverse events associated with acute marijuana use include vascular events (e.g., myocardial infarction and stroke). Nonmedical cannabinoid studies clearly indicate that long-term marijuana use is associated with neuropsychological impairment (measured during a nonintoxicated state), amotivation, other drug use, addiction, altered brain development, chronic bronchitis and other respiratory infections, increased risk of psychosis, depression, and anxiety, as well as a poorer prognosis in these disorders.[132,135]

Useful information for patient education comes from a study of typical dispensary products (e.g., baked goods, beverage, or candy).[136] THC levels of these products are highly variable and ranged from less than 1 mg to 1,236 mg when tested. The study found that only 17% of edible cannabinoid products were labeled correctly, with 23% being underlabeled and 60% being overlabeled.[136] The median ratio of THC (more active psychoactive compound) to cannabidiol (more protective compound) was 36:1, and only 1% of products had the recommended ratio of 1:1 to balance clinical benefit and adverse events.[136] The PCP and other members of the integrated team should also educate patients regarding the hazards of using cannabis while operating heavy machinery or driving. A hazardous blood level can be obtained with only one serving of a cannabinoid.

Screening and Assessment for Cannabis Use and CUD

In 2008, the USPSTF concluded that the current evidence was insufficient to assess the balance of benefits and harms of screening adolescents, adults, and pregnant women for illicit drug use.[137] In states that have legalized cannabis for recreational use, medical professionals should ask direct questions about any use of cannabis, although this has yet to be included in formal primary care recommendations.

Interventions for Cannabis Use and CUD

There are no formal recommendations for the use of brief interventions for high-risk misuse of cannabis or for CUD. It is our practice to take an educational approach, similar to that of brief interventions for high-risk alcohol use, in individuals with high-risk marijuana use. Behavioral interventions that are effective for adults and the development of interventions that reduce cost and required clinician time are ongoing.[138]

Interventions with children and adolescents are more effective if a parent is involved in the intervention, unless a more severe use disorder is present, or there is evidence of a co-occurring conduct disorder. In these cases, the patient should be referred to more specialized, intensive outpatient or dual diagnoses-capable residential treatment.[139]

Currently no FDA-approved pharmacotherapies exist for the treatment of CUD.

OTHER DRUG USE AND DRUG USE DISORDERS

Insufficient evidence exists, according to the USPSTF, for the routine screening of adolescents, adults, and pregnant women for other illicit drug use.[139] There also appears to be limited benefit from screening and brief interventions. The absence of an official recommendation simply reflects the current absence of evidence for universal SBIRT concerning illicit drugs, marijuana, and nonmedical use of other prescription drugs. As illicit drug use behaviors are mostly socially frowned upon, if not outright illegal, most drug users are already aware of the risks and of the fact that their use is nonnormative. This may help explain the ineffectiveness for illicit drug abuse of the SBIRT model, which was initially created for alcohol, then tentatively expanded to other substances. This does not lessen the importance of identifying and addressing illicit drug use, legal marijuana misuse, and misuse of prescription medications. What it does suggest is that screening using validated tools to detect unhealthy illicit drug use may not immediately lead to reduced drug use or fewer problems after a brief intervention.[140] Rather, more intensive interventions are likely required.

Despite failure to date to generalize SBIRT to other illicit drug use, the single-question screen "How many times in the past year have you used an illegal drug or a prescription medication for nonmedical reasons?" has successfully been used in various studies to identify other drug use.[38] A patient who screens positive should be evaluated for a possible SUD. If a patient meets criteria for an SUD, which are similar for all classes of substances, commencement of treatment remains the standard of care. In treatment-seeking patients, motivational interventions, CBT,[143] contingency management,[144] family and couples therapy,[145] and 12-step facilitation[64] are just a few of the psychosocial strategies that may be effective for various groups of patients, along with treatment of co-occurring medical and psychiatric conditions. All new patients, and those with demographic or clinical risks, such as male sex, behavioral problems, family members with substance use problems, those with symptoms of a psychiatric disorder, or medical issues potentially related to drug use, may be an appropriate target group for the single-question drug use screen. Given the limited interventions available to PCPs, the nonpharmacotherapeutic approach to treatment of other drug use disorders should be approached similarly to alcohol. The only additional caveat is that the general approach to the prescription of stimulants for chronic attentional problems has many parallels to the discussion of other controlled substances such as sedatives and opioids.

SUPPORTING RECOVERY EFFORTS IN AN INTEGRATED SETTING

Relapse is common with SUDs, even when the condition is being managed and the patient is compliant and motivated for treatment. Relapse does not indicate that treatment has failed but signals that it needs to be adjusted, reinstated, or changed in order to move toward recovery. Monitoring SUDs is a therapeutic intervention and should serve to inform clinical decision making. It is not a punitive measure. Through the monitoring process, integrated care teams and PCPs perform important roles in relapse prevention and can facilitate movement through the care continuum of treatments for SUDs.

During every patient visit, inquiring about substance use is important. Providers should ask about not only the patient's drug of choice but other substances, including nicotine. Due to the shame and stigma associated with SUDs and particularly relapse, patient reports may be less than forthcoming. A nonconfrontational, nonjudgmental attitude based on openness, honesty, and empathy is essential when interacting with SUD patients. Follow-up visits should include inquiries about recovery activities: 12-step meeting attendance frequency, sponsor contacts, 12-step work, or attendance at other self-help groups. A discussion of the patient's current treatment attendance and review of recovery progress often helps build the therapeutic alliance between the patient and primary care team members. In addition, a review of medical symptoms and use of medical services, hospitalizations, or emergency visits may reveal possible evidence of relapse or substance use. Asking about adherence to pharmacotherapy and confirming use of prescribed medication and review of the PDMP should occur with each visit. Disturbances in self-care, mood, anxiety, sleep, and pain often either are evidence of relapse or can trigger relapse. Such symptoms are common in the early stages of recovery and should be assessed at each visit. Since SUDs have often impacted patients' social functioning, it is important to inquire about employment, relationships, legal problems, and leisure activities.

Since reemergence of psychiatric symptoms can lead to relapse, monitoring for recurrence of depression, mood disorders, and anxiety is important. Psychiatric symptoms may be induced by a substance, but a number of mental health disorders predate the onset of the substance use. These mental health disorders are present even during extended periods of abstinence and should be addressed and treated appropriately. Substance use is sometimes difficult to differentiate from psychiatric disorders. Studies have shown that between 26% and 32% of patients with substance-induced depression were reclassified in follow-up as having independent major depressive disorders.[146]

During follow-up visits, family members, friends and other stakeholders can provide valuable information regarding the patient's recovery progress. Care must be taken to obtain appropriate patient consent in compliance with confidentiality rules and the special regulations for disclosure of information regarding substance abuse patients, 42 CFR Part 2.[148] Reviewing medical records and collaborating with other specialty providers ensures that the patient truly has integrated care.

Integrated primary care teams play a crucial role in the ongoing monitoring of medical problems that have been caused or exacerbated by a relapse of a SUD, by the toxic effects of the substance, the route of use of the substance, or the co-occurring high-risk behaviors. Regular screening for HIV, hepatitis B (if not vaccinated) and C, sexually transmitted diseases, and tuberculosis should occur in high-risk patients.

Monitoring for relapse can include detection by physical exam (e.g., alterations in vital signs, fresh track marks), following biomarkers (e.g., transaminases, MCV, GGT, CDT, PeTH), accessing the PDMP, and performing urine toxicology screening. The frequency of follow-up visits, accessing PDMP, and urine toxicology screening should be based on the assessment of risk, aberrant behavior, time in recovery, and medical and psychiatric stability, with considerations given to the financial burden on the patient. High-risk patients should be screened at least every three months if not monthly (consider this in individuals who are less likely to verbally report use, such as those who are older, female, or disabled; have legal and social problems; and have more severe drug problems); low-risk patients can be monitored twice a year.[93]

Often patients with SUD have neglected their physical health, and follow-up primary care visits serve to provide preventive care services and should complement the SUD recovery. Immunizations should be updated, and cancer screening and counseling regarding healthy dietary habits and physical activity are essential. Oral hygiene often is affected by alcohol, tobacco, methamphetamine, and opioids and should be addressed. All patients should be counseled on gun safety, seat belt use, and safe sexual practices.

Two issues affecting women with SUDs deserve particular attention in primary care. The prevalence of domestic violence is substantially increased among women with substance problems: Some studies suggest that 60% to 70% of women attending SUD treatment have been victims of abuse.[150] Routine assessment regarding domestic violence should occur for all women patients, particularly those with SUD. See Chapter 18: Violence and Suicide for additional information about screening and treatment for domestic violence.

Women with SUDs have higher rates of unintended pregnancy than the general population and, at the same time, have significantly increased maternal and neonatal morbidity and mortality. Use of reliable birth control methods in women with SUD is low; most are using condoms as their method of contraception. Traditional SUD treatments fail to address contraception or to provide adequate long-acting reversible methods such as intrauterine devices or implants. Primary care integration can have a major impact in this area.[151]

PCPs should take all precautions against prescribing addictive medications and should ensure that other providers of patient care avoid medications that may be detrimental to recovery and or may initiate the path to relapse. Mood-altering medications (stimulants) or controlled substances should be avoided unless their use is necessary. Regardless of the patient's drug of choice, extra care needs to be taken in prescribing any controlled substance. Opioids should be not be used until all nonpharmacologic therapies and nonopioid alternatives are exhausted or in the case of severe acute pain. Benzodiazepines and related benzodiazepine receptor agonists such as eszopiclone, zaleplon, and zolpidem should be avoided in the management of anxiety and insomnia. If controlled substances are prescribed for acute indications, the minimal amount should be dispensed, and close follow-up in three to seven days should accompany such prescriptions. Patients should be encouraged to discuss the medication with their SUD treatment provider, recovery support group, 12-step sponsor, and/or family members for proper oversight in administration of the short-acting medication.

CONCLUSION

Addiction and SUDs are extremely prevalent and are commonly encountered in the primary care and integrated care settings. PCPs have often felt frustrated and poorly equipped to deal with the problems presented by patients with SUDs. The traditional separation of SUD treatment programs from mainstream medicine has often not provided

BOX 14.4
EVIDENCE FOR SUBSTANCE USE DISORDERS IN INTEGRATED CARE SETTINGS

Strength of recommendation taxonomy (SOR A, B, or C)

- **Unhealthy alcohol use screening is ranked third of the top five prevention priorities for U.S. adults among preventive practices by the U.S. Preventive Services Task Force (USPSTF). Screening for unhealthy alcohol use should be offered to all primary care and integrated care patients routinely.[35,37,38] (SOR A)**
- **Single-item questionnaires, for all forms of alcohol misuse, have a sensitivity of 82% and specificity of 79%.[37,38] (SOR A)**
- **Single-item alcohol screening instruments are valid and reliable for identifying the spectrum of unhealthy alcohol use.[37,38] (SOR A)**
- **Single-item screening for substance misuse or substance use disorders can be performed in integrated and primary care settings.[39,139,140,142] (SOR C)**
- **The USPSTF finds insufficient evidence for the routine screening for substances other than tobacco and alcohol. However, providers should ask direct questions about drug use.[139] (SOR C)**
- **Brief intervention with goal setting by primary care providers and integrated care team members who are not addiction specialists decreases drinking in high-risk, unhealthy alcohol users. Brief intervention increases the proportion of adults who abstain from binging and adhere to goals. However, brief intervention is not efficacious for patients with severe alcohol use disorder. There is little evidence to support the long-term effects of brief intervention on morbidity, mortality, or quality of life.[35,50,51] (SOR A)**
- **Studies have shown higher rates of abstinence for those attending 12-step meetings. Clinicians should encourage participation in 12-step mutual help groups such as Alcoholics Anonymous.[65,66] (SOR A)**
- **Naltrexone and acamprosate are approved by the U.S. Food and Drug Administration for the treatment of alcohol dependence and have been shown to be effective in decreasing cravings and lessening the amount of alcohol used if relapse occurs. They should be considered along with counseling for the treatment of alcohol dependence.[74,75,78,79] (SOR A)**
- **Clinicians and health care delivery systems should consistently identify and document tobacco use status and treat every tobacco user seen in a health care setting. The identification and documentation of tobacco use alone may affect quit rates.[83] (SOR A)**
- **All nonpregnant adult smokers should be offered both behavioral counseling and pharmacotherapy to quit. Pregnant women should be offered counseling. Interventions should occur in all stages of change.[83] (SOR A)**
- **Multiple randomized controlled trials have shown the effectiveness and safety of office-based therapy with buprenorphine for the treatment of opioid use disorders.[112–114] (SOR A)**

effective care for SUD patients. With the development of integrated care teams, the expansion of improved screening tools, pharmacotherapy, and more effective treatment modalities, integrated care practices and primary care providers can increasingly play a role in SUD screening, assessment, treatment, and referral. The integration of SUD treatment into primary care integrated settings holds the promise of providing improved acceptability to patients, a decrease in the stigmatization of SUDs, decreased costs, enhanced satisfaction for providers, and improved outcomes for patients. A summary of recommended treatment approaches and relevant evidence in integrated settings is found in Box 14.4.

REFERENCES

1. National Center on Addiction and Substance Abuse (CASA) at Columbia University. Missed Opportunity: National Survey of Primary Care Physicians and Patients on Substance Abuse, 2000.
2. Kessler RC, Berlund P, Demler O, Jin R, Merikangas KR, Walters EE. Lifetime prevalence of DSM-IV disorders in the National Comorbidity Survey Replication. Arch Gen Psychiatry. 2005;62(6):593–602.
3. Center for Behavioral Health Statistics and Quality. (2015). Behavioral health trends in the United States: Results from the 2014 National Survey on Drug Use and Health (HHS Publication No. SMA 15-4927, NSDUH Series H-50). http://www.samhsa.gov/data/sites/default/files/NSDUH-FRR1-2014/NSDUH-FRR1-2014.pdf. Accessed July 25, 2016.
4. Vital signs: Overdoses of prescription opioid pain relievers—United States, 1999–2008. MMWR Morb Mortal Wkly Rep. 2011;60(43):1487–1492.
5. Jones CM, Logan J, Gladden RM, Bohm MK. Vital signs: Demographic and substance use trends among heroin users—United States, 2002–2013. MMWR Morb Mortal Wkly Rep. 2015;64(26):719–725.
6. Volkow N, Koob G, McLellan TA. Neurobiologic advances from the brain disease model of addiction. N Engl J Med. 2016;374:363–371.
7 Substance Abuse and Mental Health Services Administration. Results from the 2011 National Survey on drug abuse and health: Summary of national findings. Rockville, MD, 2012.
8. Friedmann PD. Effect of primary medical care on addiction and medical severity in substance abuse treatment programs. J Gen Intern Med. 2003;18(1):1–8.
9. Keyes KM, Hatzenbuehler ML, McLaughlin KA, et al. Stigma and treatment for alcohol disorders in the United States. Am J Epidemiol. 2010;172(12):1364–1372.
10. Khantzian EJ. The self-medication hypothesis of substance use disorders: A reconsideration and recent applications. Harvard Rev Psychiatry. 1997:4(5): 231–244.
11. Greenfield SF, Brooks AJ, Gordon SM, et al. Substance abuse treatment entry, retention, and outcome in women: A review of the literature. Drug Alcohol Depend. 2007;86(1):1–21.
12. The Patient Protection and Affordable Care Act, P.L. 111-148, March 23, 2010.
13. Paul Wellstone and Pete Domenici Mental Health Parity and Addiction Equity (MHPAE) Act (P.L.110-343).
14. Institute of Medicine (IOM). Crossing the Quality Chasm for Mental Health and Substance Use Disorders. Washington DC: National Academy Press, 2006.
15. Hunter SB, Schwartz RP, Friedmann PD. Introduction to the special issue on the studies on the implementation of integrated models of alcohol, tobacco, and/or drug use interventions and medical care. J Subst Abuse Treat. 2016;60:1–5.
16. Asarnow JR, Rozenman M, Wiblin J, Zeltzer L. Integrated medical-behavioral care compared with usual primary care for child and adolescent behavioral health: A meta-analysis. JAMA Pediatrics. 2015;169(10):929–937.
17. Ballesteros J, Duffy JC, Querejeta I, Ariño J, González-Pinto A. Efficacy of brief interventions for hazardous drinkers in primary care: Systematic review and meta-analysis. Alcohol Clin Exp Res. 2004;28(4):608–618.
18. Bertholet N, Daeppen JB, Wietlisbach V, Fleming M, Burnand B. Reduction of alcohol consumption by brief alcohol intervention in primary care: Systematic review and meta-analysis. Arch Intern Med. 2005;165(9):986–995.
19. Saitz R, Larson MJ, LaBelle C, Richardson J, Samet JH. The case for chronic disease management for addiction. J Addict Med. 2008;2(2):55–65.
20. Kim TW, Saitz R, Cheng DM, Winter MR, Witas J, Samet JH. Effect of quality chronic disease management for alcohol and drug dependence on addiction outcomes. J Subst Abuse Treat. 2012;43(4):389–396.
21. Saitz R, Cheng DM, Winter M, et al. Chronic care management for alcohol and other drug dependence: The AHEAD randomized trial. JAMA 2013;310(11):1156–1157.
22. Pade P, Cardon K, Hoffman R Geppert CM. Prescription opioid abuse, chronic pain, and primary care: A Co-occurring Disorders Clinic in the chronic disease model. J Subst Abuse Treat. 2012;43(4):446–450.
23. American Psychiatric Association. Diagnostic and Statistical Manual of Mental Disorders (5th ed.). Arlington, VA: American Psychiatric Publishing; 2013.
24. Demers CH, Bogdan R, Agrawal A. The genetics, neurogenetics and pharmacogenetics of addiction. Curr Behav Neurosci Rep. 2014;1(1):33–44.

25. Volkow N, Menke M. The genetics of addiction. Hum Genet 2012;131(6):773–777.
26. McLellan AT, Lewis DC, Obrien CP, Kleber HD. Drug dependence a chronic medical illness: Implications for treatment, insurance and outcomes evaluation. JAMA. 2000;284(13):1689–1695.
27. American Psychiatric Association/Academy of Psychosomatic Medicine. Dissemination of integrated care within adult primary care settings: the collaborative care model. https://www.psychiatry.org/psychiatrists/practice/professional-interests/integrated-care/collaborative-care-model. Published Spring 2016. Accessed July 25, 2016.
28. Miller B, Gilchrist E, Ross K, et al. Core Competencies for Behavioral Health Providers Working in Primary Care. Prepared from the Colorado Consensus Conference, February 2016. http://farleyhealthpolicycenter.org/wp-content/uploads/2016/02/Core-Competencies-for-Behavioral-Health-Providers-Working-in-Primary-Care.pdf Accessed July 24, 2016.
29. Unutzer J, Harbin H, Druss M. The collaborative care model: An approach for integrating physical and mental health care in Medicaid health homes. Center for Health Care Strategies and Mathematica Policy Research, May (2013). http://www.mdcbh.org/images/HH_IRC_Collaborative_Care_Model_052113.pdf Accessed July 24, 2016.
30. Academy for Integrating Behavioral Health and Primary Care. Agency for Healthcare Research and Quality, Rockville, MD. http://www.ahrq.gov/cpi/about/otherwebsites/integrationacademy.ahrq.gov/index.html. Accessed July 24, 2016.
31. Substance Abuse and Mental Health Services Administration. Health care and health systems integration. http://www.samhsa.gov/health-care-health-systems-integration. Updated March 7, 2016. Accessed July 24, 2016.
32. Scharf DM, Eberhart NK, Hackbarth NS, et al. Evaluation of the SAMHSA Primary and Behavioral Health Care Integration (PBHCI) Grant Program: Final Report, 2013. U.S. Department of Health and Human Services Assistant Secretary for Planning and Evaluation Office of Disability, Aging and Long-Term Care Policy. https://aspe.hhs.gov/basic-report/evaluation-samhsa-primary-and-behavioral-health-care-integration-pbhci-grant-program-final-report.
33. Grant BF, Goldstein RB, Saha TD, et al. Epidemiology of DSM-5 alcohol use disorder results from the National Epidemiologic Survey on Alcohol and Related Conditions III. JAMA Psychiatry. 2015;72(8):757–766.
34. Merrill J, Duncan M. Addiction disorders. Med Clin North Am. 2014;98(5):1097–1122.
35. Moyer V. Screening and behavioral counseling interventions in primary care to reduce alcohol misuse: US Preventative Task Force Recommendation Statement. Ann Intern Med. 2013;159(3):210–218.
36. Reinert DF, Allen JP. The alcohol use disorders identification test: An update of research findings. Alcohol Clin Exp Res. 2007;31(2):185–199.
37. National Institute on Alcohol Abuse and Alcoholism. Helping patients who drink too much: a clinician's guide, 2005. http://pubs.niaaa.nih.gov/publications/Practitioner/CliniciansGuide2005/clinicians_guide. Accessed July 24, 2016.
38. Smith P, Schmidt S, Allensworth-Davies D, Saitz R. Primary care validation of a single-question alcohol screening test. J Gen Intern Med. 2009;24(7):783–788.
39. McNeely J, Cleland CM, Strauss SM, Palamar JJ, Rotrosen J, Saitz R. Validation of self-administered single-item screening questions (SISQs) for unhealthy alcohol and drug use in primary care patients. J Gen Intern Med. 2015;30(12):1757–1764.
40. American College of Obstetrics and Gynecology (ACOG). Guidelines for Women's Health Care, 2nd edition. Washington, DC: ACOG; 2002. http://www.acog.org/About-ACOG/ACOG-Departments/Tobacco--Alcohol--and-Substance-Abuse.
41. Chasnoff IF, Wels AM, McGourty RF, Bailey LK. Validation of the 4 P's Plus screen for substance use in pregnancy. J Perinatol. 2007;27(12):744–748.
42. Chiodo LM, Sokol RJ, Delaney-Black V, Janisse J, Hannigan JH. Validity of the T-ACE I pregnancy in predicting child outcome and risk drinking. Alcohol. 2010;44(7):595–603.
43. Knight JR, Sherritt L, Shrier LA, Harris SK, Chang G. Validity of the CRAFFT substance abuse screening test among adolescent clinic patients. Arch Pediatr Adolesc Med. 1992;156(6):607–614.
44. Center for Substance Abuse Treatment. Substance abuse among older adults. Treatment Improvement Protocol (TIP) Series, No. 26. 1998. DHHS Publication (SMA) 98-3179. Rockville, MD: Substance Abuse Mental Health Services Administration. http://adaiclearinghouse.org/downloads/TIP-26-Substance-Abuse-Among-Older-Adults-67.pdf. Accessed July 24, 2016.
45. Grant BF, Stinson F, Dawson D et al. Prevalence and co-occurrence of substance use disorders and independent mood and anxiety disorders: Results from the National Epidemiologic Survey on Alcohol and Related Conditions. Arch Gen Psychiatry. 2004;61(8):807–816.
46. Wilcox HC, Conner KR. Association of alcohol and drug use disorders and completed suicide: An empirical review of cohort studies. Drug and Alcohol Dep. 2004;76(Supp):S11–S19.
47. Substance Abuse and Mental Health Service Administration. The role of biomarkers in the treatment of alcohol use disorders, 2012 Revision. HHS Publication No. (SMA) 12-4686. Rockville, MD. http://store.samhsa.gov/shin/content/SMA12-4686/SMA12-4686.pdf. Accessed July 24, 2016.

48. Jones A. Evidence-based survey of the elimination rates of ethanol from the blood with applications in forensic casework. Forensic Sci Int. 2010;200(1-3):1–20.
49. Nanau R, Neuman M. Biomolecules and biomarkers used in diagnosis of alcohol drinking and in monitoring therapeutic interventions. Biomolecules. 2015;5(3):1339–1385.
50. Strobbe S. Prevention and screening, brief intervention, and referral to treatment for substance use in primary care. Prim Care Clin Office Pract. 2014;41(2):185–213.
51. Substance Abuse and Mental Health Services Administration (SAMHSA). Screening, brief intervention, and referral to treatment (SBIRT). Accessed November 17, 2013.
52. Centers for Medicare & Medicaid Services, Department of Health and Human Services. Screening and behavioral counseling interventions in primary care to reduce alcohol misuse. Publication ICN 907798, 2013. http://www.integration.samhsa.gov/Screening_and_Behavioral_Counseling_Interventions_in_Primary_Care_to_Reduce_Alcohol_Misuse,_CMS,_Aug_2013.pdf. Accessed July 24, 2016.
53. Sobell MB, Sobell LC. Guided self-change model of treatment for substance use disorder. J Cogn Psychother. 2005;19(3):199–210.
54. Whitlock EP, Polen MR, Green CA, Orleans T, Klein J. Behavioral counseling interventions in primary care to reduce risky/harmful alcohol use by adults; a summary of the evidence for the US Preventative Services Task Force. Ann Intern Med. 2004;104(7): 557–568.
55. Anton RF, O'Malleey SS, Ciraulo DA, et al. Combined pharmacotherapies and behavioral intervention for alcohol dependence: The Combine study: A randomized controlled trial. JAMA. 2006;295(17):2003–2017.
56. Sullivan JT, Sykora K, Schneiderman J, Naranjo CA, Sellers EM. Assessment of alcohol withdrawal: The Revised Clinical Institute Withdrawal Assessment for Alcohol Scale (CIWA-Ar). Br J Addict. 1989;84(11):1353–1357.
57. Stephens JR, Liles EA, Dancel R, Gilchrist M, Kirsch J, DeWalt DA. Who needs inpatient detox? Development and implementation of a hospitalist protocol for the evaluation of patients for alcohol detoxification. J Gen Intern Med. 2014;29(4):587–593.
58. Amato L, Minozzi S, Davoli M. Efficacy and safety of pharmacological interventions for the treatment of the alcohol withdrawal syndrome. Cochrane Database Syst Rev. 2011(6):CD008537.
59. Daeppen JB, Gache P, Landry U, et al. Symptom-triggered vs. fixed-schedule doses of benzodiazepine for alcohol withdrawal: A randomized treatment trial. Arch Intern Med. 2002;162(10):1117–1121.
60. Myrick H, Malcolm R, Randall PK, et al. A double-blind trial of gabapentin versus lorazepam in the treatment of alcohol withdrawal. Alcohol Clin Exp Res. 2009;33(9):1582–1588.
61. Leung JG, Hall-Flavin D, Nelson S, Schmidt KA, Schak KM. The role of gabapentin in the management of alcohol withdrawal and dependence. Ann Pharmacother. 2015;49(8):897–906.
62. Kadden R, Carroll K, Donovan D, et al. Cognitive-Behavioral Coping Skills Therapy Manual: A Clinical Research Guide for Therapists Treatment Individuals with Alcohol Abuse and Dependence. NIAAA Project MATCH Monograph Series, Vol. 3, NIH Publication No. (ADM) 92-1895. Washington, DC: Government Printing Office; 1992. http://pubs.niaaa.nih.gov/publications/MATCHSeries3/Project%20MATCH%20Vol_3.pdf. Accessed July 24, 2016.
63. Miller WR, Zweben A, DiClimente C, Rychtarik R. Motivational Enhancement Therapy Manual: A Clinical Research Guide for Therapists Treating Individuals With Alcohol Abuse and Dependence. Rockville MD: National Institute on Alcohol Abuse and Alcoholism; 1992. http://lib.adai.washington.edu/pubs/match2/match2practicalstrategies.pdf. Accessed July 24, 2016.
64. Nowinski J, Baker S, Carroll K. Twelve-Step Facilitation Therapy Manual: A Clinical Research Guide for Therapists Treating Individuals With Alcohol Abuse and Dependence. Bethesda, MD: National Institute on Alcohol Abuse and Alcoholism; 1995. http://pubs.niaaa.nih.gov/publications/ProjectMatch/match01.pdf. Accessed July 24, 2016.
65. Ouimette PC, Moos R, Finney J. Influence of outpatient treatment and 12-step group involvement on one-year substance abuse treatment outcomes. J Stud Alcohol Drugs. 1998;59(5):513–522.
66. Moos R, Moos B. Participation in treatment and Alcoholics Anonymous: A 16-year follow-up of initially untreated individuals. J Clin Psych. 2006;62(6):735–750.
67. Alcoholics Anonymous. http://www.aa-intergroup.org/directory_specialty.php?code=glbt. Accessed July 24, 2016.
68 Celebrate Recovery, A Christ-Centered Recovery Program. http://www.celebraterecovery.com. Accessed July 24, 2016.
69. Smart Recovery. Self-Management and Recovery Training. http://www.smartrecovery.org. Accessed July 24, 2016.
70 LifeRing. Secular Recovery. http://lifering.org. Accessed July 24, 2016.
71. Birds of a Feather International. http://www.boaf.org. Accessed July 24, 2016.
72. International Doctors in AA. And we will know peace. https://www.idaa.org. Accessed July 24, 2016.
73. The Other Bar. Supporting recovery in the legal community. http://www.otherbar.org. Accessed July 24, 2016.

74. Garbutt JC, Kranzler HR, O'Malley SS, et al. Efficacy and tolerability of long-acting injectable naltrexone for alcohol dependence: A randomized controlled trial. JAMA. 2006; 295(17):2003–2007.
75. Rosner S, Hackl-Herrwerth A, Leucht S, et al. Acamprosate for alcohol dependence. Cochrane Database Syst Rev 2010; (9): CD004332. doi:10.1002/14651858.CD004332.pub2.
76. Skinner MD, Lajmek P, Pham H, Aubin HJ. Disulfiram efficacy in the treatment of alcohol dependence: A meta-analysis. PLoS One. 2014;9(2):e87366.
77. Blodgett JC, Del Re AC, Maisel NC, Finney JW. A meta-analysis of topiramate's effects for individuals with alcohol use disorders. Alcohol Clin Exp Res. 2014;38(6):1481–1488.
78. Volpicelli JR, Alterman AI, Hayashida M, O'Brien CP. Naltrexone in the treatment of alcohol dependence. A controlled study. Arch Gen Psychiatry. 1992;49(11):881–887.
79. Donoghue K, Elzerbi C, Saunders R, Whittington C, Pilling S, Drummond C. The efficacy of acamprosate and naltrexone in the treatment of alcohol dependence, Europe versus the rest of the world: A meta-analysis. Addiction. 2015;110(6):920–930.
80. Anton RF, Myrick H, Wright TM, et al. Gabapentin combined with naltrexone for the treatment of alcohol dependence. Am J Psychiatry. 2011;168(7):709–717.
81. Schifano F. Misuse and abuse of pregabalin and gabapentin: Cause for concern? CNS Drugs. 2014;28(6):491–496.
82. Benowitz, Neal L. Nicotine addiction. N Engl J Med 2010;362(24):2295–2303.
83. Fiore MC, Jaén CR, Baker TB, et al. Treating Tobacco Use and Dependence: 2008 Update. Clinical Practice Guideline. Rockville, MD: U.S. Department of Health and Human Services. Public Health Service. May 2008. http://bphc.hrsa.gov/buckets/treating-tobacco.pdf. Accessed July 24, 2016.
84. Fiore MC, Baker TB. Treating smokers in the health care setting. N Engl J Med. 2011;365(13):1222–1231.
85. Piper M, Baker T, Mermelstein R, et al. Recruiting and engaging smokers in treatment in a primary care setting: Developing a chronic care model implemented through a modified electronic health record. Transl Behav Med. 2013;3(3):253–263.
86. Morris CD, Morris CW, Martin L, Lasky GB. Dimensions: Tobacco Free Toolkit for Healthcare Providers, 2013. https://www.bhwellness.org/toolkits/Tobacco-Free-Toolkit.pdf. Accessed July 24, 2016.
87. Nicotine Anonymous. Offering to help those who desire to stop using nicotine. https://nicotine-anonymous.org. Accessed July 24, 2016.
88. American Lung Association. Freedom from Smoking. http://www.ffsonline.org. Accessed July 24, 2016.
89. Yeh JS, Bullen C, Glantz SA. E-cigarettes and smoking cessation. N Engl J Med. 2016;374(22):2172–2174.
90. Cerimele JM, Halperin A, Saxon A. Tobacco use treatment in primary care patients with psychiatric illness. J Am Board Fam Pract. 2014;27(3):399–410.
91. University of California, San Francisco. Smoking Cessation Leadership Center. http://smokingcessationleadership.ucsf.edu. Accessed July 24, 2016.
92. Edlund MJ, Martin BC, Russo JE, DeVries A, Braden JB, Sullivan MD. The role of opioid prescription in incident opioid abuse and dependence among individuals with chronic non-cancer pain: The role of opioid prescription. Clin J Pain. 2014;30(7):557–564.
93. Dowell D, Haegerich T, Chou R. CDC Guideline for prescribing opioids for chronic pain—United States, 2016. MMWR. 2016;65(1):1–49.
94. Muhuri PK, Gfroerer JC, Davies MC. Substance Abuse and Mental Health Services Administration. Associations of nonmedical pain reliever use and initiation of heroin use in the United States. CBHSQ Data Review. http://www.samhsa.gov/data/2k13/DataReview/DR006/nonmedical-pain-reliever-use-2013.pdf. Published August 2013. Accessed July 24, 2016.
95. Reid MC, Engles-Horton LL, Weber MB, Kerns RD, Rogers EL, O'Connor PG. Use of opioid medications for chronic non-cancer pain syndromes in primary care. J Gen Intern Med. 2002;17(3):173–179.
96. Gorlay DL, Heit HA, Almahrezi A. Universal precautions in pain medicine: A rational approach to the treatment of chronic pain. Pain Med. 2005;6(2):107–112.
97. Owen G, Burton A, Schade C, Passik S. Urine drug testing: Current recommendations and best practices. Pain Physician. 2012;15:(3 Suppl);ES119–ES133.
98. Substance Abuse and Mental Health Services Administration. Clinical Drug Testing in Primary Care. Technical Assistance Publication (TAP) 32. HHS Publication No. (SMA) 12-4668. Rockville, MD: Substance Abuse and Mental Health Services Administration, 2012. https://store.samhsa.gov/shin/content/SMA12-4668/SMA12-4668.pdf. Accessed July 24, 2016.
99. Moeller KE, Lee KC, Kissack JC. Urine drug screening: Practical guide for clinicians. Mayo Clin Proc. 2008;83(1):66–76.
100. Lee M, Silverman S, Hansen H, Vikram P. A comprehensive review of opioid induced hyperalgesia. Pain Physician. 2011;14(2):145–161.
101. Washington State Agency Medical Directors Group. AMDG 2015 interagency guideline on prescribing opioids for pain. Olympia, WA; 2015. http://www.agencymeddirectors.wa.gov/guidelines/Pain/cot. Accessed July 24, 2016.

102. Amato L, Davoli M, Minozzi S, Ferroni E, Ali R, Ferri M. Methadone at tapered doses for the management of opioid withdrawal. Cochrane Database Syst Rev. 2013; 2:CD003409.
103. Kakko J, Svanborg KD, Kreek MJ, Heilig M. 1-year retention and social function after buprenorphine-assisted relapse prevention treatment for heroin dependence in Sweden: A randomized, placebo-controlled trial. Lancet. 2003;361(9358):662–668.
104. Deaths and severe adverse events associated with anesthesia-assisted rapid opioid detoxification—New York City, 2012. MMWR Morb Mortal Wkly Rep. 2013;62:9(38)777–780. http://dy3uq8jh2v.search.serialssolutions.com/?sid=Entrez:PubMed&id=pmid:24067581.
105. Narcotics Anonymous. An introduction to Narcotics Anonymous. https://www.na.org. Accessed July 24, 2016.
106. Chronic Pain Anonymous. A fellowship for those with chronic pain or chronic illness. http://www.chronicpainanonymous.org. Accessed July 24, 2016.
107. Joseph J, Appel P, Schniedler J. Deaths during and after discharge from methadone maintenance treatment. Albany: New York State Office of Alcoholism and Substance Abuse Services; June 1981; Outcome Study Report #18.
108. Fullerton CA, Kim M, Thomas CP, et al. Medication-assisted treatment with methadone: Assessing the evidence. Psychiatr Serv. 2014;65(2):146–157.
109. Methadone Mortality—A 2010 Reassessment. Rockville, MD: Division of Pharmacologic Therapies Center for Substance Abuse and Mental Health Services Administration; 2010.
110. Substance Abuse and Mental Health Service Administration. Buprenorphine/Drug Addiction Treatment Act of 2000. http://buprenorphine.samhsa.gov/data.html. Accessed July 24, 2016.
111. Center for Substance Abuse Treatment. Clinical guidelines for the use of buprenorphine in the treatment of opioid addiction. Treatment Improvement Protocol Series 40. DHHS Publication No. (SMA) 04-3939. Rockville, MD: Substance Abuse and Mental Health Services Administration; 2004. http://store.samhsa.gov/product/TIP-40-Clinical-Guidelines-for-the-Use-of-Buprenorphine-in-the-Treatment-of-Opioid-Addiction/SMA07-3939.
112. Mattick RP, Kimber J, Breen C, Davoli M, Breen R. Buprenorphine vs placebo or methadone maintenance for opioid dependence. Cochrane Database Syst Rev 2003;(2):CD002207.
113. Ling W, Hillhouse M, Ang A, Jenkins J, Fahey J. Comparison of behavioral treatment conditions in buprenorphine maintenance. Addiction. 2013;108(10):1788–1798.
114. Fiellin DA, Barry DT, Sullivan LE, et al. A randomized trial of cognitive behavioral therapy in primary care-based buprenorphine. Am J Med. 2013;126(1):74e11–7.
115. Substance Abuse and Mental Health Service Administration. Buprenorphine Training for Physicians. http://www.samhsa.gov/medication-assisted-treatment/training-resources/buprenorphine-physician-training. Accessed July 24, 2016.
116. Kleber HD. Treatment of narcotic addicts. Psychiatr Med. 1985;3(4):389–418.
117. Krupitsky E, Nunes EV, Ling W, Illeperuma A, Gastfriend DR, Silverman BL. Injectable extended-release naltrexone for opioid dependence: A double-blind, placebo-controlled, multicentre randomised trial. Lancet. 2011;377(9776):1506–1513.
118. Jones H. Treating opioid use disorders during pregnancy: Historical, current and future directions. Subst Abuse. 2013;34(2):89–91.
119. Patrick SW, Schumacher RE, Benneyworth BD, Krans EE, McAllister JM, Davis MM. Neonatal abstinence syndrome and associated health care expenditures: United States, 2000–2009. JAMA. 2012;307(18):1934–1940.
120. Jones HE, Heil SH, Baewert A, et al. Buprenorphine treatment of opioid-dependent pregnant women: A comprehensive review. Addiction. 2012;107(Suppl 1):5–27.
121. Jones HE, Finnegan LP, Kaltenbach K. Methadone and buprenorphine for the management of opioid dependence in pregnancy. Drugs. 2012;72(6):747–757.
122. Jones HE, Kaltenbach K, Heil SH, et al. Neonatal abstinence syndrome after methadone or buprenorphine exposure. N Engl J Med. 2010;363(24):2320–2331.
123. Wiegand SL, Stringer EM, Stuebe AM, Jones H, Seashore C, Thorp J. Buprenorphine and naloxone compared with methadone treatment in pregnancy. Obstet Gynecol. 2015;125(2):363–368.
124. Ciraulo D, Knapp, C. The pharmacology of non-alcohol sedative hypnotics. In: Ries R, Fiellin D, Miller S, Saitz R, eds. The ASAM Principles of Addiction Medicine, 5th ed. Chevy Chase, MD: ASAM; 2014:117–134.
125. Park TW, Saitz R, Ganoczy D, Ilgen MA, Bohnert AS. Benzodiazepine prescribing patterns and deaths from drug overdose among US veterans receiving opioid analgesics: Case-cohort study. BMJ. 2015;350:h2698. doi:http://dx.doi.org/10.1136/bmj.h2698
126. Lader M. Benzodiazepines revisited—will we ever learn? Addiction. 2011;106(12):2086–2109.
127. Paquin AM, Zimmerman K, Rudolph JL. Risk versus risk: A review of benzodiazepine reduction in older adults. Expert Opin Drug Saf. 2014;13(7):919–934.

128. Farmer RF, Kosty DB, Seeley JR, et al. Natural course of cannabis use disorders. Psychol Med. 2015;45(1):63–72.
129. Hasin DS, Kerridge B, Saha T, et al. Prevalence and correlates of DSM-5 cannabis use disorder, 2012–2013: Findings from the National Epidemiologic Survey on Alcohol and Related Conditions–III. Am J Psychiatry. 2016;173(6):588–599.
130. Cerdá, M, Moffitt T, Meier M, et al. Persistent cannabis dependence and alcohol dependence represent risks for midlife economic and social problems: A longitudinal cohort study. Clin Psychol Sci. 2016; doi:10.1177/2167702616630958.
131. Volkow N, Baler R, Compton W, Weiss SR. Adverse health effects of marijuana use. N Engl J Med. 2014;370(23):2219–2227.
132. Whiting PF, Wolff RF, Deshpande S, et al. Cannabinoids for medical use: A systematic review and meta-analysis. JAMA. 2015; 313(24):2456–2473.
133. Mehmedic Z, Chandra S, Slade D, et al. Potency trends of Δ9-THC and other cannabinoids in confiscated cannabis preparations from 1993 to 2008. J Forensic Sci. 2010;55(5):1209–1217.
134. Lynskey M, Heath A, Bucholz K, et al. Escalation of drug use in early-onset cannabis users vs co-twin controls. JAMA. 2003;289(4):427–433.
135. Vandrey R, Raber J, Raber M, Douglass B, Miller C, Bonn-Miller MO. Cannabinoid dose and label accuracy in edible medical cannabis products. JAMA. 2015;313(24):2491–2493.
136. Polen MR, Whitlock EP, Wisdom JP, Nygren P, Bougatsos C. Screening in Primary Care Settings for Illicit Drug Use: Staged Systematic Review for the U.S. Preventive Services Task Force. Evidence Synthesis No. 58, Part 1. Prepared by the Oregon Evidence-based Practice Center under Contract No. 290-02-0024. AHRQ Publication No. 08-05108-EF-s. Rockville, MD, Agency for Healthcare Research and Quality, January 2008.
137. Budney A, Stanger C, Tilford J, et al. Computer-assisted behavioral therapy and contingency management for cannabis use disorder. Psychol Addict Behav. 2015;29(3):501–511.
138. Piehler TF, Winters K. Parental involvement in brief interventions for adolescent marijuana use. Psychol Addict Behav. 2015;29(3):512–521.
139. U.S. Preventive Services Task Force (USPSTF). Final Update Summary: Drug Use, Illicit: Screening. 2015. http://www.uspreventiveservicestaskforce.org/Page/Document/UpdateSummaryFinal/drug-use-illicit-screening.htm. Accessed July 25, 2016.
140. Saitz R, Palfai T, Cheng D, et al. Screening and brief intervention for drug use in primary care: The ASPIRE randomized clinical trial. JAMA. 2014;312(5):502–513.
141. Patnode C, O'Connor E, Rowland M, Burda BU, Perdue LA, Whitlock EP. Primary care behavioral interventions to prevent or reduce illicit drug use and nonmedical pharmaceutical use in children and adolescents: A systematic evidence review for the US Preventive Services Task Force. Ann Intern Med. 2014;160(9):612–620.
142. Smith P, Schmidt S, Allensworth-Davies D, Saitz R. A single-question screening test for drug use in primary care. Arch Intern Med. 2010;170(13):1155–1160.
143. Carroll K, Rounsaville B, Nich C, Gordon LT, Wirtz PW, Gawin F. One-year follow up of psychotherapy and pharmacotherapy for cocaine dependence. Delayed emergence of psychotherapy effects. Arch Gen Psychiatry. 1994;51(12):989–997.
144. Lussier JP, Heil SH, Mongeon JA, Badger GJ, Higgins ST. A meta-analysis of voucher-based reinforcement therapy for substance use disorders. Addiction. 2006;101(2):192–203.
145. Epstein EE, McCrady BS. Behavioral couples treatment of alcohol and drug use disorders: Current status and innovations. Clin Psychol Rev. 1998;18(6):689–711.
146. Ramsey SE, Kahler CW, Read JP, Stuart GL, Brown RA. Discriminating between substance-induced and independent depressive episodes in alcohol dependent patients. J Stud Alcohol. 2004;65(5):672–676.
147. Nunes EV, Liu X, Samet S, Matseoane K, Hasin D. Independent versus substance induced major depressive disorder in substance-dependent patients: Observational study of course during follow-up. J Clin Psychiatry. 2006;67(10):1561–1567.
148. Substance Abuse and Mental Health Services Administration. Substance Abuse Confidentiality Regulations. www.Samhsa.gov. Accessed June 26, 2016.
149. McDonell MG, Graves MC, WestII et al. Utility of point-of-care urine drug tests in the treatment of primary care patients with drug use disorders. J Addict Med. 2016;10(3)196–201.
150. George S. Boulay S, Galvani S. Domestic abuse among women who misuse psychoactive substances: An overview for the clinician. Addict Disor Ther Treat. 2011;10(2): 43–49.
151. Black K, Day C. Improving access to long-acting contraceptive methods and reducing unplanned pregnancy among women with substance use disorders. Subst Abuse. 2016;10(Suppl 1):27–33.

15

Integrated Care for Binge Eating and Other Eating Disorders

JOEL YAGER, PHILIP S. MEHLER, EILEEN D. YAGER, AND ALISON R. YAGER

BOX 15.1

KEY POINTS

- **Both fully formed and subclinical cases of eating disorders are common in primary care practices, but often go unnoticed, because patients are reluctant to disclose their eating disorder(s).**
- **Eating disorders may be missed, or often are neglected, because co-occurring medical and psychiatric disorders take precedence.**
- **Among the eating disorders, binge eating disorder is most prevalent, occurring with increased frequency in patients with more severe obesity.**
- **Establishing a trusting alliance is key to obtaining accurate information for complete assessment.**
- **For uncomplicated early cases, interventions at the primary care level may be adequate to reverse and manage these disorders.**
- **Integrated primary care practices with behavioral health specialists can also offer education, counseling, medication management, psychotherapeutic treatments, and referral to health coaches, registered dietitians, community resources, psychiatrists, and eating disorder specialists, as needed.**

INTRODUCTION

This chapter focuses on developing integrated care plans for assessing and managing the most prominent presentations of eating disorders in primary care settings. Binge eating disorder (BED) is an officially sanctioned disorder in the American Psychiatric Association's *Diagnostic and Statistical Manual of Mental Disorders,* Fifth Edition (DSM-5).[1] Since BED is the most prevalent eating disorder encountered in primary care, and is strongly connected with the obesity epidemic and its linked medical comorbidities, in this chapter we direct most discussion to this disorder. We also briefly address the management of anorexia nervosa (AN) and bulimia nervosa (BN). See Box 15.1 for some key points about eating disorders.

Primary care clinicians face many barriers when delivering care for patients with eating disorders: (1) patients often require more time than primary care can allocate to routine office visits, (2) patients with an eating disorder require demanding, perplexing, and time-consuming clinical decision making, (3) complex interpersonal and family interactions are needed for successful treatment, and (4) in many locales, patients lack access to specialized professionals or facilities. Nevertheless, primary care clinicians and their staffs have clear roles in treating patients with eating disorders.[2] Primary care providers can serve as first-responder problem identifiers, diagnosticians, patient and family educators, managers, and triage coordinators and, using a registry, can track patients' progress and outcomes throughout their clinical course.

Recognizing that considerable diversity exists in primary care practice staffing patterns, this chapter approaches the integrated treatment of eating disorders from the vantage point of staffing models currently advocated for emerging health care environments, consisting of various configurations of the following:

- Primary care clinicians (behavioral health specialists [BHSs], social workers, psychologists, health coaches)
- Medical assistants, who room patients, take vital signs and brief preliminary histories, and might write notes for the primary care clinicians
- Care coordinators, who serve as medical case managers, arrange for follow-up care with other specialists and community resources
- BHSs
- Live or telehealth consulting psychiatrists

BHSs might offer brief (typically up to three) sessions of psychotherapy, when included in the treatment plan. Integrated care practices are encouraged to employ electronic medical records and registries of patients used for systematic data collection, outcome tracking, and population management. Although they significantly contribute to managing patients with eating disorders, registered dietitians are infrequently integral to primary care practices, and are usually separately engaged.

In contrast to the well-studied collaborative care trials for depression in primary care practices,[3] no studies employing these staffing models for eating disorders have been conducted in primary care settings. Therefore, although based on considerable clinical experience, the following recommended approaches must be regarded as tentative, and to some extent aspirational.

INTEGRATED CARE FOR BED

Diagnosis

In DSM-5, BED is listed for the first time as a discrete diagnosis, requiring the presence of binge eating episodes (at least once per week for at least 3 months), consuming large quantities of food in short amounts of time, feeling out of control regarding eating, and having one's self-evaluation/self-esteem heavily influenced by one's weight and shape. Compensatory behaviors of purging, excessive exercise, laxative abuse, and diuretic abuse are not present. Before coming to clinical attention, most patients with BED experience many weekly episodes of binge eating over the course of years. Consequently, the majority present as overweight to obese. Severity is rated according to the number of discrete episodes of binge eating per week:

- Mild, average one to three episodes
- Moderate, average four to seven episodes
- Severe, average eight to 13 episodes
- Extreme, 14 or more episodes per week

Epidemiological Considerations

Whereas community prevalence rates of BED are generally noted to be in the range of about 1.4% to 2%, and as high as 5%,[4] the prevalence of BED substantially increases in specific clinical populations. Among adult obese patients seeking care in weight loss programs, rates of BED have been estimated at 8% to10%,[5] and rates are much higher among patients seeking bariatric surgery. The female-to-male ratio of roughly 3:1 is lower than for other eating disorders. Onset is ordinarily in the late teens and early 20s,[6] and coincidences with obesity increases over time. Subclinical cases of BED are thought to be even more highly prevalent.

Clinical Presentations

For patients who acknowledge difficulties, or for advanced cases, diagnosis is straightforward and no elaborate workup is required. Difficulties arise for individuals with less pronounced conditions, those who hide their eating disorders because of shame, and/or those who try to attribute their eating and weight problems to primary medical conditions (usually "endocrine problems"), or deflect attention to other medical and psychiatric conditions. Several concurrent conditions should heighten clinician concerns that clinically significant BED might be present:

1. Obesity (the more pronounced, the higher the risk of BED)
2. Higher rates of fibromyalgia and irritable bowel syndrome[6]
3. Obese patients with type II diabetes mellitus (even early adolescents), show increased rates of BED.[7]
4. About 13% of women with polycystic ovary syndrome (PCOS) reportedly have BED.[8]

In addition, patients with BED have high rates of psychiatric comorbidity. Overall, 73.8% of primary care patients with BED, had at least one additional lifetime psychiatric disorder, and 43.1% at least one current psychiatric disorder, including mood (49%), anxiety (41%), substance use (22%), personality (20–30%),[9] and posttraumatic stress (about 24%) disorders.[10]

TEAM MEMBER ACTIVITIES IN ASSESSMENT AND TREATMENT

Primary care teams can offer substantial help to the majority of patients with binge eating problems.

Medical Assistants and Front Desk Personnel

Screening for BED

Before primary care clinicians see patients, preliminary screening is likely to be done by medical assistants or front desk personnel. Standard health screening, asking about weight changes and eating concerns, as well as recorded height and weight from which body mass index (BMI) can be calculated, can alert clinicians to the need for further inquiry. The item "loss of appetite or overeating" on the Patient Health Questionaire-9 (PHQ-9)[11] might serve as a preliminary crude screener, but lacks diagnostic specificity. For obese patients, some medical practices might opt to go further, for example using the Patient Health Questionnaire Eating Disorder Module (PHQ-ED).[12] However, no published studies show definitive clinical utility for this approach. Other binge eating screeners and measures have been published, including the Binge Eating Scale (BES)[13] and the Binge Eating Disorders Test (BEDT),[14] but neither has gained traction in clinical practice.

Follow-up Activities for Medical Assistants

At follow-up visits, medical assistants will record weights and vital signs, re-administer screening measures the practice might choose to repeat, and record appropriate notes for the primary care clinicians' attention.

Primary Care Clinician

Initial Diagnostic Assessment

After assessing preliminary information, primary care clinicians should follow up with screening questions as well, such as, "Do you have any issues with your eating behavior or weight?" and "Do you think you could use some assistance in that area?" Asking obese/overweight patients these questions can uncover concerns regarding eating habits, overeating, binge eating, and self-control. If patients answer affirmatively, primary care clinicians should obtain additional history and symptoms to confirm the diagnosis. Clinicians can facilitate making the diagnosis by sensitively inquiring about eating habits, and sympathetically acknowledging how hard it is for individuals with weight issues to exert adequate control over their appetites. If clinicians inquire about weight struggles from the vantage point of a good therapeutic alliance, patients are more likely to reveal their difficulties.

Following diagnostic confirmation and severity assessment, primary care clinicians can assess BED patients for co-occurring psychiatric and behavioral difficulties and medical comorbidities. Although aspects of this assessment and patient education might be delegated to BHSs, primary care clinicians will want to be familiar with these details in order to formulate the overall treatment plan. Examples of patient details to note: patient eating and exercise patterns; self-esteem in relation to weight, shape, and appearance; functional impairments imposed by BED and obesity; and motivation to change both binge eating behaviors and weight. Similarly, assessing binge eating, obesity, and eating habits for the family as a whole is important, because family members can be treatment allies or, conversely, can sabotage treatment.

Mood, anxiety, posttraumatic stress disorder (PTSD), substance use, personality issues, and associated safety considerations (suicidal ideation or plans) require assessment. Patients who have significant comorbid psychiatric disorders or any safety concerns such as potential suicidality should be referred to specialty-trained qualified psychiatrists, clinical psychologists, or psychiatric social workers.

Medical comorbidities are straightforward, for the most part involving commonly co-occurring physical concomitants and sequelae of obesity and metabolic syndrome.

Educating Patients and Families About the Disorder

Education should begin with *naming the disorder.* Providing a specific name and telling patients that well-studied, effective, evidence-based treatments are available for BED, may help reduce feelings of shame and hopelessness. Encouraging a "recovery" model may help demoralized patients assume greater degrees of self-control and self-involvement with care. Patients are informed that with guidance toward "recovery," they can do much to facilitate remission, and many self-help tools are available. Guided self-help, based on cognitive-behavioral therapy (CBT) principles, is more effective than a wait-list or no treatment. A self-help manual entitled *Overcoming Binge Eating* has been studied in controlled trials in the United Kingdom and has been so successful at helping patients improve and recover, that this book can be "prescribed" and paid for by the National Health Service.[15]

Informing patients that BED often occurs with other psychological and psychosocial difficulties will come as no surprise to them and should reassure them that the clinician will not neglect these other issues in the course of treatment.

Next, the patient should be educated about the treated and untreated course of BED. Psychotherapy-based treatments are generally successful, with studies showing 50% to 80% response, and persistence of response for one to two years.[16] When untreated, the odds of successful weight loss management are small. Untreated, BED may diminish over a period of years but is almost always accompanied by increasing obesity. For patients who aspire to have a healthy weight, dealing specifically with binge eating is crucial. Studies show that CBT-based programs focusing on BED are generally more successful than behavioral weight management programs alone, although combining the two can be successful and might result in better outcomes.[17,18] Most evidence favors CBT, although interpersonal psychotherapy (IPT) has also been effective in randomized trials, with large effect sizes for psychotherapy treatments. For BED patients with significant psychiatric difficulty and emotional dysregulation, dialectical behavior therapy (DBT) has been effective.[19]

For patients with medically serious stage 3 obesity (BMI > 40), or with BMIs higher than 35 with significant medical comorbidities, clinicians may want to educate them about the relationship between BED and outcomes for bariatric surgery.[20] Although bariatric surgery is not absolutely contraindicated in the presence of BED, most surgeons prefer to operate on obese patients only after BED is under control and has remitted. The subsequent postoperative course of obesity is not substantially different for patients with prior histories of BED, compared to those who never had BED.

Formulating the Treatment Plan

The treatment plan should include patient education, establishment of a CBT program (through guided self-help or professionally managed self-help), consultation with a registered dietitian, working with a health coach (see Chapter 25: Health Coaching), behavioral weight loss programs where indicated, referral to community resources, including wellness and fitness programs and lay-led organizations, and, possibly, adjunctive medication. Initial decisions to offer medication usually depend on the presence of comorbid mood or anxiety disorders, or lack of response to initial psychotherapeutic treatment (further discussed below). Referrals for higher levels of behavioral care at this point are made based only on behavioral safety concerns, not for BED per se.

Follow-up with Primary Care Clinicians

Specifics will depend on the treatment plan. With regard to frequency of patient visits, for uncomplicated patients, brief visits to monitor the physiologic and clinical course and to manage medication can ordinarily be scheduled every 1 to 3 months. If medications are used, patients should be seen (or at least contacted by telephone) about two weeks after initiation of medication to assess for tolerability and adverse effects, such as activation, anxiety, or gastrointestinal side effects. If patients satisfactorily progress with the behavioral plan and become less symptomatic, primary care clinicians can schedule return visits in 3 to 6 months.

Medication Decisions for BED

CBT alone is often successful for BED. Medication alone has shown only a medium effect size (compared to large effects for CBT and IPT). Adding medications to CBT as initial treatment of BED alone, often appears to have little additional impact. However, if a patient has comorbid mood, anxiety, or substance use disorders within a primary care scope of practice, or if a patient has previously failed to respond to CBT treatment, then initiating pharmacologic (e.g., selective serotonin reuptake inhibitors [SSRIs], serotonin and norepinephrine reuptake inhibitors [SNRIs]), as well as psychosocial treatments for the comorbid disorders may be indicated.

Antidepressant medications and topiramate have both shown some effectiveness for BED. As SSRIs generally produce fewer adverse effects in clinical practice than topiramate,[21] SSRIs are often first choice.

If patients are making little or no progress after 2 months of CBT alone, SSRIs can be offered as a treatment option. Studies have shown modest efficacy in reducing binge eating for the SSRI citalopram (in studies using up to 60 mg/day, higher than the currently recommended upper level of 40 mg/day), escitalopram (up to 30 mg/day), fluoxetine (10–80 mg/day), and sertraline (25 to 200 mg/day), and even smaller effects for the SNRI duloxetine (up to 120 mg/day).[31] If SSRIs have proven ineffective, or are not tolerated, topiramate (25–400 mg/day) can be tried.

The stimulant medication lisdexamfetamine (50–70 mg/day) has received FDA approval for treating BED; however, since the major clinical trial supporting this indication excluded patients with psychiatric and medical comorbidities, potential short- and long-term adverse impacts of using this stimulant medication for individuals with such comorbidities are unknown.[22]

Follow-up Considerations

Follow-up visits should include weight and assessment of binge eating status, noting the number of episodes of binge eating per week (the DSM-5 severity measure), their intensity, estimated calories per binge, and cravings related to binge eating. Primary care practices can routinely measure BED, using the PHQ-ED.

Although recovery might be declared after 6 asymptomatic months, an asymptomatic year or two should pass for sustained confidence. Ongoing monitoring and treatment of obesity, recurrences, and concurrent psychiatric comorbidities always take longer.

When to Refer

Patients who experience substantial reductions in binge eating episodes within 2 to 3 months may be entirely managed in primary care settings. Those failing to respond, despite consultation, and CBT with affiliated behavioral specialists, should be referred to eating disorder specialists. Currently, loose, informal community-based networking arrangements among eating disorder specialists are common. These networks sometimes consolidate into interest groups of local eating disorder specialists, or affiliates of national eating disorder professional associations, through which participants may join together for mutual education, peer case supervision, journal clubs, and other professional activities.

Care Coordinator

Managing Registries

Care coordinators can enroll patients in registries, and depending on preference and resources, initiate treatment. Maintaining registries of overweight and obese patients might be useful in primary care practices for tracking progress and outcomes, with data entered at each visit. For patients with BED, adding PHQ-9 data and simple assessments of the number of binge episodes per week or month could suffice.

Practices employing quality measures might consider assessing the number of patients screened for BED among high-risk populations (e.g., those with BMI > 30 or 35), the number offered BED treatment among those who screen positive, and the number treated who recover or remit within 6 months, and at a year. If there is a sufficient population of BED patients, a BHS could offer a time-limited group treatment.[23]

Offering Resources and Referrals

Care coordinators can provide patients with resources regarding self-guided care for BEDs, CBT, community organizations, health coaching, and other referrals when needed. Resources include fact sheets, self-help books, websites, and, increasingly, apps used in self-monitoring.[24] Local community practitioners specifically interested in treating patients with eating disorders can be identified via advocacy and professional association websites as listed in Box 15.2.

Access to lay-led organizations assisting patients with BED and obesity can be found on the web via Weight Watchers, Take Off Pounds Sensibly (TOPS), and Overeaters Anonymous. Some patients with BED have reported good results and high satisfaction with some local Overeaters Anonymous groups.[25,26] BED patients should also be encouraged to participate in local exercise and wellness programs.

Since few primary care practices employ registered dietitians, BED patients should be routinely referred for consultations with dietitians who can take detailed dietary histories and offer monitored counseling.

Referrals might also be made to local or telehealth-based psychologists, social workers, psychiatrists, health coaches or other eating disorder specialists. Care coordinators can initiate and maintain ongoing contact with these specialists. Within primary care practices, patient course and ongoing

BOX 15.2
EATING DISORDERS RESOURCES

NATIONAL ASSOCIATIONS

- **Academy for Eating Disorders: http://www.aedweb.org**
- **Binge Eating Disorder Association: http://bedaonline.com**
- **International Association of Eating Disorder Professionals: http://www.iaedp.com/**
- **National Eating Disorders Association: http://www.nationaleatingdisorders.org/binge-eating-disorder**
- **National Eating Disorders Coalition: http://www.nedc.com.au/binge-eating-disorder**

REPRESENTATIVE FACT SHEETS AND PATIENT HANDOUTS

- **National Institutes of Mental Health: http://www.nimh.nih.gov/health/topics/eating-disorders/index.shtml**
- **National Health Service Foundation Trust (UK): http://www.ntw.nhs.uk/pic/leaflets/Eating%20Disorders%20A4%202015.pdf**
- **Kaiser-Permanente—Binge Eating Disorder: https://healthy.kaiserpermanente.org/health/care/!ut/p/a0/FchBCsMgEAXQs-QA8iEtNmSXUyS6GyZDRtBRilR6-7TL9xBxIBp90kU9VaP8c-BqXayvKpS7OjH-cq5NzkTYERHbm65CCFYdE6v8T0c6EXTM3j9fD7RSlrFN0w3ONdN-/**
- **Kaiser-Permanente—Eating Disorders: https://healthy.kaiserpermanente.org/health/care/!ut/p/a0/FchBCsMgEEDRs-QAw2RaQ7S7CUmv0OpuEImCmiDSXr_p6vMOnyjq_JJu_R0VMmXrQ1h_YoVyRDDJJ7xBc6dGeTvQjaeoAXH8P_SevJ54B2nVgvRimYxzsB0TYCT2yAtVHmSfNtXQjPUvSXh-EHmj1c_Q!!/**
- **Intermountain Health Care System: http://intermountainhealthcare.org/ext/Dcmnt?ncid=522602504**

EATING DISORDERS SPECIALIST BOOK SERVICE

- **http://www.edcatalogue.com/books/**

treatment needs can be reviewed during impromptu "staff huddles" or regularly scheduled team meetings. Differences of opinion regarding treatment among staff and/or outside caregivers should be resolved via open communication, prioritizing patient preferences.

Behavioral Health Specialist

Treatment for patients with BED may consist of stepped therapies, starting with guided self-help, based on CBT or IPT, medications, and lay-led group treatment referrals. BHSs can initiate behavioral weight management strategies, teaching moderate caloric restriction, suggesting increased physical activity and exercise, and offering basic nutritional counseling. BHSs might also employ evidence-based techniques, such as motivational interviewing, behavioral activation, and problem-solving treatment; track response to treatment; and facilitate treatment changes if patients fail to improve. BHSs might also work with care coordinators to offer patients additional educational resources. Practices whose BHSs are qualified to manage eating disorders can initiate formal CBT treatments, and possibly organize group therapy programs to help manage a population of BED patients.

HEALTH COACH

In some settings health coaches have been trained to assist patients with eating disorders. Strongly immersed in principles of motivational interviewing, coaches are trained to promote change through the recognition of ambivalence in the patient, reflective listening and eliciting change talk. They also encourage family members and other care givers to identify, reflect on and change their own behaviors to better assist patients. The primary role of the coach is to support family members and other caregivers in warm, non-judgmental and empathetic approaches. Lay caregivers as well as professional coaches have been successfully trained in these approaches.[26a]

CONSULTING PSYCHIATRIST

Most BED patients without significant comorbidities may not require psychiatric consultation. However, patients with significant psychiatric comorbidities or personality disorders, or patients requiring complex medication management may benefit from a telehealth or face-to-face meeting with a psychiatrist. Referral to eating disorder specialists may be required for patients with refractory BED.

When Local Resources Are Lacking

Many communities lack eating disorder specialists. Fortunately, resources are increasingly available via telehealth[27] and e-therapy.[28] Studies have demonstrated the effectiveness of telehealth treatment of BED. Some groups, such as the National Eating Disorders Association, support volunteer-staffed chat rooms for patients and families. Since the telehealth field is moving so rapidly, clinicians are advised to contact the organizations listed in Box 15.2 for updated information.

Urgent and Emergency Situations

Urgent and emergency situations encountered in patients with BED result from significant psychiatric or medical comorbidities. On occasion, mood, anxiety, and substance abuse problems escalate to suicidal, or violent threats or behaviors, beyond the scope of usual primary care management. In these circumstances, clinicians will refer patients and families for emergency or specialist care. Table 15.1 shows a clinical pathway for managing BED in primary care practice.

INTEGRATED CARE FOR ANOREXIA NERVOSA (AN) AND BULIMIA NERVOSA (BN)

Recognizing the complex interactions of medical, nutritional, and psychosocial factors in eating disorders, practice guidelines formulated in the United States, Great Britain, and elsewhere have strongly advocated for team-based care, administered by combinations of primary care clinicians, mental health professionals familiar with eating disorders (including psychiatrists, psychologists, and psychiatric social workers), registered dietitians, dentists, and, as indicated, other medical subspecialists.[29–33] The specific services to be enlisted depend on each patient's particular issues, including financial and geographic access to professionals and treatment settings.

Guiding principles differ for the care of early-onset children, adolescent patients with AN, adult patients with chronic AN (referred to as "severe and enduring AN" [SEAN]),[34] and older adolescent/adult patients with BN. That said, primary care practices, often augmented by a registered dietitian, can successfully manage a substantial number of early clinical cases without the need for specialized eating disorders professionals.[35] For all primary care team members, establishing a warm and trusting alliance with patients and families is a prerequisite for effectively assessing and treating patients with AN and BN.

Diagnosis and Clinical Presentations

DSM-5 characterizes AN by restriction of caloric intake below nutritional requirements, resulting in significantly low body weight in the context of age, sex, developmental trajectory, physical health, and body frame. Here "significantly low weight" is defined as weight less than minimally normal or, for children and adolescents, less than minimally expected. Notably, contrasting with earlier criteria, DSM-5 does not specify precise weight percentages (e.g., ≤75% or 80% of expected or "ideal" body weight) to make the diagnosis. Similarly, amenorrhea is no longer a diagnostic requirement, since the clinical course of individuals with scanty menses differs little from those of patients reporting full-blown amenorrhea.

A second key DSM-5 diagnostic criterion is intense fear of gaining weight or becoming fat ("fat phobia"), or simply persisting in behaviors that interfere with weight gain, even though the individual is at significantly low weight and doesn't consciously profess fat phobia. For example, to lose weight, patients might vigorously exercise for hours each day; in AN, excessive exercise is often the first symptom to appear and the last to disappear, in a process that might span several years.

TABLE 15.1. CRITICAL PATHWAY: PRIMARY CARE MANAGEMENT OF BED

	Initial Visit	Week 3	Week 8–10	Month 6–9	Month 9–12
Assessment Tools and Outcome Measures Team members: medical assistant, nurse	Clinical interview DSM-5 BED severity measure[a] PHQ-9 Consider PHQ-ED, BES, BEDT	Clinical interview DSM-5 severity measure[a] PHQ-9	Clinical interview DSM-5 severity measure[a] PHQ-9	Clinical interview DSM-5 severity measure[a] PHQ-9	Clinical interview DSM-5 severity measure[a] PHQ-9
Physical/Lab/Diagnostic Tests Team members: physician or adv. practice professional	Vital signs including BP, height and weight (for BMI[b]), metabolic panel	Vital signs including weight	Vital signs including weight	Vital signs including weight	Vital signs including weight; +/– metabolic panel
Differential Diagnosis Team members: physician, adv. practice professional, or behavioral health	DSM-5 for BED Assess motivation for change[c] Also assess for mood, anxiety, PTSD, substance use, personality disorder, safety assessment[e] Medically: consider obstructive sleep apnea	Assess for medications[d] If already prescribed, assess tolerability, effects, adverse effects	Monitor medication, as needed	Monitor medication, as needed	Monitor medication, as needed
Time	30 minutes	15 minutes	15 minutes	15 minutes	15 minutes
Emergency Risk Assess Team members: physician, adv. practice professional, or behavioral health	Assess for self-harm, suicidality				
Educational Materials Team members: care coordinator or others	Websites[f] Books				

(continued)

TABLE 15.1. CONTINUED

	Initial Visit	Week 3		Week 8–10	Month 6–9	Month 9–12
PCP Visit Objective	Diagnose, motivate, engage, refer	Assess medication effects; refer to psychiatrist prn		Assess progress and medication effects; refer to psychiatrist rn		Assess progress, outcome, or need for ongoing medications; refer to psychiatrist prn
	Initial Visit	Week 2	Week 3	Week 8–10	Month 6–9	Month 9–12
Treatment Planning and implementation	Treat BED prior to obesity per se. Treat comorbid psychiatric substance disorders[h] Refer to behavioral specialist for CBT. Consider adjunctive SSRI.	BHS initiates stepped care/ CBT/ITP	BHS ***weekly*** for 16–20 weeks[g]	BHS	If BED symptoms have remitted, advance to behavioral weight management	
Consultations	BHS for BED. Psychiatric consult if indicated by severity of mood, anxiety, PTSD, substance use, personality disorder, and/or behavioral risk assessment. Refer to emergency department or eating disorder services prn.	Refer to psychiatrist, psychologist, social worker prn for full assessment and treatment plan			If BMI ≤ 35 with medical complications or 40 ≤ consider consult with bariatric surgeon	

[a]After 2–3 months of CBT expect severity to be substantially reduced, for example, from extreme to moderate (from ≥14 to 4–7 episodes/week), or severe to mild (8–13 to 1–3 episodes/week) At 9–12 months, episodes of binge eating should occur only sporadically, if at all. Concomitant use of medications might hasten this improvement.
[b]Generally, for eating disorders, BMI measures have been preferred over hip/waist ratios.
[c]Assessments should be clinical. Self-report scales to assess readiness for change in eating disorders can be used, though none of them are currently recommended for routine clinical use.
[d]Depending on psychiatric comorbidities, patient preferences, and history of prior treatments, medications may be initiated at the first visit or not at all. For patients who fail to respond to CBT after 2–3 months of treatment, a medication trial should be encouraged. Medications and dosages used for BED are discussed in the text and in references 22 and 45.
[e]Rating scales used for screening and severity for these disorders can be found in appropriate chapters throughout this volume.
[f]Lists of websites and sources for educational books such as *Overcoming Binge Eating* are found in Box 15.2. See reference 16.
[g]Initial visits are ordinarily scheduled for 45–50 minutes; subsequent visits are ordinarily scheduled for 15–50 minutes, depending on specific task or treatment modalities to be accomplished.
[h]Prioritize patient problems according to potential safety risks, level of dysfunction, and in accordance with patient preferences.

A third key criterion is disturbance in how individuals experience their body weight, or their self-evaluation/self-esteem excessively influenced by weight or shape, and by a persistent lack of recognition of the serious risks imposed by the current low weight.

Two AN subtypes are recognized based on predominant eating patterns lasting at least 3 months: (a) purely restrictive eating, and (b) restricted eating interrupted by episodes of binge eating/purging. The latter subtype occurs in up to 40% to 50% of patients and usually carries much greater risks of medical morbidity and mortality than the restrictive subtype. DSM-5 further characterizes AN severity according to BMI:

Mild, BMI ≥ 17

Moderate, BMI 16–16.99

Severe, BMI 15–15.99

Extreme, BMI < 15

Diagnosing BN in DSM-5 requires episodes of binge eating large quantities of food in short amounts of time, feeling out of control regarding eating, and either purging by vomiting (most common) or other maladaptive compensatory behaviors to lose ingested calories and weight, such as excessive exercise and/or laxative or diuretic misuse. These episodes must occur at least once per week for at least 3 months. Here, too, the individual's self-evaluation/self-esteem is heavily influenced by weight and shape. Patients with BN are not thin enough to meet criteria for AN, and, technically speaking, BN per se is not diagnosed in individuals who have AN, even the binge eating and purging type. Weights in individuals with BN range from relatively normal to obese. As with BED, severity is rated according to the number of discrete binge eating and purging episodes, or inappropriate compensatory behavior episodes per week:

Mild, average one to three episodes

Moderate, average four to seven episodes

Severe, average eight to 13 episodes

Extreme, 14 or more episodes/week

Epidemiological Considerations

For AN, onset is highest for females aged 15 to 19 years, but new-onset cases also occur at later ages. Estimates of lifetime prevalence of AN in communities range from 1.2% to 2.2%, and up to 4% using relaxed screening criteria.[36] Female-to-male ratios for AN range from 10:1 to 15:1. For BN, lifetime prevalence rates of about 1.5% have been reported.[37] The female-to-male ratio for BN is estimated at 15:1 to 20:1.[38] Onset is predominantly in the late teens and early 20s.[5]

Children and Adolescents

Patients often initially deny, minimize, rationalize, and defend their attitudes and behaviors. Younger patients with AN most often come to clinical attention via concerned parents, teachers, coaches, or friends who become apprehensive and alarmed when patients start to act and eat differently, and begin to look too thin. Clinicians with access to patients' growth charts will see flattening or decline as patients fall off their growth curves. Adolescent patients who have started to menstruate will experience a decline in menstrual functioning. Often patients seem more anxious, sullen, and secretive than usual, and more driven to exercise. Although base-rates of new-onset AN are not particularly high in most primary care practices, clinicians working in middle school, high school, and college health settings, who focus on sports medicine (particularly gymnastics, track, and dance), and who assess infertility, are more likely to encounter new-onset patients. Due to social contagion in local schools, some clinicians occasionally encounter mini-epidemics.

Younger patients with BN, presenting openly with symptoms of depression and anxiety and assorted vague somatic complaints, might still be secretive about their binge eating and purging. Sensitive clinicians routinely ask such patients about their eating habits and concerns.

Young Adults

Aside from referrals by mental health professionals, obstetrician/gynecologists, or dentists (who might observe dental enamel erosion due to vomiting), young adult patients with unidentified eating disorders might present for complaints related to mood and anxiety disorders, digestive and gastrointestinal complaints, fatigue, and infertility.

Adult Patients with SEAN or Chronic BN

Patients with chronic difficulties may be more obvious and/or forthcoming, often presenting at points of physical crisis, such as fainting, seizures, or collapse associated with dehydration, electrolyte disturbance, and/or nutritional debilitation.

TEAM MEMBER ACTIVITIES IN ASSESSMENT AND TREATMENT

Medical Assistants and Front Desk Personnel

Initial Screening

Current practice suggests that eating disorder screening should generally be limited to vulnerable populations: female sex; younger age; histories of abuse; participation in dance, gymnastics or other weight-oriented sports; and positive family histories. The most widely used screen in primary care practice is the SCOFF questionnaire,[39] which takes only moments to administer either verbally or in writing. The SCOFF acronym is based on keywords of its five questions: (1) Do you make yourself **S**ick because you feel uncomfortably full? (2) Do you worry that you have lost **C**ontrol over how much you eat? (3) Have you recently lost more than **O**ne stone (14 lb) in a 3-month period? (4) Do you believe yourself to be **F**at when others say you are too thin? (5) Would you say that **F**ood dominates your life? To score, each *yes* response equals 1 point; a score of 2 indicates a likely diagnosis of AN or BN. Additionally, heights and weights (from which BMI is calculated) and vital signs should be measured.

Follow-up Activities for Medical Assistants

At follow-up visits, medical assistants record weights and vital signs, administer other applicable screening measures, and record information for the clinician's attention.

Primary Care Clinicians

Assessment

Although details of assessment and education might be delegated to BHSs, once the diagnosis is suspected, clinicians will want to obtain necessary information for initial treatment planning. The first key decisions concern potential needs for medical support and stabilization: Can this patient be managed as an outpatient? Hospitalization for medical stabilization is indicated for weight less than 70% of ideal body weight, rapid weight loss, bradycardia, significant orthostatic blood pressure changes, end-organ dysfunction, poor motivation, inability to change eating patterns and behaviors in healthy directions, or inability, despite good efforts, to reverse one's outpatient course. Decisions to hospitalize younger children for medical stabilization should be made earlier rather than later, and if possible, care should be managed by adolescent medicine specialists.

For all patients, assessments should address eating, purging, and exercise patterns; self-esteem in relation to weight, shape, and appearance; and motivation to change. For younger children and adolescents, the family's capacity to get involved with and take on substantial roles in treatment should be estimated.

General psychiatric assessment should focus on mood, anxiety (including non-eating/exercise-related obsessive-compulsive signs and symptoms), PTSD, substance use (cigarettes, alcohol, and other substances), personality (including perfectionism and impulsivity), and safety considerations (suicidal thinking or plans).

Assessing for medical complications and comorbidities is straightforward. Almost every organ system may be affected by malnutrition seen with AN.[39] For AN, assessment for the rate of weight loss, measurement of blood pressure with orthostatic changes, a cardiovascular examination, and a dental examination are necessary. For patients with AN and BN, screening laboratory tests suffice, including a complete blood count and a comprehensive metabolic panel, including electrolytes. Endocrine studies are generally not necessary, except for testosterone levels in males. An electrocardiogram is useful for patients with bradycardia or concerns about arrhythmia (e.g., complaints of palpitations). For patients with significant weight loss and menstrual irregularities lasting several months, a bone density examination (e.g., DXA scan) is useful. Dental examination should assess demineralization.[38]

Educating Patients and Families About the Disorder

Communications should center around naming the disorder and informing patients and families that AN or BN are well-understood and highly treatable conditions and that other co-occurring psychological/interpersonal difficulties will also receive attention. They should be informed about general treatment options and recommendations for AN or BN (Table 15.2).

TABLE 15.2. LEVEL OF CARE GUIDELINES FOR PATIENTS WITH EATING DISORDERS

	Level 1: Outpatient	Level 2: Intensive Outpatient	Level 3: Partial Hospitalization (Full-Day Outpatient Care)[a]	Level 4: Residential Treatment Center	Level 5: Inpatient Hospitalization
Medical status	Medically stable to the extent that more extensive medical monitoring, as defined in levels 4 and 5, is not required.			Medically stable to the extent that intravenous fluids, nasogastric feedings, or multiple daily laboratory tests are not needed.	**For adults:** Heart rate <40 bpm; blood pressure <90/60 mmHg; glucose <60 mg/dl; potassium <3 mEq/L; electrolyte imbalance; temperature <97.0°F; dehydration; hepatic, renal, or cardiovascular organ compromise requiring acute treatment; poorly controlled diabetes. **For children and adolescents:** Heart rate near 40 bpm, orthostatic blood pressure changes (>20 bpm increase in heart rate or >10–20 mmHg drop), blood pressure <80/50 mmHg, hypokalemia,[b] hypophosphatemia, or hypomagnesemia.
Suicidality[c]	If suicidality is present, inpatient monitoring and treatment may be needed, depending on the estimated level of risk.				Specific plan with high lethality or intent; admission may also be indicated in patient with suicidal ideas or after a suicide attempt or aborted attempt, depending on the presence or absence of other factors modulating suicide risk.
Weight as percentage of healthy body weight[d]	Generally >85%	Generally >80%	Generally >80%	Generally <85%	Generally <85%; acute weight decline with food refusal even if not <85% of healthy body weight.
Motivation to recover, including cooperativeness, insight, and ability to control obsessive thoughts	Fair to good motivation	Fair motivation	Partial motivation; cooperative; patient preoccupied with intrusive, repetitive thoughts[e] >3 hours/day.	Poor to fair motivation; patient preoccupied with intrusive repetitive thoughts[e] 4–6 hours a day; patient cooperative with highly structured treatment.	Very poor to poor motivation; patient preoccupied with intrusive repetitive thoughts[e]; patient uncooperative with treatment or cooperative only in highly structured environment.

(*continued*)

TABLE 15.2. CONTINUED

	Level 1: Outpatient	Level 2: Intensive Outpatient	Level 3: Partial Hospitalization (Full-Day Outpatient Care)[a]	Level 4: Residential Treatment Center	Level 5: Inpatient Hospitalization
Co-occurring disorders (substance use, depression, anxiety)	Presence of comorbid condition may influence choice of level of care.				Any existing psychiatric disorder that would require hospitalization.
Structure needed for eating/gaining weight	Self-sufficient	Self-sufficient	Needs some structure to gain weight	Needs supervision at all meals or will restrict eating	Needs supervision during and after all meals, or nasogastric/special feeding modality
Ability to control compulsive exercising	Can manage compulsive exercising through self-control	Some degree of external structure beyond self-control required to prevent patient from compulsive exercising; rarely a sole indication for increasing the level of care.			
Purging behavior (laxatives and diuretics)	Can greatly reduce incidents of purging in an unstructured setting; no significant medical complications, such as electrocardiographic or other abnormalities, suggesting the need for hospitalization.			Can ask for and use support from others or use cognitive and behavioral skills to inhibit purging.	Needs supervision during and after all meals and in bathroom; unable to control multiple daily episodes of purging that are severe, persistent, and disabling, despite appropriate trials of outpatient care, even if routine laboratory test results reveal no obvious metabolic abnormalities.

Environmental stress	Others able to provide adequate emotional and practical support and structure.	Others able to provide at least limited support and structure.	Severe family conflict or problems or absence of family so patient is unable to receive structured treatment in home; patient lives alone without adequate support system.
Geographic availability of treatment program	Patient lives near treatment setting.		Treatment program is too distant for patient to participate from home.

Source: Adapted and modified from La Via M, Kaye WH, Andersen A, Bowers W, Brandt HA, Brewerton TD, Costin C, Hill L, Lilenfeld L, McGilley B, Powers PS, Pryor T, Yager J, Zucker ML: Anorexia nervosa: criteria for levels of care. Paper presented at the annual meeting of the Eating Disorders Research Society, Cambridge, Mass, November 5–7, 1998.

Note: In general, a given level of care should be considered for patients who meet one or more criteria under a particular level. However, these guidelines are not absolute, and their application requires physician judgment.

[a]This level of care is most effective if administered for at least 8 hours/day, 5 days/week; less intensive care is demonstrably less effective. Olmsted MP, Kaplan AS, Rockert W: Relative efficacy of a 4-day versus a 5-day day hospital program. Int J Eat Disord 2003; 34:441–449.

[b]If the patient is dehydrated, whole-body potassium values may be low, even if the serum potassium value is in the normal range; determine concurrent urine specific gravity to assess for dehydration.

[c]Determining suicide risk is a complex clinical judgment, as is determining the most appropriate treatment setting for patients at risk for suicide. Relevant factors to consider are the patient's concurrent medical conditions, psychosis, substance use, other psychiatric symptoms or syndromes, psychosocial supports, past suicidal behaviors, and treatment adherence and the quality of existing physician–patient relationships. These factors are described in greater detail in the APA's American Psychiatric Association: Practice guideline for the assessment and treatment of patients with suicidal behaviors. Am J Psychiatry 2003; 160(11 suppl):1–60.

[d]Although this table lists percentages of expected healthy body weight in relation to suggested levels of care, these are only approximations and do not correspond to percentages based on standardized values for the population as a whole. For any given individual, differences in body build, body composition, and other physiological variables, may result in considerable differences as to what constitutes a healthy body weight in relation to "norms." For example, for some patients, a healthy body weight may be 110% of the standardized value for the population, whereas for other individuals, it may be 98%. Each individual's physiological differences must be assessed and appreciated. In addition, for children, consider the rate of weight loss. Finally, weight level per se should never be used as the sole criterion for discharge from inpatient care. Many patients require inpatient admission at higher weights, and should not be automatically discharged, just because they have achieved a certain weight level, unless all other factors are appropriately considered. See text for further discussion regarding weight.

[e]Individuals may experience these thoughts as consistent with their own deeply held beliefs (in which case they seem to be ego-syntonic and "overvalued"), or as unwanted and ego-alien repetitive thoughts, consistent with classic obsessive-compulsive disorder phenomenology.

For AN, consensus strongly suggests that earlier, effective interventions are more likely to prevent serious sequelae, such as cognitive deterioration associated with malnourished brains, irreversible loss of height, osteoporosis, and other enduring physiologic effects. Approximately 50% to 70% of children and adolescents treated for first-episode AN substantially improve, although complete psychological, as well as physiological recovery often takes several years. Approximately 20% of patients develop SEAN. Premature death rates, primarily in SEAN patients, vary from 5% to 10%, roughly half from medical complications due to malnutrition, and roughly half from suicide. Suicide rates for patients with chronic AN, particularly those with the binge–purge subtype, who also abuse alcohol, are high, more than 50 times comparable to community rates.[40]

For BN, little is known about the natural course of untreated conditions, although some evidence suggests modest overall improvement with time.[41,42] Treatments with CBT or IPT alone show substantial benefits,[43] and these are often improved when combined with SSRIs.[44] Systematically scheduled follow-up visits produce more sustained recovery and less relapse than as-needed visits.[45] Since most patients with BN have other comorbid psychiatric disorders, these conditions should routinely receive appropriate concurrent treatment. Up to 15% display a "multi-impulsive" type of disorder, with co-occurring borderline/cluster B personality disorder features, mood instability often meeting criteria for bipolar spectrum disorder (usually bipolar II disorder), attention-deficit/hyperactivity disorder, and frequently alcohol and substance abuse as well.[46] Such patients often require multipronged treatment approaches using DBT, medications, and substance abuse treatment.

Basic Clinical Management

Milder cases of AN in children and adolescents, marked by modest dieting, appearance concerns, and modest weight loss, can often be managed by1) primary care clinicians, offering support, education, advice, and monitoring, and 2) engaging parents as home-based treatment allies, who take responsibility for ensuring their children eat appropriately. In these scenarios, patients are followed weekly; during these visits they are weighed by staff, and are briefly seen regarding overall progress. Patients should be weighed after voiding and in gowns rather than street clothes, to make sure they are not hiding heavy objects to artificially increase recorded weights. Such plans should involve registered dietitians and BHSs responsible for counseling, psychological monitoring, and directing patients and families to additional resources as needed. The organizations and websites listed in Box 15.2 primarily address AN and BN.

Patients with more severe weight loss; intractable abnormal eating and exercise behaviors; psychological denial; significant psychiatric comorbidities; safety concerns regarding self-harm, family violence, or physiological status; family inability to actively help patients at home; or past history of significant edema formation following attempts to cease purging, may require hospitalization for medical stabilization. Some patients may need subsequent treatment in inpatient, residential, or intensive outpatient eating disorders programs prior to transitioning to usual ambulatory care. Patient preferences, insurance, and access to treatment resources dictate options. For extreme cases, highly specialized medical units may prove to be life-saving.[47]

Where available, family-based treatment (FBT) is a preferred treatment for child and adolescent patients who can be treated as outpatients. In FBT, family members are coached to firmly but lovingly assume control of the patient's feedings in home settings (while avoiding raging battles).[48–50] Although many communities lack FBT practitioners, professionals are being increasingly trained in this approach across the country. In any event, mental health clinicians willing to learn about eating disorders treatment can offer patients and families significant assistance.

For adult patients with a relatively recent onset of AN, integrated treatment usually combines medical monitoring in primary care settings, with ongoing care from eating disorders–trained mental health professionals, health coaches, and registered dietitians. These teams should address both patient and family concerns, and manage comorbid medical and psychiatric conditions.

Best practices for adult patients with SEAN, who have typically been chronically ill for a decade or more, focuses on safety planning. Patients with SEAN may be treated with harm reduction, psychosocial rehabilitation, motivational interviewing, and education of patients and families about realistic expectations for chronic mental illness, without depriving them of hope, and without unrealistically pressuring patients to fully recover.[51] Medical safety considerations entail designating team members to follow patients medically at set intervals, and deciding at what points (e.g., minimum weight, other physiologic parameters) patients should be medically treated, and if necessary, hospitalized for stabilization. Safety considerations also require having plans to deal with worrisome degrees of suicidality. Motivational interviewing and psychosocial rehabilitation are generally conducted by mental health professionals and case managers with whom patients can establish trusting relationships, and who know the patients, families, and available resources.

Whereas SSRIs (e.g., fluoxetine up to 60 mg/day, sertraline up to 200 mg/day) are effective for treating normal-weight individuals with BN (whether depressed or not), no medication has proven effectiveness for treating AN.[52] Second-generation antipsychotic medications have, at best, a modest impact on weight and outcome in AN. Most AN studies have been conducted with low-dose olanzapine.[53] Although clinicians occasionally employ other psychiatric medications to target depression, anxiety, or obsessive-compulsive symptoms, and some anecdotal reports support such practices, the overall value of these interventions for AN has not been demonstrated.

Patients with AN and BN can be considered remitted when they are behaviorally improved and physiologically healthy (usually takes several to many months) and recovered, when they are free from their disorders' plaguing and impairing thoughts, attitudes, emotions, and behaviors (ordinarily requires one to several years). Many months may be required for regained weight to redistribute normally, and for body image to become realistic. Relapse prevention is always integral to treatment planning. The American Psychiatric Association's practice guidelines for the treatment of patients with eating disorders offers recommended levels of care for various physiologic and psychiatric indications as shown in Table 15.2.

When to Refer

Patients who adequately respond within 2 to 3 months, show good motivation, gain an average of 1 to 1.5 pounds/week, while medically monitored, and reduce frequency of excessive exercise, binge eating and purging episodes, can be entirely managed at the primary care level, unless other emergent psychiatric or behavioral disorders are beyond the scope of primary care practice. Treatment-resistant patients will require consultations with a psychiatrist and, very likely, referral to an eating disorders specialist.

When Local Resources Are Lacking

Unfortunately, many communities lack accessible eating disorders specialists and programs. Studies have demonstrated effectiveness for telehealth treatment for BN, and patients with AN may also benefit.[37] As for BED, patients and families might access volunteer-staffed chat rooms through the National Eating Disorders Association, and other organizations listed in Box 15.2.

Urgent and Emergency Situations

Patients may initially present with urgent or emergency medical and/or psychiatric issues, or these may develop during ongoing treatment. Medically compromised patients, particularly those less than 70% of ideal body weight, may require initial hospitalization for medical stabilization. Decisions to hospitalize for medical safety and stabilization should be made sooner rather than later. Children and adolescents showing rapid weight loss, food refusal, orthostatic hypotension, or bradycardia with heart rates less than 40/minute may need hospitalization. Treatment guidelines for these situations have been published.[54] Adult patients with longstanding AN may be maintained in primary care practices even at low weights, so long as their weights exceed predetermined "safety" levels. However, patients whose weights fall below these levels should be hospitalized for stabilization.

Patients who purge are more likely to require urgent and emergent interventions for dehydration and/or acute electrolyte imbalance, situations ordinarily managed in emergency departments, in urgent care settings, or during brief medical hospitalizations. In general, potassium levels less than 2.8 mEq/L and bicarbonate levels greater than 36 mEq/L need higher levels of management. The care of patients with eating disorders in emergency departments, requires unique skills. Consequently, referring providers should encourage their emergency department colleagues to become familiar with the published literature on these issues.[55]

Psychiatric and behavioral urgent and emergent situations in patients with AN and BN can stem from the eating disorders themselves, and/or from associated psychiatric difficulties. Patients who simply cannot bring themselves to eat, cannot desist from exercising or purging, and/or decline, despite weeks of competent outpatient intervention, usually necessitate higher levels of care. Patients with co-occurring

BOX 15.3

SUMMARY OF RECOMMENDED TREATMENT APPROACHES AND RELEVANT EVIDENCE

Strength of recommendation taxonomy (SOR A, B, or C)

- **For BED**
  - **a. Establish alliance. (SOR A)[29,33]**
  - **b. CBT with or without SSRI for binge eating per se (SOR A)[17,20,22,45]**
  - **c. CBT may be initiated via guided self-help in stepped care treatments. (SOR B)[20,28]**
  - **d. Behavioral activation and behavioral management for medically supervised weight loss (SOR B)[19,21]**
- **For AN**
  - **a. Children and adolescents**
    - **i. Establish alliance with patient and family. (SOR A)[31]**
    - **ii. Educate, counsel, refer to lay organizations, arrange consultation with registered dietitian. (SOR A)[31]**
    - **iii. Family-based treatment programs, with professional coaching (SOR B)[31,49]**
    - **iv. For rapid weight loss and lack of response, hospitalize in children's hospital for medical stabilization, earlier rather than later. (SOR A)[29,31,55]**
    - **v. Depending on status, refer to eating disorder specialists for ongoing care. (SOR C)[29,31,33,51]**
    - **vi. Primary care clinician provides ongoing monitoring of weight, physical status, medications. (SOR C)[33,51]**
  - **b. Adult patients with relatively recent onset of AN**
    - **i. Establish alliance with patient and family. (SOR A)[29,33]**
    - **ii. Educate, counsel, refer to lay organizations, arrange consultation with registered dietitian and eating disorder specialists, as needed. (SOR A)[29,33]**
    - **iii. Coordinate monitoring and medication management with eating disorders specialists. (SOR A)[33,51]**
    - **iv. Establish medical and psychological safety parameters and refer for medical stabilization and hospital intervention, as indicated. (SOR A)[29,33,51]**
  - **c. Adult patients with SEAN**
    - **i. Establish alliance with patient and family. (SOR A)[29,33,34]**
    - **ii. Establish safety parameters, regarding weight, blood pressure, and other cardiovascular measures at which point, medical stabilization might be required. (SOR A)[29,33,34]**
    - **iii. Assign one team member to monitor patient at regular intervals (no less than monthly) for physiological status, psychiatric safety. (SOR C)[34]**
    - **iv. BHS or eating disorder specialist to engage patient in harm reduction, psychosocial rehabilitation, motivational interviewing (SOR B)[34]**
    - **v. Do not impose unrealistic expectations regarding recovery. (SOR C)[34]**

mood, anxiety, and substance use disorders, resulting in suicidal or violent threats or behaviors, require urgent or emergent psychiatric evaluation and management. Rarely, primary care clinicians might have to involve law enforcement to help involuntarily transfer patients to emergency services.

After medical and/or psychiatric stabilization, decisions can be made regarding options, such as eating disorder inpatient units, partial hospitalization/day hospitals, intensive outpatient programs, and traditional ambulatory care.

OTHER EATING DISORDERS

In addition to AN, BN, and BED, several other feeding and eating disorders have been delineated, including the newly defined "avoidant and restrictive feeding and intake disorder," night eating syndromes of various types, purging disorder (occurring without frank binge eating), and other atypical disorders. Full diagnostic criteria and associated clinical characteristics for these disorders can be found in pages 329 to 354 of the DSM-5.[1]

CONCLUSION

Eating disorders are prevalent conditions, accompanied by high rates of both medical and psychiatric comorbidities, affecting individuals throughout the life-span. Since many patients are reluctant to disclose their struggles concerning eating behaviors and the psychological difficulties associated with them, screening for these conditions in primary care treating settings is likely to reveal many previously undetected cases. Over recent decades a great deal has been learned regarding successful interventions for these conditions. See Box 15.3 for a summary of recommended treatment approaches and relevant evidence. Primary care practitioners and the many ancillary staff who work in these settings, working collaboratively with a variety of mental health professionals and consulting specialists, have much to offer these patients, alleviating acute symptoms, managing chronic conditions, and reducing risks of further complications and mortality.

REFERENCES

1. American Psychiatric Association. (2013). Diagnostic and Statistical Manual of Mental Disorders, fifth edition (DSM-5). Washington, DC American Psychiatric Association; 2013.
2. Mehler PS. Diagnosis and care of patients with anorexia nervosa in primary care settings. Ann Intern Med. 2001;134(11):1048–1059.
3. UnützerJ, KatonW, CallahanCM, et al Collaborative care management of late-life depression in the primary care setting: A randomized controlled trial. JAMA. 2002;288(22):2836–2845.
4. Kessler RC, Berglund PA, Chiu WT, et al. The prevalence and correlates of binge eating disorder in the World Health Organization World Mental Health Surveys. Biol Psychiatry. 2013;73(9): 904–914.
5. Lin HY, Huang CK, Tai CM, et al. Psychiatric disorders of patients seeking obesity treatment. BMC Psychiatry. 2013;13:1. doi:10.1186/1471-244X-13-1.
6. Javaras KN, Pope HG, Lalonde JK, et al. Co-occurrence of binge eating disorder with psychiatric and medical disorders. J Clin Psychiatry. 2008;69(2):266–273.
7. TODAY Study Group, Wilfley D, Berkowitz R, Goebel-Fabbri A, et al. Binge eating, mood, and quality of life in youth with type 2 diabetes: Baseline data from the TODAY study. Diabetes Care. 2011;34(4):858–860.
8. Kerchner A, Lester W, Stuart SP, Dokras A. Risk of depression and other mental health disorders in women with polycystic ovary syndrome: A longitudinal study. Fertil Steril. 2009;91(1):207–212.
9. Friborg O, Martinussen M, Kaiser S, et al. Personality disorders in eating disorder not otherwise specified and binge eating disorder: A meta-analysis of comorbidity studies. J Nerv Ment Dis. 2014;202(2):119–125.
10. Grilo CM, White MA, Barnes RD, Masheb RM. Posttraumatic stress disorder in women with binge eating disorder in primary care. J Psychiatr Pract. 2012;18(6):408–412.
11. Kroenke K, Spitzer RL, Williams JB. The PHQ-9: Validity of a brief depression severity measure. J Gen Intern Med. 2001;16(9):606–613.
12. Striegel-Moore RH, Perrin N, DeBar L, Wilson GT, Rosselli F, Kraemer HC. Screening for binge eating disorders using the Patient Health Questionnaire in a community sample. Int J Eat Disord. 2010;43(4):337–343.
13. Greeno CG, Marcus MD, Wing RR. Diagnosis of binge eating disorder: Discrepancies between a questionnaire and clinical interview. Int J Eat Disord. 1995;17(2):153–160.
14. Vander Wal JS, Stein RI, Blashill AJ.The EDE-Q, BULIT-R, and BEDT as self-report measures of binge eating disorder. Eat Behav. 2011;12(4):267–271.
15. Fairburn CG. Overcoming Binge Eating, Second Edition: The Proven Program to Learn Why You Binge and How You Can Stop. New York: Guilford Press; 2013.
16. Hilbert A, Bishop ME, Stein RI, et al. Long-term efficacy of psychological treatments for binge eating disorder. Br J Psychiatry. 2012;200(3):232–237.
17. Wilson GT, Wilfley DE, Agras WS, Bryson SW. Psychological treatments of binge eating disorder. Arch Gen Psychiatry. 2010;67(1):94–101.
18. Devlin MJ, Goldfein JA, Petkova E, et al. Cognitive behavioral therapy and fluoxetine as adjuncts to group behavioral therapy for binge eating disorder. Obes Res. 2005;13(6):1077–1088.
19. Wilson GT. Treatment of binge eating disorder. Psychiatr Clin North Am. 2011;34(4):773–783.
20. Apovian CM, Aronne LJ, Bessesen DH, et al. Pharmacological management of obesity: An Endocrine Society clinical practice guideline. J Clin Endocrinol Metab. 2015;100(2):342–362.
21. McElroy SL, Guerdjikova AI, Mori N, O'Melia AM. Pharmacological management of binge eating disorder: current and emerging treatment options. Ther Clin Risk Manag. 2012;8:219–241.
22. McElroy SL, Hudson JI, Mitchell JE, et al. Efficacy and safety of lisdexamfetamine for treatment of adults with moderate to severe binge-eating disorder: a randomized clinical trial. JAMA Psychiatry. 2015;72(3):235–246.

23. Wilfley DE, Welch RR, Stein RI, et al. A randomized comparison of group cognitive-behavioral therapy and group interpersonal psychotherapy for the treatment of overweight individuals with binge-eating disorder. Arch Gen Psychiatry. 2002;59(8):713–721.
24. Fairburn CG, Rothwell ER. Apps and eating disorders: A systematic clinical appraisal. Int J Eat Disord. 2015;48(7):1038–1046. doi:10.1002/eat.22398.
25. Hertz P, Addaad M, Ronel N. Attachment styles and changes among women members of Overeaters Anonymous who have recovered from binge-eating disorder. Health Soc Work. 2012;37:110–122.
26. Yager J, Landsverk J, Edelstein CK. Help seeking and satisfaction with care in 641 women with eating disorders. I. Patterns of utilization, attributed change, and perceived efficacy of treatment. J Nerv Ment Dis. 1989;177(10):632–637.
26a. Macdonald P, Hibbs R, Rhind C, et al. Disseminating skills to carers of people with eating disorders: an examination of treatment fidelity in lay and professional carer coaches. Health Psychol Behav Med. 2014;2(1):555–564.
27. Shingleton RM, Richards LK, Thompson-Brenner H. Using technology within the treatment of eating disorders: A clinical practice review. Psychotherapy (Chicago). 2013;50(4):576–582.
28. Loucas CE, Fairburn CG, Whittington C, Pennant ME, Stockton S, Kendall T. E-therapy in the treatment and prevention of eating disorders: A systematic review and meta-analysis. Behav Res Ther. 2014;63:122–131.
29. American Psychiatric Association. Treatment of patients with eating disorders, 3rd ed. Am J Psychiatry. 2006;163(7 Suppl):4–54.
30. Yager J, Devlin MJ, Halmi KA, et al. Guideline Watch (August 2012): Practice guideline for the treatment of patients with eating disorders, 3rd ed. American Psychiatric Association. http://psychiatryonline.org/pb/assets/raw/sitewide/practice_guidelines/guidelines/eatingdisorders-watch.pdf Accessed May 31, 2015.
31. Lock J, La Via MC; American Academy of Child and Adolescent Psychiatry (AACAP) Committee on Quality Issues (CQI). Practice parameter for the assessment and treatment of children and adolescents with eating disorders. J Am Acad Child Adolesc Psychiatry. 2015;54(5):412–425.
32. Hay P, Chinn D, Forbes D, et al. Royal Australian and New Zealand College of Psychiatrists clinical practice guidelines for the treatment of eating disorders. Aust N Z J Psychiatry. 2014; 48(11):977–1008.
33. National Collaborating Centre for Mental Health (UK). Eating Disorders: Core Interventions in the Treatment and Management of Anorexia Nervosa, Bulimia Nervosa and Related Eating Disorders. Leicester: British Psychological Society; 2004.
34. Hay PJ, Touyz S, Sud R. Treatment for severe and enduring anorexia nervosa: A review. Aust N Z J Psychiatry. 2012;46(12):1136–1144.
35. Sim LA, McAlpine DE, Grothe KB, Himes SM, Cockerill RG, Clark MM. Identification and treatment of eating disorders in the primary care setting. Mayo Clin Proc. 2010;85(8):746–751.
36. Smink FR, van Hoeken D, Hoek HW. Epidemiology, course, and outcome of eating disorders. Curr Opin Psychiatry. 2013;26(6):543–548.
37. Hudson JI, Jiripi E, Pope HG, Kessler RC. The prevalence and correlates of eating disorders in the National Comorbidity Survey Replication. Biol Psychiatry. 2007;61(3):348–358.
38. Keel PK, Heatherton TF, Dorer DJ, Joiner TE, Zalta AK. Point prevalence of bulimia nervosa in 1982, 1992, and 2002. Psychol Med. 2006;36(1):119–127.
39. Mehler PS, Brown C. Anorexia nervosa—medical complications. J Eat Disord. 2015;3:11. doi:10.1186/s40337-015-0040-8.
40. Keel PK, Dorer DJ, Eddy KT, Franko D, Charatan DL, Herzog DB. Predictors of mortality in eating disorders. Arch Gen Psychiatry. 2003;60(2):179–183.
41. Fairburn CG, Cooper Z, Doll HA, Norman P, O'Connor M. The natural course of bulimia nervosa and binge eating disorder in young women. Arch Gen Psychiatry. 2000;57(7):659–665.
42. Yager J, Landsverk J, Edelstein CK. A 20-month follow-up study of 628 women with eating disorders, I: Course and severity. Am J Psychiatry. 1987;144(9):1172–1177.
43. Kass AE, Kolko RP, Wilfley DE. Psychological treatments for eating disorders. Curr Opin Psychiatry. 2013;26(6):549–555.
44. Flament MF, Bissada H, Spettigue W. Evidence-based pharmacotherapy of eating disorders. Int J Neuropsychopharmacol. 2012;15(2):189–207.
45. Mitchell JE, Agras WS, Wilson GT, Halmi K, Kraemer H, Crow S. A trial of a relapse prevention strategy in women with bulimia nervosa who respond to cognitive-behavior therapy. Int J Eat Disord. 2004;35(4):549–555.
46. Fichter MM, Quadflieg N, Rief W. Course of multi-impulsive bulimia. Psychol Med. 1994;24(3):591–604.
47. Chu ES, Gaudiani JL, Mascolo M, et al. ACUTE center for eating disorders. J Hosp Med. 2012;7(4):340–344.
48. Lock J. An update on evidence-based psychosocial treatments for eating disorders in children and adolescents. J Clin Child Adolesc Psychol. 2015;44(5):707–721.
49. Månsson J, Parling T, Swenne I. Favorable effects of clearly defined interventions by parents at the start of treatment of adolescents with restrictive eating disorders. Int J Eat Disord. 2016;49(1):92–97. doi:10.1002/eat.22379.

50. Wilfahrt RP. The role of the generalist in the initial treatment of adolescent anorexia nervosa. Minn Med. 2015;98(2):37–40.
51. Yager J. Management of patients with chronic, intractable eating disorders. In: Yager J, Powers P, eds: Clinical Manual of Eating Disorders. Washington, DC: American Psychiatric Press; 2007:407–437.
52. Mitchell JE, Roerig J, Steffen K. Biological therapies for eating disorders. Int J Eat Disord. 2013;46(5):470–477.
53. Dold M, Aigner M, Klabunde M, Treasure J, Kasper S. Second-generation antipsychotic drugs in anorexia nervosa: A meta-analysis of randomized controlled trials. Psychother Psychosom. 2015;84(2):110–116.
54. Academy for Eating Disorders. Eating Disorders: Critical Points for Early Recognition and Medical Risk Management in the Care of Individuals with Eating Disorders (AED Report 2012 second edition). http://www.aedweb.org/downloads/Guide-English.pdf. Accessed May 31, 2015.
55. Mascolo M, Trent S, Colwell C, Mehler PS. What the emergency department needs to know when caring for your patients with eating disorders. Int J Eat Disord. 2012;45(8):977–981.

16

Treating Somatic Symptom Disorder and Illness Anxiety in Integrated Care Settings

ALLA LANDA, MARINA MAKOUS, AND BRIAN A. FALLON

BOX 16.1

KEY POINTS

1. **Somatic symptoms and fears about them are neurophysiologic phenomena and should not be dismissed by clinicians as "not real."**
2. **Stepped-care approach to the treatment of somatic symptom disorder (SSD) and illness anxiety (IA) is recommended.**
3. **Effective treatment requires integration of primary care and mental health at all levels of care, establishment of psychosomatic services, and reorganization of fragmented medical care to a whole-person medicine approach. These changes have been shown to be clinically effective and to reduce costs and inefficient use of health care resources.**
4. **The abandonment of mind–body dualism and an increase in biopsychosocial awareness (BPSA) are essential for the culture of the integrated care clinic.**
5. **Interventions need to be tailored to the patient's current level and stage of BPSA.**
6. **The key difference between SSD and IA is that in SSD distress is due to somatic symptoms (e.g., pain) while in IA distress is primarily due to fear of serious medical condition (e.g., mild pain elicits fear that patient has cancer).**
7. **Specialized psychotherapy and pharmacologic treatments delivered by an interdisciplinary team can be effective treatments for SSD and IA.**

INTRODUCTION

Integration of medical and mental health care is essential for the effective treatment of patients with somatic symptom disorder (SSD) or illness anxiety (IA). The world's best models of care for these disorders are based on an integrated approach. Unfortunately, in many countries, patients with SSD and IA often fall through the cracks between primary care and mental health and do not find much help in either specialty. Such a chasm is often widened by a lack of communication between disciplines, leading to increased patient suffering, disability, and ineffective use of health care resources.[1] This creates a public health problem, and in some countries, an alarming one, given the prevalence of individuals with these disorders in medical settings.[2]

A number of challenges in the diagnosis and treatment of SSD and IA contribute to this public health problem. While the diagnosis of SSD or IA rightfully motivates a primary care provider (PCP) to make a referral to a behavioral health specialist (e.g., psychiatrist, psychologist, or a clinical social worker who specializes in psychosomatic medicine), many patients will not accept a psychiatric diagnosis and therefore will not follow the PCP's recommendations, making it impossible for them to get the specialized treatment they need. Another difficulty is the continuous need for reassessment and differentiation between the symptoms that require medical treatment (e.g., cancer) and symptoms that require SSD/IA-focused treatment. Yet another challenge is clinician burnout. Patients with these disorders often present with unending suffering and complaints despite numerous investigations and treatments, making clinicians feel helpless. Patients often feel that their symptoms are not taken seriously and are dismissed as "not real" or "unimportant" by the physician, clinic staff, and/or their family and friends. This adds to their despair, further exacerbating the vicious cycle of distress and somatic symptoms. Finally, in many countries, the very organization of health care and medical education is organ- or system-focused, making the treatment of brain–body conditions quite challenging as these disorders fall through the gap in the psychiatry–medicine divide. However, patients with SSD and IA can be treated effectively, and working with these patients can be a deeply rewarding experience for both the PCP and behavioral health clinicians.

The approaches presented in this chapter are aimed at overcoming these challenges and helping multidisciplinary teams to care for SSD and IA patients in primary care or integrated care settings. They are based on the integration of (1) the best practices and available guidelines for treating these conditions in the world today, (2) evidence from research studies on diagnosis and treatment, and (3) the latest translational research relevant to the understanding of the etiology and treatment of SSD and IA. Research on SSD and IA has been expanding rapidly. Usually, it takes years for the insights from basic neuroscience to be implemented into clinical care and tested in large randomized control trials and dissemination studies. To diminish this time gap, this chapter presents approaches that are informed by the latest findings in translational neuroscience relevant to SSD and IA. Box 16.1 summarizes key points that are discussed in this chapter.

CLINICAL PRESENTATION AND ETIOLOGY

The nosology of somatic symptoms and illness fears is complex and has changed considerably in recent years. Numerous diagnostic labels are used to describe somatic symptoms somatoform, multisomatoform, abridged somatoform, bodily distress syndrome, psychophysiologic, psychosomatic, functional, or somatic symptom disorders; somatization; medically unexplained, psychogenic, or idiopathic symptoms. In a medical office, a patient with somatic symptoms may be diagnosed with fibromyalgia, irritable bowel syndrome, or chronic fatigue syndrome, as criteria for these diagnoses are based on the similar list of symptoms. Terms also periodically change to newer ones that haven't yet acquired the pejorative connotation of "not real" or "imagined," a connotation that is understandably distressing for patients.

Recently, the *Diagnostic and Statistical Manual of Mental Disorders*, Fifth Edition (DSM-5)[3] replaced the *Diagnostic and Statistical Manual of Mental Disorders*, Fourth Edition (DSM-IV)[4] diagnoses of somatoform, somatization, and pain disorders with the diagnosis of SSD. While the new criteria have some advantages (e.g., the diagnosis no longer requires a certain arbitrary number of symptoms as was the case with DSM-IV's somatization disorder), the primary disadvantage is that the criteria now include both the somatic symptoms and "excessive worry or distress about somatic symptoms," making it difficult to distinguish patients who primarily have somatic symptoms from those who primarily have a fear about what their somatic symptoms mean (e.g., pain vs. worry that pain is a sign of undiagnosed cancer, the latter being a symptom of IA). Because the distinction between these two dimensions is important for treatment planning, we focus separately on somatic symptoms and IA.

Somatic Symptoms

Clinical Presentation

Patients with somatic symptoms present with bodily symptoms (e.g., pain, fatigue, gastrointestinal [GI] symptoms) resulting in distress and impairment. If a medical problem is present, the severity of distress or disability significantly exceeds what would be expected. Estimates of lifetime prevalence of somatic symptoms depend on the diagnostic criteria used. Studies that have used more inclusive criteria report a 12-month prevalence of somatic symptoms of up to 30% in the general population[2] and up to 49% in primary care clinics.[5] Women are more frequently affected than men.[2]

Patients with somatic symptoms are often frustrated by the lack of a medical diagnosis. Because these patients consult many different physicians in pursuit of a diagnosis and treatment, the result is often fragmented patient care, unnecessary repetitive tests, and costly, potentially dangerous surgeries. Ordering multiple diagnostic tests increases the likelihood of an abnormal finding that is medically inconsequential, which, despite reassurance from the physician, leads to the patient's concern that findings are being ignored. For example, multiple studies of asymptomatic populations revealed that structural spine or knee abnormalities on magnetic resonance imaging did not predict pain.[6,7] Additional rounds of tests and procedures lead to further delays in the initiation of treatments focused on somatic symptoms.

A somatic reaction to an acute stressor usually resolves on its own or when the PCP offers psychoeducation and reassurance. Somatic symptoms associated with chronic or early developmental stressors require a specialized treatment. Because timely diagnosis and treatment are important for preventing the transformation of acute somatic symptoms into chronic ones, exploration of psychosocial stressors at the initial primary care visit is essential. Unfortunately, in most current medical practices, psychological stressors are often considered last, after all medical reasons for the symptoms have been explored, leading to significant delays in establishing the diagnosis of SSD. Clues to the diagnosis of SSD include: (1) symptoms that change bodily location from one month to the next, (2) neurologic complaints that do not follow the anatomic distribution of nerve pathways, (3) somatic symptoms that fluctuate with varying levels of stress on macro (scale of months and years) and/or micro (scale of minutes, hours, days) levels, and (4) amplified affective or experiential aspect of a symptom (e.g., report a of pain rating of "20" on a 0–10-point scale or a report of pain level that does not correspond to the patient's observed level of functioning).

Patients with chronic somatic symptoms are often disconnected from their emotions, alexithymic (i.e., have difficulty expressing emotions verbally), have problems tolerating conflicting emotions, or have difficulty differentiating between various emotions they experience. Typically, when asked about feelings in an emotional situation, these individuals either don't respond or talk about thoughts, actions, or somatic sensations. Research suggests these difficulties are often associated with a history of early interpersonal trauma, insecure attachment, or growing up in non-optimal interpersonal environments (e.g., when a parent is depressed or physically ill, emotionally abusive, or overprotective), or cultural norms that restrict emotional expression; all of these factors can impede socioemotional development.[2,8] As adults, many patients tend to feel lonely or are highly sensitive interpersonally, perceiving others as hurting, abandoning, or unavailable.[8] Though some patients may seem socially distant, this demeanor may represent the defensive stance of someone who craves interpersonal closeness but fears abandonment and rejection. Lack of help from physicians is often perceived by an emotionally fragile patient as yet another abandonment, which exacerbates the vicious cycle of interpersonal distress and somatic symptoms. In a subgroup of patients, emotional conflict kept outside of awareness can also manifest as somatic symptoms.

Comorbidity and Differential Diagnosis

An appropriate medical workup is essential for ruling out an underlying medical disorder in patients with somatic symptoms.[2,9] Although a patient may present with exclusively somatic complaints, comorbid psychiatric disorders among those with somatic symptoms are common. In one study, 54% of the patients with somatic symptoms had comorbid depression, anxiety, or both.[10] In another study, over 76% of primary care patients with depression presented somatically.[11] Careful temporal plotting of somatic and mood symptoms as well as assessment of which symptoms cause most distress and disability helps to determine which diagnosis is primary. Once the primary disorder is effectively treated, somatic symptoms may dissipate. Somatic symptoms (especially chronic pain) may be particularly comorbid with atypical depression, characterized by mood reactivity (i.e., patient's mood may be brightened by interaction with the physician) and heightened interpersonal sensitivity. Somatic symptoms should not be confused with factitious disorders (e.g., Munchausen syndrome) or malingering. Unlike malingers who manipulate society by reporting fictitious symptoms, or factitious and Munchausen patients, who unconsciously long to be treated as an ill patient, patients with somatic symptoms genuinely experience bodily distress.

Etiology

Somatic symptoms may result from different etiologic pathways. Recent research suggests that genetic predisposition, multigenerational transmission of trauma through psychological or epigenetic mechanisms, exposure to early stressors, or a non-optimal early interpersonal environment can all influence development of the nervous and immune systems. These factors can contribute to difficulty differentiating somatic and emotional cues from the body, problems with the regulation of somatic and emotional distress, and chronic hyperactivation of central neural circuits (i.e., central sensitization).[2,8] These obstacles to healthy development may predispose a person to experiencing emotional distress primarily somatically.

Illness Anxiety

Clinical Presentation

IA refers to the irrational, excessive fear or belief that one has a serious illness based on a misinterpretation of physical signs and symptoms. Individuals with IA do not experience sustained relief after being reassured by a PCP that no serious illness is present. IA can also affect a patient with an underlying medical condition if worry about a stable illness becomes so excessive as to impair the patient's well-being and functioning. In the DSM-5, IA with no or only mild somatic symptoms is referred to as illness anxiety disorder. IA, however, is also a criterion for DSM-5 SSD. Previously, in DSM-IV, IA was a distinct diagnosis known as hypochondriasis.

Issy Pilowsky in 1967 identified three central aspects of hypochondria: fear of illness, disease conviction, and bodily preoccupation. These three aspects may occur in any combination, giving the patient a distinctively different clinical presentation. For example, a patient with a high degree of illness fear may actually avoid going to see a doctor, scared that the doctor will confirm the presence of a dreaded disease. In fact, avoidance of medical care is a dangerous and often underrecognized symptom of IA that causes patients to miss available life-saving diagnostic procedures and treatments. However, in another presentation of IA, a patient with a high degree of disease conviction and lower fear may pursue a diagnosis with relentless persistence, berating physicians who fail to repeat a full battery of tests and becoming enraged by medical science's inability to help. A patient with high bodily preoccupation but lesser conviction may present to the physician with a variety of inexplicable physical complaints and appear to have SSD. Other obsessional traits may be present: a fear that terrible harm might come to loved ones; intrusive, horrific images; obsessive thoughts about dirt or germs; an anxiety-driven need for perfection, order, or symmetry; troubling sexual images; and scrupulous moral or religious concerns. Common compulsions include excessive body checking, searching for medical information, and talking about their medical symptoms and fears with others.

Transient hypochondriasis implies illness fears that last weeks or months and do not become chronic, typically abating on their own (e.g., medical students often develop transient hypochondriasis after learning about a new horrific disease). In IA, disease fears persist for at least 6 months. The course of IA may wax and wane in severity, exacerbated by various stressors in the patient's life.

Estimates of the prevalence of IA depend on the restrictiveness of the criteria. A meta-analysis of 47 independent samples suggested that IA was found in up to 13% in the general population and up to 8% in primary care settings.[12] In a study of specialty clinics in England, the prevalence of health anxiety assessed by self-report questionnaire was 25% in neurology, 21% in respiratory medicine, 19.5% in gastroenterology, 19% in cardiology, and 18% in endocrinology.[13]

Comorbidity and Differential Diagnosis

Common conditions that might present with IA include panic disorder, major depression, and generalized anxiety disorders. The similarities between IA and obsessive-compulsive disorder have important treatment implications as the methods of treating obsessive-compulsive disorder are also effective for hypochondriasis.

Etiology

The etiology of IA is unclear but likely includes psychological, cultural, and biological components. Psychologically, IA may serve as a window into unresolved emotional issues or earlier developmental conflicts. Culturally, IA and bodily concerns may be an acceptable mode of expressing emotional stress. One current theory emphasizes that hypochondriacs have a tendency to amplify, augment, and misinterpret normal bodily sensations, experiencing interoceptive cues as more intense and noxious.[14] Hypochondriacs are physiologically hyperreactive to external stimuli.[15] The neurochemical underpinnings of these constitutional differences in the IA patient may be similar to the serotonergic imbalance seen in OCD, or to the noradrenergic imbalances seen in panic disorder, with similar neural circuity abnormalities observed in all three conditions.[16]

Somatic Symptoms Versus Illness Anxiety

While somatic symptoms and IA often co-occur, most patients suffer primarily from either somatic symptoms or IA. Different treatment approaches to these conditions have been suggested (e.g., treatment studies with serotonergic pharmacotherapy typically report greater improvement in IA than in somatic symptoms).[17] To determine which treatment approach to emphasize, the clinician should determine whether somatic symptoms or obsessional anxiety about health are central. We recommend using direct questions about distress and functional interference from somatic symptoms versus from illness worries as described in the Columbia Somatic Symptoms & Illness Anxiety Ratio Scale.[18] This scale should be administered after rapport is established and after the clinician validates the patient's symptoms; posing a question about anxiety too early may communicate to the patient that the symptoms are not taken seriously.

IDENTIFICATION AND TREATMENT IN INTEGRATED HEALTH CARE SYSTEMS

Overall Approach and Principles

The following are essential principles of effective care for patients with SSD and IA in integrated settings and relevant recommendations for organization of care.

1. Complete Abandonment of Mind–Body Dualism

For centuries, the division between the body and the mind/brain has been at the core of philosophy and mentality in many cultures around the world. The biopsychosocial approach proposed by Engel in the 1970s[19] aimed to reverse this dualism by emphasizing that everything that is psychological *is* biological, and everything that is biological *is* psychological. *Bio*, *psycho*, and *social* are just different levels of inquiry at which health can be considered from molecular, through organ, individual, family, to societal levels and beyond. (For example, an emotion of anger involves fluctuation of neural circuits and neurotransmitters in the brain, muscle tension, and perhaps a behavior of clenching a fist or yelling). This paradigm shift away from dualism to full acceptance of the biopsychosocial approach is necessary for treating SSD and IA, for organizing effective care, and for explaining these diagnoses to patients. Since duality is deeply rooted in our culture, eradicating this dualism in everyday patient care is a process that will initially require an effort on the part of clinicians and health care organizations.

One example of implementation of this paradigm shift is seen in outpatient pain clinics in which all patients, regardless of the presenting complaint, are seen by both a pain physician and a pain psychologist during their first visit. (See Chapter 23: Integrated Chronic Pain and Psychiatric Management.) Some countries have institutionalized this paradigm shift. For example, in Germany many medical centers have a psychosomatic medicine service focused on patients with somatic symptoms arising from medical and/or psychological causes (e.g., SSD, mixed anxiety/depression with somatic symptoms, anxiety due to breast cancer diagnosis) where patients receive integrated multidisciplinary treatments.

2. Emotions and Stress Are Universally Experienced on a Somatic (Bodily) Level

Patients with somatic symptoms are often perceived by others (including health care professionals) as "them" versus "us," and as having mysterious, inexplicable symptoms. However, any emotion is a somatic experience, involving physiologic changes in our bodies. For example, feeling lack of energy for days after a breakup with a romantic partner, or experiencing an increase in the rate of breathing when we are anxious are natural somatic reactions to stress. There is an individual variability in the tendency to somatize, in the intensity and duration of bodily distress, as well as in the ability of a person to regulate this distress. Highlighting to patients the universality of somatization will help them feel less alienated and more accepting of the bidirectional relationship between emotions and somatic symptoms. This is a crucial component of treatment. Sincere acceptance and understanding of the patient's suffering goes a long way.

Similarly, fears of having a serious disease and of death are universal phenomena. The duration, distress, and dysfunction associated with these fears distinguish pathologic from nonpathologic IA.

3. Level and Stage of a Patient's Biopsychosocial Awareness Informs All Aspects of Care

Treatment of SSD and IA will depend on the degree to which a patient accepts the diagnosis, which, in turn, will depend to a large degree on whether the patient adopts a biopsychosocial understanding of health, disease, and his/her symptoms. We call this a biopsychosocial awareness (BPSA). Patients, health care professionals, and societies vary in the level of BPSA. In fact, full BPSA is still rare among patients, clinicians, and health care organizations in many countries around the world. BPSA is, however, not an all-or-none phenomenon; and it can increase gradually, with time and interventions, in a person or in an organization. To help conceptualize this process, we developed the Columbia Stages for BioPsychoSocial Awareness (CS-BPSA) model (Fig. 16.1) and a rating scale to track a patient's progress (Table 16.1). The CS-BPSA includes two dimensions: comprehensiveness of BPSA and the stage of readiness for BPSA. The stage of readiness dimension is based on the framework of the Trans-Theoretical Stages of Change[20] developed by Prochaska and DiClemente, who had suggested that an individual's readiness to develop new, healthier behaviors is a process that consists of five stages: (1) precontemplation, (2) contemplation, (3) preparation, (4) action, and (5) maintenance.

A patient presenting to primary care can be at any stage (temporal) and level (unidirectional vs. reciprocal concept of biopsychosocial interaction) of BPSA (see Fig. 16.1 and the example in Table 16.1). If SSD or IA is suspected, one of the primary goals of evaluation is determining the patient's current stage and level of BPSA in order to tailor appropriate interventions.

Levels of BPSA

In the CS-BPSA model levels describe the degree of awareness of the bidirectional relationship between emotions and somatic symptoms (see Fig. 16.1B). Level A indicates recognition that somatic symptoms can unidirectionally affect mood or functioning, level B indicates recognition that psychological stressors or emotions can unidirectionally influence the body and lead to somatic symptoms, and level C indicates awareness of the bidirectional relationship between "bio" and "psychosocial." If a patient presents with no BPSA, usually level A is the easiest to reach first. To facilitate this, clinician may ask: "Has your pain affected your sleep?" or "How does pain make you feel emotionally?" or "It must be difficult to pick up your two-year-old son when you have such severe back pain; how has that affected your relationship with him?" Though unidirectional, level A is a step toward full BPSA. Level B refers to awareness of the reverse relationship: stress/emotion/brain affect the body and may produce or exacerbate somatic symptoms. Level B understanding will range in depth, for example, from acknowledging that lack of sleep can increase pain, to realization that anger at a spouse leads to bouts of back pain. Stressors that are more "somatic" (sleep, appetite) are more easily integrated into Level B BPSA than emotions, blends of emotions, conflicting emotions, or interpersonal issues. Full BPSA (Level C) implies acceptance of the complete bidirectionality of *bio* and *psychosocial* factors, including the vicious circle that this relationship creates (e.g., the realization that "anger at a spouse elicits my back pain, which in turn makes my anger even stronger").

Stages of Change in BPSA

A patient at the *precontemplation stage* (see Fig. 16.1A and example in Table 16.1) presents with complete mind–body dualism. These patients are usually focused on finding only a biological explanation for somatic symptoms and are not open to considering BPSA. At this stage, the most challenging task for a clinician is to stay at the patient's level of understanding, carefully assessing whether the patient is ready to move to the contemplation stage (i.e., to consider the association between stressors and somatic symptoms). However, pushing a patient along the stages too fast may only alienate the patient and harm the doctor–patient relationship, making the patient feel misunderstood, depressed, or angry. The main tasks at the precontemplation stage are acknowledging the patient's suffering and symptoms and establishing a cooperative patient–clinician working alliance. Hearing another person (especially a clinician) reiterate the patient's main complaint can be a powerful validation. The clinician may say: "You have been in a lot of pain for many years." Open-ended questions about symptoms and stressors are more helpful than statements. Instead of saying "Your GI problems can be related to the stress of losing your job," the clinician may ask, "Did your GI symptoms increase in the last month? What else was going on in your life at that time?" Patients are more likely to incorporate new understanding of the link between stressors and symptoms into their view of the world if they arrive at those conclusions by themselves.

The clinician's best stance at the *contemplation stage* is to invite the patient to be on a team of investigators regarding his or her condition. This demonstrates interest in the patient's experience, validates the presence of somatic symptoms, and models a genuine curiosity regarding links between somatic symptoms and experiences. After all, with no laboratory findings to confirm SSD, we can never have 100% certainty about the diagnosis. However, we can

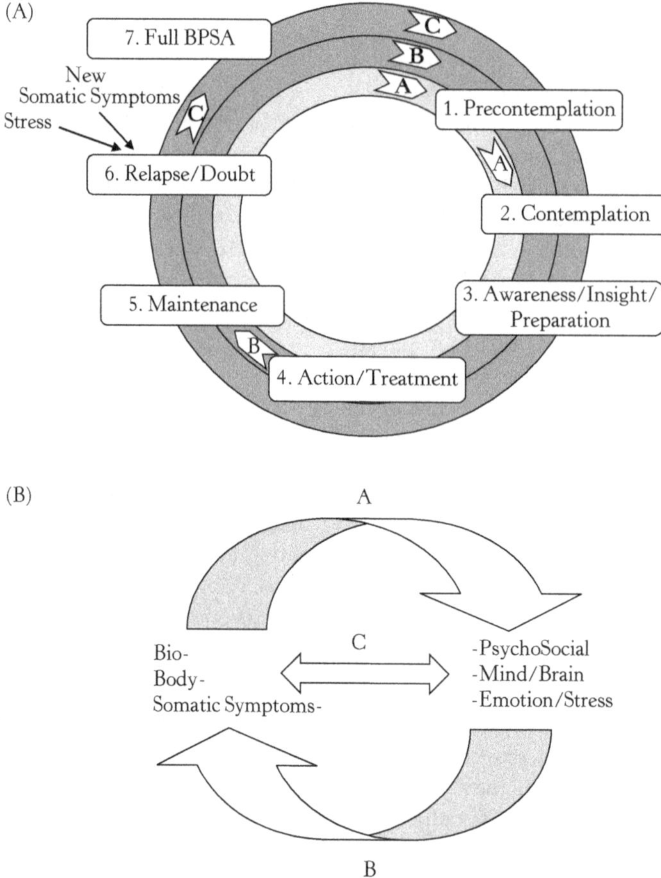

FIGURE 16.1. Columbia Stages (A) and Levels (B) of Biopsychosocial Awareness (CS-BPSA) model overview.

(A) Key for stages of BPSA.

Stages	*Description of Person's Current Views*
1. Precontemplation	Mind/brain-body dualism: there is no relationship between body and mind/brain
2. Contemplation	Considering possibility of A, B, and/or C level mind/brain-body relationships
3. Awareness/Insight/Preparation	Biopsychosocial awareness (BPSA) at A, B, and/or C level; preparation for treatment or action
4. Action/Treatment	Treatment engagement at A, B, or C levels, application of BPSA in life
5. Maintenance	Continued application of BPSA in life
6. Relapse/Doubt	Going back in stages or levels, often occurs with increase of stress or new somatic symptoms
7. Full BPSA	Level C awareness re all SS; applies level C BPSA to new SS, even under stress
(B) Key for Levels of BPSA.	
Levels	
A	Somatic symptoms can affect mood/functioning/level of stress
B	Psychosocial stress/emotion/brain can affect somatic symptoms and the body
C	Bidirectional relationship between Bio/Body/Somatic symptoms and Emotion/Mind/Brain/Stress

TABLE 16.1. COLUMBIA STAGES OF BIOPSYCHOSOCIAL AWARENESS RATING FORM (CS-BPSA-R) AND EXAMPLE OF ASSESSMENT

CS-BPSA-S—RATING FORM

Instructions: Please use the Clinician's Form below to code each symptom separately on both Stage of BPSA and Level of BPSA (only Precontemplation is not associated with a Level of BPSA). Each coding is *symptom specific*: each somatic symptom may be at a different *Stage* of BPSA and at a different *Level* of biopsychosocial integration. Level C awareness is not necessary for engagement in treatment or successful outcome. A patient may stay at level A or B awareness his/her whole life, but benefit from treatments that meet him/her at that level. Intervention for each somatic symptomhas to match current Stage and Level of BPSA. Optimal zone/focus of work during evaluation and treatment is moving one step at a time between the Levels (A, B, C) and/or Stages.

Patient's Name ____________ Date ________ Rated by ____________

	Levels of Integration				Patient's Perspective
Stages of BPSA	None	A	B	C	
1. Pre-contemplation	back pain				"Caused by disk problem," "does not have anything to do with any other aspect of wellbeing, mood, relationships". Patient denies observable correlation of back pain and moments of unexpressed anger
2. Contemplation		headaches			Considers possibility that headaches at night are contributing to insomnia and feeling tired next day
3. Awareness/Insight/ Preparation				GI symptoms	Realization that GI symptoms start with increase of anxiety, and then fear of GI cancer increases anxiety and GI symptoms
4. Action			shortness of breath during panic attack		"Caused by anxiety"—scheduled appointment with psychiatrist; but no recognition of panic attacks affecting worsening relationship with children due to avoidance of activities
5. Maintenance				fatigue and lack of energy	Aware of the following vicious cycle and acts on breaking it: fatigue and lack of energy is associated with feeling alone and memories of being abandoned by parents; fatigue leads to withdrawal from social interaction with friends and boyfriend, which leads to deepening of the feelings of aloneness. When feeling this way patient now reaches out to friends, boyfriend, and/or psychotherapist, which alleviates both feelings of abandonment and fatigue.
6. Relapse/doubt		difficulty concentrating			Presents with new fear that previously identified symptom of depression is an early sign of Alzheimer's disease
7. Full BSPA					

track temporal relationships between symptoms and life experiences, look for patterns at the macro (years, months) and micro (minutes, hours, days) levels, and integrate this knowledge with the research studies of patients with similar presentations. A comprehensive multidisciplinary evaluation (described subsequently) helps patients in the precontemplation and the contemplation stages move towards the awareness, preparation, and action stages.

Once any level of BPSA (A, B, or C) is reached, the patient moves into the *awareness, insight, and preparation stage,* which involves considering putting BPSA into action. A collaborative approach to treatment planning increases the likelihood of the plan implementation by a patient. Inquiring about the patient's thoughts, feelings, and expectations provides an opportunity to dispel myths about treatments that are often not accurate. The *action/treatment stage* involves starting a psychosomatic treatment or implementing BPSA in everyday life (see examples in Table 16.1).

Once a person reaches BPSA regarding a symptom, the *maintenance stage* usually requires an active approach to supporting patient's BPSA (e.g., continued assessment by clinicians, or participation in BPSA-promoting activities). *Relapse* back to a lack of BPSA can happen at any stage and regarding one or all symptoms. New symptoms or stressors are particularly susceptible to relapse. For example, a patient who already learned that his GI symptoms are associated with anxiety may present in the precontemplation stage with the new onset of back pain. Therefore, ongoing work on relapse prevention in the maintenance stage is important.

Using the CS-BPSA Model

The CS-BPSA Rating form (see Table 16.1) can be used during diagnosis and treatment planning and for tracking the patient's progress. The optimal zone of intervention during the moment-to-moment interactions with patients is usually one level or stage away from the patient's current BPSA. Jumping over a level or stage can alienate a patient and lead to a rupture in the patient–clinician relationship. A patient may be at different levels and stages of BPSA regarding different symptoms (see the examples in Table 16.1). Progress in treatment and symptom alleviation, however, often happens before a full BPSA is achieved, and some patients may become asymptomatic without ever achieving compete BPSA.

4. A Multidisciplinary Team Approach Is Essential

"It takes a village . . ." An ideal team may include a variety of primary care providers (e.g., physician, physician assistant, nurse practitioner), nurses, behavioral health specialists (e.g., psychiatrist, psychologist, clinical social worker), a care manager, a mind–body therapist, a physical therapist, a nutritionist, and/or a sleep specialist. The team may be permanent (i.e., a core team of the clinic is preferred), or, if that is not feasible, the team can be created as a "team without walls" in which specialists relevant to treating a particular patient (e.g., GI, infectious disease, pain physician) collaborate via phone, electronic medical records, telebehavioral health, and so forth. (See Chapter 9: Telehealth in an Integrated Care Environment for discussion about virtual teams.) Regular multidisciplinary team case conferences are essential.

For patients, the very fact of primary care and behavioral health integration communicates the biopsychosocial approach to health and disease. Mind–body dualism might, however, still creep in. For example, a common view of a medical care as *primary* and mental health as *supplementary/optional* can be perceived by patients as implicit communication of *biological* being much more important than *psychological*. Genuine respectful collaboration, as seen in an integrated care team, validates the unity of biopsychosocial factors for the patient.

Many patients with somatic symptoms or IA feel a lack of control over their bodies and lives, which increases their distress and exacerbates somatic symptoms. Engaging patients as part of an integrated care team is essential, as it restores their feelings of agency and promotes self-awareness and responsibility. Asking open-ended questions (e.g., "What are your goals?" "What treatments do you believe will help?" "What are your fears?"), inviting the patient's feedback, and developing a treatment plan in an interactive way is therapeutic. It is also important to let patients know that they can and will see different members of an integrated care team.

5. Changing the Culture of a Clinic and Health Care Organization to Adopt Full BPSA

Moving organizations along BPSA stages of change and implementing the principles described herein requires commitment at the team and organization (e.g., clinic, hospital) levels. The following methods may facilitate this change: (1) create a BPSA-informed organizational structure (e.g., by including the primary care and behavioral health professionals in the team and by organizing regular multidisciplinary team meetings); (2) train all staff in the BPSA model and its clinical applications; (3) disseminate information about the latest research on the diagnosis and treatment of somatic symptoms and IA; and (4) develop interactive trainings, including role plays of clinical scenarios, that help the team learn how colleagues from other disciplines think, and how they interact with patients, in order to develop a unified and cohesive way of treating patients as a team.

A BPSA culture also includes recognition of the burnout and stress among health care professionals. Patients suffering from somatic symptoms or IA are particularly difficult to treat. Professionals caring for these patients often develop feelings of helplessness and frustration, as well as empathic emotional and bodily reactions. Processing these reactions with colleagues, in a group setting, can prevent burnout, contribute positively to clinicians' heath, and promote BPSA-informed self-awareness. Onsite training for clinic staff in mind–body techniques (e.g., mindfulness training or relaxation techniques) helps their well-being and enhances the BPSA culture of the clinic.

Language is an integral aspect of culture. It is important to explore which terms for somatic symptoms and IA are currently best accepted by the local community of patients and health care professionals. At the same time, patients and providers need to be educated about the actual meaning of the terms they may hear (e.g., that *psychosomatic* does *not* mean "it's all in your head"). While adopting acceptable terms, it is important to not avoid or be apologetic about using the term *psychological*, as doing so indirectly communicates that the term has derogatory meaning and implicitly promotes mind–body dualism. In fact, it is best not to divide factors into *medical/biological* and *psychological*. Currently, in many cultures, referring to the "brain" and the "nervous system" provides an easily understandable bridge between the "bodily" and "psychological" as people tend to readily accept that the brain is involved in psychological processes, yet at the same time is an organ of our body, which controls other bodily functions.

6. The Quality of Patient–Clinician Relationship Is an Essential Treatment Component

Patients with somatic symptoms and IA often crave care and interpersonal connection. Many of them grew up in challenging interpersonal environments and continue to experience interpersonal distress and loneliness, expecting others to hurt, ignore, or abandon them.[8] Repeated experiences of having their symptoms discredited as imaginary reinforce their distrustful interpersonal worldview and exacerbate interpersonal sensitivity and somatic symptoms. Continuously fearing rejection, they are particularly attuned to nonverbal and implicit interpersonal cues. Unfortunately, clinicians often react negatively to patients suffering with somatic symptoms and IA. One study reported that the single greatest factor that led a physician to suspect hypochondriasis in a patient was the degree of frustration in treating that patient.[21] Videotapes of PCPs interviewing somatoform pain patients revealed split-second facial expressions of disgust. Breaking the vicious cycle of interpersonal distress and exacerbation of somatic symptoms is highly therapeutic. In fact, a recent study showed that a physician's patient-oriented interview style affected activity in pain-modulating brain regions.[22]

Patient–clinician communication styles vary by team member and country. If maintaining professional distance with a patient is a cultural norm, it might be advisable to modify this enculturated style toward a more personable, warm, and engaged approach, as professional distance might be perceived as lack of care by a sensitive patient. Being listened to and validated by all team members (i.e., front desk to medical and specialist staff) are vital human needs that frequently are unmet among patients with somatic symptoms and IA. Giving patients their voices, as much as possible, will start reversing their experience of feeling invalidated/not heard by physicians, team members, friends, and family.

Primary care clinicians, and ultimately the team, are advised to be transparent with somatic symptoms or IA patients about what diagnoses were ruled out and why, and to cite specific research that is being considered when thinking about the patient. Sharing the team's reasoning and treatment plan with the patient shows the thoughtfulness that went into making a recommendation, helps a patient experience being cared for, and models the biopsychosocial way of thinking.

7. Including Translational Research Findings in Education of Patients and Clinicians

Symptoms of SSD and IA are often surrounded by a mystique and raise the questions "Are they real? How do they magically appear in the absence of any detectable peripheral damage or disease?" Unfortunately, in many cultures *psychosomatic* still means "not real" or "imagined." Neuroscience research indicates that validity of somatic symptoms should no longer be questioned: Musculoskeletal pain, GI, neurologic, and other bodily symptoms can be experienced without findings of peripheral abnormalities. Numerous studies showed that somatic symptoms are associated with dysregulation of neural circuits in the brain; changes in brain neurochemistry and immune functions; emotions and stress that can modulate physical pain on a neural level and can affect health in humans and animals; and the quality of the early environment, which affects development of the brain and other systems of the organism.[8,23,24] These findings help demystify SSD and IA syndromes, providing both patients and their treatment teams tangible information that can decrease anxiety caused by "unexplained symptoms, for unknown reasons, with uncertain future," as well as increase the clinician's confidence when recommending psychosocial (i.e., neuromodulating) treatments for somatic symptoms, as these treatments affect neural circuits and neurotransmitter systems in the brain. Research-based psychoeducation is critical.

Organization of Care

The current state of SSD and IA treatment varies among countries.[2] While several countries have guidelines for the treatment of specific symptoms (e.g., chronic pain or fibromyalgia), specialized guidelines for the organization of care and treatment of SSD and IA patients are rare. Germany[25] and the Netherlands[26] issued comprehensive guidelines based on the systematic review of the latest evidence. The Dutch Multidisciplinary Guideline for Medically Unexplained Symptoms, commissioned by the Dutch Ministry of Public Health, Welfare, and Sport, was published in 2011.[26] In 2012, the third edition of the Guidelines for Management of Patients with Non-specific, Functional, and Somatoform Bodily Complaints was issued in Germany.[25] It was developed by a special taskforce organized by the German College of Psychosomatic Medicine and the German Society of Psychosomatic Medicine and Medical Psychotherapy, which consisted of the representatives of 28 medical and psychological societies who reached a multidisciplinary consensus on assessment and treatment guidelines. Recommendations presented here are based on the integration of those guidelines and research conducted since they were published.

Systems Approach to Establishing Integrated Care for SSD and IA

Overwhelming evidence points to the need for radical reorganization of fragmented health care approaches to SSD and IA. This reorganization needs to be in accord with the evidence from neuroscience for the crucial role of the central nervous system in health and disease. International consensus suggests that the following organization of care is essential for the effective identification, diagnosis, and treatment of SSD and IA: (1) creation of specialized psychosomatic clinics, (2) integration of primary care and specialty psychosomatic/behavioral health care, and (3) a stepped-care approach to treatment.[2,14,25,26] The following steps (or levels) of care are suggested: (1) multidisciplinary collaborative care within the primary care clinic; (2) multidisciplinary care in primary care clinic in combination with outpatient psychosomatic/BHS treatment (e.g., individual and/or group psychotherapy); and (3) intensive psychosomatic day-treatment and inpatient programs in collaboration with primary care.

Implementation of these changes may seem unrealistic in the current climate of the primary care medicine/mental health divide, especially given the shortage of health care resources in many countries. However, the new model of integrated care offers hope. Studies demonstrate that an integrated approach not only results in effective treatment of somatic symptoms and IA, but also dramatically decreases health care costs and disability, as well as inefficient use of resources and physician–patient time. Patients with somatic symptoms and IA represent a large proportion of visits in primary care, neurology, pain, GI, other medical clinics, and emergency departments. The cost of such inefficient care is enormous. For example, medical care costs of SSD in the United States in 2002 were estimated at $256 billion, an amount nearly double the $132 billion cost of diabetes care that year.[1] The overall societal costs almost double health care costs as they include disability and decreased productivity, which are highly prevalent among untreated SSD and IA patents.[27]

The cost and resource effectiveness of providing specialized psychosomatic care was documented in a number of studies in several countries.[27] For example, in Chile, a randomized controlled trial of Brief Family Intervention (one to three sessions) among 256 somatoform patients decreased health care cost at the 1-year-follow-up by 97% versus no change in the treatment-as-usual control group ($p < .0001$, $d = .8$).[28] (See Chapter 27: Best Practice for Family-Centered Health Care: A Three-Step Model for additional information about a family therapy approach.) Among 216 patients with fibromyalgia in Spain, psychoeducation intervention significantly decreased pain, improved global and physical functioning, and demonstrated cost utility of the intervention versus usual care.[29] In a Canadian emergency department study, treating 50 patients with medically unexplained symptoms with a short-term dynamic therapy (averaging 3.8 sessions and $438/patient) reduced emergency department visits by 69% and costs by $910/patient.[30] In Germany, treatment for somatic symptoms comprising 10 weekly group sessions conducted by the PCP and psychosomatic specialists/BHS decreased the severity of somatic symptoms, psychosocial distress, and the number of visits to a PCP.[31] (See Chapter 28: Group Interventions in Integrated Care Settings for additional information about groups.) In the Netherlands, a randomized controlled trial of a collaborative-care model, which included training for primary care clinicians and a psychiatric consultation for patients with persistent medically unexplained symptoms, showed a 58% decrease in somatic symptoms and a significant reduction in health care use.[32]

In a number of countries, including the United States, the health care payers (e.g., Medicare and private health insurance companies) have initiated and promoted transition to accountable care models (enabling collaborative multidisciplinary care as opposed to the traditional fee-for-service model), which are being rewarded financially.[33] (See Chapter 6: Financing Integrated Care Models.) This shift makes the resource-intensive in-depth multidisciplinary assessments described in this chapter not only financially feasible but advantageous.

Specialized psychosomatic services that collaborate with other medical and psychiatric departments in a hospital are essential. Has this been done? In Germany, almost every university hospital has a specialized psychosomatic department. In 2007, there were 151 of them throughout the country, treating about 50,000 patients.[2] Psychosomatic clinic staff members provide education to other medical specialties regarding the diagnosis and treatment of somatic symptoms and IA, which contributes to implementation of a BPSA culture in a hospital or health care system and helps move patients along the steps of care. In Denmark, the staff of the Research Clinic for Functional Disorders and Psychosomatics gradually educated their medical colleagues throughout the hospital in recognizing the somatic symptoms and IA and facilitating somatic symptoms/IA-focused treatments.[34] An innovative collaborative care program in Germany brings psychosomatic care to the workplace, which increases early detection and intervention for somatic symptoms and IA.[35]

While transition to electronic medical records may have increased efficiency in providing health care for many other diagnoses, this is not yet the case with SSD and IA. Providers tend not to enter SSD and IA diagnoses into the electronic medical record. Those who do may enter any of the terms used to described somatic symptoms and IA, hindering reliable tracking of these conditions. Reluctance to enter a diagnosis of SSD or IA into the electronic medical record may occur for many reasons, one of which is the limited availability of specialized treatments for these disorders. Systematic reorganization of care for SSD and IA should include educating providers about the importance of accurately documenting and tracking these patients' diagnosis and treatment progress.

At a primary care clinic level, the implementation of a stepped-care approach would include the following:

1. Creating a multidisciplinary team of a PCP, a BHS, a physical therapist, a mind–body clinician, and a care manager
2. Establishing collaboration with a psychosomatic and/or behavioral health specialist in the area
3. Training all staff in the BPSA model and in effective clinician–patient communication
4. Developing regular multidisciplinary case conferences
5. Identifying psychoeducational materials about somatic symptoms and IA (handouts, videos, internet resources)
6. Organizing time-limited or ongoing psychoeducational groups
7. Setting up mind–body therapy groups or establishing collaboration with existing ones
8. Setting up a system for periodic check-ins with patients by a care manager.

Necessary steps include establishing close collaboration between primary care and a specialized psychosomatic clinic/other BHS providers. Psychosomatic medicine/behavioral health clinicians can participate in multidisciplinary evaluations in primary care to (1) contribute to diagnosis and treatment planning, (2) facilitate continuity of care if transition to specialized treatment is needed, and (3) provide additional expertise in treating particularly challenging cases.

Care Pathways

The level of care recommended for a particular patient depends on (1) the severity of somatic symptoms and illness anxiety; (2) the level and stage of the patient's BPSA; (3) medical and psychiatric comorbidities; (4) acute versus chronic stressors (e.g., bereavement within a month of death of a loved one vs. years of loneliness); and (5) developmental predisposing factors (e.g., well-developed emotional awareness and no early developmental traumas vs. a profound lack of emotional awareness and growing up in an emotionally abusive environment). The PCP's involvement at every step is crucial for the continuity of care (see Fig. 16.2 for an overview of the care pathways).

Evaluation for Somatic Symptoms and Illness Anxiety

Up to 49% of visits to primary care clinics are associated with somatic symptoms,[5] and other patients may have psychosocial factors contributing to their medical conditions. Therefore, any initial visit to primary care would benefit from psychosomatic assessment. Self-report somatic symptoms screening scales (Tables 16.2 and 16.3) can be administered to all patients presenting to a clinic, and patients scoring high on these measures can then be seen by both primary care and behavioral health practitioners at an early stage of evaluation. As there is no clear consensus that any one or several screening instruments are better than other(s), individual practices will need to make their own choices depending on their context and goals. These scales are particularly helpful in picking up multiple somatic symptoms that are common is SSD and help differentiate between SSD and IA, for which patients usually present with one primary complaint.[25,36,37] Box 16.2 summarizes the issues to be addressed during the initial evaluation by the interdisciplinary team. Because somatic symptoms often require additional medical workup or review of medical records, the initial evaluation may take more than one visit. Evaluation visits to rule out other medical causes and arrive at an SSD or IA diagnosis should be closely spaced.

Somatic symptoms and IA occurring exclusively in the context of another psychiatric disorder usually dissipate once the underlying condition is treated. When referring a patient to psychiatry/psychology, it is important to stress a collaborative team-oriented treatment plan, saying: "Dr. B and other members of the team will work together to help you; you will see Dr. B and other members of the team on a regular basis" to minimize the chance that the patient will feel dismissed or handed over. If somatic symptoms and anxiety persist beyond successful treatment of the other neuropsychiatric condition, the steps recommended for primary SSD/IA should be followed.

In the case of mild somatic symptoms/anxiety, acute stressors, and/or a high stage of BPSA, patients can be effectively treated in primary care with psychoeducation (by a BHS, primary care clinician, or nurse), with reassurance from the PCP, time-limited individual or group sessions by the BHS, and/or a mind–body group. In the case of moderate to severe symptoms, a chronic or complicated course, developmental predisposition, and/or a low BPSA level or stage, a comprehensive multidisciplinary evaluation is recommended (Fig. 16.2).

Comprehensive Multi-Disciplinary Evaluation (CMDE)

Usually, the CMDE is conducted in a primary care clinic or in an integrated practice. If it occurs in a psychosomatic clinic, the primary care team takes part in the evaluation. The CDME is both assessment and the first stage of treatment. Headed by a PCP and BHS, a team relevant to the patient's somatic symptoms is assembled, and a care manager is assigned. A thorough critical review of medical records for any potentially missed diagnoses or necessary diagnostic assessments is conducted.[9] Fragmented care by multiple physicians actually puts somatic symptoms and IA patients at risk for missed diagnoses. In a semistructured diagnostic interview with the patient (see Table 16.2), the clinician comprehensively reviews all symptoms and systems and then conducts a Comprehensive Symptoms and Experiences Timeline (CSET) interview (Box 16.3). If it is not feasible for the PCP and the BHS to interview a patient together, one clinician conducts parts of CDME, the other team members are informed about the details of the interview, and the patient is made aware of this.

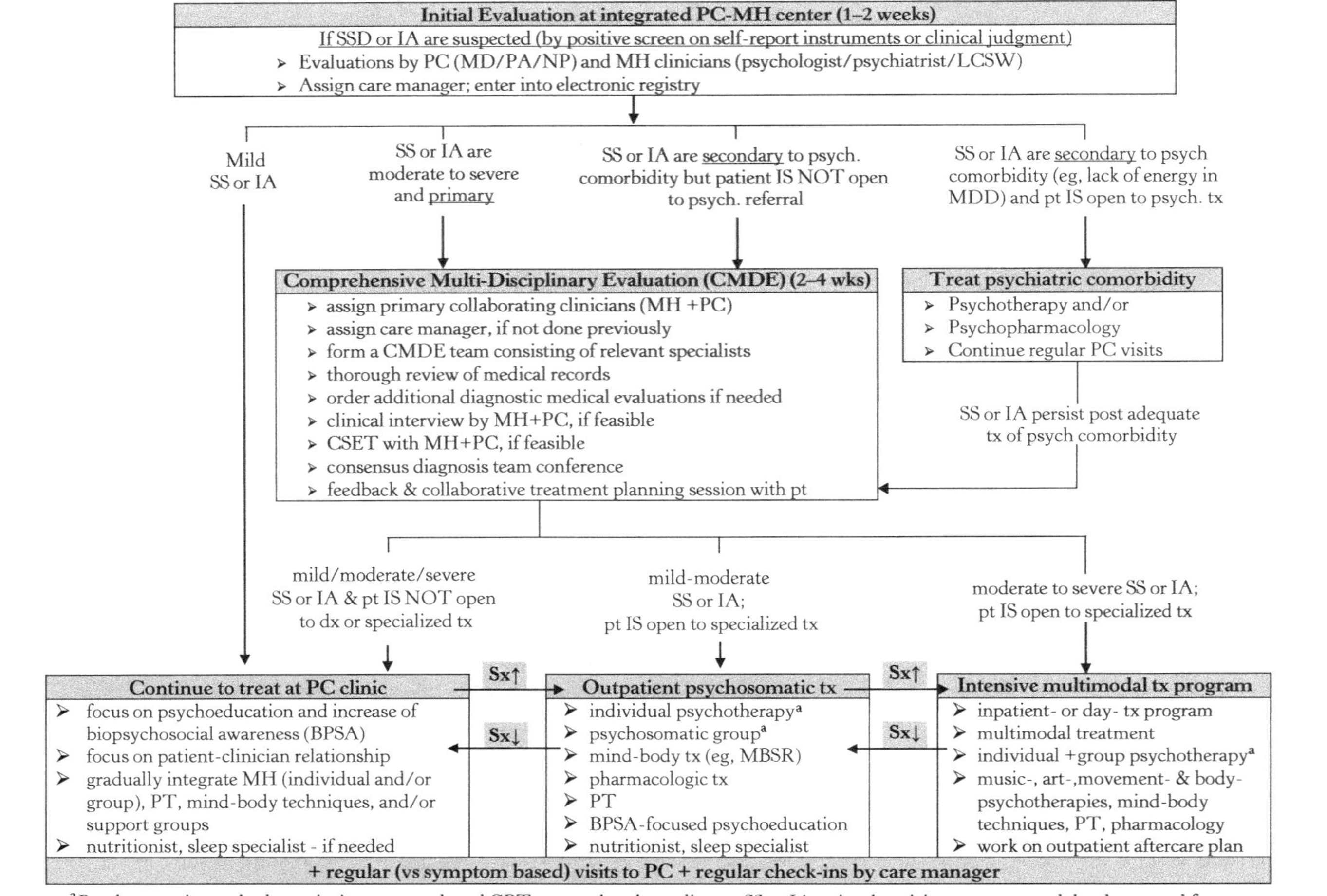

[a]Psychosomatic psychodynamic, interpersonal, and CBT approaches depending on SS vs IA ratio, chronicity, stressors, and developmental factors

Abbreviations: CBT, cognitive behavioral therapy; CSET, comprehensive symptoms and experiences timeline; IA, illness anxiety; LCSW, licensed clinical social worker; MBSR, mindfulness-based stress reduction; MD, doctor of medicine; MDD, major depressive disorder; MH, mental health; NP, nurse practitioner; PA, physician assistant; PC, primary care; pt, patient; PT, physical therapy; SS, somatic symptoms; sx, symptoms; tx, treatment

FIGURE 16.2. Critical pathways for stepped-care treatment approach to SSD and IA.

TABLE 16.2. SELECTED RELEVANT ASSESSMENT INSTRUMENTS

Purpose/Domain	Time Points	Instruments	Time to Administer	Completed by
Screening for somatic symptom disorder (SSD) and illness anxiety (IA)[a]	Intake	Patient Health Questionnaire (PHQ-15)[38]	1–2 min	Patient
		Screening for Somatoform Symptoms-7 (SOMS-7 or SOMS-2)[39]	3–5 min	Patient
		Bodily Distress Syndrome (BDS) Checklist[40]	3 min	Patient
		Whiteley Index for hypochondriasis[41] (WI-14, WI-7)	5 min	Patient
		Fibromyalgia Screening Scale[42]	3 min	Patient
Diagnosis of SSD & IA	Comprehensive Multidisciplinary Evaluation (CDME), mental health evaluation	Structured Clinical Interview (SCID) for DSM-5[43]		Clinician
		-- SSD and IA modules only	5–15 min	
		-- Comprehensive DSM-5 diagnosis	30–90 min	
		Schedules for Clinical Assessment in Neuropsychiatry (SCAN) for ICD-10 & DSM-IV[44b]		Clinician
		-- SS and IA modules only	5–15 min	
		-- Comprehensive psychiatric diagnosis	30–90 min	
		MINI for DSM-IV[45]		Clinician
		-- Somatoform disorders module	5–10 min	
		-- Comprehensive DSM-IV diagnosis	20–40 min	
Somatic symptoms type and severity	Initial visit; CMDE; periodic assessments during treatment	PHQ-15[38]	1–2 min	Patient
		SOMS-2 or SOMS-7[39]	3–5 min	Patient
		Brief Pain Inventory (BPI)[46 c]	5 min	Patient
IA severity, dimensions, and insight into illness	CMDE; periodic assessments during treatment	WI-14, WI-7[41]	3 min	Patient
		Hypochondriasis Yale-Brown Obsessive Compulsive Scale Modified (H-YBOCS-M): semistructured interview & self-report[47]	20–45 min	Clinician & patient
SSD vs. IA differential diagnosis	Initial visit; CMDE	Columbia Somatic Symptoms vs Illness Anxiety Ratio (CSS-IAR)[18 d]	3 min	Clinician or patient
Current biopsychosocial awareness (BPSA)	Initial visit; CMDE; throughout treatment	Columbia Stages of BioPsychoSocial Awareness Rating (CS-BPSA-RS)[48 d]	3 min	Clinician

Early life environment and stressors[a]	CMDE	Childhood Trauma Questionnaire (CTQ)[49a]	3 min	Patient
		Parental Bonding Instrument (PBI)[50]	5 min	Patient
Lifelong trauma[a]	CMDE	Life Events Checklist (LEC)[51a]	5 min	Patient
Current interpersonal well-being[a]	CMDE	UCLA Loneliness Scale[52a]	3 min	Patient
Developmental trajectory; association of life stressors and somatic symptoms; family history of somatic symptoms	CMDE; beginning of treatment	Comprehensive Symptoms and Experiences Timeline (CSET) [d]	45 min to several sessions	Clinician with patient

[a]Multiple other relevant measures are available or may be in development.
[b]Available at http://whoscan.org/wp-content/uploads/2014/10/xinterview.pdf
[c]Contact Dr. Charles S. Cleeland at symptomresearch@mdanderson.org
[d]Contact Dr. Alla Landa at AL2898@cumc.columbia.edu

TABLE 16.3. CRITICAL CARE PATHWAYS FOR SOMATIC SYMPTOMS AND ILLNESS ANXIETY

Stages and Steps of Care	Patient Characteristics	Team Members and Timeline	Helpful Instruments[a,b]	Goals of Integrated Team	Issues/Questions
Screening for SSD and IA at primary care	All primary care intakes	Part of initial intake paperwork given by office receptionist 10 min, pre-evaluation visit	PHQ-15[38] SOMS-2 or SOMS-7[39] Whiteley Index for hypochondriasis (WI-14, WI-7)[41]	Identification of patients with possible somatic symptoms or IA	Positive screens to be flagged and followed up by primary care clinician
Initial evaluation for SS/IA at primary care	Patients who screened positive on self-report measures and those with suspected SSD or IA during clinical evaluation	PCP, BHS, care manager 1 or 2 visits	CSS-IA Ratio Scale[18] BPI (body image for pain localizations; visual analog scale for pain; Pain Disability Index)[46] Symptom checklists (WHO-5, BSI, SCL-90R) H-YBOCS-M[47] Mood & somatic symptoms diary Functioning: SF-36, 12, 8	Diagnosis Evaluation of BPSA Begin psychoeducation Begin treatment planning	Was a thorough medical workup competed? Relative somatic symptoms vs. IA contribution? Acute vs. chronic? Recent stressors? Are somatic symptoms/IA primary or secondary to depression or anxiety disorder? Severity? Is CMDE warranted?
Comprehensive Multidisciplinary Evaluation (CMDE)	Somatic symptoms or IA are (1) suspected to be primary; OR (2) are secondary to psychiatric comorbidity but patient is NOT open to psychiatric referral; OR (3) persist after adequate treatment of psychiatric comorbidity	PCP, BHS, care manager, medical specialists relevant to somatic symptoms; consider including a specialist in psychosomatics 2–4 visits over 2–4 weeks	PHQ15,[38] SOMS-2 or SOMS-7,[39] WI-14 or WI-7[41] if not done during screening; Diagnostic Interview (SCID,[43] SCAN,[44] MINI[45]) Brief Pain Inventory[46] Symptom checklists (WHO-5, BSI, SCL-90R) Mood & somatic symptoms diary Functioning: SF-36, 12, 8 Loneliness scale[52] CTQ, PBI[50] CSET	Diagnosis Evaluation of BPSA CSET to increase BPSA Psychoeducation Increase in BPSA Collaborative treatment planning	Was thorough medical workup completed? Relative somatic symptoms vs. IA contribution? Acute vs. chronic? Recent and lifetime stressors? Are somatic symptoms/IA primary or secondary to depression or anxiety disorder? Severity? CSET and MSET interventions to increase BPSA and motivate for treatment Collaborative treatment planning
Referral to treat psychiatric comorbidity	Somatic symptoms or IA are secondary to psychiatric comorbidity (e.g., lack of energy due to depression) and patient IS open to psychiatric treatment	PCP; psychiatrist and/or psychologist or clinical social worker 1 session after initial evaluation or during CMDE	Mood & somatic symptoms diary SOMS-2, SOMS-7[39] WI-14/7[41] BPI[46] General symptom measure (BSI, SCL90, WHO5) to monitor progress	Treatment of other underlying neuropsychiatric disorder	Primary care and mental health specialists continue to work as a team. If somatic symptoms or IA persist after depression or anxiety is treated, reconsider SSD/IA as primary; consider CMDE.

Treat SSD/IA at primary care clinic	1. Mild SSD or IA; OR patient is NOT open to diagnosis or specialized treatment 2. Patient is in remission after specialized psychosomatic treatment	PCP, BHS, care manager; psychotherapy and mind–body clinicians; physical therapist; nutritionist and sleep specialist, if needed At least 6 months, then reassess; work on relapse prevention is ongoing	Mood & somatic symptoms diary SOMS-2, SOMS-7[39] WI-14/7[41] BPI[46] General symptom measure (BSI, SCL90, WHO5) to monitor progress	Psychoeducation Increase in BPSA Engage in physical therapy, mind–body treatments, psychotherapy	Primary care and mental health specialists continue to work as a team. Care manager is involved in care. Regular multidisciplinary team rounds
Outpatient psychosomatic treatment with regular primary care visits	1. Mild or moderate 2. SSD/IA & patient is open to specialized treatment	PCP, care manager, specialists in psychosomatic clinic At least 30 sessions	Mood & somatic symptoms diary SOMS-2, SOMS-7[39] WI-14/7[41] BPI[46] General symptom measure (BSI, SCL90, WHO5) to monitor progress	Primary care support Maintain continuity of care once psychosomatic treatment stops. Relapse prevention	Integrated primary care/mental health team works together with psychosomatic program.
Intensive multimodal psychosomatic treatment program (day treatment or inpatient program)	1. Moderate to severe SSD or IA, patient is open to specialized treatment	PCP, care manager, multidisciplinary psychosomatic treatment team 2–3 months	Mood & somatic symptoms diary SOMS-2, SOMS-7[39] WI-14/7[41] BPI[46] General symptom measure (BSI, SCL90, WHO5) to monitor progress	Primary care support Maintain continuity of care once psychosomatic treatment stops. Relapse prevention	Integrated primary care/mental health team works together with psychosomatic program.

[a]Names of many of these instruments are given in full in Table 16.2.
[b]Instruments to use in a particular setting to be chosen with both usefulness and feasibility in mind.
Additional abbreviations: BPI, Brief Pain Inventory; BPSA, biopsychosocial awareness; BSI, Brief Symptom Inventory; CMDE, Comprehensive Multidisciplinary Diagnostic Evaluation; H-YBOCS-M, Hypochondriasis-Yale Brown Obsessive Compulsive Scale—Modified; MINI, International Neuropsychiatric Interview; PBI, Parental Bonding Index, SCAN, Schedules for Clinical Assessment in Neuropsychiatry; SCID, Structured Clinical Interview for DSM; SCL-90, Symptom Checklist; MOS SF-36, Medical Outcomes Study Short Form; WHO, World Health Organization.

BOX 16.2

ISSUES TO BE ADDRESSED DURING INITIAL EVALUATION BY THE INTERDISCIPLINARY TEAM

- **Have all medical problems been thoroughly evaluated and ruled out?**
- **Is the SSD or IA of recent onset? Can the triggering stressor(s) be identified?**
- **Are somatic symptoms or IA occurring exclusively in the context of another neuropsychiatric disorder?**
- **If yes, is the patient in treatment or willing to receive treatment for this disorder? (Guidelines for treating that neuropsychiatric disorder are to be followed, while educating the patient that somatic symptoms are common symptoms of that disorder.)**
- **What is the relative contribution of SSD versus IA? (Columbia Somatic Symptoms Versus Illness Anxiety Ratio [CSSIAR] scale, Table 16.1)**
- **Is the IA patient avoidant of medical tests or care?**
- **What is the patient's current level and stage of BPSA? (See Fig. 16.1.)**
- **Is IA or SS a culturally syntonic mode of affect expression?**
- **Conduct a thorough review of all systems and symptoms, including a symptom checklist (Table 16.1). SS patients often come in with one most distressing symptom (e.g., pain), but when questioned directly reveal other symptoms (e.g., gastrointestinal disturbance, sensitivity to sensory stimuli, fatigue, or insomnia) that significantly contribute to functioning and well-being. This information may also provide additional evidence for a central sensitization syndrome.**
- **Assess which symptoms limit functioning and cause most distress in order to choose the initial focus of treatment.**
- **Schedule regular follow-up appointments (not symptom-dependent).**

While a time-consuming procedure, CSET is both a diagnostic tool and a powerful intervention to enhance BPSA, identify stressors and developmental factors, and engage the patient in treatment planning. Though devoting so much time to one patient is not customary for PCPs in many countries, this investment of time actually proves time saving for future primary care visits.[31] While ideally CSET is done by medical staff (physician or nurse practitioner) and BHS together, in many settings this it is not feasible. In this case, after the physician or nurse practitioner goes over medical aspects of evaluation, the BHS can do the CSET part, making sure that the patient is aware that the medical staff will be informed of the data collected and that the diagnosis and treatment plan will be made by the multidisciplinary team.

CSET consists of plotting all somatic symptoms and life experiences on a whole-life timeline in order to explore, together with the patient, the patterns of temporal relationships between them (see details in Box 16.3). CSET helps unaware patients discover links between somatic symptoms and stressors, which is a fundamental step in treatment of somatic symptoms and IA.

CMDE involves continuous exploration of the biopsychosocial interactions on macro (whole life), intermediate (daily/weekly), and micro (moment-to-moment) levels. Conducting CMDE over several visits allows exploration of changes in somatic symptoms and the patient's thoughts and feelings since the previous appointment. Sharp changes in somatic symptoms (e.g., increase or decrease of pain) during a session should be immediately followed up with exploration of what the patient has been feeling or thinking. The Micro Symptoms and Experiences Timeline (MSET) (see Box 16.3) provides unique in-the-moment opportunities for increasing BPSA insight, which often takes priority over collecting information. Additionally, self-report measures of early life and current life stressors (see examples of measures in Table 16.2, such as the Childhood Trauma Questionnaire,[49] Life Events Checklist,[53] and Parental Bonding Index[54]) can help

BOX 16.3

COMPREHENSIVE SYMPTOMS AND EXPERIENCES TIMELINE (CSET) AND MICRO SYMPTOMS AND EXPERIENCES TIMELINE (MSET)

CSET

- **CSET to be completed after a clinical interview (once rapport is established), completed in 2 hours or more (in one or two sessions), by the PCP and a BHS together if possible.**
- **Collaboratively developed with the patient: "We are going to do this together"**
- **The interviewer helps the patient feel in control of the timeline process and does not make BPSA interpretations that reveal any preconceived notions. The most profound BPSA intervention is the patient's own discovery of the temporal associations between symptoms and life stressors.**
- **Together interviewer and patient review the patient's whole life and plot all health problems and life experiences, including early and current environment and relationshipson a chalkboard/dry erase board.**
- **First the interviewer draws a vertical line symbolizing time from the patient's birth until today.**
- **Names of important people in patient's early life (parents, siblings, grandparents, nannies) are written above the line, symbolizing importance of familial processes that happened before the patient was born.**
- **The interviewer asks about these people's health and medical problems now and when the patient was growing up and records this information next to the names.**
- **All somatic symptoms from early childhood to now are placed on the right of the timeline; the interviewer carefully asks about the onset and ending of each somatic symptom, and about any other health issues through life starting at birth.**
- **Once onset of a symptom is mentioned, the interviewer may ask: "What was going on in your life at that time?" and record the answer on the other side of the line.**
- **Both positive and negative life experiences are recorded.**
- **The patient's own words are used as much as possible. If a word actually has a slightly different meaning or is a metaphor, the interviewer records the words used by the patient and puts them in quotes—for example, "I felt my world was crashing."**
- **The interviewer pays particular attention to and plots any changes in somatic symptoms or their severity, overall health, life stressors, life transitions, relational changes, and emotional states, always periodically inquiring about others in the patient's life: parents, siblings, romantic relationships, friendships, community, and social roles (e.g., engaged with church, left football team, started peer-support group, moved to different town).**
- **Usually the patient starts noticing temporal patterns. The interviewer clarifies these observations, makes a note of them, and continues exploration.**
- **If this does not occur spontaneously, the interviewer invites the patient to look at the full timeline together and to notice any patterns, first by asking, "What do you see? What jumps out at you?"**
- **The timeline is always a work in progress.**
- **At the end of the session the interviewer makes a photo of the timeline, sends it to the patient, and invites the patient to refer to it during treatment.**

MSET

- **Apply principles of CSET to moment-to-moment or hours-to-days changes in somatic symptoms to assess BPSA and alexithymia, and clarify the diagnosis.**
- **If the patient describes changes in somatic symptoms severity since the last visit, the interviewer asks what the patient was thinking or feeling when the changes occurred. If the patient has difficulty recalling it, the interviewer can help the patient recall the experience by further questioning (e.g., when, where, who were you with), and by exploring feelings and thoughts.**
- **If changes in somatic symptoms occur during the session the interviewer can ask about thoughts and feelings (e.g., "What else are you feeling in your body right now? Show me where you feel it in your body."). This may help identify emotions that were preceding the change in somatic symptoms.**

assess stressors and convey the importance of these factors for health.

The team case conference for consensus diagnosis and treatment planning is followed by a feedback and treatment planning session with the patient. Presenting SSD and IA diagnoses to a patient in a BPSA-sensitive way is challenging. In addition to BPSA-informed communication (previously described), the following components of feedback session are recommended:

1. Validation of symptoms (somatic symptoms and/or anxiety regarding somatic symptoms)
2. Delivery of the diagnosis with a clear explanation of the meaning of SSD or IA labels
3. Asking the patient to explain his or her understanding of the diagnosis to catch any misunderstanding (repeat this during treatment, as relapses in misunderstanding are common)
4. Conveying that treatments exist and getting better is possible, though it may take time
5. A metaphor coined by Dr. Stanley Fahn, a neurologist at Columbia University, of "computer hardware problem versus software problem" is helpful in explaining to a patient that his or her symptom is a result of a problem in the functioning ("software") of the nervous system versus structural ("hardware") damage or disease.
6. Communicate the team's commitment to help the patient and highlight the value of a multidisciplinary approach.

Interactive treatment planning facilitates the patient's commitment to the plan. Practical steps might include the following:

1. Writing out the patient's goals (e.g., decrease pain and loneliness)
2. Clarifying known ways to achieve these goals (e.g., increase activity, decrease opioids, learn to cope with interpersonal stressors)
3. Describing treatments that can help achieve the goals (e.g., favorite physical activity; medication adjustment, initiation of psychotherapy)
4. Outlining the specific steps the patient chooses to take

Treatment for Somatic Symptoms and Illness Anxiety

Treating Somatic Symptoms

Though challenging to treat, somatic symptoms can be alleviated. The quality of life of patients can be improved by multidisciplinary care, specialized individual and group psychotherapies, and medications.[2] Effective pharmacologic interventions focus on central sensitization and regulation of related neurotransmitter systems.[25] Medications that target noradrenergic pathways, such as the tricyclics (e.g., amitriptyline [10–150 mg/day] or cyclobenzaprine [immediate-release 10 tid or extended-release 15–30 mg/day]) or serotonin–norepinephrine reuptake inhibitors (SNRIs; e.g., venlafaxine [150–225 mg/day], duloxetine [60–120 mg/day], or milnacipran [100–200 mg/day]), have been shown to be helpful for fibromyalgia, chronic pain syndromes, and/or neuropathic pain. Medications that target GABA pathways (e.g., pregabalin [300–600 mg/day] and gabapentin [900–3,600 mg/day]) have also been shown to be helpful in reducing centrally mediated pain. Opioids should be avoided as they are not helpful for central pain and can lead to opioid-induced hyperalgesia.[55] There is no unbiased consistent evidence to support the use of selective serotonin reuptake inhibitors (SSRIs) for the treatment of chronic pain syndromes.[56]

Both psychodynamic/interpersonal psychotherapy[36,57,58] and cognitive-behavioral therapy (CBT)[59] have been shown to alleviate somatic symptoms to various degrees,[25] with some evidence pointing to psychodynamic therapies in particular leading to functional improvement.[60] Psychotherapeutic strategies shown to be most helpful are those that focus on emotions and interpersonal relationships, teaching the individual to read somatic emotion cues from the body and to express and regulate emotions in the interpersonal environment. Working through developmental traumas and stress has also been shown to be a key element of treatment.[60] Initial engagement might employ expressive psychotherapies, such as music, art, and/or dance/movement psychotherapies, as these are powerful ways to engage the patient's emotions at a nonverbal level, enhancing the development of self-awareness, symbolization, expression, and regulation of emotions. Because patients with somatic symptoms often have a detached relationship with their own bodies, therapeutic techniques that help develop nonthreatening bodily awareness can be particularly helpful, such as relaxation techniques, breathing therapies, mindfulness meditation (e.g., Mindfulness-Based Stress Reduction), or biofeedback. The combination of individual and group psychotherapy may be particularly helpful for those who suffer from somatic symptoms. Patients with more severe somatic symptoms may require intensive multimodal day-treatment or inpatient programs that incorporate these approaches.[25,61,62] These programs were shown to be effective and to help normalize the functioning of neural circuits in patients with somatic symptoms, as measured by functional magnetic resonance imaging.[61,63]

Treatment Approaches to IA

Optimal treatment consists of integrated care, psychotherapy, and pharmacotherapy.[14] Both individual CBT and group CBT have been shown to be effective in number of studies.[64] A dose–response relationship was observed in CBT treatments, with a greater number of sessions associated with greater improvement. This suggests that the relationship with the therapist might be an important factor that facilitates change.[64] Acceptance and commitment group therapy can reduce IA symptoms.[65] Mindfulness-based interventions, such as deep breathing, progressive muscle relaxation, and meditation, are helpful in reducing symptoms and learning new ways to relate to one's body.[66] SSRIs (fluoxetine, paroxetine) can alleviate IA,[67,68] with higher doses of fluoxetine (40–80 mg) and of paroxetine (40–50 mg) considered to be more effective than lower doses. While there haven't been any controlled trials comparing the efficacy of an SSRI versus an SNRI for illness anxiety, one study of depressed patients[69] that compared an SNRI and an SSRI revealed that the SNRI duloxetine had greater efficacy for symptoms of psychomotor retardation, general somatic symptoms, and sexual problems, while the SSRI sertraline led to greater improvement in agitation, anxiety symptoms, and hypochondriasis. Long-term follow-up studies suggest that improvement in IA is sustained comparably for those treated with either CBT or SSRI therapy.[70]

Organization of Treatment of SSD and IA in Integrated Care Model

For patients with mild somatic symptoms or IA, for those resistant to psychosomatic care, or if there are no BHS/psychosomatic providers in the area, multidisciplinary SSD/IA treatment can be arranged in integrated care settings. Regular (as opposed to symptom-based) appointments, as determined by individual patient needs, are recommended.[2,25] A team of clinicians relevant to the patient's somatic symptoms and level of BPSA is assembled (e.g., PCP, individual and/or group psychotherapists, physical therapist, expressive psychotherapists, mind–body psychotherapists; nutritionist and sleep specialists, if needed). A group intervention conducted by the PCP and BHS/psychosomatic specialist together was shown to be effective for somatic symptoms[31] and is an efficient way of using clinicians' time. Ideally, treatment would involve a combination of individual and group treatment. Continuous psychoeducation delivered in a BPSA-sensitive way is an integral component of treatment. Psychoeducation has to be both general (up-to-date evidence-based information about SSD and IA should be given to all these patients) and personally tailored (information relevant to the patient's current concerns and level of readiness). The following are examples of psychoeducational resources that may be used throughout the treatment:

1. Bodily Distress Syndrome Brochure for Patients. The Research Clinic for Functional Disorders and Psychosomatics at Aarhus University Hospital. http://funktionellelidelser.dk/fileadmin/www.funktionellelidelser.au.dk/patient_Pjecer/7_BDS_information.pdf. Published 2011. Accessed May 25, 2016
2. Educational videos. New South Wales Ministry of Health for and on behalf of the Crown in right of the State of New South Wales. http://www.hnehealth.nsw.gov.au/Pain/Pages/Educational-videos.aspx Accessed May 25, 2016.
3. FibroGuide. Chronic Pain and Fatigue Research Center (CPFRC) at the University of Michigan. http://fibroguide.med.umich.edu Accessed May 25, 2016
4. Retrain Pain Foundation. http://www.retrainpain.org/ Accessed May 25, 2016.

The care manager keeps the treatment team in communication with one another, helps the patient stay engaged in treatment, and tracks the patient's symptoms in a practice registry.

In all modalities of care, the main components of treatment are as follows:

1. Increasing BPSA and understanding of the diagnosis

BOX 16.4
SUMMARY OF RECOMMENDED TREATMENT APPROACHES AND RELEVANT EVIDENCE

Strength of recommendation taxonomy (SOR A, B, or C)

- **Patients with *mild* somatic symptoms/IA can be treated in primary care or integrated care environments. (SOR A).[25,71–75]**
- **Patients with *moderate* somatic symptoms/IA can and should be treated by primary or integrated care and outpatient psychosomatic treatments. (SOR A)[25,26,59,74–81]**
- **Patients with *severe* somatic symptoms/IA benefit from a multimodal inpatient or day-treatment program. (SOR B)[25,26,61,62,82–85]**
- **Close collaboration between all multidisciplinary clinicians is valuable at all steps of care. (SOR A)[25,32,75,86]**
- **The collaborative team care should be coordinated by the primary care providers following a structured treatment plan. (SOR B)[25,87]**
- **Shared decision making regarding treatment planning is helpful. (SOR B)[88]**
- **An attentive, accepting, and empathic stance in verbal and nonverbal communication with a somatic symptoms patient is therapeutic. (SOR A)[89,90]**
- **Ordering additional medical tests for the purpose of reassuring patients with IA is not helpful. (SOR B)[91]**
- **Specialized psychotherapy is an effective treatment for SSD and IA. (SOR A)[25,92]**
- **Patients with somatic symptoms particularly benefit from multimodal treatments that have a developmental approach and focus on emotions, interpersonal relationships, and the association between somatic symptoms and psychosocial distress—for example, psychosomatic psychodynamic psychotherapies (SOR A),[36,57,58,93,94] psychotherapies that change the patient's relationship with his or her body (mind–body progressive muscle relaxation, mindfulness meditation) (SOR A),[95-97] psychoeducation (SOR A),[86] glutamatergic medications for chronic pain (SOR A), and SSRIs or SNRIs (SOR A).[25]**
- **IA patients benefit from CBT (SOR A)[64,98] and SSRIs (SOR A).[68,99]**
- **SSD and IA patients benefit from both individual and group treatments. (SOR A)[25]**

2. Helping the patient change the relationship with his or her body from fear and avoidance to awareness and acceptance
3. Increasing emotional awareness and learning effective ways of emotional expression and regulation
4. Learning to recognize emotional cues from the body
5. Increasing level of physical activity (in physical therapy, mind–body groups, and so forth)
6. Improving functioning and interpersonal well-being, and decreasing isolation

Psychosomatic interventions can continue beyond symptom alleviation to minimize the risk of somatic symptoms/IA relapse. When somatic symptoms flare up, previously successful treatments may be restarted.

For patients with moderate to severe somatic symptoms/IA, referral for specialized outpatient or inpatient psychosomatic treatment is warranted. In the multidisciplinary approach, the primary care team stays involved, following up with the patient and participating in the psychosomatic center case conferences.

CONCLUSIONS

SSD and IA are challenging yet possible to treat. See Box 16.4 for a review of the evidence which support our approach. Integrating primary care and psychosomatic/mental health treatment, using a stepped-care approach, helping patients develop full BPSA, meeting their relational needs, and changing the culture of the primary care clinics to promote full BPSA can lead to significant relief of patients' suffering. Implementation of this approach within health care systems will also decrease burnout and increase the sense of fulfillment among health care professionals. Reorganization of health care systems to adopt the BPSA-informed multidisciplinary model is needed to improve treatment of SSD and IA and to increase the cost-effectiveness of health care at both hospital and societal levels. These approaches have been used successfully in several countries. Given the personal and financial burden of SSD and IA on individuals, health care providers, and society, and the fact that integrated care has been demonstrated to be feasible and effective, it behooves health care policy planners and health care system leaders to accept the challenge to reshape the approach to care of those with SSD and IA.

REFERENCES

1. Barsky AJ, Orav E, Bates DW. Somatization increases medical utilization and costs independent of psychiatric and medical comorbidity. Arch Gen Psychiatry. 2005;62(8):903–910.
2. Creed F, Henningsen P, Fink P. Medically Unexplained Symptoms, Somatisation and Bodily Distress: Developing Better Clinical Services. Cambridge, UK: Cambridge University Press; 2011.
3. American Psychiatric Association. Diagnostic and Statistical Manual of Mental Disorders, Fifth Edition (DSM-5). Arlington, VA: American Psychiatric Publishing; 2013.
4. American Psychiatric Association. Diagnostic and Statistical Manual, text revision (DSM-IV-TR). Arlington, VA: American Psychiatric Association; 2000.
5. Haller H, Cramer H, Lauche R, Dobos G. Somatoform disorders and medically unexplained symptoms in primary care: A systematic review and meta-analysis of prevalence. Dtsch Arzteblatt Int. 2015;112(16):279–287.
6. Borenstein DG, O'Mara JW, Jr., Boden SD, et al. The value of magnetic resonance imaging of the lumbar spine to predict low-back pain in asymptomatic subjects: a seven-year follow-up study. J Bone Joint Surg Am. 2001;83(9):1306–1311.
7. Jensen MC, Kelly AP, Brant-Zawadzki MN. MRI of degenerative disease of the lumbar spine. Magn Reson Quart. 1994;10(3):173–190.
8. Landa A, Peterson BS, Fallon BA. Somatoform pain: A developmental theory and translational research review. Psychosom Med. 2012;74(7):717–727.
9. Schildkrout B. Masquerading Symptoms: Uncovering Physical Illnesses That Present as Psychological Problems. Hoboken, NJ: Wiley; 2014.
10. Löwe B, Spitzer RL, Williams JBW, Mussell M, Schellberg D, Kroenke K. Depression, anxiety and somatization in primary care: syndrome overlap and functional impairment. Gen Hosp Psychiatry. 2008;30(3):191–199.
11. Dworkind M, Yaffee M. Somatization and the recognition of depression and anxiety in primary care. Am J Psychiatry. 1993;150(5):734–741.
12. Weck F, Richtberg S, MB Neng J. Epidemiology of hypochondriasis and health anxiety: Comparison of different diagnostic criteria. Curr Psychiatry Rev. 2014;10(1):14–23.
13. Tyrer P, Cooper S, Crawford M, et al. Prevalence of health anxiety problems in medical clinics. J Psychosom Res. 2011;71(6):392–394.
14. Starcevic V, Noyes R. Hypochondriasis and Health Anxiety: A Guide for Clinicians. New York: Oxford University Press; 2014.
15. Gramling SE, Clawson EP, McDonald MK. Perceptual and cognitive abnormality model

of hypochondriasis: Amplification and physiological reactivity in women. Psychosom Med. 1996;58(5):423–431.

16. Van den Heuvel O, Mataix-Cols D, Zwitser G, et al. Common limbic and frontal-striatal disturbances in patients with obsessive compulsive disorder, panic disorder and hypochondriasis. Psychol Med. 2011;41(11):2399–2410.
17. Fallon BA. Pharmacotherapy of somatoform disorders. J Psychosom Res. 2004;56(4):455–460.
18. Landa A, Fallon BA. Columbia Somatic Symptoms & Illness Anxiety Ratio Scale. Unpublished Scale. 2014. Contact Dr. Alla Landa at AL2898@cumc.columbia.edu
19. Engel GL. The clinical application of the biopsychosocial model. J Med Phil.1981;6(2):101–124.
20. Prochaska JO, DiClemente CC. Toward a Comprehensive Model of Change. Berlin/Heidelberg: Springer; 1986.
21. Barsky AJ, Wyshak G, Latham KS, Klerman GL. Hypochondriacal patients, their physicians, and their medical care. J Gen Intern Med.1991;6(5):413–419.
22. Sarinopoulos I, Hesson AM, Gordon C, et al. Patient-centered interviewing is associated with decreased responses to painful stimuli: An initial fMRI study. Patient Educ Couns. 2013; 90(2):220–225.
23. Lane RD, Waldstein SR, Chesney MA, et al. The rebirth of neuroscience in psychosomatic medicine, Part I: Historical context, methods, and relevant basic science. Psychosom Med. 2009;71(2):117–134.
24. Lane RD, Waldstein SR, Critchley HD, et al. The rebirth of neuroscience in psychosomatic medicine, Part II: Clinical applications and implications for research. Psychosom Med. 2009; 71(2):135–151.
25. Schaefert R, Hausteiner-Wiehle C, Häuser W, Ronel J, Herrmann M, Henningsen P. Non-specific, functional, and somatoform bodily complaints. Dtsch Arzteblatt Int. 2012;109(47):803–813.
26. van der Feltz-Cornelis CM, Hoedeman R, Keuter EJ, Swinkels JA. Presentation of the Multidisciplinary Guideline Medically Unexplained Physical Symptoms (MUPS) and Somatoform Disorder in the Netherlands: Disease management according to risk profiles. J Psychosom Res.2012;72(2):168–169.
27. Konnopka A, Schaefert R, Heinrich S, et al. Economics of medically unexplained symptoms: A systematic review of the literature. Psychother Psychosom. 2012;81(5):265–275.
28. Schade N, Torres P, Beyebach M. Cost-efficiency of a brief family intervention for somatoform patients in primary care. Fam Syst Health.2011;29(3):197–205.
29. Luciano JV, Sabes-Figuera R, Cardenosa E, et al. Cost-utility of a psychoeducational intervention in fibromyalgia patients compared with usual care: An economic evaluation alongside a 12-month randomized controlled trial. Clin J Pain. 2013;29(8):702–711.
30. Abbass A, Campbell S, Hann SG, Lenzer I, Tarzwell R, Maxwell R. Cost savings of treatment of medically unexplained symptoms using intensive short-term dynamic psychotherapy (ISTDP) by a hospital emergency department. Arch Med Psychol. 2010;2(1):34–44.
31. Schaefert R, Kaufmann C, Wild B, et al. Specific collaborative group intervention for patients with medically unexplained symptoms in general practice: a cluster randomized controlled trial. Psychother Psychosom. 2013;82(2):106–119.
32. van der Feltz-Cornelis CM, van Oppen P, Ader HJ, van Dyck R. Randomised controlled trial of a collaborative care model with psychiatric consultation for persistent medically unexplained symptoms in general practice. Psychother Psychosom. 2006;75(5):282–289.
33. Rittenhouse DR, Shortell SM, Fisher ES. Primary care and accountable care—two essential elements of delivery-system reform. N Engl J Med. 2009;361(24):2301–2303.
34. Fink P, Rosendal M. Functional Disorders and Medically Unexplained Symptoms: Assessment and Treatment. Aarhus, Denmark: Aarhus University Press; 2015.
35. Rothermund E, Kilian R, Hoelzer M, et al. "Psychosomatic consultation in the workplace"—a new model of care at the interface of company-supported mental health care and consultation-liaison psychosomatics: Design of a mixed methods implementation study. BMC Public Health. 2012;12(1):780.
36. Sattel H, Lahmann C, Gündel H, et al. Brief psychodynamic interpersonal psychotherapy for patients with multisomatoform disorder: Randomised controlled trial. Br J Psychiat. 2012;200(1):60–67.
37. olde Hartman TC, Borghuis MS, Lucassen PL, van de Laar FA, Speckens AE, van Weel C. Medically unexplained symptoms, somatisation disorder and hypochondriasis: Course and prognosis. A systematic review. J Psychosom Res. 2009;66(5):363–377.
38. Spitzer RL, Kroenke K, Williams JB. Validation and utility of a self-report version of PRIME-MD: The PHQ primary care study. Primary Care Evaluation of Mental Disorders. Patient Health Questionnaire. JAMA. 1999;282(18):1737–1744.
39. Rief W, Hiller W. A new approach to the assessment of the treatment effects of somatoform disorders. Psychosomatics. 2003;44(6):492–498.
40. Budtz-Lilly A, Fink P, Ornbol E, et al. A new questionnaire to identify bodily distress in primary care: The "BDS checklist." J Psychosom Res. 2015;78(6):536–545.
41. Pilowsky I. Dimensions of hypochondriasis. Br J Psychiat. 1967;113(494):89–93.
42. Wolfe F, Clauw DJ, Fitzcharles M-A, et al. Fibromyalgia criteria and severity scales for clinical and epidemiological studies: A modification of the ACR Preliminary Diagnostic Criteria for Fibromyalgia. J Rheumatol. 2011;38(6):1113–1122.

43. First MB. User's Guide to Structured Clinical Interview for DSM-5 Disorders-SCID-5: Clinician Version. Arlington, VA: American Psychiatric Association; 2015.
44. Wing JK, Babor T, Brugha T, et al. SCAN. Schedules for Clinical Assessment in Neuropsychiatry. Arch Gen Psychiatry. 1990;47(6):589–593.
45. Sheehan DV, Lecrubier Y, Sheehan KH, et al. The Mini-International Neuropsychiatric Interview (M.I.N.I.): The development and validation of a structured diagnostic psychiatric interview for DSM-IV and ICD-10. J Clin Psychiatry. 1998;59(Suppl 20):22–33; quiz 34–57.
46. Daut RL, Cleeland CS, Flanery RC. Development of the Wisconsin Brief Pain Questionnaire to assess pain in cancer and other diseases. Pain.1983;17(2):197–210.
47. Skritskaya NA, Carson-Wong AR, Moeller JR, Shen S, Barsky AJ, Fallon BA. A clinician-administered severity rating scale for illness anxiety: Development, reliability, and validity of the H-YBOCS-M. Depress Anxiety. 2012;29(7):652–664.
48. Landa A. Columbia Stages of BioPsychoSocial Awareness Scale 2015 Contact Alla Landa at AL2898@cumc.columbia.edu.
49. Bernstein DP, Fink L, Handelsman L, et al. Initial reliability and validity of a new retrospective measure of child abuse and neglect. Am J Psychiatry. 1994;151(8):1132–1136.
50. Parker G, Tupling H, Brown LB. A parental bonding instrument. Br J Med Psychol. 1979;52(1):1–10.
51. Blake DD, Weathers FW, Nagy LM, et al. The development of a clinician-administered PTSD scale. J Trauma Stress.1995;8(1):75–90.
52. Russell DW. UCLA Loneliness Scale (Version 3): Reliability, validity, and factor structure. J Pers Asses.1996;66(1):20–40.
53. Blake DD, Weathers FW, Nagy LM, et al. The development of a clinician-administered PTSD scale. J Trauma Stress. 1995;8(1):75–90.
54. Parker G, Tupling H, Brown L. A parental bonding instrument. Br J Med Psychol. 1979;52(1):1–10.
55. Mao J. Opioid-Induced Hyperalgesia. Boca Raton, FL: CRC Press; 2009.
56. Walitt B, Urrútia G, Nishishinya MB, Cantrell SE, Häuser W. Selective serotonin reuptake inhibitors for fibromyalgia syndrome. São Paulo Med J. 2015:133(5):454–454.
57. Abbass A, Kisely S, Kroenke K. Short-term psychodynamic psychotherapy for somatic disorders. Psychother Psychosom. 2009;78(5):265–274.
58. Monsen K, Monsen JT. Chronic pain and psychodynamic body therapy: A controlled outcome study. Psychother Theor Res Pract Train. 2000;37(3):257.
59. Kroenke K. Efficacy of treatment for somatoform disorders: A review of randomized controlled trials. Psychosom Med. 2007;69(9):881–888.
60. Koelen JA, Houtveen JH, Abbass A, et al. Effectiveness of psychotherapy for severe somatoform disorder: meta-analysis. Br J Psychiat. 2014;204(1):12–19.
61. de Greck M, Scheidt L, Bölter AF, et al. Multimodal psychodynamic psychotherapy induces normalization of reward related activity in somatoform disorder. World J Biol Psychiatry. 2011;12(4):296–308.
62. Beutel ME, von Heymann F, Bleichner F, Tritt K, Hardt J. [Efficacy of psychosomatic inpatient treatment for somatoform disorders: results of a multicenter study]. Z Psychosom Med Psyc. 2014;60(1):17–24.
63. De Greck M, Bölter AF, Lehmann L, et al. Changes in brain activity of somatoform disorder patients during emotional empathy after multimodal psychodynamic psychotherapy. Frontiers Hum Neurosci. 2013;7:410. doi:10.3389/fnhum.2013.00410.
64. Olatunji BO, Kauffman BY, Meltzer S, Davis ML, Smits JA, Powers MB. Cognitive-behavioral therapy for hypochondriasis/health anxiety: A meta-analysis of treatment outcome and moderators. Behav Res Ther. 2014;58:65–74.
65. Eilenberg T, Fink P, Jensen J, Rief W, Frostholm L. Acceptance and commitment group therapy (ACT-G) for health anxiety: A randomized controlled trial. Psychol Med. 2015:1–13.
66. McManus F, Surawy C, Muse K, Vazquez-Montes M, Williams JMG. A randomized clinical trial of mindfulness-based cognitive therapy versus unrestricted services for health anxiety (hypochondriasis). J Consult Clin Psychol. 2012;80(5):817–828.
67. Greeven A, van Balkom AJ, Visser S, et al. Cognitive behavior therapy and paroxetine in the treatment of hypochondriasis: A randomized controlled trial. Am J Psychiatry. 2007;164(1):91–99.
68. Fallon BA, Petkova E, Skritskaya N, et al. A double-masked, placebo-controlled study of fluoxetine for hypochondriasis. J Clin Psychopharmacol. 2008;28(6):638–645.
69. Mowla A, Dastgheib SA, Jahromi LR. Comparing the effects of sertraline with duloxetine for depression severity and symptoms: A double-blind, randomized controlled trial. Clin Drug Investig. 2016:1–5.
70. Greeven A, van Balkom AJ, van der Leeden R, Merkelbach JW, van den Heuvel OA, Spinhoven P. Cognitive behavioral therapy versus paroxetine in the treatment of hypochondriasis: An 18-month naturalistic follow-up. J Behav Ther Exp Psychiatry. 2009;40(3):487–496.
71. Hoedeman R, Blankenstein AH, van der Feltz-Cornelis CM, Krol B, Stewart R, Groothoff JW. Consultation letters for medically unexplained physical symptoms in primary care. Cochrane Database Syst Rev. 2010;12.
72. Reid S, Wessely S, Crayford T, Hotopf M. Frequent attenders with medically unexplained

symptoms: Service use and costs in secondary care. Br J Psychiat. 2002;180(3):248–253.
73. Rosendal M, Blankenstein AH, Morriss R, Fink P, Sharpe M, Burton C. Enhanced care by generalists for functional somatic symptoms and disorders in primary care. Cochrane Database Syst Rev. 2013;10.
74. Burton C, Weller D, Marsden W, Worth A, Sharpe M. A primary care symptoms clinic for patients with medically unexplained symptoms: Pilot randomised trial. BMJ Open. 2012;2(1):e000513.
75. Zonneveld LN, van Rood YR, Timman R, Kooiman CG, Van't Spijker A, Busschbach JJ. Effective group training for patients with unexplained physical symptoms: A randomized controlled trial with a non-randomized one-year follow-up. PLoS One. 2012;7(8):e42629.
76. McBeth J, Prescott G, Scotland G, et al. Cognitive behavior therapy, exercise, or both for treating chronic widespread pain. Arch Intern Med. 2012;172(1):48–57.
77. Henningsen P, Zipfel S, Herzog W. Management of functional somatic syndromes. Lancet. 2007;369(9565):946–955.
78. Kleinstäuber M, Witthöft M, Hiller W. Efficacy of short-term psychotherapy for multiple medically unexplained physical symptoms: A meta-analysis. Clin Psychol Rev. 2011;31(1):146–160.
79. Sumathipala A. What is the evidence for the efficacy of treatments for somatoform disorders? A critical review of previous intervention studies. Psychosom Med. 2007;69(9):889–900.
80. Haggarty JM, O'Connor BP, Mozzon JB, Bailey SK. Shared mental healthcare and somatization: Changes in patient symptoms and disability. Prim Health Care Res Dev. 2015:1–10.
81. Schröder A, Rehfeld E, Ørnbøl E, Sharpe M, Licht RW, Fink P. Cognitive–behavioural group treatment for a range of functional somatic syndromes: Randomised trial. Br J Psychiat. 2012;200(6):499–507.
82. Haase M, Frommer J, Franke G-H, et al. From symptom relief to interpersonal change: Treatment outcome and effectiveness in inpatient psychotherapy. Psychother Res. 2008;18(5):615–624.
83. Huber D, Albrecht C, Hautum A, Henrich G, Klug G. [Effectiveness of inpatient psychodynamic psychotherapy: a follow-up study]. Zeitschrift fur Psychosomatische Medizin und Psychotherapie. 2008;55(2):189–199.
84. Liebherz S, Rabung S. Do patients' symptoms and interpersonal problems improve in psychotherapeutic hospital treatment in Germany? A systematic review and meta-analysis. PloS One. 2014;9(8):e105329.
85. Wunner C, Reichhart C, Strauss B, Söllner W. Effectiveness of a psychosomatic day hospital treatment for the elderly: A naturalistic longitudinal study with waiting time before treatment as control condition. J Psychosom Res. 2014;76(2):121–126.
86. Luciano JV, Martínez N, Peñarrubia-María MT, et al. Effectiveness of a psychoeducational treatment program implemented in general practice for fibromyalgia patients: A randomized controlled trial. Clin J Pain. 2011;27(5):383–391.
87. Pols RG, Battersby MW. Coordinated care in the management of patients with unexplained physical symptoms: Depression is a key issue. Med J Austr. 2008;188(12):S133–S137.
88. Bieber C, Müller KG, Blumenstiel K, et al. A shared decision-making communication training program for physicians treating fibromyalgia patients: Effects of a randomized controlled trial. J Psychosom Res. 2008;64(1):13–20.
89. Anderson M, Hartz A, Nordin T, et al. Community physicians' strategies for patients with medically unexplained symptoms. Fam Med. 2008;40(2):111.
90. Aiarzaguena JM, Grandes G, Gaminde I, Salazar A, Sanchez A, Arino J. A randomized controlled clinical trial of a psychosocial and communication intervention carried out by GPs for patients with medically unexplained symptoms. Psychol Med. 2007;37(02):283–294.
91. Rolfe A, Burton C. Reassurance after diagnostic testing with a low pretest probability of serious disease: Systematic review and meta-analysis. JAMA. 2013;173(6):407–416.
92. Sharma MP, Manjula M. Behavioural and psychological management of somatic symptom disorders: An overview. Int Rev Psychiatr. 2013;25(1):116–124.
93. Selders M, Visser R, van Rooij W, Delfstra G, Koelen JA. The development of a brief group intervention (Dynamic Interpersonal Therapy) for patients with medically unexplained somatic symptoms: A pilot study. Psychoanal Psychother. 2015;29(2):182–198.
94. Fjorback LO, Arendt M, Ørnbøl E, et al. Mindfulness therapy for somatization disorder and functional somatic syndromes—Randomized trial with one-year follow-up. J Psychosom Res. 2013;74(1):31–40.
95. Röhricht F, Elanjithara T. Management of medically unexplained symptoms: Outcomes of a specialist liaison clinic. Psychiatr Bull. 2014;38(3):102–107.
96. Lahmann C, Nickel M, Schuster T, et al. Functional relaxation and guided imagery as complementary therapy in asthma: A randomized controlled clinical trial. Psychother Psychosom. 2009;78(4):233–239.
97. Lahmann C, Röhricht F, Sauer N, et al. Functional relaxation as complementary therapy in irritable bowel syndrome: A randomized, controlled clinical trial. J Altern Complement Med. 2010;16(1):47–52.
98. Barsky AJ, Ahern DK. Cognitive behavior therapy for hypochondriasis: A randomized controlled trial. JAMA. 2004;291(12):1464–1470.
99. Louw K-A, Hoare J, Stein D. Pharmacological treatments for hypochondriasis: A review. Curr Psychiatry Rev. 2014;10(1):70–74.

17

Working with Personality Disorders in an Integrated Care Setting

ROBERT E. FEINSTEIN AND JOSEPH V. CONNELLY

BOX 17.1

KEY POINTS

- **Patients with a personality disorder (PD) are common in primary care and medical settings.**
- **Patient with borderline personality disorder (BPD) may present with suicidal ideation or threat, or problems related to stormy interpersonal relationships. Lifetime prevalence of BPD patients having one comorbid psychiatric disorder approaches 100%. Mood disorders, bipolar disorder, anxiety, substance use, and schizotypal and narcissistic personality disorders all have high co-occurrence rates with BPD.**
- **Patients with antisocial personality disorder (ASPD) often present in an integrated care practice seeking secondary gain. Substance use is the most common co-occurring disorder.**
- **Patient with a narcissistic personality disorder (NPD) typically present with co-occurring substance abuse, mood, anxiety disorders, and other comorbid personality disorders. They subsequently may reveal their entitlement, devaluing attacks, and demanding style.**
- **Patient with obsessive-compulsive personality disorder (OCPD) should be differentiated from patients with obsessive-compulsive disorder (OCD). OCPD patients typically present with co-occurring anxiety/panic disorders, affective disorders, or substance abuse problems, and often there is a high comorbidity rate of OCPD with OCD. Patients with OCPD may subsequently reveal their perfectionistic, hypercritical, overly detailed personality features, which may need management by the practice.**
- **PD patients can be successfully managed using the personality disorder schema, which describes clinician reactions, patient core beliefs, fears, behaviors, ways of coping, use of specific defense mechanisms, and characteristic patterns of adherence and medical utilization.**
- **An integrated care team can use a care pathway for diagnosis, management, brief treatment, and long-term planning for PD patients.**
- **PD patients should be referred for their primary psychiatric treatment to a PD specialist or to a program specializing in the treatment of PDs. Patients should be followed and supported by the integrated care practice.**

INTRODUCTION

Patients with personality disorders (PDs) are common in medical settings. They can elicit intense reactions from members of an integrated care team, which can affect the team's evaluation, diagnoses, choices of diagnostic testing, medical orders, prescribed medication, suggested treatment, and referrals. See Box 17.1 for a summary of the key points for managing these four personality disorders.

In general, patients with PDs show rigid extremes of personality traits, display maladaptive coping, are damaging to themselves or others, and have a functional impairment in interpersonal, social, or occupational functioning. They often have difficulties with employment, have multiple interpersonal and family problems, and may have excess morbidity and mortality, especially in relation to cardiovascular disease.[1] Many patients have chronic behavioral problems such as suicidal ideation, and some may complete a suicide. Patients with PDs also may have an increased risk for violence.[2] Some patients with PDs have difficulty adhering to medical recommendations and may be a high utilizer of medical care or "treatment seeking" while others misuse or underuse medical care and are "treatment resisting."[3] As with other psychiatric illnesses, PDs are probably the result of multiple interacting biological, genetic, and environmental factors. Twin studies suggest a heritability of personality traits and personality disorders ranging from 30% to 60%.[2] A psychosocial view suggests that family and early childhood experiences (e.g., emotional, physical, and sexual abuse; neglect; bullying), family upbringing, and culture are also important contributors to the development of a PD.[2]

Patients with chronic medical and substance use illnesses may be more difficult to manage and treat if they also have comorbid PDs. In addition, the outcomes of treatment of major psychiatric disorders (e.g., depression, anxiety, trauma) can be substantially worse when comorbid PDs go unrecognized or are excluded from a focus during treatment of the primary psychiatric disorder. For all these reasons, this is an important group of patients to recognize, manage, briefly treat, and refer for long-term treatments.

In this chapter, we will limit our discussion to an integrated care team's approach to the diagnosis, management, treatment, and referral of borderline, antisocial, narcissistic, and obsessive-compulsive PDs. We are limiting this chapter to these four disorders because they have the highest prevalence rates and present the greatest challenges to an integrated care team. Review Box 17.2[4] for a description of these PDs. A full review of diagnoses and management of all other PDs disorders is available elsewhere.[5,6]

BOX 17.2
DESCRIPTION OF FOUR PERSONALITY DISORDERS

BORDERLINE PERSONALITY DISORDER

Interpersonal relationships can be unstable, chaotic, and rapidly changing.
Attaches or detaches quickly or intensely.
Lacks a stable image of herself or himself.
Dysregulated emotions include intense and inappropriate anger, hostility, depression, anxiety, sadness, rage, excitement.
Sensitive to rejection, abandonment, criticism.
Makes suicidal threats or gestures.
May engage in cutting or burning.
Needs approval or reassurance.
Acts impulsively.
Elicits extreme reactions/feelings in others.
May feel empty or bored.
Fears and avoids being alone.
May be needy or dependent.

ANTISOCIAL PERSONALITY DISORDER

Takes advantage of others, manipulates others' emotions to get what is wanted.
Often is cruel, seeking power over others, angry, or hostile.
Lacks moral values.

Lack empathy and shows little remorse for harm/injury caused to others
Engages in unlawful/criminal behavior
Lies, cheats, or misleads
Unreliable and irresponsible
Little concern for the consequences of his or her actions
Feels immune or invulnerable
Acts impulsively, regardless of the consequences
Exaggerated sense of self-importance
May abuse alcohol or other drugs
Gets into power struggles
Believes his or her problems are caused by others or external events

NARCISSISTIC PERSONALITY DISORDER

Feels privileged and entitled
Expects preferential treatment
Has an exaggerated sense of self-importance
Has little empathy
Has difficulty understanding or responding to others' needs and feelings
Treats others as an audience. Asks others to witness his/her importance, brilliance, or beauty.
Seeks appreciation and associations with people who are of high status, superior, or "special"
Has fantasies of unlimited success, power, beauty, talent, brilliance
Arrogant, haughty, or dismissive
Reacts to criticism with feelings of rage or humiliation, holds grudges, dwells on insults, slights, or criticism for long periods
Seeks power or influence over others
Seeks to be the center of attention
Can manipulate others' emotions to get what is wanted
Thinks others are envious of him or her
Believes his or her problems are caused by other people or by external factors
Feels envious and/or competitive with others
Fantasizes about finding ideal, perfect love
Critical and/or controlling of others

OBSESSIVE-COMPULSIVE PERSONALITY DISORDER

Conscientious, responsible, can be self-righteous or moralistic
Overly concerned with details, rules, procedures, order, organization
Perfectionistic and intolerant of human frailties
Rigid in daily routine and anxious if it is altered
Excessively devoted to work and productivity; difficulty with leisure and relationships
Difficulty throwing things away
Can be controlling
Self-critical and sets unrealistically high standards for self
Preoccupied with concerns about dirt, cleanliness, contamination
Stingy and withholding
Inhibited or constricted with difficulty acknowledging or expressing wishes and impulses
Indecisive
Has obsessive thoughts
Has high moral and ethical standards and strives to live up to them

Abridged Prototype Description of Personality Disorder, Shedler-Westen Assessment Procedure (SWAP). Reprinted by permission by Jonathan Shedler, PhD.[4]

CLASSIFICATION, EPIDEMIOLOGY, BIOLOGICAL BASIS, AND PSYCHOSOCIAL FORMULATION OF FOUR PERSONALITY DISORDERS

In a community sample of people, 9.1% have a PD.[7] The American Psychiatric Association's *Diagnostic and Statistical Manual of Mental Disorders*, fifth edition (DSM-5) [8] divides the PDs into three groups described as Cluster A, B, or C. Cluster A patients are classified as "odd or eccentric" and include paranoid, schizoid, and schizotypal PDs. Cluster B patients are classified as "dramatic, emotional, or erratic" and include the antisocial, histrionic, borderline, and narcissistic PDs. Cluster C patients are classified as "anxious or fearful" and include dependent, obsessive-compulsive, and avoidant PDs. Patients with Cluster A represent 5.7%[7], Cluster B 4.5% to 6.1%,[9] and Cluster C 6.0%[7] of the population. People often meet criteria for more than one cluster and PD.

Borderline Personality Disorder; Cluster B Group

Prevalence

The community prevalence rate of borderline personality disorder (BPD) is 0.7%[10] and the lifetime prevalence ranges from 0.5%[11] to 5.9% (99% confidence interval, 5.4–6.4).[12] It is equally prevalent in men and women.[12] BPD is associated with substantial mental and physical disability, especially among women. It is prevalent in younger patients, in separated/divorced/widowed adults, in people with lower socioeconomic incomes and education, and in Native American men. [12] It is less prevalent among Hispanic men and women, and Asian women.[12]

Common Co-occurring Disorders

The lifetime incidence of BPD patients experiencing one comorbid psychiatric disorder approaches 100%.[11] Mood disorder, bipolar disorder, anxiety, schizotypal and narcissistic personality disorders (NPD), and substance use have high co-occurrence rates with BPD.

Biological Basis

A consistent finding is that BPD individuals have a decrease in volume in the anterior cingulate gyrus, hippocampus, amygdala, and surrounding areas of the temporal lobe compared with healthy individuals. Some studies have raised the possibility that the smaller volumes in BPD may relate to comorbidity with posttraumatic stress disorder (PTSD), a history of serious trauma affecting hippocampal volume, or the effects of comorbid major depressive disorder on amygdala volume.[13] Patients with BPD also show prefrontal neuropsychological dysfunction that may cause dysregulation of emotions and aggression.[13]

Patients with BPD show substantial heritability scores of 0.65 to 0.76. There is a strong genetic correlation between BPD traits and neuroticism, and an inverse relationship with conscientiousness and agreeableness.[13]

Psychosocial Formulation

There appears to be a high prevalence of a history of sexual, physical, and/or emotional abuse. The borderline syndrome is formulated by some as a frequent comorbidity or a variant of PTSD.[14]

Antisocial Personality Disorders; Cluster B Group

Prevalence

The lifetime prevalence of antisocial personality disorders (ASPDs) in the general population is 3.6%, adult antisocial behavior is 12.3%, and conduct disorder without adult antisocial behavior is 1.1%.[15]

Common Co-occurring Disorders

Substance use is the most common disorder co-occurring with ASPD, with a 30.3% lifetime prevalence of any alcohol use disorder and a 10.3% lifetime prevalence rate of any drug use disorder.[15] For all substances, abuse was more common than dependence. All substance disorders were more common among men than women. The most common illicitly abused drugs are marijuana, cocaine, amphetamines, hallucinogens, opioids, sedatives, tranquilizers, and inhalants.[15]

Biological Basis

Family, twin, and adoption studies suggest that antisocial spectrum disorders and psychopathy are heritable. Some research suggests reduced prefrontal volumes,[13] serotonergic dysregulation in the septohippocampal system, developmental or acquired abnormalities in the prefrontal brain systems, and reduced autonomic activity in ASPD. These deficits may be responsible for low arousal, poor fear conditioning, and decision-making deficits.[16]

Psychosocial Formulation

Early neglect, abuse, and maltreatment are common in patients with ASPD. The childhoods of these patients are filled with insecurity, chaos, harsh discipline, overindulgence, and neglect. Clinicians report there is an absence of consistent loving and protective influences that has led to a failure in the capacity for human attachment.[17]

Narcissistic Personality Disorders; Cluster B Group

Prevalence

The prevalence of narcissistic personality disorders (NPDs) varies from 0% to 6% in the general population, 1.3% to 17% in the clinical population, and 8.5% to 20% in outpatient psychiatric private practice.[18] The lifetime prevalence of NPD is 6.2%.[19] NPD is more common in men (7.7%) than in women (4.8%). NPD was significantly more prevalent in separated/divorced/widowed and never-married adults, younger adults, black men and women, and Hispanic women. [19] NPD is associated with considerable disability among men, whose rates exceed those of women.[19]

Common Co-occurring Disorders

Substance use, mood, anxiety, and other personality disorders commonly co-occur in patients with NPD. Less common comorbidities include bipolar I disorder, PTSD, schizotypal, and BPD. In women with NPD, additional co-occurring disorders include specific phobias, generalized anxiety disorder, and bipolar II disorder. Men with NPD are more likely to experience alcohol abuse, alcohol dependence, drug dependence, and co-occurring histrionic and obsessive-compulsive personality disorders (OCPD).

Biological Basis

There are no data available on the biological features of this disorder.

Psychosocial Formulation

Patients who develop NPD may be more sensitive to nonverbal or unstated affects, attitudes, and expectations from others.[19] The child's natural abilities, capacities, or talents are often exploited by his or her caregivers (who may also be narcissistic) for the maintenance of their self-esteem. These children are not sure if they are loved for their abilities or for who they are. These repeated experiences can lead to the development of a grandiose self (because of excessive praise) unintegrated with a devalued and worthless sense of self (because the child never felt loved).[17]

Obsessive-Compulsive Personality Disorder; Cluster C Group

Prevalence

The prevalence of OCPD in the general population is 7.9%, making it the most common of all personality disorders.[20] In an outpatient psychiatric population, OCPD was identified as the third most common PD, with a point prevalence rate of 8.7%. In a psychiatric inpatient population, OCPD is the second most prevalent PD, with a rate of 23.3%.[21] OCPD is equally common in males and females. Younger patients are less likely to carry the OCPD diagnosis. Blacks, Asians/Pacific Islanders, and Hispanics were less likely to carry the OCPD diagnosis compared to whites.[20] OCPD is associated with at least moderate impairment in psychosocial functioning, reduced quality of life, and a considerable economic burden.[21] Obsessive-compulsive disorder (OCD) can be distinguished from OCPD because OCD patients experience marked subjective distress caused by obsessions and compulsions and significant time lost in performing these repetitive symptoms; these features are not typically present in patients with OCPD.

Common Co-occurring Disorders

Studies from nonclinical populations indicate that a lifetime diagnosis of OCPD is moderately common in individuals with annual prevalence rate of anxiety disorders (23– 24%), affective disorders (24%), and/or substance-related disorders (12–25%).[21] There is evidence of higher comorbidity rates between OCPD and OCD than between other personality disorders and OCD.[21]

Biological Basis

OCPD has a heritability rate of 0.78. Genetic effects account for 27% of the variance of OCPD symptoms.[22]

Psychosocial Formulation

Psychoanalysts hypothesize that anality and obsessionality (e.g., related to rigid toilet-training practices) are caused by parental dominance, overcontrol, and intrusiveness,[17] although no studies have confirmed or disproved this hypothesis. Two studies[21] suggest that patients with OCPD have "not formed secure attachments, received less care, and experience more overprotection during their childhood and fail to develop emotionally and empathetically."[21]

PERSONALITY DISORDER SCHEMA

Patients with a PD characteristically elicit both common and specific reactions, based on the specific PD disorder, in integrated care team members. They also have characteristic core beliefs, fears, behaviors, and ways of coping and use specific defense mechanisms. Patients with each specific PD also have characteristic patterns of adherence to medical recommendations and demonstrate typical patterns in their use of medical services. An overview of the features and management of patients with BPD, ASPD, NPD, and OCPD is provided as a schema of personality disorders in Tables 17.1 and 17.2.

Observed Personality Traits May Suggest the Diagnosis

While the prototypic PD descriptions in Box 17.2 and the DSM-5 are useful aids to making a diagnosis, the members of the integrated care team may first notice a personality trait before they can make a PD diagnosis. For example, a patient with BPD may be noticed because some staff members like and support this patient while others are angry with or intensely dislike the same patient. Patients who lie about their history and manipulate the team to get disability benefits suggests a patient has ASPD. A patient who idealizes the doctor but denigrates the front office staff may suggest a patient with NPD. A patient who keeps asking for more details about his or her care and treatment and is highly critical whenever the practice is not functioning perfectly suggests a patient with OCPD.

Team Member Reactions (Countertransference) to Patients with a Personality Disorder

A patient with a PD can engender feelings, reactions, and behaviors in the integrated care team that need to be recognized, understood, and used for the patient's benefit. Patients can provoke feelings in the care team members through the interpersonal interaction that the patient has with individual team members. Typically intense experiences and emotional reactions to a patient are the first warning signs of a possible diagnosis of a PD. Team members' reactions to a patient are often referred to as "patient-generated countertransferences." These describe unusual intense feelings, uncharacteristic fantasies, or atypical behaviors enacted by team members.

Intense Feelings

Intense team feelings (e.g., frustration, annoyance, anger, fury, and hate toward the patient) can be elicited by interpersonal interactions with a patient with a PD. Alternatively, strong feelings of love, sexual arousal, or a desire to rescue the patient or give "exceptionally" good care may occur in some staff members. Team members may wish to avoid the patient, terminate the relationship, or transfer the patient to another team member or colleague. In extreme cases, intense feelings aroused in a team member, can become a source of team conflict or a focal point leading a staff member into a boundary violation with the patient. These enactments can be extremely damaging to team functioning and all individuals involved. They can result in poor care delivery for the patient.

Team Members' Thoughts and Fantasies

Members of the integrated care team may also recognize that certain patients elicit unusual thoughts or fantasies. These include excessive worry about a patient after normal work hours, dreaming about a patient, or experiencing exaggerated and/or intrusive, angry, sexual, or curious fantasies about the patient during personal times. A list of common reactions that are associated with each of the four PDs is given in Table 17.1.

Atypical Team Member Behaviors

Some patients have the uncanny and destructive ability to involve team members in atypical medical behaviors that deviate markedly from the normal customary care and treatment offered within the scope of the integrated care team practice. Common atypical team member behaviors may include ordering tests to placate a patient; asking for more than the usual number of consults on a patient whose case does not seem medically complicated; suggesting increasingly aggressive diagnostic testing or procedures when the yield of these tests is likely to be low; repeatedly extending the time spent with a particular patient and/or family; lowering or waiving the customary fees; offering free psychotherapy or other treatments; or developing a personal (not professional) relationship with a patient. These

TABLE 17.1 SCHEMA FOR PERSONALITY DISORDERS

Prototype Personality Disorders	Clinician Reactions	Patient Core Beliefs	Patient Fears	Patient Health Behaviors	Patient Coping Style	Patient Defenses
Borderline	feels manipulated, angry, impotent, depleted, self-doubting; wish to rescue or get rid of the patient; guilty	I am very bad or very good; Who am I?; I can't be alone.	separations, loss; emotional abandonment; not being loved and cared for; fluctuating self-esteem	impulsive behaviors, suicidal actions, cutting, anger/violence, panic; anxiety, poor reality testing, stormy relationships	emotional coping using tears, anger, or fear to help solve problems; help seeking: asking others for help	splitting, projection, projective-identification, dissociation, regression, acting out, omnipotence, idealization/devaluation, mini-psychotic experiences
Antisocial	feels used, exploited, or deceived; anger; a wish to uncover lies, punish, or imprison	People are there to be used and exploited; I come before all others.	boredom; loss of prestige, power, or esteem	lies, deceit, cheating, and manipulation; violence; seeks secondary gain	action oriented: taking an action to immediately rectify the problem	acting out, splitting
Narcissistic	feels devalued or overvalued; inferior or superior; fearful of patient's criticism or anger; wish to retaliate, devalue, or get rid of the patient	I am special; I am important; I come first; The world should revolve around me.	loss of prestige, image, power, or self-esteem	self-aggrandizement; inflated or deflated/depressed view of self; entitled; devalue/idealize; viciousness; envious, competitive	controlling others; denial: can be adaptive depending on the situation	splitting, projection, projective-identification, acting out, regression, denial
Obsessive-Compulsive Personality Disorder	control of negative reactions to patient stinginess, need for order, details, and stubbornness; distanced from feelings; bored	People should do better; try harder; I must be perfect; make no errors or mistakes; details, not feelings, rule.	disorder, mistakes, imperfection; fears, avoids feelings, especially rage/anger, anxiety, self-doubt, dependency	perfectionism, driven, orderliness; logical, compulsions, controlling, critical; stubbornness/stinginess; workaholic, rational	informational: gathering information then deciding; logical/rational; reasoned, logical, deductive	isolation of affect, intellectualization, reaction-formation, undoing, controlling, displacement, dependent, inhibition, phobias, repression

TABLE 17.2 SCHEMA FOR PERSONALITY DISORDERS			
Prototype Personality Disorders	Adherence	Medical Utilization	Team Member Management
Borderline	Patients show inconsistent adherence, as adherence is influenced by emotional storms, interpersonal conflicts, or chaotic lifestyles	Misuse or overuse of medical services; overuse of a wide variety of psychiatric services	1. Empathize with patient's fear of abandonment/separation and plan for absences by arranging coverage. 2. Express a wish to help, and satisfy reasonable needs. 3. Ask the patient to monitor impulsive behaviors with a diary/log. 4. Set firm limits and do not punish. 5. Correct reality distortions and unreasonable patient expectations. 6. Gently question irrational thoughts and suggest more rational ones. 7. Teach adaptive coping skills and interpret splitting and other defences. 8. Negotiate safety plans. If acutely suicidal, the patient must go to the emergency department. If the patient refuses, let the patient know that this therapeutic breach may end the relationship.
Antisocial	Patients may be treatment resistant, problematic, or intolerant of the need for adherence	Underuse of medical and psychiatric resources; may misuse medical/ psychiatric resources for secondary gain	1. Empathize with patient's fear of exploitation & low self-esteem. 2. Determine if you are being used for a secondary gain. 3. Should you suspect dishonesty, verify symptoms and illness progression with others. 4. Don't moralize. Explain that deception results in your giving the patient poor care. 5. Correct reality distortions and unreasonable patient expectations. 6. Gently question irrational thoughts and suggest more rational ones. 7. Teach adaptive coping skills and interpret defenses.
Narcissistic	Patients are treatment resisting, as they know better; often intolerant of need for ongoing adherence	Underuse of care when they suspect they are ill; may feel entitled to special care once diagnosed or may abuse care team	1. Empathize with patient's vulnerability and low self-esteem. 2. Don't mistake patient's superior attitude for *real* confidence and don't confront entitlement. 3. When devalued or attacked, acknowledge the patient's hurt and your mistakes, and express your continued wish to help. 4. If devaluing continues, offer a referral as an option, not as punishment. 5. Correct reality distortions and unreasonable patient expectations. 6. Gently question irrational thoughts and suggest more rational ones. 7. Teach adaptive coping skills and interpret splitting and other defenses.

TABLE 17.2 CONTINUED

Prototype Personality Disorders	Adherence	Medical Utilization	Team Member Management
Obsessive-Compulsive	Patients rigidly and inflexibly follow the adherence rules; anxious if unexpected changes are required	Conflicted: fear of losing control when ill may lead to underuse, but fear of uncertainty may lead to overuse. Frequent treatment seekers.	1. Empathize with patient's logical, detailed, unemotional style of thinking. 2. If obsessive thoughts are interfering with medical care, ask about the patient's feelings. 3. Don't struggle or confront patients with issues of perfectionism, control, critical judgments. 4. Set limits on excessive demands. 5. Avoid abandoning the patient. 6. Correct reality distortions and unreasonable patient expectations. 7. Gently elicit irrational thoughts and suggest more rational ones. 8. Teach adaptive coping skills and interpret specific defenses.

atypical behaviors should trigger consideration that the patient may have a PD that needs attention, a different management strategy, consultation with the behavioral health specialist (BHS), or referral to a mental health professional who specializes in PDs. For example, patients with BPD often leave in their wake many care providers who are exhausted and worried about their patients' suicidal threats. Team members who recognize a variety of provoked feelings can learn to use this information to help identify the PD subtype according to the feelings elicited. More importantly, team members who recognize their own and other team members' unusual reactions and atypical behaviors will focus on making appropriate medical decisions and avoid the use of inappropriate management, medical care, treatment, and referral recommendations.

Patient Core Beliefs, Irrational Thoughts, Fears, and Behaviors

Team members can apply principles of cognitive-behavioral therapy (CBT) to facilitate the management of patients with PDs. CBT describes a patient's core beliefs and worldview, personality-specific fears, irrational thoughts, and behaviors. Table 17.1 describes these for four common PDs. Understanding the core beliefs and fears of each specific PD can facilitate empathy with patients and can be used to plan interventions. A stressor often interacts with a core belief and fear. This leads to irrational thinking, negative moods, and emotions that ultimately trigger maladaptive behaviors and/or physical symptoms. Behaviors or symptoms often feed back directly to confirm a core belief and fear. Core beliefs and fears are readily activated during a routine medical visit when a patient feels sick and vulnerable. These can be addressed, if evident and problematic, during the medical encounter.

For example, a patient with NPD and diabetes typically acts entitled, demeaning, and demanding. NPD patients have a core belief that they are special, important, and unusually talented, and that the world should revolve around them. When patients with NPD become medically ill, they may be verbally abusive and denigrating to the medical staff for not giving them the special care and attention they feel they deserve. If staff members understand the patient's core beliefs and associated fears, the patient's offensive behaviors can be managed, not by confronting this bombastic presentation, but rather by acknowledging that the patient may feel vulnerable, inconvenienced, or depressed and that it is no fun to be sick.

Adherence and Medical Utilization

Patients with specific PDs display predictable adherence and medical utilization behaviors. Patients with BPD are inconsistently adherent to medical recommendations and may overuse, underuse, or misuse medical services.[3] They are excessively "treatment seeking" of psychiatric services.[23] Patient with ASPD typically do not adhere to medical recommendations[3] but are known to overuse medical services when they are seeking secondary gain.[23] Patients with NPD are typically nonadherent because they do not want to need medical expertise. They can be over or underutilizers of medical services[3] but they are underutilizers of psychiatric services.[23] Patients with OCPD tend to be rigidly adherent but are variably over or underutilizers of medical service.[3] They are treatment seeking of psychiatric services.[23]

Patient Coping Styles and Defense Mechanisms

Using a crisis intervention, problem-solving, and psychodynamic approach (see Chapter 26: Crisis Intervention in Integrated Care) a primary care provider, a BHS, and/or a psychiatrist can attempt to relieve a range of problems interfering with patients receiving optimal medical care. A problem-solving approach recognizes that patients have coping styles, which are characteristic ways of dealing with the external environment. Common coping styles associated with each PD and relevant interventions are described in Table 17.1.

Members of the integrated care team can attempt to relieve the "core problem/symptom" interfering with medical care by fostering the patient's awareness of his or her defenses. Defenses are unconscious psychological processes used to resolve internal conflicts, manage moods, mediate external dangers, and facilitate adaptations to reality. By understanding the constellation of specific defenses used with each PD, the physician may be able to modify (by confrontation, clarification, and interpretation) the pathologic functioning of the defense(s) interfering with the patient–physician or team alliance and necessary medical care. Table 17.1 lists common defenses associated with each PD.

For example, a BPD patient feels hurt and abandoned by her physician, who is leaving for a medical conference. She accuses the physician of not caring and expresses suicidal ideation. This patient uses devaluation (she deprecates the physician as uncaring) and acting out (she expresses suicidal ideation or intent). With this understanding, the physician can begin to help the patient. First, he must not take the patient's devaluing and manipulation personally. The physician can empathize with the patient's fears of abandonment. He can use a *confrontation*, telling the patient that his going to a conference is being incorrectly experienced as a personal abandonment. He can use a *clarification*, stating that his absence does not communicate anything about his wish to care for her, nor does it say anything about his future availability. The patient can be reassured of the dates of the physician's return and make an appointment, which will set the expectation of his future availability. He can also be sensitive to the patient's fear of transitions and have her preemptively meet his medical coverage or other team members before his departure. In some circumstances, where the provider is knowledgeable about the patient's psychosocial history and has a good working alliance, the provider might add an *interpretation*—for example, "unlike your mother . . . I am not leaving you. I am going to a conference and I will see you soon."

The BHS can understand the coping strategies and characteristic defenses of difficult patients and teach them, in advance, the use of more adaptive coping skills. The BHS can also help patients develop effective self-management and stress-reduction strategies.

INTEGRATED CARE TEAM OFFICE MANAGEMENT, INTERVENTIONS AND REFERRALS

General Principles

The management, brief treatment, and long-term treatment of patients with a PD are primarily psychological. The initial goal in an integrated care setting is to deliver needed medical care. If this goes smoothly, there is no immediate need to identify patients with PDs. The three reasons to identify these patients and develop a systematic approach to their care are (1) the patient presents with symptoms or problems related to the PD (i.e., a BPD patient is suicidal or an ASPD patient is using the practice for secondary gain); (2) the patient presents with a co-occurring disorder in which the PD is complicating the treatment; and (3) the patient is creating problems within the practice. In these circumstances, the team members can perform different roles and develop a pathway for integrated care. The general team management intervention strategies for treating the wide scope of PDs in an integrated care practice is described in Box 17.3.

BOX 17.3

TEN INTERVENTIONS FOR MANAGING PERSONALITY DISORDERS

1. **Stabilize the external environment: noise, privacy, light.**
2. **Stabilize the internal environment: basic needs, reality testing, medication.**
3. **Empathize with the patient's worldview.**
4. **Focus on improving the capacity to test reality.**
5. **Accept the patient's limitations.**
6. **Describe and confront unreasonable patient expectations and set limits.**
7. **Question irrational thoughts or behaviors related to care.**
8. **Discuss coping style and interpret defense mechanisms affecting care.**
9. **Use family support.**
10. **Use psychopharmacology.**

Team Meetings

Team conferences and regular meetings to review patients with PDs are especially helpful when new patients enter the practice. Letting the entire team know of potential issues can preemptively address possible management problems. Different team members can be assigned tasks, while remembering that the BHS and psychiatrist may be most helpful in developing a practice management strategy, assessing risk, or referring patients for long-term treatment with a PD specialist outside the practice. The team will need to keep in touch with the patients and monitor their progress. Patients should be followed in a practice registry that includes emergency contact information, list of medications, list of co-occurring disorders, problem list, names and contact information for the PD specialist or program, and names of other medical providers. Progress, new needs, or new co-occurring diagnoses should be regularly updated. Regular subteam (often called a "teamlet") management meetings (any combination of the BHS, psychiatrist, care coordinator, and health coach) can be mixed with occasional large-team updates. A care pathway detailing the roles and tasks of integrated team members is summarized in Table 17.3.

Front Desk Staff and Medical Assistants

Front desk staff members are in an excellent position to report interactions that suggest a patient may have a PD. A medical assistant may routinely administer mental health and substance use screeners (Patient Health Questionnaire [PHQ-9][24] or an Alcohol Use Disorders Identification Test [AUDIT]),[25] which may offer added clues suggesting BPD (e.g., a positive screen for suicidal ideation) or comorbid conditions (e.g., alcoholism) associated with other PDs. The medical assistant should communicate such observations and reactions to these patients, to other team members. Recording emergency contact information and other basic health data in the registry is helpful. Medical assistant should alert the nurse to any issues they identify.

Nurse

The nurse's observations and reactions to the patient should be brought to the team. With a more detailed awareness of a patient's interactions and interpersonal style, the nurse can administer additional mental health, substance abuse, or PD screeners. The nurse could review Box 17.2 or the DSM-5 criteria for PDs or use one or more of the three PD screeners: the Personality Assessment Screener (PAS, a 22-item self-report measure),[26] Standardized Assessment of Personality[27] (eight items from a standardized interview), and the Iowa Personality Disorder Screen[28] (five-minute standardized interview). Use of these screeners requires some training, and they could alternatively be used by the BHS. The nurse can also obtain the basics of the patient's psychosocial, occupational, and legal history. It is important to convey this information to the primary care provider (PCP) and document additional information in the practice registry.

PCP

The PCP reviews the results of the screeners and focuses on the patient's chief complaint and relevant

TABLE 17.3 PATHWAY OF CARE FOR PD PATIENTS	
Front office staff and medical assistant	1. Administer mental health and substance abuse screeners (e.g., Patient Health Questionnaire [PHQ-9] and CAGE, QPD [See Chapter 10 Automated Mental Health Assessment for Integrated Care: The Quick PsychoDiagnostics (QPD Panel) Panel Meets Real-World Clinical Needs] 2. Be aware of and note reactions to patient to be discussed with the team. 3. Record emergency contact information. 4. Alert nurse and primary care provider to any core issues identified. 5. Document in the registry.
Nurse	1. Administer any additional mental health, substance abuse, or personality disorder screeners. 2. Be aware of and note reactions to patient to be discussed with the team. 3. Screen for safety (suicide and violence risk), as needed. 4. Take additional psychosocial, occupational, legal history. 5. Alert primary provider to core issues. 6. Document in the registry.
Primary care provider/ advanced practice nurse	1. Attend to medical complaints and illnesses. 2. Review screeners. 3. Establish the working alliance. 4. Do safety assessment, as needed. 5. Use personality disorder schema in Table 17.1 to facilitate preliminary personality diagnosis and management, as needed. 6. Diagnosis co-occurring psychiatric diagnoses. 7. Develop short-term goals (e.g., acute plan and level of care needed). 8. "Warm handoff" to behavioral health specialist or psychiatrist as needed.
Behavioral health specialist (BHS)/ therapist	1. Receive "warm handoff" or referral from primary care provider. 2. Establish the working alliance (partnership with the patient, keeping the patient involved in problem solving, maximizing patient autonomy). 3. Use personality disorder schema in Table 17.1 to facilitate preliminary personality diagnosis and management. 4. Confirm the specific personality disorder diagnosis (Box 17.2 or DSM-5 criterion). 5. Review and expand the psychosocial, interpersonal, occupational, and legal histories. 6. Confirm diagnosis of co-occurring disorders. 7. Short term: help patient decide on new life choices (dealing with daily living, interpersonal, occupational, legal challenges) and consequences of new life choices made. 8. Short term: diagnose, address, and develop plans for treatment of co-occurring disorders. 9. Short term: use crisis intervention or problem-solving approach for acute problems. 10. Short term: work with the team to identify problematic team reactions, teach staff how these help with diagnosis, and suggest adaptive staff management strategies. 11. Long term: counsel about family, educational, occupational, or legal. issues and decide on treatment plan. 12. Long term: teach self-management, interpersonal, and stress management skills. 13. Long term: anticipate and plan for helping the patient with transition or endings (e.g., vacations, absences, change in providers, referral). 14. Long term: consult with the psychiatrist, care coordinator, or health coach. 15. Long term: refer the patient to personality disorder specialist or specialized program. 16. Follow and coordinate care with personality disorder specialist. 17. Update the registry for progress, problem lists, medication changes.

TABLE 17.3 CONTINUED

Consulting psychiatrist	1. Use approaches of the BHS (as above). 2. Review and confirm personality disorder and other co-occurring diagnoses. 3. Suggest, facilitate, or arrange appropriate level of urgent care. 4. Assess for safety, as needed. 5. Assist the team (in a team meeting) in managing staff reactions and developing patient management strategies. 6. Prescribe pharmacotherapy for primary personality disorder or co-occurring disorders. 7. Develop population-based standard of care for subgroups of patients with personality disorders. 8. Update the registry for medication, new problems or diagnoses, progress.
Care coordinator/case manager	1. Meet the patient to determine any needs for care coordination. 2. Support and refer to a personality disorder specialist or specialty program. 3. Refer the patient for educational, employment, or legal resources. 4. Mobilize system, community, or family support. 5. Collect and facilitate communication and reports from other providers. 6. Update the registry, as needed.
Health coach, if available	1. Motivate the patient to make better life choices and help reorganize educational and occupational life goals to be compatible with his or her values. 2. Review wellness needs as recommended by primary care provider. 3. Offer nutrition, weight, exercises, sleep, and substance use harm-reduction approaches, and teach stress management techniques. 4. Implement wellness plan and assess wellness goals using outcome measures.

medical, psychiatric, or substance use issues. It is essential to develop a good working alliance focusing on a positive relationship with the patient, one that is hopeful and optimistic, open and engaging, nonjudgmental, consistent, and reliable.[9,10,29,30] The PCP can assess for suicide or violence risk (see Chapter 18: Violence and Suicide) as needed and can use the PD schema (see Tables 17.1 and 17.2, Box 17.3) to guide diagnosis, assessment, and management strategies. He or she should preliminarily confirm the PD diagnosis and make the initial decision about the immediate level of care that is needed: emergency department, inpatient mental health, substance abuse treatment, or outpatient care. At some point, a "warm handoff" to the BHS or psychiatrist is generally warranted.

BHS

The BHS will receive a "warm handoff" or a referral from the PCP. The first goal is to establish a working alliance with the patients that keep them involved in problem solving while maximizing their autonomy.[10,29] The BHS can also use the PD schema (see Tables 17.1 and 17.2) to facilitate preliminary PD diagnosis and assessment, and for assistance on some basic intervention strategies. The BHS should confirm the specific PD diagnosis by using the prototype model (see Box 17.2), the DSM-5[8] criteria, a personality disorder screener[26–28] or by referring the patient to a PD specialist. Confirming co-occurring diagnoses is also important. Reviewing and delving more deeply into the patient's psychosocial, occupational, and legal history is also essential to create a short-term treatment plan.

Short-Term Treatment Plan

The BHS should use a crisis intervention (See Chapter 26: Crisis Intervention in Integrated Care) or problem-solving approach. The initial session should focus on building the alliance, diagnosing any co-occurring disorders, helping the patient to decide on new life choices (e.g., dealing with substance abuse; issues of daily living; and interpersonal, occupational, and legal challenges), and anticipating the consequences of any new life choices that are made.

The BHS can also assist members of the integrated care team with working through their reactions to the patient, explaining how their reactions can be a useful aid to diagnosis, and suggesting adaptive strategies for managing the patient within the practice.

Long-Term Management

For patients who are not seeing a PD specialist, the BHS should continue to focus on family, interpersonal, educational, employment, and legal issues.[9,10,29] Teaching self-management (for suicidal impulses), interpersonal, and stress management skills[10,29] may help patients function better in their lives. It is also important to make plans for helping the patient with transition or endings[10,29] (e.g., vacations, absences, change in providers, referrals).[10,29] It is often advisable to consult with the psychiatrist and refer the patient to the care coordinator or health coach, as needed. The optimal treatment goal for all PD patients with unresolved issues is to refer them to a PD specialist or specialized program.[10,29–31] Evidence-based psychological treatments[10,29–31] for specific PDs can be reviewed in Table 17.4.

Since definitive treatment can take years, the role of the BHS is to continue to support and follow the patient while coordinating care with the PD specialist or program. The BHS should update the team and the registry on the patient's progress, problem lists, and upcoming transitions.

Psychiatrist

The psychiatrist can assume roles and strategies similar to the BHS and can clarify the PD diagnosis and co-occurring disorders, provide treatment, or refer the patient to a PD specialist or other mental health service. He or she should assess for safety and substance abuse; assess and manage suicidal BPD patients; reduce the risk of potentially violent patients with ASPD; develop a management strategy for entitled, demanding, substance-using patients with NPD; or work with staff in the management of hypercritical, perfectionistic, anxious, or depressed patients with OCPD. The psychiatrist can also help the BHS and the team develop strategies for patient management within the practice and should update the registry with any new medications, problems, or diagnoses, and patient progress. Developing population-based standards of care for a subgroup of BPD patients can be useful. Psychiatrists can also initiate psychopharmacologic treatment.

Medications should be viewed as adjunctive to the primary psychological treatment and should only be prescribed by a knowledgeable PCP or psychiatrist. Patients with PDs may need treatment with medication when cognitive, affective, or impulsive symptoms are contributing to acute problems or when there is a co-occurring mental health or substance abuse problem. Table 17.4 lists medication choices and doses.

Patients with BPD may benefit from medication targeting acute problematic symptoms; these include cognitive perceptual symptoms (minipsychotic symptoms such as a thought disorder, hallucinations, or other breaks with the sense of reality); mood, irritability, or affect dysregulation symptoms; or impulsivity.[32–36] Medication should be used briefly since there is no evidence of long-term benefits for BPD.[32–38] Since lifetime co-occurring psychiatric diagnosis (e.g., bipolar, depression, anxiety, or substance use) is extremely likely, many patients with BPD are maintained on long-term medications.

Medications for patient with ASPD (see Table 17.4) may be used to target violence or impulsivity. Lithium and phenytoin have limited evidence for decreasing violence and impulsivity.[10,15,37] Since substance abuse commonly co-occurs with ASPD, it may be helpful to prescribe medications used to treat addictions, which are also listed in Table 17.4: Treating Substance Use Disorders in Integrated Care Setting for additional information about the use of medically assisted treatments for addictions.

There are no medications that are useful for the primary treatment of NPD.[19] In this group, medications are used to treat the most common co-occurring disorders of substance use, and anxiety or mood disorders.

Limited evidence exists for effective pharmacologic treatment of OCPD. There is weak evidence that carbamazepine and fluvoxamine may have some benefit.[20] There is better evidence for the use of citalopram in patients with OCPD and co-occurring depression[20] (see Table 17.4). In patients with OCPD, medications are frequently used to treat co-occurring problems such as anxiety or mood disorders, and substance abuse.

Care Coordinator

The role of the care coordinator is to (1) support and refer the patient to a PD specialist or program; (2) coordinate referrals for acute housing, food, or insurance benefits or for educational, employment, or legal resources; (3) mobilize a system of care and family support; (4) collect and facilitate communication and reports from other providers; and (5) update the registry.

TABLE 17.4 TREATMENT OF FOUR PERSONALITY DISORDERS

	Evidence-Based Psychotherapy	Medications[32–38]	Referrals
Borderline Personality Disorder (BDP)	• Dialectical Behavioral Therapy (DBT)[a] • Mentalization-Based Therapy (MBT)[b] • Transference-Focused Psychotherapy (TFP)[c] • Cognitive Analytic Therapy (CAT)[d] • Schema-Focused Therapy (SFT)[e] • General psychiatric management/structured clinical management[31] • Supportive psychoanalytic psychotherapy • Supportive group therapy	To be used short term unless also treating a co-occurring disorder. **Cognitive Perceptual Symptoms** *Atypicals* Olanzapine 2.5–10 mg Risperidone 1–4 mg Clozapine 75–550 mg *Typical Antipsychotics* Haloperidol 1–4 mg Perphenazine 12–16 mg Trifluorperazine 2–6 mg Thiothixene 2–40 mg Loxapine 13.5–14.5 mg Chloropromazine 105–120 mg **Mood, Irritability/Affect Dysregulation** *Selective Serotonin Reuptake Inhibitors (SSRIs)* Fluoxetine 20–80 mg Sertraline 100–200mg Venlafaxine 75–225 mg *Monoamine Oxidase Inhibitor (MAOI)* Tranylcypromine 60 mg **Anger** *Low-Dose Antipsychotics* *Mood Stabilizers* Divalproex 1,000–2,000 mg Omega-3 fatty acid 1,000 mg *Other Antidepressants* Amitriptyline 100–300 mg Miansarin 30 mg Amoxapine 200–250 mg **Impulsivity** *SSRIs* Fluoxetine 20–80 mg OD Sertraline 100–200 mg OD Venlafaxine 75–225 mg *Low-Dose Antipsychotics* *Mood Stabilizers (Check levels)* Divalproex 1,000–2,000 mg Lithium 3000–1,800 mg	• Community providers with specialized specific personality disorder psychotherapy skills • Community mental health team management • Emergency department or crisis interventions service for suicidality, violence risk • Intensive outpatient treatment with specialized BPD providers • Short-term partial hospitalization • Acute psychiatric inpatient admissions for acute suicidal risk or treatment of BPD with a co-occurring condition • Specialized (personality disorder-specific) long-term inpatient or residential psychiatric care for BPD with specialized BPD providers • Involve family. • Referral for long-term education or employment goals

(continued)

	TABLE 17.4 CONTINUED		
	Evidence-Based Psychotherapy	Medications[32–38]	Referrals
Antisocial Personality Disorder (ASPD)	• MBT individual and group • Cognitive and behavioral group-based therapies	To be used short term unless also treating a co-occurring disorder **For Violence Prevention** Lithium 300–1,500 mg Phenytoin 300–400 mg Follow blood levels. **Alcohol Addiction** Disulfiram 125–500 mg Acamprosate 666 tid Naltrexone 25–50 mg Naltrexone IM 380 mg/month **Opiate Addiction** Naltrexone PO 25–50 mg Naltrexone IM 380 mg/month Buprenorphine/naloxone 2 mg/0.5–24 mg/6 mg/ Methadone 15–100 mg/day in a methadone treatment program	• Referral for co-occurring substance abuse treatment • Referral for long-term training or education programs or employment • National Institute for Health and Care Excellence (NICE) guideline[10] for ASPD
Narcissistic Personality Disorder (NPD)	• Psychoanalysis • Psychodynamic psychotherapy • TFP • SFT • Metacognitive Interpersonal Therapy (MIT) • Group therapy • Couples therapy	No meds except if treating a co-occurring disorder	• Community providers with specialized specific personality disorder psychotherapy skills • Community mental health
Obsessive Compulsive Personality Disorder (OCPD)	• Cognitive therapy • Cognitive-behavioral therapy (CBT) • Group CBT • Interpersonal therapy (ITP) if depressed • SFT • Supportive/expressive dynamic therapy • Modified DBT	**OCPD Alone** Carbamazepine 800–1,600 mg in divided doses Carbamazepine XR 400–1,600 mg in divided doses Fluvoxamine 25–300 mg **OCPD and Depression** Citalopram 10–40 mg	• Community providers with specialized specific personality disorder psychotherapy skills • Community mental health

[a] *Dialectical Behavior Therapy:* Developed as a modified version of cognitive-behavioral therapy, it also incorporates the concept of "mindfulness" drawn from Buddhist philosophy. The treatment focuses on emotional regulation, distress tolerance, and interpersonal effectiveness through individual therapy, group skills training, and telephone coaching.[31]

[b] *Mentalization-Based Therapy:* An adaption of psychodynamic psychotherapy grounded in attachment theory, which emphasizes improving patients' ability to "mentalize"—that is, to understand their own and other people's mental states and intentions. The treatment is delivered in a twice-weekly individual and group therapy format or as part of daily attendance at a treatment center.[31]

[c] *Transference-Focused Psychotherapy:* A form of psychodynamic psychotherapy derived from Otto Kernberg's theory of object relations, which describes contradictory internalized representations of self and others. It focuses intensely on the therapy relationship and is delivered as twice-weekly individual sessions aimed at the integration of split-off aspects of the personality.[31]

[d] *Cognitive Analytic Therapy:* Brief focused therapy that integrates ideas from psychoanalytic object relations theory and cognitive-behavioral therapy. A collaborative therapy that uses diagrams and letters to help people to recognize and revise confusing patterns and mental states, it is delivered individually over 24 weeks with follow-ups.[31]

[e] *Schema-Focused Therapy*: A development of cognitive-behavioral therapy founded by Jeffrey Young, it blends elements of Gestalt therapy, object relations, and constructivist therapies. It identifies and modifies dysfunctional patterns (schemata) made up of patients' memories, feelings, and thoughts about themselves and others. It is usually delivered as once- or twice-weekly individual therapy.[31]

Health Coach

Health coaches can support the BHS by motivating PD patients to make better life choices and help reorganize their educational, occupational, and life goals in conjunction with their core values. Coaches trained in wellness activities can review the wellness needs of the patient and wellness recommendations made by the PCP. Health coaches with appropriate training can counsel about nutrition, weight, exercise, sleep, and substance harm reduction and can teach stress management. The coach should enter the wellness plan in the registry and track progress and wellness outcomes.

SPECIFIC INTERVENTIONS

The schema for personality disorders (see Tables 17.1 and 17.2) provides some useful information and interventions. Additional information for the integrated care team follows.

BPD

Common Experiences for the Integrated Care Team

BPD patients often become dependent on members of the integrated care team and may become extremely demanding, clinging, or helpless, or act in a self-destructive manner. Team members typically feel manipulated, angry, depleted, exhausted, or self-doubting. Teams may wish either to get rid of the patient or to rescue the patient from himself or herself. Patients with BPD often fear separation or abandonment and may react to potential losses with panic, emotional instability, anger, or impulsive (suicidal or self-destructive) actions. They often react to medical care with an aggressive and dependent clinging to their physicians and other team members. They may idealize some team members while devaluing others and may make entitled demands for special treatment when they get frustrated. They tend to relate to staff as "all good or all bad," which significantly contributes to their poor life functioning and can create problems within the team.

Under stress, patients may temporarily lose reality testing and manifest severe distortions in perceptions or sense of reality. Low-dose antipsychotic medications[34] may be useful in these circumstances. BPD patients may misunderstand the physician's or team member's intentions or instructions. They may also experience episodes of derealization or depersonalization, or brief psychotic episodes. BPD patients may have extreme fluctuations in self-perception, vacillating from a grandiose overestimation of their capabilities to an excessively harsh underestimation of their talents. They may also experience stormy and chaotic relationships with others. They rely heavily on defenses of splitting, projective identification, projection, and overvaluation and devaluation.

Initial Evaluation and Management

The diagnosis of a BPD patient may be suspected by the way the patient treats the staff. The diagnosis may also be suspected by positive results on general mental health screening (e.g., PHQ-9 positive screen for suicidal ideation). A PD diagnosis should be considered in patients with substance abuse since it so commonly co-occurs with all PDs. Personality diagnosis can be accomplished by using the prototype PD (Box 17.2), the DSM-5, or one of the PD screeners.[26–28] More sophisticated PD assessments, administered by PD specialists, include the Shedler-Westen Assessment Procedure (SWAP)[3] and the Minnesota Multiphasic Personality Inventory (MMPI-22).[38]

Obtaining additional psychosocial and occupational history may be suggestive as well because patients with BPD often report intense unstable relationships, work problems, confusion in their identity (finding a meaningful sustained focus in their lives), as well as a history of co-occurring substance abuse.

The goal of the integrated care team during the patient's initial visit to the practice is to stay focused on the medical questions at hand. If features of BPD are affecting the team's ability to deliver medical care, then the management strategies and interventions described in Tables 17.1 through 17.4 are suggested. If the presenting complaint is related to the BPD diagnosis (suicidal threats or behaviors, cutting/burns noticed during a physical examination, or other psychosocial or occupational dysfunction), then developing a short-term treatment plan is advisable.

Short-Term Treatment Goals

In the integrated care setting, BPD patients with acute issues should be seen by the BHS, psychiatrist, and care coordinator, depending on the issue. The focus of a more detailed mental health assessment by the BHS should be to develop a working alliance, to ensure the patient is actively involved in finding solutions, and to encourage the patient to consider the need for new acute life choices and treatment.[10]

Often a short-term problem-solving approach or crisis intervention (see Chapter 26: Crisis Intervention in Integrated Care) is the preferred focus. During a brief short-term therapy, the BHS should focus on acute suicidal or violence risk and establish safety as the first priority (see Chapter 18: Violence and Suicide).

Often the first decision is to determine the level of care needed. Patients with severe BPD and acute risks may need referral to an emergency department, inpatient psychiatric or substance abuse service, partial hospitalization, or intensive outpatient treatment. These are short-term measures that should evolve into a long-term outpatient plan. Once safety is ensured and outpatient care is possible, it is important for the BHS to obtain a full psychosocial, occupational, and legal history and an understanding of the patient's support network. This includes getting emergency contact information from the patient. It is important to double-check the accuracy of the BPD diagnosis. The care coordinator or BHS should be involved in bringing the family or other supports to aid the patient and/or to secure a referral to an individual specialist or program for treatment.

Long-Term Treatment Goals

Most patients with BPD will need long-term treatment and should be referred to a BPD specialist or specialized program.[10,29,30] There are many evidence-based psychotherapy[10,29–31] treatments for BPD patients, as detailed in Table 17.4. Successful evidence-based mental health treatment is typically twice per week for a mean duration of two years.[23] Because of the need for long-term psychotherapy, the integrated practice will need to carefully coordinate its medical care with the treating specialist. All medical and mental health providers and members of the patient's support network should be alerted when the patient's therapist is away on vacation or out for illness. These are transitional times when a BPD patient may present with an acute crisis. The patient's progress and treatment plan should be tracked in the patient registry.

ASPD

Common team reactions to a patient with ASPD are feelings of being used, exploited, or deceived. This can lead to anger in team members, wishes to punish or uncover lies, or a desire to imprison or be free of the patient. Patients with ASPD fear they will become vulnerable, lose respect or admiration from others, and become easy prey to manipulation when they become ill. They expect to be exploited, demeaned, or humiliated. Like the narcissistic patient, they often have low self-esteem, excessive self-love, compensatory feelings of superiority, grandiosity, recklessness, emotional shallowness, and a lack of concern for others. They often react to medical care with entitled demands for special treatment. When caught in dishonesty they may angrily attack or devalue team members. They may resort to other psychopathic manipulations of deception, lying, cheating, or stealing. Often their intelligent appearance and friendly, facile, slick, superficial charm is beguiling for team members. They can lose reality testing when stressed by the potential of getting caught in their deceptive practices. This is manifested by impulsive actions that reveal severely impaired or even psychotic judgments. When they are receiving medical care for a legitimate illness, they typically function at the same level and often appear to have the same characteristic issues as NPD patients. They can often be managed similarly to an NPD patient.

The team's goal for the initial visit is to stay focused on the medical questions at hand. If this is possible, there is no need to confirm this diagnosis. If features of ASPD are affecting the team's ability to deliver needed medical care, than the suggested approach would be to use the management strategies and interventions as described in Tables 17.1 through 17.4.

Sometimes the presenting complaints of the patient to an integrated care team are specifically related to the ASPD and are related to his or her efforts at a secondary gain. For example, ASPD patients may seek (1) documentation for an illness, which is now resolved, that excuses them from work; (2) help and documentation to obtain disability benefits when a true disability is not present; (3) letters and support to document substance abuse treatments to resolve "driving under the influence" proceedings when the patient is not actively involved in substance use treatment; and (4) medications for pain, anxiety, or attention-deficit/hyperactivity disorder (ADHD), including requests for medical marijuana, opiates for pain, benzodiazepines for alleged anxiety disorder, or stimulants for purported ADHD.

If there is dishonesty in a patient's communication in the form of partial truths, misinformation, outright lying, cheating, or stealing, it is important to avoid the common reaction of moralizing and not to confront the lies directly. Instead, grant patients the reality that they have the ability to fool all their physicians if they choose to do so. The team can suggest that the result of any deception is that the team may make poorly informed medical decisions, which will ultimately result in the patient receiving inadequate or poor medical care. Patients may need to be reminded that the team's role is to help with medical problems and not to pass judgments or help the patient obtain unwarranted medical or social service benefits. It is also important not to inadvertently collude with the patient's plans for secondary gain. For example, if the physician thinks a patient's request for disability is fraudulent or unwarranted, the patient should not be referred for additional disability evaluations. When secondary gain requests appear, it is important to not feel pressured to satisfy the patient's request on the initial visit. Take the time, over several visits, to clinically evaluate the merits and needs related to the patient's complaints. Other recommendations include the following:

- Take an extensive psychosocial, legal, forensics, and occupational history.[10]
- Perform focused physical examinations and testing as appropriate.
- Check state Schedule II prescribing information, if available.
- Consider a urine toxicology screen before prescribing medications that can be abused.
- Use rating scales to document a mental health disorder over repeated visits.
- Obtaining collateral information from the patient's family.
- Get releases of information from other providers to provide supportive documentation.

Clinically, it is most helpful to be positive, to offer hope and optimism about the patient's engagement, to not be punitive, and to continue helping the patient look for more adaptive solutions. Medications targeting violence or impulsivity have limited effectiveness but may be occasionally prescribed by a psychiatrist. Medication for co-occurring substance use is often helpful for patients with ASPD; Table 17.4 provides medication and dosing options.

If the patient has acute problems that need additional resolution, referral to the BHS, psychiatrist, and care coordinator may be warranted. The BHS should use a solution-oriented or crisis-intervention approach. Priorities include focusing on safety issues, especially prevention of domestic, child, or elder abuse; harm reduction if substance use is a problem; or referral for substance use treatment. Criminal or legal problems, substance use, custody issues, and financial problems may be helped by various interventions. These can include conversations with the patient's probation officer, referral to a lawyer or other legal services, referral to debt reduction services, or enrolling the patient in a substance use treatment program. The care coordinator might refer the patient to an educational or training program or assist the patient with pursuit of employment. Referral to alternative levels of general mental health care is rarely useful. Specialists using mentalization-based psychotherapy or group-based CBT can treat some motivated patients with ASPD.

NPD

Patients with NPD may come to the attention of the care team because of the way they treat medical staff. They can be insulting and demeaning when they are not treated as "special."

Reactions to the narcissistic patient are often difficult to manage. The superior, critical, entitled, self-loving, arrogant attitude of these patients can be intimidating. Team members may feel that they are being devalued, feel inferior, or may be fearful of the patient's anger and criticism. Patients with NPD, with their lapses in empathy and a tendency to be interpersonally exploitative, can readily provoke members of the care team to respond with anger, harsh criticism, or belittlement, or with an effort to rid the practice of such a difficult patient.

The core fears of these patients are due to their fragile self-esteem. They fear loss of power, beauty, and success. They fear they will be exploited if they ever show vulnerability. They cope with an underlying low self-esteem (typically not visible or apparent) by seeking power and control. They often make demands for constant approval and praise from others. Any perceived insult to their self-esteem makes them feel rejected, deflated, and criticized, and frequently results in feelings and expressions of rage, shame, or humiliation. In medical settings they can appear gracious and charming when they are well, and are often experienced as leaders. When ill, they may challenge the authority of the medical staff, insulting or denigrating them and treating them as if they were servants; this belittling attitude tends to generate conflict and resentment. Narcissistic patients find it difficult to adhere to medical recommendations since the need for medical care makes them feel weak and inferior, as though they are no longer in a position of authority. Their need to be superior may lead them to look for their own solutions, underuse appropriate medical care, or doctor shop for the "real expert."

As with all PDs, the team's goal during the initial visit is to stay focused on the medical questions at hand. Without problems in care there is no need to search for or confirm a PD diagnosis. If features of NPD are affecting the team's ability to deliver needed medical care, then patient management may be required.

Patients with NPD don't come to integrated care practices because of their PD; they do, however, seek treatment for many other issues that would be easier to treat if they did not have NPD. Substance use, suicidal complaints, and depression are the most common presentations for patients with NPD. Between 24% and 64.2% of NPD patients meet criteria for substance use disorder, one of the most prevalent comorbid disorders in NPD patients.[19,40] Suicidal preoccupation in NPD has a number of unique characteristics, such as the absence of an association with depression, lack of communication about being suicidal, self-esteem dysregulation, and a history of traumatic life events that have assaulted their self-esteem.[40] Events that may precipitate substance use, suicidal ideation, or depression include project or financial failures, major difficulties with school or work, sudden unemployment, or legal or disciplinary problems related to fraud, marriage, child custody, or physical illness.[40] These events can assault their narcissistic equilibrium, grandiose self-esteem, self-importance, and self-perceived image of success or brilliance. Depression, precipitated by negative life events, is deeply shaming for patients with NPD. They are likely to feel defeated and trapped by depressive experiences that are at odds with their excessive self-esteem and expectations of exceptional functioning.

OCPD

According the prototypic descriptions (see Box 17.2) patients with OCPD are characterized by eight personality traits: preoccupation with details, perfectionism, excessive devotion to work and productivity, over-conscientiousness, inability to discard worthless objects, inability to delegate tasks, miserliness, rigidity, and stubbornness. These traits are ego-syntonic lifelong patterns that many patients view as personal strengths that they can use adaptively in their professional life. OCPD patients do not experience the severe obsessions and compulsions, the significant time lost obsessing or in performing repetitive tasks, or the marked subjective distress that are the common characteristics of OCD. There is evidence of higher comorbidity rates between OCPD and OCD than between other PDs,[21] suggesting that these disorders are on the same spectrum and may have some common neurobiological origins. OCPD patients' attention to detail leads them to a perfectionistic belief and/or worry that they must not make mistakes or be imperfect. They can interpret rules, regulations, and values rigidly and stubbornly. Patients with OCPD are often uncomfortable with feelings and emotions. They may fear disorderliness and dirt. The compulsive, orderly, obstinate, stingy, critical, controlling, self-righteous side of their personalities often creates difficulty in relationships with coworkers, friends, and family. As the most common PD in the general population, it is associated with at least moderate impairment in psychosocial functioning,[41,42] reduced quality of life,[43,44] and a considerable economic burden.[45]

The goal of the initial contact with these patients is to address their medical issues. In general, OCPD is generally not the primary focus of the patient's visit. Medical illness or medical complications often represent a dangerous threat to the patient's sense of self-control. The team should understand and empathize with this perceived loss of self-control and offer detailed information and care plans. Discussing disease self-management strategies, tracking of symptoms, and developing medication adherence strategies may help the OCPD patient regain some sense of control in the management of his or her illness or problem.

Struggle or conflict with the patient over control should be avoided. Reality distortions, including perfectionistic demands, excessive criticism, or questioning, may respond to limit setting. Gentle exploration of the patient's feeling and fears can be helpful.

From a mental health point of view, patients with OCPD seek treatment for co-occurring anxiety disorders (panic attack and generalized anxiety), mood disorders, and substance use disorders. In the process of treating these disorders the personality features of OCPD may become apparent and troublesome. Patients with OCPD may demand excessive precision and details when describing a diagnosis, treatment recommendations, or use of

BOX 17.4
SUMMARY OF RECOMMENDED TREATMENT APPROACHES AND RELEVANT EVIDENCE

Strength of recommendation taxonomy (SOR A, B, or C)

- Twin studies suggest heritability of personality traits and PDs ranging from 30% to 60% (SOR A).[2]
- 9.1% of a community sample has a PD (SOR A).[7]
- The lifetime prevalence of borderline personality disorder (BPD) ranges from 0.5% to 5.9%. Lifetime prevalence of a BPD patient having one comorbid psychiatric disorder approaches 100%. Mood disorders, bipolar, anxiety, schizotypal and narcissistic personality disorders, and substance abuse have high co-occurrence rates (SOR A).[7,11,12]
- Lifetime prevalence of antisocial personality disorder (ASPD) in the general population is 3.6%, adult antisocial behavior is 12.3%, and conduct disorder without adult antisocial behavior is 1.1%. Substance use is the most common co-occurring disorder with ASPD with a 30.3% lifetime prevalence of any alcohol use disorders and a 10.3% lifetime prevalence rate of any drug use disorder (SOR A).[7,15]
- Lifetime prevalence of narcissistic personality disorder (NPD) is 6.2%. Substance use, mood and anxiety disorders, and other PDs commonly co-occur in patients with NPD (SOR A).[19]
- The prevalence of obsessive-compulsive personality disorder (OCPD) is 7.9%, making it the most common PD. Studies from nonclinical populations indicate that a lifetime diagnosis of OCPD is moderately common in individuals with anxiety disorders (23–24%), affective disorders (24%), and/or substance-related disorders (12–25%) (SOR A).[20,21]
- There are three PD screeners that can assist in diagnosis: Personality Assessment Screener (a 22-item self-report measure), Standardized Assessment of Personality (eight-item self-report), and Iowa Personality Disorder Screen (five-minute standardized interview) (SOR B).[26–28]
- Shedler-Westen Assessment Procedure (SWAP) and the Minnesota Multiphasic Personality Inventory (MMPI-22) are definitive tests that can be used by PD specialists to diagnose a PD (SOR A).[3,28]
- Practice guidelines for the management and treatment of PDs are useful (SOR B).[10,29–31]
- The management, brief treatment, and long-term treatment of patients with PDs are primarily psychological (SOR A).[10,29–31]
- Regular integrated care team planning and use of a care pathway are helpful in the management and treatment of patients with BPD and ASPD (SOR B).[10,29–31]
- The first treatment goal is to establish a working alliance—a partnership with the patient that keeps the patient involved in problem solving and maximizes his or her autonomy (SOR A).[10,29–31]
- There are now many viable evidence-based psychotherapies that are effective for the treatment of BPD, ASPD, NPD, and OCPD (SOR A).[10,19,21,29–31]
- Patients with BPD will need long-term psychological treatment and should be referred to a BPD specialist or a specialized program (SOR A).[10,29–31]
- Medications for patients with BPD can be used short term to target cognitive perceptual symptoms; mood, irritability, or affect dysregulation symptoms; or impulsivity (see Table 17.4. (SOR B).[32–35]
- Medications to target violence or impulsivity for patients with ASPD, such as lithium and phenytoin, have limited evidence for efficacy in this patient group (SOR C).[10,15,36]
- Carbamazepine and fluvoxamine may be helpful for the primary treatment of OCPD (SOR C).[20] Citalopram is useful for patients with OCPD and a co-occurring depression (SOR B).[20]

medications and potential side effects. Their questions may be repetitive, with requests for greater and greater detail. Patients can be annoyed, critical, or hostile about problems in scheduling, delays in being seen, the care team not having read prior records, billing or insurance issues, or other perceived imperfections in the way a practice is run. The office management of these issues is the same as previously described and can be can be reviewed in Tables 17.1.

CONCLUSION

Patients with PDs contribute significantly to wear and tear on the integrated care team, and frequently this results in poor-quality medical care for this difficult yet all-too-common patient population. This chapter described the diagnosis, management, intervention, and referral strategies for working with patients who have four common PDs seen in medical settings. The PD schema is a useful management tool that can help guide the care offered by the integrated care team. We also present a care-management strategy for all members of the integrated care team and describe the typical presentations and issues common in each disorder. See Box 17.4 to review the prevalence and evidence-based treatment for these four common personality disorders.

REFERENCES

1. Athanassios D, Tsopelas C, Tzeferakos G. Medical comorbidity of cluster B personality disorders. Curr Opin Psychiatr. 2012;25(5):398–404.
2. Gask L, Evans M, Kessler D. Personality disorder. Br Med J. 2013;347(7924):28–32. doi:http://dx.doi.org/10.1136/bmj.f5276.
3. Tyrer P, Mitchard S, Methuen C, Ranger M. Treatment-rejecting and treatment-seeking personality disorders: Type R and Type S. J Pers Disord. 2003;17(3):263–268.
4. Shedler-Westen Assessment Procedure (SWAP). http://www.SWAPassessment.org Published 2015. Accessed March 26, 2016.
5. Feinstein RE, Connelly J. Difficult clinical encounters: Patients with personality disorders. In: Rakel R, ed. Textbook of Family Medicine, 9th ed. Philadelphia: W. B. Saunders; 2015:1074–1089.
6. Feinstein RE. Personality traits and disorders. In: Blumenfield M, Strain J, eds. Psychosomatic Medicine. Philadelphia: Lippincott Williams & Wilkins; 2006:843–865.
7. Crawford TN, Cohen P, Johnson JG, et al. Self-reported personality disorder in the children in the community sample: Convergent and prospective validity in late adolescence and adulthood. J Pers Disord. 2005;19(1):30–52.
8. American Psychiatric Association. Diagnostic and Statistical Manual of Mental disorders, Fifth ed. Arlington, VA: American Psychiatric Publishing: 2013.
9. Grant BF, Stinson FS, Dawson DA, Chou SP, Ruan WJ. Co-occurrence of DSM-IV personality disorders in the United States: Results from the National Epidemiologic Survey on Alcohol and Related Conditions. Compr Psychiatry. 2005;46(1):1–5.
10. Kendall T, Pilling S, Tyrer P, et al. Borderline and antisocial personality disorders: Summary of NICE guidance. Br Med J. 2009;338(7689):293–295.
11. Leichsenring F, Leibing E, Kruse J, New AS, Leweke F. Borderline personality disorder. Focus. 2014;11(2):249–260.
12. Grant BF, Chou SP, Goldstein RB, et al. Prevalence, correlates, disability, and comorbidity of DSM-IV borderline personality disorder: Results from the Wave 2 National Epidemiologic Survey on Alcohol and Related Conditions. J Clin Psychiatry. 2008;69(4):533–545.
13. Perez-Rodriguez MM, Zaluda L, New AS. Biological advances in personality disorders. Focus. 2013;11(2):146–154.
14. Stein DJ. Borderline personality disorder: toward integration. CNS Spectr. 2009;14(7):352–356.
15. Compton WM, Conway KP, Stinson FS, Colliver JD, Grant BF. Prevalence, correlates, and comorbidity of DSM-IV antisocial personality syndromes and alcohol and specific drug use disorders in the United States: Results from the National Epidemiologic Survey on Alcohol and Related Conditions. J Clin Psychiatry. 2005;66(6):1–478.
16. Raine A, Lencz T, Bihrle S, LaCasse L, Colletti P. Reduced prefrontal gray matter volume and reduced autonomic activity in antisocial personality disorder. Arch Gen Psychiatry. 2000;57(2):119–127.
17. McWilliams N. Psychoanalytic Diagnosis: Understanding Personality Structure in the Clinical Process. New York: Guilford Press; 2011.
18. Russ E, Shedler J, Bradley R, Westen D. Refining the construct of narcissistic personality disorder: Diagnostic criteria and subtypes. Am J Psychiatry. 2008;165(11):1473–1481.
19. Stinson FS, Dawson DA, Goldstein RB, et al. Prevalence, correlates, disability, and comorbidity of DSM-IV narcissistic personality disorder: Results from the Wave 2 National Epidemiologic Survey on Alcohol and Related Conditions. J Clin Psychiatry. 2008;69(7):1033–1045.
20. Grant JE, Mooney ME, Kushner MG. Prevalence, correlates, and comorbidity of DSM-IV obsessive-compulsive personality disorder: Results from the National Epidemiologic Survey on Alcohol and Related Conditions. J Psychiatr Res. 2012;46(4):469–475.
21. Diedrich A, Voderholzer U. Obsessive–compulsive personality disorder: A current review. Curr Psychiatry Rep. 2015;17(2):1–10.

22. Reichborn-Kjennerud T, Czajkowski N, Neale MC, et al. Major depression and dimensional representations of DSM-IV personality disorders: A population-based twin study. Psychol Med. 2010;40(09):1475–1484.
23. Bender DS, Dolan RT, Skodol AE, et al. Treatment utilization by patients with personality disorders. Am J Psychiatry. 2001;158(2):295–302.
24. Kroenke K, Spitzer RL, Williams JB. The PHQ-9: Validity of a brief depression severity measure. J Gen Intern Med. 2001;16(9):606–613.
25. Saunders JB, Aasland OG, Babor TF, de la Fuente JR, Grant M. Development of the Alcohol Use Disorders Identification Test (AUDIT): WHO Collaborative Project on Early Detection of Persons with Harmful Alcohol Consumption—II. Addiction. 1993;88(6):791–804.
26. Morey LC. Personality Assessment Screener. Odessa, FL: Psychological Assessment Resources Inc., 1991.
27. Moran P, Leese M, Lee T, Walters P, Thornicroft G, Mann A. Standardised Assessment of Personality–Abbreviated Scale (SAPAS): Preliminary validation of a brief screen for personality disorder. Br J Psychiatry. 2003;183(3):228–232.
28. Langbehn DR, Pfohl BM, Reynolds S, et al. The Iowa Personality Disorder Screen: Development and preliminary validation of a brief screening interview. J Pers Disord.1999;13(1):75–89.
29. Bateman AW, Gunderson J, Mulder R. Treatment of personality disorder. Lancet. 2015;385 (9969):735–743.
30. Oldham JM. Guideline watch: Practice guideline for the treatment of patients with borderline personality disorder. Focus. 2005;3(30):396–400.
31. Gunderson JG, Weinberg I, Choi-Kain L. Borderline personality disorder. Focus. 2014; 11(2):129–145.
32. Feurino III L, Silk KR. State of the art in the pharmacologic treatment of borderline personality disorder. Curr Psychiatry Rep. 2011;13(1):69–75.
33. Crawford MJ, MacLaren T, Reilly JG. Are mood stabilisers helpful in treatment of borderline personality disorder? Br Med J. 2014; 349:g5378.
34. Soloff PH. Psychopharmacology of borderline personality disorder. Psychiatric Clin North Am. 2000;23(1):169–192.
35. Paton C, Crawford MJ, Bhatti SF, Patel MX, Barnes TR. The use of psychotropic medication in patients with emotionally unstable personality disorder under the care of UK mental health services. J Clin Psychiatry. 2015;76(4):1–478.
36. Ripoll LH, Triebwasser J, Siever LJ. Evidence-based pharmacotherapy for personality disorders. Focus. 2013;11(2):225–248.
37. Markovitz PJ. Recent trends in the pharmacotherapy of personality disorder. J Pers Disord. 2004;18(1):90–101.
38. Hathaway SR, McKinley JC, and MMPI Restandardization Committee. MMPI-2: Minnesota Multiphasic Personality Inventory-2: Manual for administration and scoring. Minneapolis: University of Minnesota Press; 1989.
39. Fowler JC, Oldham JM. Co-occurring disorders and treatment complexity within personality disorders. Focus. 2013;11(2):123–128.
40. Ronningstam E, Weinberg I. Narcissistic personality disorder: progress in recognition and treatment. Focus. 2013;11(2):167–177.
41. Mancebo MC, Eisen JL, Grant JE, Rasmussen SA. Obsessive compulsive personality disorder and obsessive compulsive disorder: Clinical characteristics, diagnostic difficulties, and treatment. Ann Clin Psychiatry. 2005;17(4):197–204.
42. Pinto A, Steinglass JE, Greene AL, Weber EU, Simpson HB. Capacity to delay reward differentiates obsessive-compulsive disorder and obsessive-compulsive personality disorder. Biol Psychiatry. 2014;75(8):653–659.
43. Skodol AE, Gunderson JG, McGlashan, et al. Functional impairment in patients with schizotypal, borderline, avoidant, or obsessive–compulsive personality disorder. Am J Psychiatry. 2002;159(2):276–283.
44. Soeteman DI, Hakkaart-van Roijen L, Verheul R, Busschbach JJ. The economic burden of personality disorders in mental health care. J Clin Psychiatry. 2008;69(2):259–265.

18

Violence and Suicide

ROBERT E. FEINSTEIN

BOX 18.1

KEY POINTS

- **Intimate partner violence, violence toward others, and suicide risk, frequently seen in a group of difficult patients, can be managed effectively in a primary care environment by a team composed of a primary care provider, a behavioral health specialist, a care manager, and a consulting psychiatrist.**
- **Risk is best assessed by using screening instruments in combination with a clinical approach. This population of patients should be tracked in a high-risk registry.**
- **Treatment of these high-risk patient populations often requires different levels of care at different points in time.**
- **The critical pathway presented in Table 18.2 describes a clinical approach to evaluating and managing violence and suicidal patients over one year. The pathway focuses on screening, measuring progress, and outcomes. It can be used in conjunction with the patient high-risk registry.**
- **Integrated medical and psychiatric care is focused on treating the underlying diagnosis or problem using problem solving, crisis intervention, family therapy, cognitive/behavioral therapy, or a psychodynamic approach.**
- **Medications are an adjunctive treatment approach.**
- **Criteria for psychiatric commitment and confidentiality and duty to warn/duty to protect are determined by local state laws.**
- **Diagnosis and treatment for intimate partner violence requires a multidisciplinary integrated team comprising at minimum a primary care provider, a behavioral health specialist, a care manager, and a psychiatric consultant. Care for intimate partner violence patients can be accomplished by using a clinical approach (especially working with patient ambivalence, awareness of reporting requirements, use of network support, and community resources).**

INTRODUCTION

Patients exhibiting violent or suicidal behavior have dangerous psychiatric symptoms. Symptoms expressed as feelings, thoughts, fantasies, or destructive behaviors are often associated with psychiatric disorders (e.g., psychosis, depression, substance abuse), trauma, impulsivity, anger, or feelings of hopelessness. The intensity of symptoms and behaviors varies along a spectrum of risk, ranging from minimal to fatal.

Clinical work with violent or suicidal patients is often anxiety-provoking and extremely challenging. Using a practice registry and critical pathway organizes and maximizes care offered in integrated medical and behavioral environments. The registry and critical pathway are designed to track the patient's progress and ability to connect with referrals; they are focused on outcomes. To recognize and manage violent and suicidal patients optimally, a primary care clinician should work with an interdisciplinary team composed of a behavioral health specialist, a care team manager, and a psychiatric consultant. The team should use a specific biopsychosocial-cultural approach to assess risk, avoid harmful outcomes, and organize care, while tracking patient progress. See Box 18.1 for a summary of the key points to keep in mind when dealing with potentially violent or suicidal patients.

DEFINITIONS

Violence

Violence is defined as the use of physical force or power, threatened or actual, with the intent of causing intimidation, harm, injury, death, or property damage. Medical and psychiatric treatment is required when violence is related to biological or genetic factors, psychiatric illnesses, or social problems, such as intimate partner violence (IPV). Violence as a focus of medical or psychiatric intervention and treatment should be distinguished from crime, such as homicide, or institutionalized violence, such as war or terrorism.

Suicide

Suicide is defined as intentional self-inflicted death. A suicide attempt is a potentially self-injurious act committed with a wish to die. People with suicidal ideation have thoughts about killing themselves. Deliberate, nonsuicidal self-harm is the willful self-infliction of painful, destructive, or injurious acts without the intent to die.

PRESENTATION OF VIOLENCE, INTIMATE PARTNER VIOLENCE, AND SUICIDE

Violence, IPV, and suicide present as medical phenomena on a spectrum from minor symptoms to high-risk events. All warning signs and symptoms of violence and suicide require some level of intervention. The spectrum of violence ranges from violent ideations, verbal aggression, verbal abuse or threats, damage to property, minor physical violence, dangerous assaults, to death. Suicide risk also presents on a spectrum from suicidal ideation, suicide intent, deliberate nonsuicidal self-harm, suicide attempt, to successful suicide. Dangerousness risk for both violence and suicide markedly increases with the use of weapons, especially guns. Interventions to treat these issues range from screenings and individual or family assessment of risk, to outpatient therapy with or without medication, partial hospitalization, inpatient psychiatric commitment, substance abuse treatment, and in rare cases prison. As medical issues, these symptoms rarely present in isolation and are typically associated with a specific psychiatric diagnosis or other psychosocial stressors, such as marital problems.

DIFFERENTIAL DIAGNOSIS

Violence

Patients with schizophrenia, schizoaffective disorder, or other psychotic illnesses comorbid with substance abuse have approximately a 0.3% risk of committing homicide.[1] Comorbid substance abuse accounts for most of this risk. People with paranoia, paranoid delusions, or command hallucinations may respond violently to a perceived threat. The risk of aggression increases with a depression that is accompanied by irritability, hostility, or psychosis. Patients with bipolar disorder who present in manic, hypomanic, or mixed state often display irritability, angry outbursts, or overt psychosis, which can lead to impulsive aggression. Those with antisocial, borderline, narcissistic, or histrionic personality disorder and substance use disorders, whether intoxicated or in withdrawal, may also show signs of aggression. An underlying delirium, dementia, traumatic brain injury, neurologic illness, and developmental delays are part of the differential diagnosis of aggressive disinhibited behavioral changes. In the absence of these conditions, consider intermittent explosive disorder in the differential.

Suicide

Most patients with suicidal symptoms have at least one psychiatric diagnosis. Mood disorders increase the risk of suicide during a depressive episode. Patients who seem to be recovering from depression may be just well enough to plan and carry out a suicide, which they see as the solution to their problems. Patients with depression are more likely to commit suicide if they have panic attacks or insomnia or abuse alcohol or drugs.

Compared with the general population, people with schizophrenia are 8.5 times more likely to commit suicide and have a lifetime risk of about 4.9%.[2] During the early years of this illness, suicide is frequent in hopeless patients who have depressive symptoms or insight into the extent of their mental disability. There is also a heightened period of suicide risk immediately after a hospital discharge. Although psychotic symptoms are often present at the time of an attempted or completed suicide, suicide can also occur during periods when psychotic symptoms are improving.

Alcoholism and drug abuse carry a 10% lifetime risk of suicide.[3] This risk increases further with depressive symptoms, impending interpersonal losses, other comorbid psychiatric disorders, and chronic medical disabilities.

People with borderline personality disorder have a much higher suicide risk than the general population. Other mixed personality disorders have been frequently identified in people who commit suicide.

EPIDEMIOLOGY OF VIOLENCE, IPV, AND SUICIDE

The actual number of patients presenting with risk of violence, IPV, or suicide in primary care settings is not reliably available. However, community-based statistic are available, as shown in detail in Box 18.2 and Box 18.3.

There are no reliable statistics of imminent violence risk within general outpatient primary care settings. In inpatient medical environments, over a lifetime, 100% of nurses and 24% to 57% of physicians experience aggression or violence from patients.[11] Annually, 5% to 21% of physicians experience assaults in all settings.[11] Over a lifetime, 72% to 96% of mental health workers are verbally threatened, and 35% to 56% have been assaulted at least once.[11] The most common sites for violence are emergency departments, geriatric care facilities, psychiatric and substance abuse facilities, hospital pharmacies, and outpatient practices in high-crime areas. Because violent events are highly traumatic, even if rare in primary care practice, outpatient practices should make a special effort to train staff in verbal de-escalation techniques (Table 18.1), to enable clinicians to assess and intervene to prevent immediate harm. In addition, a comprehensive violence prevention program for ambulatory outpatient settings can be developed as needed and is described elsewhere.[15]

ETIOLOGY OF VIOLENCE, IPV, AND SUICIDE

Neurobiological Factors

The serotonin neurotransmitter system is involved in the complex neurobiological processes that underlie violent and suicidal behavior.[16–18] Evidence suggests that serotonin deficiency is associated with impulsivity, aggressive behavior, and a risk of suicide.[16,17] Impulsivity seems to be an inherited trait that makes people more vulnerable to violent[18] and suicidal behaviors.[16,17] First-degree relatives of suicidal people have a four- to 10-fold increase in suicidal behavior.[3,17] Ongoing research is trying to identify genetic markers for such vulnerability.

Societal Influences

Cultural influences vary widely and can greatly affect attitudes toward violence and suicide. Media, including the Internet, television, film, and popular music, have become increasingly violent in content, and may be responsible for encouraging the likelihood of violence. However, to date, insufficient evidence exists to confirm this association.

The Japanese traditionally have viewed suicide as an honorable solution to a disgraceful situation, whereas many other cultures and religions consider suicide a dishonorable act. Media reports of celebrity suicides have been known to precipitate "copycat" suicides. Suicide as a contagion can spread through a school system or community. To prevent this phenomenon, it is customary for schools or media to downplay suicide reports.

Economic Conditions

Rates of violence and suicide are related to economic downturns and periods of high crime and occur most frequently among the poor and socioeconomically disadvantaged. Conversely, rates of violence and suicide decrease during times of economic prosperity and war.

CLINICAL APPROACH

Screening

Initial screening for suicide risk and IPV should be conducted.[6,7,14] Integrated practices need to make choices about the kind and methods of initial screening tools used, on the basis of patient population and available resources. The Patient Health Questionaire-2 (PHQ-2)[19] screens for depression, whereas the PHQ-9[20] assesses depression and suicide risk. Clinicians can use a variety of methods to screen for IPV. SAFE[21] questions are helpful:

S: Are you **S**tressed or do you feel **S**afe in your relationships?

A: Do you feel **A**fraid or have you been **A**bused by anyone?

BOX 18.2

EPIDEMIOLOGY OF VIOLENCE IN THE UNITED STATES

ADULTS AND VIOLENCE[4–7]

- **Prevalence of violence in primary care setting is unknown.**
- **People with severe mental illnesses, schizophrenia, bipolar disorder, or psychosis are 2.5 times more likely to be the victims of violence (attacked, raped, or mugged than the general population).[4–6]**

INTIMATE PARTNER VIOLENCE (IPV), 2009[7–9]

- **One in four women and one in seven men experienced severe physical IPV.**
- **20% of couples report IPV.**
- **Approximately 1.3 to 5.3 million women in the United States experience IPV each year.**
- **Lifetime estimates of IPV range from 22% to 39%.**
- **Lifetime, 30% of women experience physical violence, 9% rape, 17% sexual violence other than rape, and 48% psychological aggression from their intimate partners.**

ECONOMIC COST[7]

- **Annual health care cost of IPV ranges from $2 to $7 billion.**

SEXUAL VIOLENCE, 2009[8]

- **Lifetime risk of rape was one in four for women and one in 71 for men.**
- **Lifetime risk of stalking was one in six for women and one in 19 for men.**

YOUTH HOMICIDES, 2010[10]

- **4,828 deaths occurred.**
- **Youth homicide was the second leading cause of death for ages 10 to 24 (86% male, 14% female).**

SCHOOL VIOLENCE, 2011 (GRADES 9–12)[10]

- **12% of students were involved in a physical fight.**
- **5.9% of students did not go to school in the preceding 30 days for fear of violence.**
- **5.4% carried a weapon (gun, knife, club) once in the preceding 30 days.**
- **7.4% were injured by a weapon once or more in the previous 12 months.**

PATIENT AND VISITOR VIOLENCE IN GENERAL HOSPITAL SETTINGS, 2011[11]

- **Patients are more violent than visitors.**
- **9% to 25% of staff experienced verbal aggression each year.**
- **5% to 21% of physicians were assaulted each year.**
- **100% of nurses and 24% to 57% physicians experienced aggression or violence from patients each year.**
- **33% of psychiatrists were assaulted at least once in their lifetime.**
- **72% to 96% of psychiatric physician residents were verbally threatened.**
- **35% to 56% of psychiatric physician residents were physically assaulted.**

BOX 18.3

EPIDEMIOLOGY OF SUICIDE*

STATISTICS

- **The suicide rate in primary care settings is unknown.**
- **Suicide is the 10th leading cause of death in the United States, accounting for 36,897 deaths, with an age-adjusted rate of 11.8 deaths per 100,000 individuals.**
- **Suicide is the third leading cause of death in both males and females ages 15 to 24. Only accidents and homicides occur more frequently in this age group (approximately 10 suicides per 100,000 persons, 13 homicides per 100,000 persons, and 37.4 accidents per 100,000 persons).**
- **79% of all suicides are males.**
- **Men complete suicide at a rate four times that of women.**
- **The suicide rate for women typically peaks in middle adulthood (ages 45–49) and declines slightly after age 60.**
- **Older white men (age 65 years or older) are at the highest risk of suicide (approximately 31 suicides per 100,000 persons each year).**
- **20% of all known suicides in the United States occur among current or former military personnel. U.S. soldiers' suicide deaths outnumber all combat deaths in Afghanistan.**
- **Non-Hispanic whites are twice as likely to commit suicide as are members of other racial/ethnic groups.**
- **Less religious people, unmarried people, and those with severe illnesses have higher suicide rates.**
- **Firearms, pills, and substance use are the most common means for successful suicides.**

SUICIDE ATTEMPTS AND IDEATION

- **1 million suicide attempts occur annually (25 attempts for every one completion) in the general U.S. population.**
- **Past suicidal behavior is the strongest predictor of future attempts.**
- **79% of all suicides are males, but females attempt suicide three times more often than males.**
- **Older persons attempt suicide less often than younger persons but are more often successful (approximately four suicide attempts for one completed suicide).**

*American Association of Suicidology. http://www.suicidology.org/resources/facts-statistics. Accessed June 20, 2015; Centers for Disease Control and Prevention. Suicide facts at a glance 2012. http://www.cdc.gov/violenceprevention/pdf/suicide-datasheet-a.pdf. Accessed June 20, 2015; O'Connor E, Gaynes BN, Burda BU, Soh C, Whitlock EP. Screening for and treatment of suicide risk relevant to primary care: A systematic review for the US Preventive Services Task Force. Ann Intern Med. 2013;158(10):741–754.

F: Are *F*riends and *F*amily aware and/or can you tell them about it?

E: Do you have an *E*mergency plan?

Asking additional questions is helpful:

Can you get to an emergency room or a domestic violence shelter?

Do you have friends or a social worker to help you?

Currently, the value of routine population screening for violence risk, has yet to be demonstrated for primary care practices.

Clinical Interview

The main purpose of the clinical interview is to help patients verbalize feelings and problems to prevent them from taking dangerous actions. Interviewing should begin when frightened patients and apprehensive clinicians feel safe. Staff, security, or police should be nearby and able to intervene.

TABLE 18.1 BEHAVIORAL PHASES OF IMMINENT VIOLENCE OR SUICIDAL RISK IN PRIMARY CARE SETTINGS

Phase	Observed Patient Behavior	Suggested Intervention
Calm Phase	• Relaxed, alert, fully conscious, good self-care, and normal social interaction • Evidence of weapons, knives, pills, intoxication or withdrawal?	• Observe all patients at a remote distance for 30 seconds. • Assess during all phases.
Psychomotor Agitation (nonaggressive, nonverbal: mild violence risk)	• Physical movement (e.g., restless/pacing) • Psychic agitation (e.g., anxiety or confusion) approach–avoidance behaviors (vigilant or paranoid approach then walking away) • Suicidal: withdrawn, anxious, restless, vague statements about suicide, mute; face looks mad or sad	• Empathy/supportive: "How can I help?" • Assume a relaxed body stance, hands visible, good eye contact. Sit or stand at a 45-degree angle to the patient. • Set expectations; the time and length of the patient's visit. • Validate patient's experience. • Understand the current situation. • Medications prn: atypical antipsychotic and/or benzodiazepines
Mild Verbal Aggression (approach/avoidance behaviors have moderate violence risk)	• Patient expresses annoyance, anger, hopelessness, suicidal ideation, or helplessness. • Impulsive behaviors?	• Empathy/supportive: "How can I help?" • Name the affect ("You look upset"). • "How can I help?" • "What's happened?" • Ask: suicidal/violent? • Apologize prn. • Suggest a solution. • Appreciate patient's comments. • Medications prn
High Verbal Aggression (approach/avoidance behaviors have high violence risk)	• Impulsive behaviors, arguing, questioning authority; is insistent, defensive, yelling, or cursing • Threatens suicide	• Empathy, nonthreatening, directive, commanding, calm, or firm statements (e.g., "Sit down!" "Calm down!"). Use staff support. • Use counter-projective statements (e.g., describe the patient's feeling, and direct emotions towards others). • Maintain a distance of 1.5 leg lengths. Sit/stand at a 45-degree angle to patient. Suspect weapons. • Use time out, prn meds, end the interview, call police.
Physical Aggression (highest risk)	Patient with aggressive action (e.g., throwing things) or violence, suicidal gestures or attempts	• Show of force with additional staff present • Suspect weapons. • Call security/police. • Use medications, prn.
Post-Violence Phase (mild to moderate risk)	Patient may fear punishment or retaliation or feel guilty or ashamed.	• Reassure patient there will be no retaliation or punishment. • Review coping styles to prevent future episodes.

Establish the Working Alliance

An unruffled clinician, using calm questioning and interviewing, helps troubled patients remain engaged and in control. The interview can help patients understand their stressors and current problems with the goal of resolving anger or suicidal feelings.

Many violent or suicidal patients are defensive and deny their true intentions or the seriousness of events. If the patient cannot discuss feelings and the relevant events, the clinician can invite supportive friends or family to tell their versions of the events. A crisis intervention approach (see Chapter 26: Crisis Intervention in Integrated Care) or a family approach (see Chapter 27: Best Practice for Family-Centered Health Care: A Three-Step Model) may ameliorate the patient's denial, allowing feelings and problem solving.

Clinician Reactions to Dangerous Patients

Violent or IPV patients are often irritable, angry, and impatient and may threaten violence to gain control. Unfortunately, clinicians may react with excessive anger, hate, moralizing, retaliation, or a wish to press charges or imprison a patient. Recognizing common reactions and consulting with behavioral specialists can prevent clinicians from making emotional decisions that can lead to poorly conceived treatment plans.

Suicidal patients may feel hopeless and act helpless and use suicide threats as a means of manipulating others or of dealing with a situation they feel unable to change. Suicidal patients can elicit rescue fantasies in clinicians or, conversely, feelings of anger or a wish that the patient will die or succeed in a suicide attempt. Using behavioral health consultants to manage physician reactions is often necessary.

Obtaining History and Establishing a Focus for Care

The interview should focus on the details of the crisis. It should identify stressors and all contributory issues. Developing a specific timeline of events, beginning with "Why now?" and working backward from the present (i.e., events in the past six weeks) keeps the interview focused on problem solving and resolution instead of focusing on taking a comprehensive history (see Chapter 26: Crisis Intervention in Integrated Care Settings). Understanding the meaning and context of the crisis will suggest the focus of care and the approach to problem solving. Obtaining the details of the patient's support network, including family, friends, neighbors, other medical providers, and all useful community supports, may give insight into the nature of the current crisis. Supportive networks can/should be mobilized to assist with problem resolution.

Clinical Assessment of Violence and Suicide Risk

Long-term predictions of when, where, how, or with whom future violent or suicidal events may occur is not possible. The best approach to assess potential risk, which combines clinical assessment of violence and suicide risk with standardized risk-assessment tools. When combined, assessments can be systematized, outcomes can be improved, and careful documentation can be an essential part of a risk-management strategy. A clinical approach to imminent risk determinations can be accomplished by assessing the following eight variables.[22]

Current Violent or Suicidal Ideation

Violent and suicidal ideation ranges in risk from high to low probability of imminent danger. At highest risk are patients with violent or suicidal ideation and a plan associated with specific timing. High-risk patients may also be suffering with command auditory hallucinations or delusions of killing or hurting someone or themselves, especially in the presence of substance use. Moderate risk occurs in patients who express a nonspecific threat of violence or suicide. Ambivalence to hurting others, damaging property, or committing suicide carries lesser risk. Patients without thoughts of violence or homicide or suicide have the lowest risk.

Recent Violent, Aggressive, or Suicidal Behavior

A similar continuum of recent behaviors may correlate with imminent risk. The spectrum of imminent risk, from highest to lowest probability for dangerous behavior, is as follows:

(A) High-risk patients describe recent impulsive or intentional assaultive behavior or a serious suicide attempt, often have a specific violence or suicide plan, may have a major psychiatric illnesses and access to weapons

(B) Less imminently dangerous are patients with ambivalence, who either have hit someone without serious sequela or made less lethal suicide attempts

(C) Patients who damage property or who feel depressed or hopeless carry even less risk but still require much clinical involvement.
(D) Patients who have never demonstrated any tendency toward action are in the lowest risk group.

Past History of Aggressive/Violent and Suicidal Ideation and Behavior

A history of past violence or suicide attempts is the best predictor of future dangerousness but does not predict the timing of future events. Obtaining a detailed history of the lifetime pattern of anger or violence and suicidal tendencies is essential for understanding the patient's potential for dangerous behavior. Precipitating factors, intent, intensity, frequency, nature, and context of ideation and risky behaviors require special inquiry. Collecting information from collateral sources is essential and should include family members, victims, court records, medical records, and previous providers.

Support System

A healthy family and support network can be mobilized to reduce risk. Supportive people provide a buffer against stressors, help resolve problems, and offer concrete resources. Unfortunately, some networks can cause the problem (as in IPV situations) by covertly inciting violence or unconsciously encouraging the patient to commit suicide. Some family members may be enablers of substance abuse. Excluding hostile, angry, unsupportive, or toxic people in the patient's network is often necessary.

It is important to map the support network (see Chapter 26: Crisis Intervention in Integrated Care) and assess the network for interest, competence, and availability. Families and competent available helpers, who are interested in the patient, can provide excellent support for high-risk patients. Sometimes, excluding pathological support (e.g., hostile, angry, toxic family members) is required. Assessing the abilities of the patient's network to support a patient is most helpful when deciding if outpatient care is possible or if hospitalization is required.

Substance Abuse

Substance abuse is the largest amplifier of dangerousness. Alcoholism and drug abuse are associated with approximately a six times increased risk for suicide, compared with the general population. Interpersonal losses and comorbid psychiatric disorders may precipitate suicide in an alcoholic. Suicide is more likely in intoxicated patients or in substance use withdrawal patients and in alcoholics who have depressive episodes.

Some drugs of abuse (e.g., alcohol, stimulants) significantly increase dangerous risk, whereas other drugs, such as marijuana, have varied effects. Chronic substance abusers or compulsive binge abusers are at greater long-term risk of imminent danger than recreational users.

Ability to Cooperate with Treatment

The clinician's perception of the patient's ability to cooperate with treatment should guide decisions of the types of treatment offered. Patients who agree to take an active role in participating, planning, and arranging their own treatment are most likely to become outpatients. Patients who have limited capacity, weak motivation for treatment, or prior nonadherence to treatment recommendations may need intensive outpatient services or inpatient treatment. Patients who are dangerous to themselves or others or who cannot participate in treatment may require admission and/or commitment to an inpatient psychiatric or substance abuse facility.

Clinician Reactions During the Patient Interview

Predicting who is imminently dangerous is often possible by using behavioral observations (see Table 18.1). However, clinicians also must listen to their subjective sense of a patient's potential risk, and these feelings should also be considered when making treatment decisions.

Neurologic and Medical Issues

Some neurologic and medical disorders increase the risk for violence and suicide. Evaluation and treatment of these disorders should be a routine part of care for the high-risk patient. Neurologic disorders associated with violence risk include disorders involving damage to the frontal lobe and deep brain structures. These include traumatic brain injury, stroke, delirium, dementia, seizure disorder, brain tumors, and personality changes due to medical causes. Chronic severe medical illnesses causing significant disabilities are associated with an increased suicide risk. These include multiple sclerosis, amyotrophic lateral sclerosis, chronic pain syndromes, renal failure leading to dialysis, pancreatic cancer, other cancers, and thyroid illnesses.

Risk Assessment Tools for IPV, Violence, and Suicide

Risk assessment tools for IPV and suicide can be used in a primary care setting.

In a reversal of previous studies, the Institute of Medicine and others are recommending screening for IPV in primary care practices. IPV assessment tools include (1) Screening: Hurt, Insult, Threaten, and Scream,[23] (2) The Humiliation, Afraid, Rape, Kick Tool,[24] and (3) Partner Violence Screen.[25]

The most commonly used suicide risk assessment tool is the PHQ-9.[20] The PHQ-9 self-report asks about depressive symptoms and provides a suicide inquiry: "[Have you had] thoughts that you would be better off dead, or of hurting yourself in some way?" The Columbia-Suicide Severity Rating Scales (C-SSRS)[26] are additional suicide risk assessment tools that measure the severity and intensity of suicidal ideation, suicidal behavior, and the lethality of actual suicide attempts. This scale has predictive validity but cannot provide a definitive risk estimate. It remains essential to use the C-SSRS in combination with clinical assessments and judgments. Other suicide assessment tools include the Revised Beck Depression Inventory,[2] the Beck Scale for Suicidal Ideation,[28] and the Beck Hopelessness Scale.[29]

The Violence and Suicide Risk Assessment Scale (VASA)[30] is a short suicide and violence risk assessment and decision tool that can guide decisions about the need for inpatient versus outpatient care.

A specialized violence risk assessment tool for patients, prisoners or forensic patients is the Historical Clinical Risk-20 (HCR-20).[31] The HCR-20 has 20 items designed to aid in the judgment of violence risk, but it is not predictive of violence.

Neurologic and Medical Evaluation

A neurologic evaluation should be part of every assessment of violent or suicidal patients. Optimizing treatment of neurologic conditions linked to violence (e.g., traumatic brain injury, dementia) or medical conditions linked to suicide (e.g., thyroid, renal failure, cancer) may help prevent future episodes.

INTEGRATED HEALTH CARE TEAM AND PATIENT RISK REGISTRY

In primary care settings, integrated health care teams may be composed of a primary care and behavioral health specialist, a care or case manager, and a psychiatric consultant. In most practices the primary care provider will do the initial screening, identify the risk, and do a "warm handoff" to a case manager or behavioral health specialist. The psychiatrist may be called for a consultation about acute risk, immediate need for medication, or hospitalization. If the patient can remain in the primary care setting, the behavioral health specialist will decide how to manage the patient, and a care manager may arrange follow-up appointments and community supports. The psychiatrist may conduct a patient interview or curbside consultations with the team. Psychiatric nurse practitioners or nurses with psychiatric training can also assume advanced mental health practice roles. Regular team management meetings with flexible time commitment, variable membership (depending on patients discussed), and a management strategy (often a critical pathway) for specific populations of patients will be necessary to secure optimal outcomes (see Chapter 4: Team-Based Integrated Primary Care).

A patient registry, describing all patients with a particular problem or diagnosis, can be used to track, manage, and establish treatment algorithms for a population of patients. A risk registry is especially useful for the care of high-risk patients. Case managers or nurses can facilitate coordination of care. Patients referred for additional psychiatric or substance abuse treatment need follow-up contact within one week to make sure the patient is stable and has connected with all needed community resources. This initial after-office visit or contact can be guided using the Violence and Suicide Safety Checklist (Box 18.4) as part of the follow-up. Thereafter, regular contact with the patients, their providers of mental health or substance abuse outpatient treatment, and their support networks will provide the continuity of care needed to ensure their safety.

MANAGEMENT AND TREATMENT

Decision Algorithm for Level of Care

After the clinical interview, history, and risk assessment have been completed, the clinician can decide on the optimal treatment location, guided by the level of care options described in the decision algorithm in Figure 18.1. Clinicians who decide to let a patient with some risk leave the treatment setting should review all items on the Violence and Suicide Safety Checklist (see Box 18.4) with the patient before releasing the patient.

BOX 18.4

VIOLENCE AND SUICIDE SAFETY CHECKLIST

- **Make sure that patients have no access to guns, knives, razor blades, pills, or other means to hurt themselves or others.**
- **Review and anticipate all current and expected stressors likely to occur in the first week after discharge.**
- **Review the warning signs of increased risk, such as substance use, psychosis, mood/anxiety disorders, and posttraumatic stress disorder, that require the patient to call for help.**
- **Review the patient's use of coping styles that will reduce risk (e.g., use of relaxation techniques, exercise, distraction, self-help meetings, calls for help).**
- **Develop and review the patient's use of his or her support network and all community resources.**
- **Give the patient information about how to contact and use a local mobile crisis hotline.**
- **Review how to use medications to relieve acute new symptoms that might emerge after discharge.**
- **Review the need for psychiatric follow-up care.**
- **Review the detailed discharge plan (e.g., referral to Alcoholics Anonymous, primary care, intensive outpatient treatment, partial hospitalization, outpatient).**
- **Review/list all contact information for all of the patient's health care providers or support program referrals. Specify for the patient how the clinician can be reached in case of an emergency.**
- **Call the patient a few days (no more than one week) after discharge to confirm that the patient has connected to all needed services.**

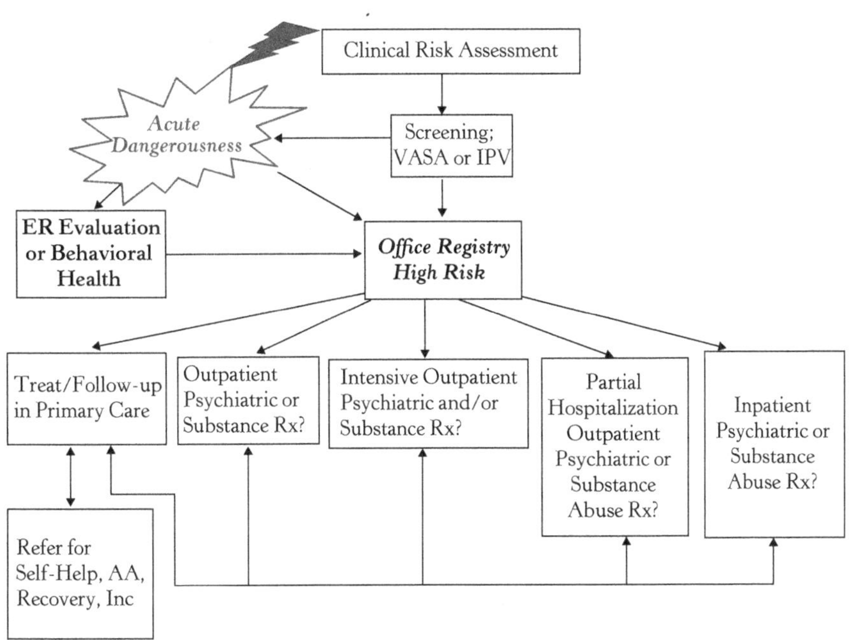

FIGURE 18.1. Decision algorithm for levels of care.

Critical Pathway

A critical pathway is an outline of the clinical approach to evaluating and managing violent and suicidal patients over a one-year period. The pathway focuses on screening, measuring progress, and outcomes (Table 18.2). The pathway can best be used in conjunction with the patient high-risk registry.

Motivation for Treatment

Assessing a patient's motivation and readiness to change is useful. Rollnick[32] describes the patient's readiness to change as based on two factors: importance of change and confidence in the patient's ability to change. Clinicians can use a scale from 0 to 10, where 10 is rated highest importance and most confident for change, and 0 is the lowest. Patients can learn to rate their own motivation for change. Patients with high importance and high confidence are most likely to change. Patients with low motivation benefit from psychoeducation to increase their motivation to change, followed by specific skills training to help boost their confidence in their ability to make a change. Some high-risk violent or suicidal patients may be sent involuntarily to emergency departments and committed to inpatient psychiatric or substance abuse care settings where they may receive treatment against their will. Various options for psychiatric care based on a patient's motivation and capacity to participate in treatment are illustrated in the decision algorithm in Figure 18.1.

A biopsychosocial-cultural formulation will help clinicians formulate a problem-solving or crisis intervention approach (see Chapter 26: Crisis Intervention in Integrated Care). This approach first considers imminent risk factors and problem solving, followed by other psychotherapeutic treatments that may require a long-term approach.

Treatment Settings

The treatment setting should be the least restrictive that will prevent patients from harming others or themselves. The VASA scale[30] can guide decisions about the level of care needed. Regardless of the treatment setting, clinicians should use the patient's support system, provide psychoeducation, address substance abuse, involve the police (if needed), provide follow-up care, and coordinate care with all providers, especially the patient's primary care provider.

Inpatient Psychiatric or Substance Abuse Hospitalization

Psychiatric hospitalization should be considered if violent or suicidal ideation or behaviors is present in a patient with a psychosis, a substance abuse disorder, a mood disorder, a serious disability, or other history of mental illness associated with violence or suicidal risk. Inpatient substance abuse treatment may be the preferred option when substance abuse is driving the symptoms and behaviors and when there is no acute violence or suicidal risk. Hospitalization may be necessary, even in the absence of violence or a suicide attempt, if a patient describes a premeditated or specific plan with a specific timeline, suggesting a high lethality risk, or when a suicide attempt includes precautions to avoid rescue or discovery, regrets about surviving, or persistent suicidal ideation.

Hospitalization may be the safest option in patients with psychiatric or substance abuse disorders who have contributing unstable neurologic or medical conditions, and for patients who have not responded to other major efforts at outpatient treatment.

Hospital admission should also be considered for patients with milder violence or suicidal risk if their support network is unavailable, not interested, or incompetent.

When creating the discharge plan from hospital and inpatient substance abuse facilities, it is essential to prevent immediate after-discharge recurrence or hospital readmission. Safety plans should include a safety checklist (see Box 18.4). Discharge plans should no longer include contracting for safety, because this does not prevent new episodes. Prior to discharge, it is important to review the safety plan with the patient and support network.[33] Best outcomes are associated with the safety plan (see Box 18.4) in combination with after-discharge follow-up within 7 days and the provision of 24-hour acute crisis teams in the community.[34] A practice registry, for use by the case manager, behavioral health specialist, or nurse, will help in monitoring the patient's progress and facilitate tracking of referrals to needed community resources. The primary care provider also may find it helpful to consult with a psychiatrist.

Partial Hospitalization Programs and Intensive Outpatient Psychiatric and Substance Abuse Treatments

Outpatient programs vary from high-intensity partial hospitalization programs with multiple daily meetings to intensive outpatient programs that

TABLE 18.2 CRITICAL PATHWAY: INTIMATE PARTNER VIOLENCE, VIOLENCE, AND SUICIDE

	Initial Visit	Week 1	Week 2–4	Week 5–10	Month 6–9	Month 9–12
Assessment & Screening Designate responsible team member: nurse, physician, advanced practice professional, behavioral health specialist (BHS), psychiatrist	• Screening and assessment • Intimate partner violence (IPV) risk assessment SAFE screening • Suicide risk assessment: PHQ-2, PHQ-9, C-SSRS-Columbia Scale • Violence & Suicide Risk Assessment Scale (VASA)	• Repeat/add relevant assessment scales.	• Repeat/add relevant assessment scales.	• Repeat/add relevant assessment scales.	• Repeat/add relevant assessment scales.	• Repeat/add relevant assessment scales.
Clinical Issues Designate responsible team member: nurse, physician, advanced practice professional, BHS psychiatrist, etc.	• Restrict weapon access (guns, etc.). • Assess for substance use. • Enter patient in risk registry. • Treat in primary care? • Refer to emergency department? • Refer for substance abuse treatment? • Refer to an IPV shelter? • See Figure 18.1 for referral options. • Refer to self-help (e.g., Alcoholics Anonymous)? • Offer medications? • Schedule follow-up.	• Encourage phone access/telehealth with patient. • Restrict weapon access. • Current stressors? • Current safety issues? • Current substance use? • Psychiatric/medical comorbidities? • Offer medications/ assess response? • Contact collaterals for information. • Establish connection to all referral resources?	• Emergencies? • Suicidal/violent; ideation/ behaviors? • Depressive/ hopeless symptoms? • Substance abuse? • Address comorbidities. • Assess medication response. • Connected to all referral resources?	• Evaluate treatment response. • Adjust treatment plan.	• Emergencies? • Dangerous behaviors? • No injuries/ deaths? • Improved functioning? • Improved quality of life? • Improved health status?	• Emergencies? • Dangerous behaviors? • No injuries/ deaths? • Improved functioning? • Improved quality of life? • Improved health status?

(continued)

TABLE 18.2 CONTINUED

	Initial Visit	Week 1	Week 2–4	Week 5–10	Month 6–9	Month 9–12
Diagnosis Designate responsible team member.	• Psychiatric: Rule out mood, psychosis, personality disorder. • Substance abuse: Rule out ETOH, opiates, marijuana. • Medical: Rule out thyroid, neurologic, chronic illness/ disability. • Social causes (e.g., poverty, financial)	• Confirm diagnosis. • Explore for other psychiatric, substance, medical comorbidities.	Explore for other comorbidities.	Explore for other comorbidities.	Explore for other comorbidities.	Explore for other comorbidities.
Physical/Lab Diagnostic Tests Designate responsible team member.	Complete physical examination, complete blood count, Chem 20 panel, drug screen, EKG, TSH, other neurologic/ psychiatric testing, as needed?	• Consider CT scan, MRI, EEG as needed. • Drug screen?	Drug screen?	• Re-evaluate diagnosis, prn? • Drug screen? • Other labs?	• Re-evaluate diagnosis, prn? • Drug screen? • Other labs?	• Re-evaluate diagnosis, prn? • Drug screen? • Other labs?
Time	45 min	30 min	Call patient as needed?	30 min	15 min	15 min
Educational Materials Designate responsible team member.	• IPV education • Education about suicide prevention, violence prevention, substance use, and medications.	• IPV education • Education about suicide and violence prevention, substance abuse, medication, comorbidity, self-help information.	• Comorbidity education • Self-help information • Medication education	• Education, prn • Self-help	Relapse prevention	Relapse prevention

Treatment Team Designate responsible provider.	• Refer to ER? • Refer for additional care. Outpatient vs. inpatient treatment? (See Fig. 18.1) • Safety checklist (Box 18.4) • Add self-help (e.g., Alcoholics Anonymous). • Emphasize practice phone availability. • Referral to crisis community service?	• Review safety checklist (Box 18.4). • Coordinate with other providers. • Review progress and outcome measures.	• Review safety checklist (Box 18.4). • Medication check • Coordinate with other providers. • Reduced symptoms and improved functioning? • Review outcome measures. • Add treatment resources, prn.	• Review safety checklist (Box 18.4). • Medication check • Get mental health substance use updates? • Reduced symptoms and improved functioning? • Review outcome measures. • Add treatment resources, prn.	• Review safety checklist (Box 18.4). • Medication check • Get mental health substance use updates? • Reduced symptoms and improved functioning? • Review outcome measures. • Recovery? • Review relapse prevention. • Add treatment resources, prn.	• Review safety checklist (Box 18.4). • Medication check • Get mental health substance use updates? • Reduced symptoms and improved functioning? • Review outcome measures. • Recovery? • Review relapse prevention. • Add treatment resources, prn.
Practice-Based Interventions Designate responsible provider.	• The practice should outreach the patient. Direct practice person to • Improve treatment adherence by direct person-to-person contact, via telehealth, phone, or email.	• Update IVP status via phone? • Violent/suicidal? • Contact collaterals. • IPV shelter, family, etc.? • Connected to resources?	Update clinical status, prn	Update clinical status, prn	Update clinical status, prn	Update clinical status, prn
Psychotherapy Designate responsible provider.	• Psychotherapy • Crisis intervention, problem solving, behavioral treatments, family interventions	Connected for psychotherapy or other psychiatric care?	• Psychotherapy progress update • Coordinate care with mental health, substance abuse.	• Progress update • Coordinate care with mental health, substance abuse.	• Progress update • Coordinate care with mental health, substance abuse.	• Progress update • Coordinate care with mental health, substance abuse.

(continued)

TABLE 18.2 CONTINUED

	Initial Visit	Week 1	Week 2–4	Week 5–10	Month 6–9	Month 9–12
Medications	Treat target symptoms or comorbid disorders.	Taking medication?	Medication follow-up/ adherence?	Medication follow-up/ adherence?	Medication follow-up/ adherence?	Medication follow-up/ adherence?
Intimate Partner Violence	• Report IPV if required by law. • Discuss safety/cycles of violence.	• Safety checklist (Box 18.4) • Ambivalent? • Referral? (Fig. 18.1)	• Safety checklist (Box 18.4) • Ambivalent? • Referral? (Fig. 18.1)	• Safety checklist (Box 18.4) • Ambivalent? • Referral? (Fig. 18.1)	• Safety checklist (Box 18.4) • Ambivalent? • Referral? (Fig. 18.1)	• Safety checklist (Box 18.4) • Ambivalent? • Referral? (Fig. 18.1)
Refer for Relevant Consultations Designate responsible team member.	• Mental health/substance abuse consultations? • Police/social agencies required? • Referral to self-help, community IPV victims' services (e.g., rape, shelter, child care).	• Review consult reports. • Family session? • Decide next steps for consultations, if any.	• Family session? • Psychiatric/ substance consultation?	• No response? • Psychiatric/ substance referral? • Re-evaluate all options.	• Re-evaluate treatment response. • Psychiatric/ substance referral?	• Re-evaluate treatment response. • Psychiatric/ substance referral?

meet several times per week. Outpatient programs typically include some combination of group therapy, patient education, occupational or vocational rehabilitation, family support, and attendance at self-help groups (e.g., Alcoholics Anonymous) combined with individual psychotherapy and psychopharmacology. Programs can be tailored to the patient's acuity, work needs, and family considerations.

Many patients will step down to the traditional one to two hours a week of psychotherapy, medications, and continuation of self-help. This is the typical plan for long-term treatment and follow-up.

Pharmacotherapy

No drugs are specifically designed to reduce violent or suicidal tendencies. However, medications targeting the primary diagnosis often reduce these risky symptoms. In emergency violent or suicidal situations patients can be treated with haloperidol and lorazepam or other fast-acting atypical antipsychotics (olanzapine, risperidone, aripiprazole, ziprasidone) in oral, sublingual, or intramuscular preparations. Antipsychotic medications, combined with a benzodiazepine, are used for rapid tranquilization. If a patient is experiencing withdrawal from sedative-hypnotics, antipsychotics are contraindicated because of seizure risk.

Long-term pharmacotherapy for violence and suicidal tendencies relies on treatment of a primary diagnosis and routinely involves the use of antidepressants, antipsychotics, mood stabilizers, benzodiazepines, or other psychotropic medications.

Antidepressants

The selective serotonin reuptake inhibitors (SSRIs) are useful for the long-term treatment of aggressive, impulsive, and violent symptoms in people with traumatic brain injuries and other impulse-control disorders. Treatment typically begins with low doses while observing for exacerbation of aggressive symptoms. In one recent study, amantadine 100 mg twice a day also decreased irritability and aggressive episodes secondary to traumatic brain injury.[35]

SSRIs are often first-line treatments for suicidal symptoms associated with depressive disorders. However, the U.S. Food and Drug Administration (FDA) has issued a black-box warning for SSRIs stating that people under 25 years of age who take SSRIs may experience increased suicidal ideation or behavior, particularly in the first month of use. Although this has raised some concern about using SSRIs for suicidal patients, recent studies[36] have shown the risk of SSRI-induced suicidal ideation is quite low and much smaller than the risk of not treating a depressed suicidal patient. Baseline levels of anxiety, agitation, and sleep disturbance should be determined at the start of antidepressant medication treatment. The FDA recommends weekly visits for the first month, biweekly for the second month, and at least one visit in the third month for patients 25 years of age or younger. This careful approach ameliorates the risk associated with SSRIs.

Depression may also be responsive to selective noradrenergic reuptake inhibitors such as venlafaxine or duloxetine. Sedating antidepressants, such as mirtazapine or trazodone, can assist in the treatment of insomnia, an independent risk factor for suicide.

Mood-Stabilizing Agents

Lithium may reduce the risk of suicide attempts in patients with mood disorders and may be useful for some aggressive or violent patients.[37] Some patients refuse to take this medication because blood level monitoring is required. The risk of lithium overdose must be monitored in suicidal patients.

Mood-Stabilizing Anticonvulsants

There is evidence that anticonvulsants may directly reduce violence or suicide risk in psychotic patients. Anticonvulsants may also be helpful in treating the violent behavior caused by traumatic brain injury, dementia, intermittent explosive disorder, manic excitement or irritability, the impulsivity associated with personality disorders, and impulse-control disorders.

Antipsychotics

Second-generation atypical antipsychotics are additional options for treating conditions associated with aggression or suicide.[38] Clozapine can reduce psychosis associated with violent and suicidal behavior.[39] Results of a systematic review lend support for the use of benzodiazepines combined, if necessary, with antipsychotic drugs, as part of a short- and long-term maintenance regime for psychotic patients acting aggressively.[40] Quetiapine may be useful in treating suicidal or violent tendencies in patients with borderline personality disorder.[41]

Benzodiazepines

Benzodiazepines have no clear short-term anti-suicide or anti-violence efficacy when used alone.[42] However, they can reduce acute violence or suicide risk that is comorbid with severe anxiety, panic attacks, agitation, or severe insomnia. Lorazepam can be offered in an oral or intramuscular form. Patients with borderline personality disorder or head injury who need benzodiazepines also need monitoring for worsening depression, disinhibition, and aggression. Benzodiazepines are the treatment of choice in agitation and violence due to withdrawal from sedative-hypnotics.

Electroconvulsive Therapy

Evidence exists that electroconvulsive therapy reduces suicidal ideation and psychosis. Electroconvulsive therapy may be particularly helpful in the treatment of psychotic highly suicidal patients, or pregnant patients who have not responded to antidepressant medication and other less invasive treatments.

Psychotherapy

Psychotherapy can play a vital role in the management of violent and suicidal behavior.

Crisis Intervention/Problem-Solving Treatment

The clinician may use and teach a problem-solving or crisis resolution strategy for ameliorating violent or suicidal symptoms (see Chapter 26: Crisis Intervention in Integrated Care). Problem solving helps the patient find more adaptive and flexible ways to feel, think, behave, and respond to provocative situations.

Behavioral and Cognitive-Behavioral Therapies

Behavior therapies constitute the single largest group of non-medication interventions used in the treatment of violence and can also be helpful in decreasing suicidal ideation and behaviors. Behavior therapy is often used with institutionalized patients and patients with chronic psychotic or severe neuropsychiatric impairment. Behavior change is understood within a specific context, and observations and interventions are made by considering antecedents, behaviors, and consequences (the ABC approach):

> Identifying and modifying Antecedents (stressors, triggers, precipitants) can help reduce risks. Antecedents (e.g., triggers, precipitants) of the behavior sometimes can be avoided.
>
> The dangerous **B**ehavior itself can be analyzed and modified.
>
> The **C**onsequence of a behavior (positive or negative) can be also modified by use of new positive reinforcements designed to foster positive adaptive behavior.

Cognitive-behavioral therapy (CBT) uses various techniques to treat violent and suicidal patients: journal or diary entries of significant events and associated feelings, thoughts, and behaviors; questioning and testing irrational thoughts, assumptions, evaluations, and beliefs; facing activities that have been avoided; and trying out new ways of behaving and reacting. Relaxation training (e.g., variations of breathing, mindfulness) and distraction techniques are adjunctively used with CBT.

Anger management (often combined with relaxation training) represents a modification of CBT for individual, family, or group treatments. Anger regulation can be achieved by interpersonal skill development, examination and use of coping strategies, and a patient-developed reflective diary.

Dialectical behavioral therapy, which is useful for borderline patients, uses diary or journal cards, mindfulness techniques, and interpersonal skills training. Patients are taught skills to decrease suicidal and angry behaviors and impulsivity, manage strong emotions, and increase their effectiveness in meeting interpersonal needs.

Other Therapies

Focal psychodynamic psychotherapy can improve reality testing, dysfunctional views of others, and pathologic defenses. This type of brief treatment can be used to identify current and past dysfunctional life patterns and improve coping, adaptation, and functional behavior patterns. Confrontations (e.g., pointing out the discrepancies between feelings, thoughts, and behaviors) can decrease patient resistance by getting feelings, thoughts, and behavioral all moving in the same positive and desired direction. Clarifications sharpen the patient's understanding of complex situations. Interpretations help foster the patient's understanding of the meaning(s) of the events contributing to dangerous behaviors.

Family therapy (see Chapter 27: Best Practice for Family-Centered Health Care: A Three-Step Model) can be effective in treating suicidal symptoms or violent behaviors occurring between two or several family members. Family therapy for violent and suicidal patients usually combines psychoeducational, behavioral, strategic, and structural approaches. Integration of a crisis intervention approach (see Chapter 26: Crisis Intervention in Integrated Care) with family therapy can help maintain focus on acute problems. Families may need education about causes of high-risk behaviors and relevant treatments for psychiatric illness, medication use, how to call for help, and encouragement to stop or decrease substance use. Family therapy may also help address pathologic patterns of communication or help families renegotiate changing roles (e.g., when a family member dies and there is a new family structure). Family members can learn how to listen, express their feelings, interpret messages, and negotiate disagreements.

CHRONIC PATTERNS OF SUICIDAL AND VIOLENT BEHAVIOR

For patients who develop a lifelong daily pattern of violence and suicidality, the clinician should focus on treating the underlying personality features, psychosis, mood disorder, or substance use that drives high-risk symptoms. Episodic, brief, and problem-focused interventions can be effective in a primary care environment. However, long-term and multimodal treatment in psychiatric outpatient settings may be required for many of these complex patients. This treatment typically involves psychotherapy in the least restrictive setting combined with medications and community support.

LEGAL ISSUES

Commitment

All states recognize the need for involuntary hospitalization. Such action is taken when patients present a danger to themselves or others or are so severely disabled that they are unable to care for themselves. In most states, any physician and most medical and mental health professionals can involuntarily detain a patient for admission to a mental health facility. Patients initially may protest but usually come to appreciate receiving appropriate psychiatric care and treatment. Committed patients retain all of their civil rights with regard to participating in treatment decisions, including taking or not taking medication.

Confidentiality

Most states recognize that protecting the patient or others takes precedence over patient confidentiality. In emergency situations, the Health Insurance Portability and Accountability Act (HIPAA) exemption rule[43] permits emergency collateral conversations with police, other doctors, family members, friends, or other affected parties, without patient consent. The decision to speak with collateral informants against the patient's wishes is a risk-benefit assessment that weighs the effects of disclosing confidential patient information against fostering the safety of others.

Duty to Warn and Duty to Protect

Clinicians are usually exempt from confidentiality requirements when they become aware that a patient is likely to commit homicide or other violence. State laws vary widely, but the 1974 Tarasoff 1 [44] decision has become a national standard for clinical practice. In this case, a former lover confided his intention to a University of California therapist and then murdered Tatania Tarasoff. The court found the university and the therapist guilty of failure to warn Ms. Tarasoff or her family that her life was in imminent danger. This case was the precedent for the therapist's "duty to warn" potential victims of life-threatening danger from a homicidal patient. Tarasoff 1 declared, "The protective privilege ends where the public peril begins." The 1976 Tarasoff 2 [45] ruling gave therapists an additional responsibility of a "duty to protect." This ruling said, "When a therapist determines, or should determine, that his patient presents a serious danger of violence to another, he incurs an obligation to use reasonable care to protect the intended victim from danger." Reasonable care means that the clinician must try to prevent the violence by taking action, such as hospitalizing the violent patient or prescribing appropriate outpatient care (see Fig. 18.1). In addition, the clinician can warn all intended victims and suggest they obtain an order of protection.

Duty-to-protect statutes have been passed in all but 13 states; however, many state laws reflect ambivalence. Some states require that a violent threat be clearly foreseeable and that the duty be extended only to "reasonably foreseeable victims" and not to the general public. Other states have "Tarasoff-limiting statutes," prescribing specific criteria that typically include a requirement of a credible threat made against an identifiable victim or location. New York is one of 13 states that has neither a specific duty-to-warn or duty-to-protect law. However, two statutes in New York state laws give clinicians the authority to warn but not the duty or responsibility to warn.

IPV

Violence between partners represents a special class of abuse that crosses all boundaries of social class, race, age, and sexual orientation. IPV occurs when a partner establishes coercive control of another partner through physical, psychological, or sexual abuse or by denying resources for self-support such that the partner is unable to leave. Statistics regarding the frequency and impact of intimate partner abuse can be reviewed in Box 18.2.

Screening for IPV

Multiple sources[46–48] recommend screening for IPV in primary care (see the risk assessment section above). In addition to standardized screening, primary care clinicians can routinely ask about partner abuse and should be alert to signs of abuse detected during physical examination. Battered patients often present with traumatic injuries, pelvic discomfort or pain, a high miscarriage rate, history of rape or incest, headaches, chronic pain, functional gastrointestinal disorders, a history of substance abuse (in the patient or partner), chronic complaints of stress, insomnia, suicide attempts, depression, or anxiety.

Clinicians can help a suspected victim of partner abuse by openly asking the patient about these suspicions. Research has shown that patients overwhelmingly want to be asked about IPV;[46] however, only 7% of physicians incorporate domestic violence questions into their routine medical care.[47]

Phases of IPV

The three phases of the partner abuse cycle[48] have been described as

1. Verbal abuse and hostility, where the abuser systematically isolates and verbally abuses the victim, undermining the partner's self-esteem
2. The violent stage, where assault and battery occur
3. The honeymoon period, where the offender is remorseful and promises that violence will never occur again

Many patients repeat this cycle many times before accepting care.

Physician/Behavioral Health Specialist Interventions for IPV

When attempting to intervene when IPV is suspected, a primary care clinician should carefully consider seven clinical domains.[7]

Establish an Alliance

Establishing an alliance with an IPV victim involves listening, asking questions, and communicating intense concern without blaming the victim. Victims of IPV are often intensely ambivalent about their partners. It is not uncommon for a victim to return to live with the abuser. In the interview, focus on the patient's ambivalence and confusion about the situation without making any judgments. Offer immediate protection and assure the victim that you will be available in the future. In addition, try to foster the patient's independent thinking, decision-making ability, and healthy coping styles, while developing clear contingency plans for dealing with any new episodes.

Provide All Necessary Medical Care

Initially, the physician must attend to acute medical problems related to abuse, which typically are injuries and physical trauma, miscarriage, sexual abuse, or rape. If IPV involves sexual violence, the clinician should follow a standardized medical protocol for collecting evidence, providing necessary medical treatment, and reporting IPV as required by local and state laws.

Review Treatment Options with the Patient

Patients experiencing IPV typically need additional support. At a bare minimum, refer the patient to the National Domestic Violence Hotline (800-799-7233). Encourage the patient to seek additional treatment with a local domestic violence treatment service, a victims' service program, a mental health clinic, or refer the patient to a specialized IPV clinician. Some patients will benefit from group treatment, whereas others can benefit from couples or family treatment with the abusing partner present.

Some patients who experience IPV may have comorbid psychiatric conditions, such as depression, suicidal tendencies, substance abuse, anxiety, or posttraumatic stress disorder. A primary care clinician needs to be alert to these additional complexities and treat or refer the patient for appropriate psychiatric evaluation and treatment.

Develop an Acute Intervention Plan and an Exit Plan

If the patient is asking for immediate protection and shelter, review the patient's options for staying with friends or extended family or in an IPV shelter. The only safe location is one where the abusing partner cannot find the victim. If the patient is ambivalent about leaving a partner, it is especially useful to develop a future exit plan. Advise the patient to put aside an extra set of keys, emergency money, some clothing, crucial documents (e.g., social security card, driver's license, immigration papers) and to have available emergency telephone numbers of people who can help.

Advise the Patient of Her or His Legal Rights

Remind the patient that IPV is against the law. Some patients may increase their personal safety and improve their psychological recovery if they press charges and their partners are prosecuted for committing a felony crime. Inform a patient how to obtain an order of protection. You can also suggest that the victim seek legal assistance for separation, divorce, child custody issues, or other civil litigation. In some states, physicians have legal requirements to report IPV to local authorities or agencies. Be aware of state reporting requirements and follow local and state laws.

Follow-up Plan

After the initial IPV diagnosis and treatment, follow the patient by using a practice registry, and arrange for follow-up contact within one week. Arrange for several options for contacting the patient, encouraging liberal telephone contact. If unable to reach the patient, notify appropriate family members, designated friends, the appropriate social service agency, or the police.

Recordkeeping

Clinicians need to document carefully all IPV-related biopsychosocial-cultural history, a comprehensive medical and physical examination, and plans and results for follow-up meetings. Medical record subpoenas of IPV patients are common for court hearings. It is best to avoid legal language in the medical record such as the "alleged beating." Instead, report event details with specific physical findings and discharge plans.

VIOLENCE AND SUICIDE PREVENTION

The most effective immediate interventions to prevent violence and suicide include: using evidence-based screenings, assessing risk, focusing on emotional distress and chronic pain, reducing access to the means of harm (especially reducing access to firearms, other weapons, pills, razor blades, and so forth), and providing treatment and needed services. See Box 18.5 for a detailed summary of evidence-based treatment approaches for reducing dangerousness. Prevention in the primary care setting includes screening for risk factors, treating comorbid psychiatric disorders, and focusing on patients with emotional distress and chronic pain. Community prevention includes public health awareness, media support, and following domestic violence laws. Specific vulnerable populations may need focused program development to prevent violence and suicide. Programs need to deal with a wide array of social, economic, and psychiatric services. High-risk populations include people with HIV/AIDS; women and children living with domestic violence or in unsafe neighborhoods; survivors of violence, sexual abuse, and rape; substance abuse populations; old and young populations; traumatized people; lesbian, gay, bisexual, and transgender people; indigenous peoples; immigrants; and others with severe socioeconomic distress.

Self-Help, Support, Web Information

Most cities have an emergency crisis call center, mobile crisis teams, respite/crisis beds, domestic violence services, substance abuse treatment centers, and community mental health centers. Hospital emergency departments can provide assessment, brief treatment, and referral to inpatient psychiatric and substance abuse facilities. Internet resources include the following:

National Domestic Violence Hotline: 800-799-SAFE; http://www.thehotline.org

National Suicide Prevention Lifeline: 800-273-8255; http://www.suicidepreventionlifeline.org

Suicide Helpline: http://psychcentral.com/helpme.htm

Teen Suicide Hotline: https://teenlineonline.org/?gclid=CMPBnvG06cQCFZE1aQodLmkA1Q

Intervention Treatment—Help Your Loved One with Addiction: http://www.intervention911.com/?cpao=111&cpca=Campaign%20Began%20Jan%202011&cpag=Top%20Drug%20Intervention%20Words&kw=intervention&gclid=CP_wy5K26cQCFZE1aQodLmkA1Q

BOX 18.5

SUMMARY OF RECOMMENDED TREATMENT APPROACHES AND RELEVANT EVIDENCE

Strength of recommendation taxonomy (SOR A, B, or C)

- **Screening for intimate personal violence (IPV) and suicide risk is recommended. (SOR A)[13,18,20,21,45]**
- **Optimal long-term treatment for these high-risk patients is psychotherapy and medications. (SOR A)[4,5,13,31]**
- **Violence and suicide risk after discharge can often be prevented in the short term by making sure that patients are connected to resources within one week of discharge and that they can access a 24-hour community crisis intervention service. (SOR A)[30,31]**
- **The best approach to prevent IPV, violence toward others, and suicide is using a risk assessment tool and clinical evaluation while determining the appropriate level of care. (SOR A)[43–45]**
- **In emergency violent or suicidal situations, patients can be treated with haloperidol and lorazepam or other fast-acting atypical antipsychotics (olanzapine, risperidone, aripiprazole, ziprasidone) in oral, sublingual, or intramuscular preparations. (SOR B)[37]**
- **The selective serotonin reuptake inhibitors (SSRIs) are useful for the long-term treatment of aggressive, impulsive, and violent symptoms in people with traumatic brain injuries and other impulse-control disorders. (SOR B)[31]**
- **Amantadine 100 mg twice a day decreases irritability and aggressive episodes secondary to traumatic brain injury. (SOR B)[32]**
- **Lithium may reduce the risk of suicide attempts in patients with mood disorders and may be useful for some aggressive or violent patients. (SOR B)[34]**
- **There is some evidence that anticonvulsants may directly reduce violence or suicide risk in psychotic patients. (SOR B)[35]**
- **Clozapine can reduce psychosis associated with violent and/or suicidal behavior. (SOR B)[36]**
- **Quetiapine may be useful in treating suicidal or violence tendencies in patients with borderline personality disorder. (SOR B)[38]**
- **A critical pathway may be useful for tracking the care needed during a one-year period. (SOR C)[17]**

REFERENCES

1. Fazel S, Gulati G, Linsell L, Geddes JR, Grann M. Schizophrenia and violence: Systematic review and meta-analysis. PLoS Med. 2009;6(8):e1000120. doi:10.1371/journal.pmed.1000120.
2. Palmer BA, Pankratz VS, Bostwick JM. The lifetime risk of suicide in schizophrenia: a reexamination. Arch Gen Psychiatry. 2005;62(3):247–253.
3. Inskip HM, Harris EC, Barraclough B. Lifetime risk of suicide for affective disorder, alcoholism, and schizophrenia. Br J Psychiatry. 1998;172(1):35–37.
4. Hiday VA. Putting community risk in perspective: a look at correlations, causes and controls. Int J Law Psychiatry. 2006;29(4):316–331.
5. Hiroeh U, Appleby L, Mortensen PB, Dunn G. Death by homicide, suicide, and other unnatural causes in people with mental illness: A population-based study. Lancet. 2001;358(9299):2110–2112.
6. Hockenhull JC, Whittington R, Leitner M, et al. A systematic review of prevention and intervention strategies for populations at high risk of engaging in violent behaviour update: 2002–8. Health Tech Assess. 2012;16(3):1–152. doi:10.3310/hta16030.
7. Bair-Merritt MH, Lewis-O'Connor A, Goel S, et al. Primary care–based interventions for intimate partner violence: A systematic review. Am J Prev Med. 2014;46(2):188–194.
8. Acierno R, Hernandez MA, Amstadter AB, et al. Prevalence and correlates of emotional, physical, sexual, and financial abuse and potential neglect in the United States: The National Elder Mistreatment Study. Am J Public Health. 2010;100(2):292–297.

9. Breiding MJ, Ziembroski JS, Black, MC. Prevalence of rural intimate partner violence in 16 US states, 2005. J Rural Health. 2009;25(3):240–246.
10. Eaton DK, Kann L, Kinchen S, et al. Youth risk behavior surveillance—United States, 2011. MMWR Surveill Summ. 2012;61(4):1–162.
11. Hahn S, Hantikainen V, Needham I, Kok G, Dassen T, Halfens RJ. Patient and visitor violence in the general hospital, occurrence, staff interventions and consequences: A cross-sectional survey. J Adv Nurs. 2012;68(12):2685–2699.
12. American Association of Suicidology. http://www.suicidology.org/resources/facts-statistics. Accessed June 20, 2015.
13. Center for Disease Control and Prevention. Suicide facts at a glance 2012. http://www.cdc.gov/violenceprevention/pdf/suicide-datasheet-a.pdf. Accessed June 20, 2015.
14. O'Connor E, Gaynes BN, Burda BU, Soh C, Whitlock EP. Screening for and treatment of suicide risk relevant to primary care: A systematic review for the US Preventive Services Task Force. Ann Intern Med. 2013;158(10):741–754.
15. Feinstein RE. Violence prevention education program for psychiatric outpatient departments. Acad Psychiatry. 2014;38(5):639–646.
16. Mann JJ. Neurobiology of suicidal behaviour. Nat Rev Neurosci. 2003;4(10):819–828.
17. Oquendo MA, Sullivan GM, Sudol K, et al. Toward a biosignature for suicide. Am J Psychiatry. 2014;171(12):1259–1277.
18. Umukoro S, Aladeokin AC, Eduviere AT. Aggressive behavior: A comprehensive review of its neurochemical mechanisms and management. Aggress Violent Beh. 2013;18(2):195–203.
19. Kroenke K, Spitzer RL, Williams JB. The Patient Health Questionnaire-2: Validity of a two-item depression screener. Med Care. 2003;41;(11)1284–1292.
20. Kroenke K, Spitzer RL. Williams JB. The PHQ-9. J Gen Intern Med. 2001;16(9):606–613.
21. Feldhaus KM, Koziol-McLain J, Amsbury HL, Lowenstein SR, Abbott JT. Accuracy of 3 brief screening questions for detecting partner violence in the emergency department. JAMA. 1997;277(17):1357–1361.
22. Feinstein RE. Clinical guidelines for the assessment of imminent violence. In: Praag HM, Plutchik R, Apter A, eds. Violence and Suicidality. Perspectives in Clinical and Psychobiological Research. New York: Brunner/Mazels; 1990:3–18.
23. Chen PH, Rovi S, Vega M, Jacobs A, Johnson MS. Screening for domestic violence in a predominantly Hispanic clinical setting. Fam Pract. 2005;22(6):617–623.
24. Sohal H, Eldridge S, Feder G. The sensitivity and specificity of four questions (HARK) to identify intimate partner violence: A diagnostic accuracy study in general practice. BMC Fam Pract. 2007;8:49.
25. Houry D, Feldhaus K, Peery B, et al. A positive domestic violence screen predicts future domestic violence. J Interpers Violence. 2004;19(9):955–966.
26. Posner K, Oquendo MA, Gould M, Stanley B, Davies M. Columbia Classification Algorithm of Suicide Assessment (C-CASA): Classification of suicidal events in the FDA's pediatric suicidal risk analysis of antidepressants. Am J Psychiatry. 2007;164(7):1035–1043.
27. Beck AT, Steer RA, Ball R, et al. Comparison of Beck Depression Inventories-IA and-II in psychiatric outpatients. J Pers Assess. 1996;67(3):588–597.
28. Beck AT, Weissman A, Lester D, et al. The measurement of pessimism: The hopelessness scale. J Consult Clin Psychol. 1974;42(6):861–865.
29. Beck AT, Kovacs M, Weissman A. Assessment of suicidal intention: The Scale for Suicide Ideation. J Consult Clin Psychol. 1979;47(2):343–352.
30. Feinstein R, Plutchik R. Violence and suicide risk assessment in the psychiatric emergency room. Compr Psychiatry. 1990;31(2):337–343.
31. Douglas KS, Webster CD. Predicting violence in mentally and personality disordered individuals. In: Roesch R, Hart SD, Ogloff JRP, eds. Psychology and Law: The State of the Discipline. Perspectives in Law & Psychology, Vol. 10. New York: Springer; 1999:175–239.
32. Rollnick S, Miller WR, Butler C. Motivational Interviewing in Health Care: Helping Patients Change Behavior. New York: Guilford Press; 2008.
33. Valenstein M, Kim HM, Ganoczy D, et al. Higher-risk periods for suicide among VA patients receiving depression treatment: prioritizing suicide prevention efforts. J Affective Disord. 2009;112(1–3):50–58.
34. Matheson SL, Shepherd AM, Carr VJ. Management of suicidal behaviour—a review of evidence for models of care: an evidence check rapid review brokered by the Sax Institute for the NSW Ministry of Health. www.saxinstitute.org.au. Accessed June 20, 2015.
35. Giacino JT, Whyte J, Bagiella E, et al. Placebo-controlled trial of amantadine for severe traumatic brain injury. N Engl J Med. 2012;366(9):819–826.
36. Leon AC, Solomon DA, Li C, et al. Antidepressants and risks of suicide and suicide attempts: A 27-year observational study. J Clin Psychiatry. 2011;72(5):580–586.
37. Cipriani A, Hawton K, Stockton S, Geddes JR. Lithium in the prevention of suicide in mood disorders: Updated systematic review and meta-analysis. Br Med J. 2013;346:f3646.
38. Fazel S, Zetterqvist J, Larsson H, Långström N, Lichtenstein P. Antipsychotics, mood stabilizers, and risk of violent crime. Lancet. 2014;384(9949):1206–1214.

39. Frogley C, Taylor D, Dickens G, Picchioni M. A systematic review of the evidence of clozapine's anti-aggressive effects. Int J Neuropsychopharmacol. 2012;15(9):1351–1371.
40. Dold M, Li C, Gillies D, Leucht, S. Benzodiazepine augmentation of antipsychotic drugs in schizophrenia: A meta-analysis and Cochrane review of randomized controlled trials. Eur Neuropsychopharmacol. 2013;23(9):1023–1033.
41. Villeneuve E, Lemelin S. Open-label study of atypical neuroleptic quetiapine for treatment of borderline personality disorder: Impulsivity as main target. J Clin Psychiatry. 2005;66(10):1298–1303.
42. Gillies D, Sampson S, Beck A, Rathbone J. Benzodiazepines for psychosis-induced aggression or agitation. Cochrane Database of Systematic Reviews. 2013:4:CD003079.doi: 101002?14651858.
43. Health Insurance Portability and Accountability Act of 1996. Public Law 104-191, 104th Congress. https://www.cms.gov/.
44. *Tarasoff v. Regents of the University of California*, 529 P.2d 553 (1974) http://en.wikipedia.org/wiki/Tarasoff_v._Regents_of_the_University_of_California. Accessed June 20, 2015.
45. *Tarasoff v. Regents of the University of California*, 17 Cal.3d 425, 551 P.2d 334, 131 Cal.Rptr.14 (Cal.1976). http://en.wikipedia.org/wiki/Tarasoff_v._Regents_of_the_University_of_California. Accessed June 20, 2015.
46. U.S. Preventive Services Task Force Recommendation Summary. Intimate partner violence and abuse of elderly and vulnerable adults: screening. http://www.uspreventiveservicestaskforce.org/Page/Topic/recommendation-summary/intimate-partner-violence-and-abuse-of-elderly-and-vulnerable-adults-screenin g?ds=1&s=intimatepartner. Published January 2013. Accessed June 20, 2015.
47. Gremillion DH, Kanof EP. Overcoming barriers to physician involvement in identifying and referring victims of domestic violence. Ann Emerg Med. 1996;27(6):769–773.
48. Institute of Medicine. Clinical preventive services for women: Closing the gaps. http://www.nap.edu/catalog/13181/clinical-preventive-services-for-women-closing-the-gaps. Accessed June 20, 2015.
49. Ebell MH, Siwek J, Weiss BD, et al. Simplifying the language of evidence to improve patient care. J Fam Pract. 2004:53(2):111–120.

PART III

Integrated Care for Medical Subspecialties and Behavioral Medicine in Primary Care

19

Integrative Care Model for Neurology and Psychiatry

Non-Epileptic Seizures Project

LYNNE FENTON, BRIAN ROTHBERG, LAURA STROM, ALISON M. HERU, AND MESHA-GAY BROWN

BOX 19.1
KEY POINTS

- **Non-epileptic seizures (NES) are very common in epilepsy centers, accounting for 20% to 30% of intractable epilepsy cases.**
- **Between 5% and 10% of NES patients also have epileptic seizures, complicating treatment.**
- **Video-electroencephalography (VEEG) is required for diagnosis of NES.**
- **Sensitive delivery of the diagnosis to patients may improve outcome.**
- **The majority of patients have at least one comorbid psychiatric diagnosis.**
- **Treatment of NES requires psychiatric interventions.**
- **Patients may be more likely to participate when psychiatric interventions take place within the neurology service.**
- **Family dysfunction is commonly associated with NES and should be screened for and treated.**
- **Group psychotherapy provides many therapeutic advantages in the treatment of NES. It is feasible to embed a group treatment within a neurology outpatient clinic.**
- **Like other complex diagnoses, NES is best treated by a team of health care providers. Because this condition spans the fields of both neurology and psychiatry, the ideal NES team is composed of members from both disciplines.**

INTRODUCTION

Non-epileptic seizures (NES), formerly called pseudo-seizures, resemble epileptic seizures but lack epileptiform activity on an electroencephalogram (EEG) and presumably have psychopathological origins. Whereas community prevalence is estimated to be 2 to 33 per 100,000,[1] NES accounts for 25% to 30% of cases referred to epilepsy centers for intractable epilepsy.[2] Between 5% and 10% of NES patients also have epileptic seizures, complicating their treatment.[3]

NES has been described since antiquity. In the 19th century, when Jean-Martin Charcot studied "hysteria," NES episodes were referred to as hysterical seizures and were thought to occur only in women. When clinicians realized that men could also have these symptoms, especially in the aftermath of war trauma, the preferred term shifted to pseudo-seizures. Currently, the term *pseudo-seizure,* considered to be derogatory, is gradually being replaced by *non-epileptic seizure* or *psychogenic non-epileptic seizure.*

NES significantly impacts health care costs and inflicts harm on patients through unnecessary treatments such as intubations and medications. A 2007 study found average costs for patients in the United States prior to being properly diagnosed with NES to be $15,000.[4] A 2003 study reported that 75% of NES patients visited emergency departments (EDs), averaging six ED visits at ~$3,400/visit prior to diagnosis. NES patients were treated in intensive care settings as frequently as patients with epileptic seizures (27.8% vs. 23.3%). Forty percent of patients with NES alone were taking at least one antiepileptic drug even 10 years after diagnosis.[5]

Most NES patients have comorbid psychiatric illnesses, particularly depression, anxiety, posttraumatic stress disorders, and other conversion symptoms. Effective treatment requires not only addressing the NES but also treating these comorbid conditions. Unfortunately, many patients fear that seeing a psychiatrist implies that their episodes are not being taken seriously, and that their neurologist might perceive them as producing their symptoms willfully, experiencing a factitious disorder, or malingering. Patients might feel abandoned if their neurologist refers them to a psychiatrist and indicates that they no longer need to be seen by the neurologist. Consequently, patients often resist undergoing psychiatric evaluation and treatment.

According to internationally recognized experts, the four steps in the management of NES are (1) making the diagnosis, (2) presenting the diagnosis, (3) gaining control of the seizures, and (4) managing seizures and life activities.[6] This chapter reviews what is known about each of these aspects of NES and discusses our integrated care team approach to managing these conditions. See Box 19.1 for a summary of important points regarding NES.

CLINICAL PRESENTATION

NES can take the form of any type of epileptic seizure. Accompanying alteration of consciousness can occur, ranging from mild to complete. Patients most frequently present to emergency, primary care, or neurology departments with a seizure or history of seizure(s). Most NES patients are eventually referred to an epilepsy center for further diagnosis and treatment. Between 10% and 20% of patients referred to epilepsy centers for drug-resistant epilepsy will go on to be diagnosed with NES rather than epileptic seizures.[1] These patients account for 20% to 30% of patients diagnosed with intractable epilepsy.[2] Between 5% and 10% of NES patients also have epileptic seizures, which complicates their treatment.[3]

Prior to the advent of video-electroencephalography (VEEG), NES was diagnosed based on seizure characteristics and other clinical factors. Several studies have sought to determine clinical predictors that can reliably distinguish NES from epileptic seizures.[7,8] Clinical signs reported to have high specificity and sensitivity for NES include asynchronous movements, eyes being forced closed during the episode, and memory/recall of the event. Pelvic thrusting was reported to have 100% sensitivity and 20% specificity for NES in one study, but this feature cannot reliably distinguish between frontal lobe epileptic seizures and NES.[8] NES events also tend to last considerably longer than epileptic seizure events and at times have a "stop-and-go" characteristic rather than the more continuous synchronous movements seen in generalized convulsive seizures.

PSYCHIATRIC COMORBIDITIES

Most NES patients have at least one other psychiatric diagnosis; only 5% of patients with NES do not have an identified comorbid psychiatric disorder or stressor.[9] The estimated prevalence of psychiatric diagnoses comorbid with NES varies widely, likely due to different study methodologies, for example the use of clinician-rated versus self-report instruments. Comorbid depression has been reported to occur in 21% to 60% of NES patients, similar to rates in epileptic seizures and far more common than in the general populations. Similarly, rates of most anxiety disorders are about equal in NES and epileptic seizure patients, both much higher than rates in the general population.[10]

Conversion disorders are conditions in which psychological stress emerges as pseudo-neurologic symptoms. NES is considered to be a type of conversion disorder. Other conversion symptoms such as weakness, numbness, pain, and disturbances of vision or hearing are also quite common in patients with NES, with reported rates of 21%[11] to 60%.[12]

Histories of traumatic events are much more common in NES patients than the general population.[13] While rates of premorbid and comorbid trauma and abuse are higher in patients with epileptic seizures than in general populations, rates in NES patients are higher still. Recent studies report frequent histories of sexual (30%), nonsexual

(73–86%), and overall (44–90%) trauma in NES patients.[14,15] Not surprisingly, posttraumatic stress disorder (PTSD) is also significantly more common in patients with NES than in the general population.[13]

Certain personality disorders have been found to be prevalent in patients with NES; reported rates vary in part due to whether self-report instruments such as the Minnesota Multiphasic Personality Inventory (MMPI) or clinician-scored instruments such as the Structured Clinical Inventory for DSM-IV Axis II Diagnoses (SCID II) are used. Compared to populations of patients with epilepsy, studies using SCID II or similar instruments have found high rates of Cluster B personality disorders (i.e., antisocial, narcissistic, histrionic, borderline), especially borderline personality disorder. Reported rates of Cluster A personality disorders (i.e., paranoid, schizoid, schizotypal) were low. Compared to the general population, Cluster C personality disorders (i.e., avoidant, dependent, obsessive-compulsive) were more common in patients with epilepsy and in those with mixed epileptic and non-epileptic seizures, but not in patients with NES alone.[10]

NES patients frequently report alterations in consciousness associated with their episodes. These alterations are usually classified as dissociative episodes, which the *Diagnostic and Statistical Manual of Mental Disorder*, 5th Edition (DSM-5) defines as "a disruption of and/or discontinuity in the normal integration of consciousness, memory, identity, emotion, perception, body representation, motor control, and behavior."[16] Dissociative symptoms are often associated with exposure to traumatic events and are thought to represent defensive reactions to overwhelming affect.

Somatic complaints are also very common in NES patients. Studies have found that 14% to 77% of NES patients have comorbid somatoform pain disorder,[17] with chronic unexplained headaches in 61% to 73% of NES patients.[18] DSM-IV somatization disorder (primarily encompassed by somatic symptom disorder in DSM-5) has been reported in 13% of NES patients[18] compared to 0.38% of the general population.[19] See Chapter 16: Somatic Symptom Disorders and Illness Anxiety in Integrated Care Settings for additional information.

SUBGROUPS OF NES PATIENTS

Many studies have attempted to subcategorize the heterogeneous population of NES patients into subgroups that might better predict outcome or guide treatment, for example by gender, age of onset, comorbid epileptic seizures, alteration in consciousness, comorbid personality disorder, history of trauma, and/or presence of brain injuries or intellectual disabilities.[20] Although definitive treatments have not yet been linked to particular subgroups, this line of investigation might further the understanding of the pathogenesis of NES and assist in designing useful treatment approaches.

DIFFERENTIAL DIAGNOSIS OF NES

The differential diagnosis of NES includes not only epilepsy but also other physiologic etiologies that can cause similar-looking events, most commonly syncope, especially convulsive syncope. Syncope may be vasovagal or caused by cardiac arrhythmias and is often accompanied by tonic movements. Epilepsy monitoring units record patients' electrocardiograms (ECGs) along with their VEEGs to screen for potential cardiac etiologies.

Other physiologic conditions in the differential diagnosis are dysautonomia, non-epileptic myoclonus, and hallucinations secondary to delirium or psychotic disorders; neurologic phenomena including transient ischemic attacks; complex migraines with motor or sensory symptoms; sleep disorders (parasomnias) such as sleepwalking and rapid eye movement (REM) sleep behavior disorders; and confusional arousals.

CLASSIFICATION OF NES

Experts debate whether NES is best described as a somatoform disorder or as a dissociative disorder. The DSM-5 classifies NES as a conversion disorder (functional neurologic symptom disorder) with a disturbance of voluntary movement or sensation in the chapter on Somatic Symptom and Related Disorders.[16] The International Classification of Diseases, Tenth Revision (ICD-10) classifies NES under the category of dissociative and conversion disorders: "conversion disorder with seizures or convulsions," with the code F44.5.[21] Overall, NES is probably better thought of as a symptom rather than as a disorder in and of itself.

EPIDEMIOLOGY AND COURSE

Population-based studies estimate the incidence of NES to be 1.4 to 4.9 per 100,000 per year, and the prevalence to be 5% that of epilepsy.[22] In epilepsy monitoring units this number is higher, between 25% and 30% of admissions.[2] Women account for 70% to 80% of individuals with NES. Most cases present in adolescence or young adulthood.[23]

Significant diagnostic delay is common in NES, with time to NES diagnosis averaging 7.2 years after onset.[24] During this delay, costs and potential harms to the patient may occur. Once the diagnosis is made, reductions in ED utilization usually occur, even in patients who continue to have episodes.[25]

Among patients with recent onset of NES, 15% to 50% were seizure-free 6 months after diagnosis.[22,25,26] One study reported that most seizures stop shortly after the diagnosis.[25] However, others suggest this improvement may not persist, and one study found that 87% of NES patients continued to have seizures at the one-year follow-up.[26] Unfortunately, the long-term prognosis is generally poor, with 71% still experiencing events at a mean of 11 years after diagnosis.[27] No reliable predictors of outcome have yet been identified.

ETIOLOGY

In the context of acute and/or chronic psychological distress and conflict, certain individuals are prone to develop functional neurologic sensory and/or motor symptoms (e.g., NES) not attributable to known brain or peripheral neurologic processes or to known disturbances in the motor or other effector systems. Some of these symptoms have been labeled as "conversion" symptoms, in which psychological conflicts are presumably channeled and "converted" into physical (somatoform) symptoms. To some extent, somatoform symptoms can be understood as a form of indirect distress communication. Griffith et al[28] explored this idea by examining 14 videotaped family interviews with patients with NES. The investigators identified "unspeakable dilemmas," such as ongoing sexual abuse, domestic violence, or school failure, in 13 patients.[28]

Childhood traumatic experiences, particularly physical and sexual abuse, are well recognized as playing a role in the development of many cases of NES[27, 29–31] and can be considered to have a predisposing role. Although the mechanisms leading from trauma to NES are unknown, one study suggests that childhood trauma might lead to NES through the development of a fearful attachment style.[32]

Current life events frequently trigger NES, possibly following a resurgence of emotions associated with current life problems or past traumas.[19] Current interpersonal conflicts and other aversive life events can be considered to have precipitating roles in the onset of NES.

Concurrent anxiety, depression, PTSD, or other psychiatric illnesses, overuse of avoidance strategies, reliance on dissociation, and a lack of mature coping strategies can perpetuate NES. Other theoretical models based on learning theory have also been postulated. The etiology and pathogenesis of NES are currently best considered to be multifactorial and primarily of psychological/traumatic origins.

MAKING THE DIAGNOSIS OF NES

Making the diagnosis of NES requires a VEEG and evaluation by a neurologist. Although one or a group of characteristic clinical signs may help distinguish non-epileptic from epileptic seizures, long-term VEEG with concurrent ECG recording remains the "gold standard" for distinguishing the two.[8] These procedures usually entail admitting the patient to an epilepsy monitoring unit for several days to a week. A diagnosis of NES can be confirmed when no epileptic activity or cardiac rhythm abnormality is identified during a characteristic event recorded with simultaneous EEG, ECG, and video recording. Occasionally, false-negative results occur in patients with focal seizures with deep or small seizure foci. Similarly, frontal lobe seizures may not show up on scalp EEG; therefore, with seizure episodes consistent with this type, the VEEG should be critically appraised so as not to lead to misdiagnosis.[8]

The interictal routine EEG, a widely available diagnostic tool, has a high false-negative rate. There are no specific interictal EEG findings that can confirm or exclude a diagnosis of NES.

TREATMENT OF NES

Very few high-quality studies exist to guide treatment of NES. Nonetheless, it is generally agreed that treatment actually begins with the delivery of the diagnosis to the patient and family. This is followed by a psychiatric evaluation and one or more psychotherapeutic interventions.[6]

Delivery of the Diagnosis

Reluctance to accept the diagnosis constitutes a significant barrier to the management of patients with NES. Typically, the diagnosis is presented by the neurologist and usually comes as a surprise to the patient. Reactions often range from anger to despair mixed with disbelief and distrust.

Once the diagnosis is delivered, outcomes may vary from reduction or resolution of events to worsening of symptoms.[34] Studies reporting a decrease in seizure frequency have described this improvement occurring as quickly as within the first 24 hours after presentation of the diagnosis. Although one study reported that most seizures stop shortly after the diagnosis,[26] others suggest this improvement may, unfortunately, not persist.[35]

Such a broad range of outcomes following diagnosis strongly suggests that unmeasured or unreported factors are influencing outcome. Experience suggests that a clinician's style of explaining NES can impact patient and family acceptance. Strategies for maximizing positive outcomes have been studied, but no published data suggest the superiority of one method over another. Common approaches include (1) an explanation of the technology used to ascertain the non-epileptic nature of the seizures, (2) assurance that the patient is not purposely having NES, (3) presentation of some of the underlying etiologies for the events, (4) reassurance that the diagnosis is common, (5) a discussion about possible discontinuation of antiepileptic drugs, and (6) open and frank discussion that the definitive treatment is psychological and directed to reducing stress and conflict.[6] In fact, studies have shown that even if seizure frequency decreases after receiving the diagnosis of NES, in the absence of psychiatric treatment no changes occur in psychological distress, function, or health-related quality of life.[34]

Psychiatric Evaluation

The NES patient should also be evaluated by a psychiatrist or other behavioral health specialist to screen for comorbid psychiatric conditions, coping styles, current and past traumas, and stressors and to make appropriate plans for psychotherapeutic and psychiatric interventions.[8,36] Special attention should be paid to childhood development, especially traumatic occurrences and difficulties with attachment. Similarly, establishing temporal relationships between current stressors and NES will facilitate the acceptance of the NES diagnosis. As comorbidities are more likely to be present than not, investigating for the presence of depression, anxiety, and PTSD is imperative.

Psychotherapeutic treatment options can be introduced beginning with the initial evaluation. Patients often feel overwhelmed by their diagnosis, so providing information about effective treatment is helpful. Exploring the patient's beliefs about the causes of the seizures helps to determine the patient's readiness for psychiatric treatment. Following the diagnosis, the patient and family may feel confused or uncertain. The psychiatrist must be prepared to answer questions about NES that have not previously been asked or have been inadequately explained. The patient and family will likely be more amenable to psychiatric treatment if the psychiatrist's description and explanation of NES parallels the discussion given by their neurologist. While some patients may still have doubts about the etiology of their seizures, most accept the need to improve coping skills and reduce stress, and will usually accept the need for treatment of depression or anxiety. Providing written material that supports psychiatric treatment is also helpful.

Ongoing Treatment by Neurology

After the diagnosis of NES has been established, if the patient does not have co-occurring epileptic seizures, antiseizure medications may be safely withdrawn.[36] While medications are likely to be useful for comorbid epileptic seizures or psychiatric diagnoses, they have not been shown helpful for NES itself.

With respect to the postdiagnostic role of the neurologist in patients with NES, 69% of neurologists report continuing to follow patients after the diagnosis of NES.[37] One study found that NES patients have better outcomes when they continue to see their neurologists.[38]

Psychotherapeutic Options

At present, the highest-quality evidence for treating NES effectively is associated with individual cognitive-behavioral therapy (CBT), as described below.[39] However, since NES is very much a social phenomenon, occurring in the context of relationships, a strong possibility exists that group therapy and family interventions may offer therapeutic benefits over and above those of individual therapy. Lower-quality but promising evidence exists for these modalities.[40–43]

Group Psychotherapy

In behavioral health settings, group interventions, an expanding treatment modality in all forms of health care, have often proven to be as efficacious as individual psychotherapy.[44] (See Chapter 28: Group Interventions in Integrated Care Settings.) Several pilot studies for NES have shown group interventions to be feasible and efficacious. For example, a 24-session weekly psychoeducational group intervention lowered the frequency of events in six out of nine completers.[40] In another NES study using 10 weekly psychoeducational group sessions, Zaroff et al[41] noted a decrease in posttraumatic and dissociative symptoms and a trend toward improved quality of life. Using group psychodynamic psychotherapy for 32 weekly sessions, Barry et al[42] demonstrated a statistically significant decline in NES frequency as well as improvement in scores on the Beck Depression Inventory (BDI) and the Global Severity Index of the Symptom Checklist-90. Follow-up after two years found that five of seven completers were seizure-free. Lastly, a four-session weekly CBT group intervention showed significant improvements in emotional domains of quality of life.[43]

Group therapists can be physicians, nurses, psychologists, social workers, health coaches, or other behavioral health specialists with experience facilitating groups. Ideally, at least one of the clinicians on an NES treatment team will have experience in or will receive training in order to provide individual or group psychotherapy to patients with this diagnosis.

Family Psychotherapy

Family dysfunction, common in patients with NES, contributes to symptoms of depression and reduces the overall quality of life in patients with NES.[45] Family treatment is a useful adjunctive treatment that can easily be combined with other therapeutic modalities such as medication management, group therapy, or individual therapy. Trained family therapists may be social workers, psychologists, nurses, or physicians.

All families merit and benefit from psychoeducation, but some families may need more intensive treatment. See Chapter 27: Best Practice for Family-Centered Health Care: A Three-Step Model for further information about options for family interventions. To determine which families need more intensive treatment, the Family Assessment Device (FAD) can serve as a self-report screening tool.[46] Associated with the McMaster Model of family-systems therapy, the FAD consists of 60 items that screen for six dimensions of family functioning; a validated 12-item version that screens for general family functioning is also available. These tools can be administered by anyone, but the results should be evaluated by a clinician trained in family treatment. The McMaster Model has been used successfully in treating patients with NES and their families. However, the specific model of family therapy to be used is often determined by the training of the family therapists available.

General principles of family therapy that apply to all systemic models are (1) conceptualizing the problem in relational terms, (2) disrupting dysfunctional relational patterns, (3) expanding the treatment system to include family members, and (4) expanding the therapeutic alliance to include family members.[47] Most family therapy capitalizes on family strengths identified during the family assessment.

Individual Psychotherapy

A 2014 Cochrane review of psychological and behavioral treatments for adults with NES found little reliable evidence to guide clinicians.[39] The review identified 12 studies, totaling 343 participants, that met the inclusion criteria. Only four were randomized controlled trials; the others were pre–post uncontrolled studies. Five involved generic psychotherapy, three CBT, two hypnosis, and one paradoxical intention. No meta-analysis was conducted due to the heterogeneity of the studies.

Only one of the 12 studies was found to be free of bias (Goldstein et al, published in 2010).[48] This single-treatment-center randomized controlled trial randomized 66 patients with NES (50 female, 16 male) to CBT plus standard medical care or standard medical care alone. The CBT intervention consisted of 12 weekly one-hour individual sessions. At the end of treatment a significant reduction in median monthly seizure frequency was observed for the CBT arm versus standard medical care ($p = .002$).

Following publication of the Cochrane review, an additional three-center randomized controlled trial on the treatment of NES was published.[49] In this study, 38 patients were randomized to four treatment arms: sertraline only, manualized CBT-informed psychotherapy (CBT-ip) only, CBT-ip plus sertraline, or treatment as usual. One trained therapist per site administered CBT for 12 one-hour weekly sessions. At the end of the study (week 16), patients in both the CBT-ip and the CBT-ip plus sertraline arms showed significant reductions in seizure frequency (51.4% and 59.3%) as well as improvement in global functioning. The patients in the medication-only and treatment-as-usual arms showed no significant improvement in seizure frequency or secondary outcome measures.

Self-Help and Support Options

Online resources available for patients with NES are listed in Box 19.2. A Facebook support group and several online mailing lists are also available.

INTEGRATED NEUROLOGY-PSYCHIATRY NES PROJECT: UNIVERSITY OF COLORADO SCHOOL OF MEDICINE EXPERIENCE

A discussion of the development of our NES project may be useful in two ways. First, our program may be useful for other centers wishing to create similar programs. Second, our program is a general example of integrating psychiatry with a specialty clinic, specifically how to do this with neurology services. Using our own processes as examples, we describe steps to be taken by others wishing to integrate behavioral health services with medical specialty programs. See Box 19.3 for an overview of recommendations for others who wish to develop behavioral health programs embedded within specialty medical service.

Convene Stakeholders

The University of Colorado School of Medicine NES Project began with a meeting of stakeholders from the departments of psychiatry and neurology and an administrative representative from ambulatory services at the University of Colorado Hospital (UCH). Ambulatory services at UCH asked the psychiatry department to develop a pilot program to demonstrate a model of feasibility and functioning of integrated behavioral health services with a specialty clinic in the hospital system. Psychiatry and neurology seemed a natural first choice; the disciplines overlap significantly, as evidenced by the subspecialties of neuropsychiatry and behavioral neurology, and by the neuroscience research collaborations on multiple projects between our two departments.

The first step in developing a large interdepartmental collaboration is to engage stakeholder leadership in the process. Appropriate stakeholders need to be identified and presented with the reasons driving the need for change. Early involvement and buy-in from these stakeholders will help ensure that

BOX 19.2

SELF-HELP AND SUPPORT OPTIONS FOR PATIENTS WITH NON-EPILEPTIC SEIZURES

- **The Truth about Psychogenic Nonepileptic Seizures: http://www.epilepsy.com/article/2014/3/truth-about-psychogenic-nonepileptic-seizures. Published March 2014. Accessed May 24, 2016.**
- **Psychogenic Nonepileptic Seizures: A Guide for Patients and Families: http://health.usf.edu/medicine/neurology/epilepsy/~/media/Files/Medicine/Neurology/Comprehensive%20Epilepsy%20Program/PNESbrochure.pdf. Accessed May 24, 2016.**
- **Psychogenic Nonepileptic Events: http://www.aafp.org/afp/2005/0901/p849.html. Published September 1, 2005. Accessed May 24, 2016.**
- **Psychogenic Nonepileptic Seizures: Diagnosis, Aetiology, Treatment and Prognosis: http://www.sanp.ch/docs/2005/2005-02/2005-02-046.pdf. Published March 2005. Accessed May 24, 2016.**
- **Living with Nonepileptic Seizures: http://night-light.org/index/disability-and-chronic-illness-resources/epilepsy-resources/nonepileptic-seizures/. Accessed May 24, 2016.**
- **Functional Neurologic Disorder patient website: www.fndhope.org. Accessed May 24, 2016.**
- **TED Talk, "The Hypnotic Power of Words": http://tedxtalks.ted.com/video/The-hypnotic-power-of-words-Kri;search%3Athe%20hypnotic%20power. Published January 14, 2014. Accessed May 24, 2016.**
- **Institute for Healthcare Improvement website: www.ihi.org. Accessed May 24, 2016.**

BOX 19.3

RECOMMENDATIONS FOR OTHERS DEVELOPING BEHAVIORAL HEALTH EMBEDDED WITHIN A SPECIALTY MEDICAL SERVICE

- **Convene stakeholders: Identify appropriate stakeholders and get early buy-in.**
- **Target population: Identify patients who will receive the intervention, and conduct literature reviews to identify both the behavioral health issues of the target population and any information about treating them within specialty clinic settings.**
- **Consultants: Recruit a consultant with expertise with the identified patient population as a valuable asset to the team.**
- **Multidisciplinary project team: Develop transdisciplinary and multidisciplinary teams to encourage buy-in from both departments and bring multiple perspectives to team discussions.**
- **Quality and safety expertise: Find and employ programs at your hospital or university to assist in project development.**
- **Location of care: Locate integrated behavioral health services within the medical specialty clinic.**
- **Care pathways: Develop a treatment algorithm to standardize screenings, patient education, and clinician training and to clarify each clinician's role on the treatment team.**
- **Develop group and family-focused approaches: Focus on group and family treatment while reserving individual treatment for the most difficult cases.**
- **Referrals: Construct registries to allow the program to locate suitable patients for group referral in order to maintain a steady flow of patients into the treatment groups.**
- **Outcome measures: Choose screening, process, and outcome measures based on literature reviews and/or feedback from consultants.**
- **Financial viability: Develop a viable business case that takes into consideration the current billing structure and allows adaptation to upcoming changes in the health care market.**

THE LONG TERM

- **Plan for continued training and supervision of clinicians to provide specialized group therapy.**
- **Develop protocols for transition of care and periodic checkups in the patient's medical home.**
- **Track screening, process, and outcome measure in registries to quantify how interventions result in multiple better patient outcomes.**

resources are available, obstacles can be lowered or removed, and needed alterations can be made to keep the project on identified timelines.

Target Population

Our neurology department identified patients with NES as their preferred patient population for this project since the needs for treating this population were overwhelming their clinics. Our large epilepsy center with an epilepsy monitoring unit makes about 200 new diagnoses of NES per year. Once diagnosed, these patients have had no formalized treatment options, creating significant disappointment and stress for patients and clinicians. Many of these patients were referred to the outpatient psychiatric clinic, but many did not accept referrals or would make appointments but fail to show up for intake. Once we settled on this population, since neither our psychiatrists nor epileptologists had much experience with NES treatment specifically, we reviewed the literature to look at interventions for the disorder.

It is important for the medical specialties to identify a target population through a combination of clinical experiences, needs assessment surveys, and feedback from patients and/or providers, using written questionnaires/surveys, focus groups, or patient data reports from electronic medical records. For example, an endocrinology practice might wish to offer behavioral health services to patients with diabetes because significant behavioral and mental health issues are associated with this chronic illness. Literature reviews should focus on identifying behavioral and mental health issues for these special populations and their treatment within specialty clinic settings. For example, a pain clinic might focus on patients with opiate addiction, an obstetrics clinic might identify a target population with postpartum depression, or a pulmonary clinic might note the high prevalence of patients with panic disorder.

Consultants

When launching our initiative, we invited an NES expert, W. Curt LaFrance Jr., MD, MPH, director of neuropsychiatry and behavioral neurology at Rhode Island Hospital, to visit and advise us. Dr. LaFrance is board certified in both neurology and psychiatry and could therefore speak clearly to the concerns of each discipline. He presented the history of NES and his pioneering work with NES patients. For example, he had recently completed a randomized clinical trial for NES patients and found significant seizure reduction and improved comorbid symptoms and global functioning with CBT-ip with and without sertraline. He visited with both departments and provided invaluable advice about assessment, treatment, and follow-up for our NES patients.

Identification and engagement with a consultant/expert can offer the objective views of an leader who has previous experience with projects of this kind, who has developed expertise with the identified patient population, and who can help connect the team with similar projects in other centers nationally and internationally.

Multidisciplinary Project Team

Concurrently, we selected core team members for the project: two epileptologists, two neurology nurses working in the epilepsy clinic, and three psychiatrists. Our first meetings focused on initial priorities: understanding the flow of patients through the epilepsy monitoring unit and its diagnostic processes, learning to work across disciplines and across departments, drafting a rough timeline for the project, and considering treatment options after diagnosis. We chose descriptive language for the patient population that the whole team could agree upon—for example, *non-epileptic seizures* rather than *psychogenic non-epileptic seizures, pseudo-seizures*, or *non-epileptic events or attacks*. We discussed how the stigma of these alternative names might impact all facets of diagnosis and treatment.

First and foremost, projects of this size require teamwork. A cross-departmental multidisciplinary team requires buy-in from both departments and all staff levels, and team members should bring diverse perspectives into team discussions. Also, since momentum can wane during program implementation, a team is better equipped than an individual to keep the project on task. Specialty medical physicians should lead and initiate pilot programs in collaboration with psychiatry and should jointly develop treatment algorithms and work out all the logistics. Discussing and making small changes first, before big ones, fosters team communication and collaborations. Next, considering the behavioral health interventions needed and relevant training for collaborating staff professionals should begin as soon as feasible. This can proceed in conjunction with other practice transformation activities that will be needed to enable the project.

Quality and Safety Expertise

As we were embarking on our project, our NES team was one of 13 programs accepted into a certificate training program (CTP) sponsored by the Institute for Healthcare Quality, Safety, and Efficiency on our campus. This is a quality and safety partnership between several of the University of Colorado School of Medicine professional schools, UCH (our hospital), Children's Hospital Colorado, and UCHealth (our health care system). The program's mission is to improve clinical outcomes, value, and patient experience across our multisite care-delivery system. The CTP year-long course focuses on developing and enhancing highly functioning clinical leadership teams capable of transforming the quality, safety, operational efficiency, and experience of care for patients. Being part of this program really cemented our team and the NES project.

We recommend finding and using local quality and safety development and improvement programs and staff to assist in project development. If internal resources are not available, national organizations may offer training opportunities similar to those of the Institute for Healthcare Improvement.

Location of Care

In developing comprehensive treatment for NES our team wanted to lower barriers to care. We were sensitive to the fact that many NES patients would not agree to get their care in our outpatient psychiatry clinic located at a distance from the main hospital. Since we knew that psychiatric treatment co-located within a neurology clinic significantly increases the likelihood that NES patients will attend psychological treatments,[50] our group chose to embed our integrated care clinic within the neurology outpatient clinic.

Whenever possible, integrated behavioral health services should be co-located within the medical specialty clinic for a variety of reasons: (1) patients prefer "one-stop shopping," (2) patients do not want to lose their specialists, and (3) patients often struggle to accept behavioral health diagnoses or treatment and want to avoid referral to a mental health clinic because of stigma.

Care Pathways

Initially, our team met weekly to develop a treatment algorithm. We decided on the following:

1. Start NES patient evaluation and treatment while the patient was still in the epilepsy monitoring unit.
2. Develop an educational video for patients and families receiving the diagnosis featuring explanations of NES and its treatment by an epileptologist, a psychiatrist, and a successfully treated patient. This educational video is presented by one of the neurology nurses, who shows this video to patients and families shortly after the neurologist delivers the diagnosis, while the patient is still in the epilepsy monitoring unit. The nurse is available to answer any questions.
3. Include family evaluation in our psychiatric evaluation and offer family therapy as needed.
4. Use group-based treatment as the primary intervention.

Figure 19.1 illustrates the critical pathway we developed for our NES patients.

After the NES diagnosis is made and the patient is told of the diagnosis, the psychiatrist on the team evaluates the patient in the epilepsy monitoring unit using a comprehensive psychiatric screen and assessment of family functioning as previously described. After psychiatric evaluation, one of several plans may be recommended: (1) the patient may be referred to the NES group in the neurology clinic, (2) patients requiring treatment of comorbid psychiatric conditions may be referred for individual treatment in our psychiatric outpatient service, (3) patients with significant family dysfunction are referred for family treatment to our psychiatry outpatient clinic, and (4) all patients continue care with their neurologist until a transition plan can be developed and implemented to transfer care back to a primary care provider and, if needed, a mental health provider.

Developing a critical pathway or a formal treatment algorithm can standardize care, including patient flow, team tasks, and treatments offered across the program, while accommodating a variety of procedures (e.g., how patients are given the diagnosis and how routinely to use group-based psychotherapies). Critical pathways and algorithms can also help clarify each clinician's role, diagnostic screening procedures, and patient education, as well as diagram how comprehensive evaluations will be used in case formulation and treatment planning.

Developing the Group Therapy

Because group psychotherapy has been shown to benefit NES patients, and groups can also accommodate larger volumes of patients as evaluated and diagnosed in our epilepsy monitoring unit, we chose to develop a group therapy approach, which we embedded in the neurology clinic. Group therapy was the primary psychiatric treatment modality; the staff comprised two psychiatrists and a neurology nurse. To help us design an effective treatment approach, we invited eight patients with a diagnosis of NES to participate in a one-time focus group. Patient feedback concerned the isolating nature of NES, helpful concepts to include in our group structure, and how to keep a therapy group running while a member is actively having an NES.

We developed our group model based on several foundational elements: (1) pilot data from previous NES groups, (2) our knowledge of group stages of development (see Chapter 28: Group Interventions in Integrated Care Settings), and (3) the topics and education we planned to cover during the group.

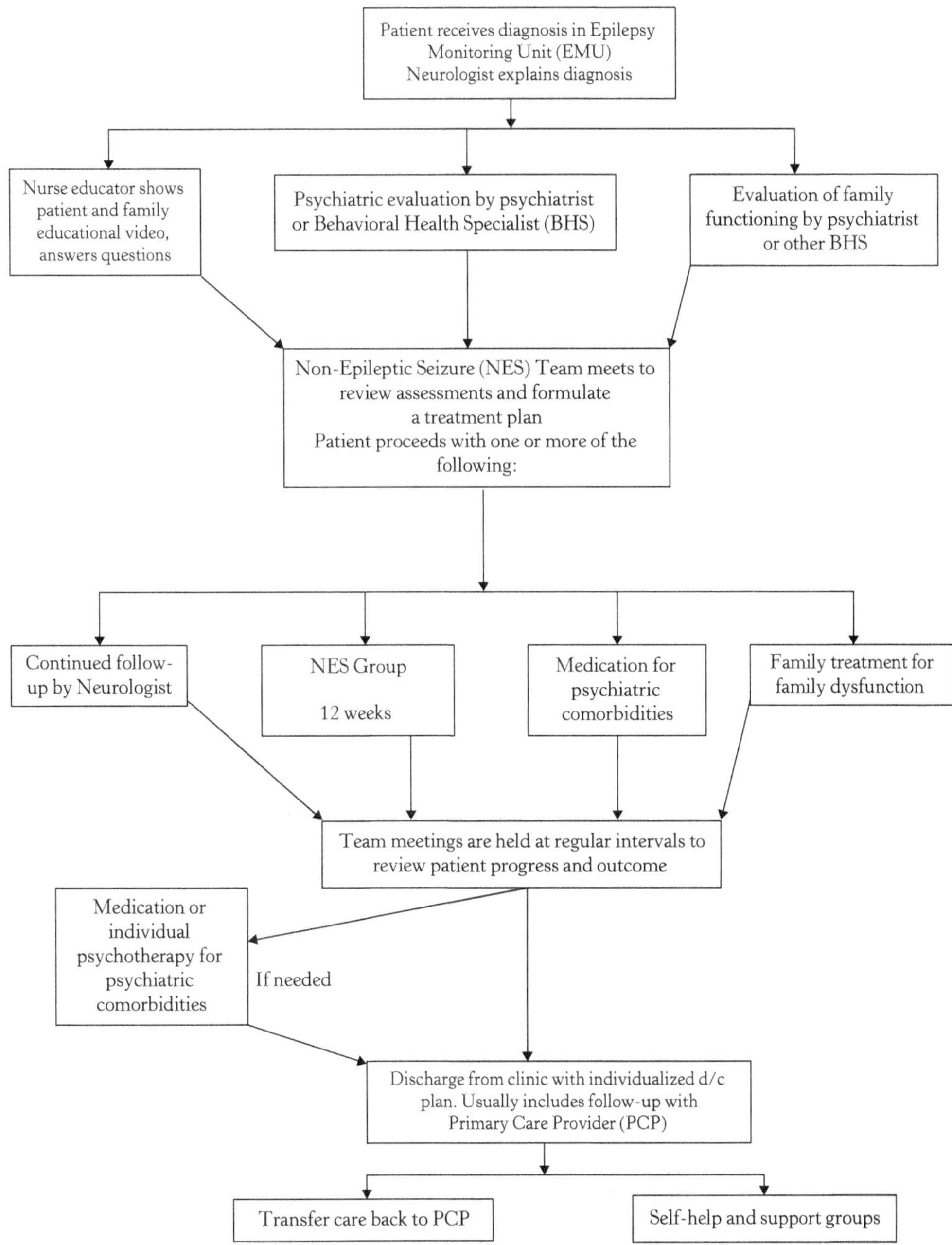

FIGURE 19.1. Non-epileptic seizures critical pathway.

The group needed to meet long enough to build trust and rapport between the members, but not so long as to incur multiple dropouts. We elected to run our pilot group for 12 weekly sessions, each session lasting for 80 minutes. The team decided that the group would need to balance fostering emotional insight, learning about NES, and developing practical tools (e.g., mindfulness exercises and relaxation techniques). We hoped to deliver sufficient care so that automatic referrals to psychiatry would not be necessary for every patient participating in our program. Since histories of childhood and adulthood trauma are prevalent in NES patients and are thought to play important roles in pathogenesis,[51] the team decided to explicitly address the patients' trauma. Discussions were balanced to meaningfully address the traumatic experiences of our NES patients without being emotionally overwhelming. Supporting discussions of traumatic events in generalities may help promote healing of emotional wounds, but too much trauma-informed discussion can lead to dissociation and increased symptomatology in patients with NES. We also identified that recognizing "triggers" for NES (usually factors such as increased stress, poor sleep, and interpersonal tensions in important relationships) needed to be explored and discussed many times during the 12-week group program. Understanding the meaning of their NES events permits members to begin constructing narratives concerning their experiences that may include recalling past events in their lives, adopting certain roles in the family, and identifying and naming strong emotions. An additional theme explored in later group sessions is the "grief for the loss of past identities or roles," such as a group member who strongly identifies as a caretaker having to uncharacteristically learn to ask for help from others.

We recommend group therapy for integrated NES programming and the use of groups for other specialty populations. There are many therapeutic advantages to using group interventions in integrated care settings, including employing the unique therapeutic factors of groups.[52] Groups can provide supportive, educational, and healing environments that cannot be duplicated in individual treatment. Groups can also help individual group members establish focused and well-defined goals, such as identifying their specific triggers and increasing their self-care management strategies and behaviors. Also, groups can enable specialty medical services to handle larger patient volumes, increase patient access to psychiatric care, lower the cost of care, and offer reasonable reimbursements for group providers. Short-term group theory principles, and techniques[53,54] can easily be incorporated into groups run in medical specialty or primary care clinics. Similarly, since closed-ended groups run more effectively when leaders adopt an active and directive stance, we recommend this type of group leadership style in medical specialty environments. For new programs, we recommend a focus-group session to assist in developing the group structure and themes to be developed over the span of treatment. The length of each session, number of sessions to be scheduled, and content of the therapy meetings will vary depending on goals for the group treatment, the types of patients attending, and the clinic's resources. Since short-term groups have defined endings, patients are encouraged to develop additional resources outside and beyond the life of the group, which may include community resources, religious supports, support from friends and family, and further behavioral health treatment, if indicated.

Individual treatment such as individual psychotherapy should be reserved for the more difficult nonresponding and psychiatrically complex cases. Individual treatment can occur in concert with ongoing group treatment. Some patients may not be appropriate for group therapy and are better handled with one-on-one care, at least initially. Later on in the course of individual treatment, if indicated, such patients can subsequently join a therapy group and still maintain individual treatment.

Referrals

Our pilot group required approximately eight patients. Most of the patients were referred by neurologist members of our project team and were also initially screened by them. Prior to the start of the group, one psychiatrist screened all referrals for seizure frequency. He also provided all referrals with an initial explanation of NES, explored their feelings about participating in a group, and discussed how patients might handle intense feelings that may emerge in the group.

We ran reports from our electronic health record to identify patients with a diagnosis of NES to begin a registry for current and future referrals. We discovered that the list was not complete due to the diagnoses used to identify these patients: Some NES patients received the diagnosis of NES, some were diagnosed with somatoform disorder, and some received both diagnoses. We worked with the entire epilepsy practice to standardize the diagnosis and select our target population.

Registries should be constructed to follow the progress of all group patients. Registries should also be used in specialty practices to help identify future patients as part of a future referral pool, which will assist in making all groups sustainable. Standardization of the diagnosis for patients is crucial to ensure accuracy of the registries. Education aimed at clinicians may be necessary to align providers in diagnostic coding. Patients may be referred from select clinicians for initial groups, but later groups can be constructed from well-developed registries.

Outcome Measures

We selected the process and outcome metrics to be assessed at the beginning and end of the intervention and modeled them after scales used in a previous study.[49] These included NES event frequency, the World Health Organization Disability Assessment Scale (WHODAS 2.0),[55] Brief COPE (measures ways of coping with stress),[56] Quality of Life in Epilepsy 31(QOLIE-31),[56758] Symptom Checklist 90 (SCL-90),[59,60] Dissociative Experiences Scale-II (DES-II),[61] and Brief Assessment of Family Functioning (BAFFS-6).[62] We also chose event frequency and the "thermometer" from QOLIE-31 to be followed weekly.

Process and outcome measures can be chosen from a literature review and/or feedback from consultants to the project. Patient self-report measures need to fit the time allotted for patients to fill them out and should not become onerous. Also, patients need to be taught to fill out forms properly, such as daily logs of seizure frequency. Clinician outcome measures should be available to all members of the team. Assigning this responsibility to one team member will help with tracking and organizing of the patient registry.

Observations about the NES Group

After the pilot group ran for 12 weeks, we reviewed notable events to help guide our clinicians in future planning. To help bridge the gap from their somatic complaints to psychological experiences, the patients frequently assigned meanings to NES, which often led to recollections of traumatic experiences in their backgrounds. Connections to trauma came up sooner than the clinicians had predicted. In future groups, the timing and intensity with which trauma material will likely emerge will undoubtedly vary depending on the unique makeup and personalities of each group. We noted a phenomenon[38] in which patients feel their families and providers don't believe they have "true" epilepsy, paralleling how they earlier felt disbelieved or disregarded when they reported being abused. Our group experienced and weathered a major life event for one group member who confronted a family member about abuse that had happened 20 years before.

Although traditional group facilitation uses only one or two clinician group leaders, we experimented with having three clinician facilitators to allow more providers to learn the model. One clinician was designated to accompany any patients who might need to step out temporarily, while the other two continued to run the group. At the beginning of sessions we invited patients to step out of the room if they were feeling particularly overwhelmed. Several did this at different times and reported they found it helpful. Patients also used mindfulness and relaxation exercises learned during the course of group to help with overstimulation. Notably, even though we discussed highly charged topics, no patients experienced NES during the 12 sessions. Towards the end of the 12 scheduled sessions, we encouraged participants to plan for ongoing support after termination of the group intervention. They elected to start a private Facebook page for patients with NES, to be maintained by the patients themselves, affirming that social media can be a powerful tool to help patients stay connected and supported. Of note, only a few members required referral to our psychiatric clinic for continued care after the group completed the 12 weeks. Post-group discharge plans, including reviews of current and potential resources, were developed with each member for potential future use.

Although our data are preliminary, we were encouraged that four of the eight group patients were subjectively improved at the end of the 12-week treatment. Those who improved changed their coping styles, generally to include more active strategies. All patients voiced how helpful it was to realize that others suffered from the same condition, and that at last they had found people who really understood what they were experiencing.

Financial Viability

Adequate reimbursement for behavioral services that are embedded in other medical clinics is a challenge. Many hospital programs, such as neurosurgical or oncology clinics, choose to pay a salary to psychologists or part-time psychiatrists in order to meet patient care needs. For our project, we chose to ask for, and received, direct psychiatric funding for a psychiatrist position in the neurology clinic. In order to justify this funding, we laid out the costs to the neurology department in maintaining the status quo. These costs included metrics such as the substantial length of time to the next available neurology appointment, and the number of psychiatric patients in the neurology clinic. We are actively working with our billing department and insurance companies to maximize billing and show our financial viability. Future directions will include developing bundled payments, at-risk contracts, or pay-for-performance arrangements with insurance

BOX 19.4

SUMMARY OF RECOMMENDED TREATMENT APPROACHES AND RELEVANT EVIDENCE

Strength of recommendation taxonomy (SOR A, B, or C)

- **Sensitive delivery of the diagnosis of non-epileptic seizure (NES) may improve outcomes. (SOR B)[33]**
- **Treatment of NES includes psychiatric interventions. (SOR B)[6]**
- **Patients may be more likely to participate when psychiatric interventions take place within the neurology service. (SOR B)[48]**
- **Treatment of family dysfunction may improve outcomes. (SOR B)[43]**
- **Group psychotherapy for patients with NES provides many therapeutic advantages over individual treatment and may improve outcomes. (SOR B)[39–42]**
- **Patients may do better after the diagnosis of NES when they continue to see their neurologist. (SOR B)[36]**

companies to include behavioral health care that will take the patients from the epilepsy monitoring unit back to their medical homes in the community.

It is important to present a viable business case to stakeholders and financial staff. This is difficult to do in the current fee-for-service environment, especially when a hospital, such as ours, does not take medical cost offsets into account when deciding on the financial viability of our programs. Changes in health care billing and compensation (to support population health and team-based care) toward value-based billing, at-risk contracts, shared bundled billing, and pay-for-performance arrangements will likely allow more creative models for financing in the future.

Long-Term Sustainability of the NES Project

The sustainability of the NES program depends on many factors, which include (1) the continued training of behavioral health specialists to provide this specialized group therapy, (2) the development of protocols for transition-of-care appointments and periodic checkups in the patient's medical home, and (3) indications that our intervention results in better patient outcomes using ongoing quality metrics and requiring a health care system that monitors and measures quality outcomes. With the move toward population health, our work with NES and other medical specialties will allow us to show that behavioral health is a viable and necessary component of good-quality health care.

CONCLUSION

NES is a condition that spans two medical specialties and is best treated with an integrated program and a team of clinicians. In describing our treatment program and its development, we hope to provide a model by which other services and institutions might develop programs not only for NES but for other conditions that can benefit from a behavioral health treatment program embedded within a medical specialty practice. See Box 19.4 for a summary of treatment recommendations and associated evidence.

REFERENCES

1. Benbadis SR, Allen Hauser W. An estimate of the prevalence of psychogenic non-epileptic seizures. Seizure. 2000;9(4):280–281.
2. Bodde NM, Brooks JL, Baker GA, et al. Psychogenic non-epileptic seizures—definition, etiology, treatment and prognostic issues: a critical review. Seizure. 2009;18(8):543–553.
3. Martin R, Burneo JG, Prasad A, et al. Frequency of epilepsy in patients with psychogenic seizures monitored by video-EEG. Neurology. 2003;61(12):1791–1792.
4. Binder LM, Salinsky MC. Psychogenic nonepileptic seizures. Neuropsychol Rev. 2007;17(4):405–412.
5. Reuber M, Pukrop R, Bauer J, Helmstaedter C, Tessendorf N, Elger CE. Outcome in psychogenic nonepileptic seizures: 1 to 10-year follow-up in 164 patients. Ann Neurol. 2003;53(3):305–311.
6. LaFrance WC, Jr., Reuber M, Goldstein LH. Management of psychogenic nonepileptic seizures. Epilepsia. 2013;54(Suppl 1):53–67.

7. Hoerth MT, Wellik KE, Demaerschalk BM, et al. Clinical predictors of psychogenic nonepileptic seizures: a critically appraised topic. Neurologist. 2008;14(4):266–270.
8. LaFrance WC Jr., Baker GA, Duncan R, Goldstein LH, Reuber M. Minimum requirements for the diagnosis of psychogenic nonepileptic seizures: A staged approach: A report from the International League Against Epilepsy Nonepileptic Seizures Task Force. Epilepsia. 2013; 54(11):2005–2018.
9. Moore PM, Baker GA. Non-epileptic attack disorder: A psychological perspective. Seizure. 1997;6(6):429–434.
10. Schachter SC, LaFrance WC, Gates JR. Gates and Rowan's Nonepileptic Seizures, 3rd ed. Cambridge, UK, and New York: Cambridge University Press; 2010.
11. Lempert T, Schmidt D. Natural history and outcome of psychogenic seizures: A clinical study in 50 patients. J Neurol. 1990;237(1):35–38.
12. Meierkord H, Will B, Fish D, Shorvon S. The clinical features and prognosis of pseudoseizures diagnosed using video-EEG telemetry. Neurology. 1991;41(10):1643–1646.
13. Bowman ES, Markand ON. Psychodynamics and psychiatric diagnoses of pseudoseizure subjects. Am J Psychiatry.1996;153(1):57–63.
14. Lacey C, Cook M, Salzberg M. The neurologist, psychogenic nonepileptic seizures, and borderline personality disorder. Epilepsy Behav. 2007;11(4):492–498.
15. Arnold LM, Privitera MD. Psychopathology and trauma in epileptic and psychogenic seizure patients. Psychosomatics. 1996;37(5):438–443.
16. American Psychiatric Association. Diagnostic and Statistical Manual of Mental Disorders, 5th ed. Washington, DC: American Psychiatric Association; 2013.
17. Harden CL. Pseudoseizures and dissociative disorders: A common mechanism involving traumatic experiences. Seizure. 1997;6(2):151–155.
18. Bowman ES, Markand ON. The contribution of life events to pseudoseizure occurrence in adults. Bull Menninger Clin. 1999;63(1):70–88.
19. Escobar JI, Burnam MA, Karno M, Forsythe A, Golding JM. Somatization in the community. Arch Gen Psychiatry. 1987;44(8):713–718.
20. Bodde NM, van der Kruijs SJ, Ijff DM, et al. Subgroup classification in patients with psychogenic non-epileptic seizures. Epilepsy Behav. 2013;26(3):279–289.
21. World Health Organization. The ICD-10 Classification of Mental and Behavioural Disorders: Clinical Descriptions and Diagnostic Guidelines. Geneva: World Health Organization; 1992.
22. Duncan R, Razvi S, Mulhern S. Newly presenting psychogenic nonepileptic seizures: Incidence, population characteristics, and early outcome from a prospective audit of a first seizure clinic. Epilepsy Behav. 2011;20(2):308–311.
23. Asadi-Pooya AA, Sperling MR. Epidemiology of psychogenic nonepileptic seizures. Epilepsy Behav. 2015;46:60–65. http://dx.doi.org/10.1016/j.yebeh.2015.03.015
24. Reuber M, Fernandez G, Bauer J, Helmstaedter C, Elger CE. Diagnostic delay in psychogenic nonepileptic seizures. Neurology. 2002;58(3): 493–495.
25. McKenzie P, Oto M, Russell A, Pelosi A, Duncan R. Early outcomes and predictors in 260 patients with psychogenic nonepileptic attacks. Neurology. 2010;74(1):64–69.
26. Mayor R, Howlett S, Grunewald R, Reuber M. Long-term outcome of brief augmented psychodynamic interpersonal therapy for psychogenic nonepileptic seizures: Seizure control and health care utilization. Epilepsia. 2010;51(7):1169–1176.
27. Akyuz G, Kugu N, Akyuz A, Dogan O. Dissociation and childhood abuse history in epileptic and pseudoseizure patients. Epileptic Disord. 2004;6(3):187–192.
28. Griffith JL, Polles A, Griffith ME. Pseudoseizures, families, and unspeakable dilemmas. Psychosomatics. 1998;39(2):144–153.
29. Fleisher W, Staley D, Krawetz P, Pillay N, Arnett JL, Maher J. Comparative study of trauma-related phenomena in subjects with pseudoseizures and subjects with epilepsy. Am J Psychiatry. 2002;159(4):660–663.
30. Brown RJ, Schrag A, Trimble MR. Dissociation, childhood interpersonal trauma, and family functioning in patients with somatization disorder. Am J Psychiatry. 2005;162(5):899–905.
31. Roelofs K, Keijsers GP, Hoogduin KA, Naring GW, Moene FC. Childhood abuse in patients with conversion disorder. Am J Psychiatry. 2002;159(11):1908–1913.
32. Holman N, Kirkby A, Duncan S, Brown RJ. Adult attachment style and childhood interpersonal trauma in non-epileptic attack disorder. Epilepsy Res. 2008;79(1):84–89.
33. LaFrance WC Jr., Alper K, Babcock D, et al. Nonepileptic seizures treatment workshop summary. Epilepsy Behav. 2006;8(3):451–461.
34. Farias ST, Thieman C, Alsaadi TM. Psychogenic nonepileptic seizures: acute change in event frequency after presentation of the diagnosis. Epilepsy Behav. 2003;4(4):424–429.
35. Wilder C MA, Farias ST, Gorelik M, Jorgensen J, Connor M. Long-term follow-up study of patients with PNES. Epilepsia. 2004;45(Suppl 7):349.
36. Oto M, Espie C, Pelosi A, Selkirk M, Duncan R. The safety of antiepileptic drug withdrawal in patients with non-epileptic seizures. J Neurol Neurosurg Psychiatry. 2005;76(12):1682–1685.
37. LaFrance WC, Jr., Rusch MD, Machan JT. What is "treatment as usual" for nonepileptic seizures? Epilepsy Behav. 2008;12(3):388–394.

38. Aboukasm A, Mahr G, Gahry BR, Thomas A, Barkley GL. Retrospective analysis of the effects of psychotherapeutic interventions on outcomes of psychogenic nonepileptic seizures. Epilepsia. 1998;39(5):470–473.
39. Martlew J, Pulman J, Marson AG. Psychological and behavioural treatments for adults with non-epileptic attack disorder. Cochrane Database Syst Rev. 2014;2:CD006370.
40. Prigatano GP, Stonnington CM, Fisher RS. Psychological factors in the genesis and management of nonepileptic seizures: Clinical observations. Epilepsy Behav. 2002;3(4):343–349.
41. Zaroff CM, Myers L, Barr WB, Luciano D, Devinsky O. Group psychoeducation as treatment for psychological nonepileptic seizures. Epilepsy Behav. 2004;5(4):587–592.
42. Barry JJ, Wittenberg D, Bullock KD, Michaels JB, Classen CC, Fisher RS. Group therapy for patients with psychogenic nonepileptic seizures: A pilot study. Epilepsy Behav. 2008;13(4):624–629.
43. Conwill M, Oakley L, Evans K, Cavanna AE. CBT-based group therapy intervention for non-epileptic attacks and other functional neurological symptoms: A pilot study. Epilepsy Behav. 2014;34:68–72.
44. McRoberts C, Burlingame G, Hoag M. Comparative efficacy of individual and group psychotherapy: A meta-analytic perspective. Group Dyn. 1998;2(2):101–117.
45. LaFrance WC, Jr., Alosco ML, Davis JD, et al. Impact of family functioning on quality of life in patients with psychogenic nonepileptic seizures versus epilepsy. Epilepsia. 2011;52(2): 292–300.
46. Epstein NB, Baldwin LM, Bishop DS. The McMaster Family Assessment Device. J Marital Fam Ther. 1983;9(2):171–180.
47. Sprenckle DH, Lebow J, Davis SD. Common Factors in Couple and Family Therapy: The Overlooked Foundation for Effective Practice. New York: Guilford Press; 2009.
48. Goldstein LH, Chalder T, Chigwedere C, et al. Cognitive-behavioral therapy for psychogenic nonepileptic seizures: A pilot RCT. Neurology. 2010;74(24):1986–1994.
49. LaFrance WC, Jr., Baird GL, Barry JJ, et al. Multicenter pilot treatment trial for psychogenic nonepileptic seizures: A randomized clinical trial. JAMA. 2014;71(9):997–1005.
50. Chen DK, Maheshwari A, Franks R, Trolley GC, Robinson JS, Hrachovy RA. Brief group psychoeducation for psychogenic nonepileptic seizures: A neurologist-initiated program in an epilepsy center. Epilepsia. 2014;55(1):156–166.
51. Fiszman A, Alves-Leon SV, Nunes RG, D'Andrea I, Figueira I. Traumatic events and posttraumatic stress disorder in patients with psychogenic non-epileptic seizures: A critical review. Epilepsy Behav. 2004;5(6):818–825.
52. Yalom ID, Leszcz M. The Theory and Practice of Group Psychotherapy, 5th ed. New York: Basic Books; 2005.
53. Klein RH. Some principles of short-term group therapy. Int J Group Psychother. 1985;35(3):309–330.
54. Poey K. Guidelines for the practice of brief, dynamic group therapy. Int J Group Psychother. 1985;35(3):331–354.
55. Üstün TB. Measuring Health and Disability: Manual for WHO Disability Assessment Schedule WHODAS 2.0. Geneva: World Health Organization; 2010.
56. Carver CS. You want to measure coping but your protocol's too long: Consider the brief COPE. Int J Behav Med. 1997;4(1):92–100.
57. Devinsky O, Vickrey BG, Cramer J, et al. Development of the Quality of Life in Epilepsy Inventory. Epilepsia. 1995;36(11):1089–1104.
58. Cramer JA, Perrine K, Devinsky O, Bryant-Comstock L, Meador K, Hermann B. Development and cross-cultural translations of a 31-item Quality of Life in Epilepsy Inventory. Epilepsia. 1998;39(1):81–88.
59. Lipman RS, Covi L, Shapiro AK. The Hopkins Symptom Checklist (HSCL)—factors derived from the HSCL-90. J Affect Disord. 1979;1(1):9–24.
60. Ruis C, van den Berg E, van Stralen HE, et al. Symptom Checklist 90-Revised in neurological outpatients. J Clin Exp Neuropsychol. 2014;36(2): 170–177.
61. Alper K, Devinsky O, Perrine K, et al. Dissociation in epilepsy and conversion nonepileptic seizures. Epilepsia. 1997;38(9):991–997.
62. Mansfield AK, Keitner, GI, Dealy J. The family assessment device: An update. Fam Process. 2015;54(1):82–93.

20

Women's Mental Health Across the Reproductive Lifespan

NOA HEIMAN, ABBY SNAVELY, AND LIZA FREEHLING

BOX 20.1

KEY POINTS

- **There are epidemiological differences between men and women when it comes to mental health due to reproductive, hormonal, and societal differences, to name a few. The integrative care team should always keep in mind the hormonal life cycle phase of the women they treat.**
- **Common mental health struggles in premenstrual disorder include affective instability, irritability or anger, depressed mood, anxiety, and/or a sense of being overwhelmed or out of control.**
- **Premenstrual dysphoric disorder is often a significant risk factor for postpartum depression or perimenopausal depression and should be monitored and recorded in the patient registry and addressed as thoroughly as possible.**
- **Pregnancy, the postpartum period, miscarriages, abortions, stillbirth, and infertility treatments are times of extreme hormonal, emotional, relational/interpersonal, and financial transition. The integrative care team should be vigilant about assessing a woman's well-being, personal history, and family history during these times.**
- **Common mental health struggles during pregnancy and postpartum are depression, anxiety, and bipolar disorder. Postpartum psychosis is rare, but very dangerous when it occurs.**
- **The relapse rate for bipolar disorder is higher in the postpartum period than for any other form of mental illness. It should be closely monitored and may be preventable by the integrative care team.**
- **Common mental health struggles during perimenopause and menopause may be depression, a sense of a "midlife crisis," and empty-nest syndrome.**
- **Perimenopausal depression may present in a qualitatively different way than depression at other phases.**

INTRODUCTION

This chapter intends to make providers, medical and behavioral alike, more cognizant of the unique properties of women's mental health across the reproductive lifespan. For example, from puberty through menopause, depression is the most frequently encountered women's mental health problem. Women all over the world have double the rate of depression than men and increased rates of almost all anxiety disorders as compared with men.[1] On the other hand, men tend to experience more alcohol dependence and antisocial personality.[2]

Women experience monthly hormonal fluctuations, significant hormonal shifts with pregnancy and the postpartum phase, and enormous fluctuations during perimenopause. Women may suffer miscarriages, undergo fertility treatments, and take exogenous hormones, which also influence the hormonal system and psychological equilibrium. Mental health problems peak for women around these transitional times. For example, a history of depression at any time is a risk factor for depression during times of reproductive hormonal fluctuation. Psychiatric hospital admissions are highest for women during pregnancy and the postpartum phase. Although much is still unknown about the complicated interplay between mental health and hormonal fluctuations, the treating team must always be aware of the hormonal life phase of female patients. Box 20.1 presents an overview of the key elements of women's mental health issues across the reproductive lifespan.

In addition, socially constructed differences between women and men in gender roles, expectations, and psychosocial stressors contribute to the unique properties of women's mental health. In our culture, women often report feeling that they are expected to perfectly juggle having a career, raising children, and maintaining a household. When a woman becomes a mother, she is expected to immediately bond, love, and be joyous with her baby. For some women, feeling that they do not meet societal expectations may make them more vulnerable to experiencing depression, anxiety, or exacerbation of an existing mental disorder.

Aside from general screening tools such as the Patient Health Questionnaire depression rating scale (PHQ-9)[3] or the Generalized Anxiety Disorder scale (GAD-7),[4] more specific screening tools based on the woman's reproductive life cycle phase may be given and will be reviewed later in this chapter. For women of reproductive age, the interplay between hormones and mental health should be addressed by compiling a multifaceted profile of medical testing along with behavioral health measures. For example, thyroid disorders may mimic mood and anxiety disorders and should be ruled out to ensure proper treatment. A discussion of women's sexual health issues may be found in Chapter 21: Assessing and Treating Sexual Problems in an Integrated Care Environment.

OVERVIEW OF WOMEN'S REPRODUCTIVE LIFE CYCLE

The menstrual cycle comprises four distinct phases: follicular, ovulatory, luteal, and menstrual. The phases of the menstrual cycle coincide with marked changes in hormone levels. Progesterone levels stay relatively stable for the first half of the cycle (follicular), then rise steadily (ovulatory), followed by a steep drop (luteal) just prior to menstruation. Comparatively, estrogen levels briefly peak in the middle of the cycle (ovulatory), drop a bit, and then rise steadily before dropping dramatically (luteal) along with progesterone just before menses. Many women will report feeling fatigued, irritable, sad, or bloated during the premenstrual phase. For some women these symptoms may be so severe or disruptive that they start dreading "that time of month." Approximately 3% to 8% of women have symptoms that are severe enough to disrupt their functioning at work, socially, or at home.[5]

A woman's attitude toward trying to conceive, being pregnant, or choosing not to have children, is never void of emotions. For women who become pregnant, the context of a pregnancy—whether it was a wanted or an unwanted pregnancy, whether it is her first or 10th child, whether there is a supportive partner and social network or not, whether she is psychologically and financially stable or not—can greatly influence a woman's feelings toward her pregnancy and newborn. Pregnancy is a time of extreme hormonal transition, psychological transition (the woman gives birth to a child, while being born herself as a mother), financial transition, and transition in societal expectations. It is not surprising that pregnancy and the postpartum stage increase the risk for the onset or exacerbation of a mental health condition. Psychiatric hospital admissions are highest for women during pregnancy and the postpartum period. However, it is important not to pathologize this phase either: For many women, even with all the challenges that come along with pregnancy (having a newborn, adjusting to motherhood and a new family structure), the childbearing period is a time of personal growth.

During the postpartum period, there are several factors that affect a woman's well-being, such as sleep loss, major role changes, and the enormous responsibility of raising a baby. Additionally, there are hormonal factors involved that make some women emotionally vulnerable to these extreme changes. After the steady rise of hormones throughout pregnancy, the immediate postpartum period involves a sharp and sudden decline in both estrogen and progesterone levels. After the delivery of the placenta, estrogen and progesterone levels fall so dramatically that by the fifth postpartum day, they are equal to prepregnancy levels.[6]

Perimenopause refers to a time period of approximately 15 years (ages 35–50) when a woman's body is transitioning toward menopause.[7] During this phase, ovarian follicle production decreases. The follicles that do develop are not as responsive to follicle-stimulating hormone (FSH), and decreased levels of estradiol, progesterone, and androgens are produced by the ovaries. The lower level of circulating estrogen and progesterone results in decreased production of gonadotropic-releasing hormone by the hypothalamus and continued production of FSH and luteinizing hormone.[7] These hormonal changes can lead to lengthening or shortening menstrual cycles, changes in the amount of menstrual blood flow, intermittent amenorrhea, and worsening or new onset of premenstrual symptoms. Over time, estrogen and progesterone levels will remain low, FSH and luteinizing hormone levels will remain high, the ovaries will stop producing follicles, and menstruation will cease.[7]

Menopause is defined by the absence of menses (amenorrhea) for 12 consecutive months and marks the end of reproductive ability. The average age of menopause in the Western world is 51 years.[7] Symptoms such as hot flashes, insomnia, and vaginal dryness are common during this time.

MAJOR ISSUES OF WOMEN'S MENTAL HEALTH

Depression Spectrum Disorders in Women

Premenstrual Dysphoric Disorder

In the *Diagnostic and Statistical Manual of Mental Disorders*, Fifth Edition (DSM-5),[8] premenstrual syndrome (PMS) has been renamed premenstrual dysphoric disorder (PMDD). According to DSM-5, PMDD is characterized by at least five symptoms in the final week before the onset of menses, an improvement within a few days after the onset of menses, and minimal or absent symptoms in the week after menses. The five symptoms of PMDD include marked affective instability, irritability, anger, depressed mood, or anxiety. One additional symptom must be present from a list that includes decreased interest, problems with concentration, lethargy, appetite disturbances, sleep disturbances, a sense of being overwhelmed or out of control; or one physical symptom, including breast tenderness, joint or muscle pain, bloating, or weight gain. Many women with PMDD may have an underlying mood disorder.

It is unclear what exactly contributes to PMDD, but medically speaking, it has traditionally been suspected that the symptoms of PMS and PMDD are related to the steep decline in hormone levels seen in the luteal phase of the menstrual cycle. Some women may be more biologically sensitive to these hormonal changes;[9] most likely a complex interaction between hormones and neurotransmitters in the central nervous system contributes to premenstrual mood disorders.[9]

While PMDD is found in women worldwide, there has been debate over the years whether PMDD is a culture-bound syndrome or a distinct disorder with a genetic or biological component. The feminist movement and others have argued that PMS is strictly a social construct of Western society. In a 1987 paper, Thomas Johnson[10] claimed that PMS is an expression of "conflicting societal expectations" on women. Support for this argument may come from studies showing more pronounced rates of PMS in Western cultures.[11] However, the question of whether or not it is a social construct per se, or the result of confounding factors, is still unresolved. Some studies suggest that other environmental factors, such as trauma, contribute to PMDD. Several studies have found a higher rate of PMDD in women with a trauma history or a stressful event within the past year. Others have shown a psychological component to PMDD, suggesting that perceived stress tends to exacerbate PMDD.[5] The interplay between genetic/biological, societal, or psychological variables is still quite unclear.

Peripartum Depressive Symptoms and Depression

Women who are pregnant or undergoing fertility treatments have increased levels of hormones and associated symptoms that may be difficult to distinguish from depression (e.g., weight gain, sleep changes, fatigue). It is important to remember that half of postpartum depressions (PPDs) begin during pregnancy. Diagnosis of depression in the perinatal period uses the same criteria as major depressive disorder, though it can be difficult to distinguish, as discussed above.

Negative effects of untreated peripartum depression on a child include insecure attachment, behavioral problems, cognitive dysfunction, increased risk of abuse and neglect, childhood psychiatric problems, sleep problems, or infanticide.[12] Negative effects on a mother include preterm delivery, impaired self-care, increased substance abuse, increased postnatal complications, increased risk of cesarean section, increased health care costs, refractory depression, or suicide.

Half of pregnant women with a history of depression relapse in the first trimester and 90% by second trimester. Sixty-eight percent of pregnant women who stop taking their medications have a depression relapse. Twenty-six percent relapse even while taking medications.[13] This may be due to the increased metabolism of the antidepressant medication during pregnancy, which may warrant an increase in dose.[14]

Postpartum Depression

The postpartum phase is a high-risk time for the onset or recurrence of severe mood disorders. Depression is the most common medical complication of childbirth, with a prevalence of 13%. There is a greater increase in psychiatric admissions postpartum than at any other time in a woman's life. Previous episodes of depression or bipolar disorder are a major risk factor for the development of PPD. Women should also be screened for a history of PMDD or PMS symptoms, as this increases the risk for PPD.[15] Other risk factors for PPD include depression or anxiety during pregnancy, poor social support, intimate partner violence,[15] family history of mental illness, single motherhood, having more than three children, cigarette smoking, low income, and age younger than 20 years.[16]

PPD is diagnosed according to the major depressive disorder criteria in the DSM-5. However, symptoms specific to PPD may include lack of interest or enjoyment in the baby, difficulty sleeping when the baby is sleeping, excessive guilt related to mothering, impaired concentration/decision making, agitation/restlessness, and, with suicidal thinking, a belief that the baby would be better off with another mother. Of women experiencing PPD, 41% to 57% also have ego-dystonic obsessive thoughts (thoughts that conflict with or are contrary to the person's ideal self-image), though women are unlikely to reveal these unless specifically asked.[17]

Women presenting with their first depressive episode in the postpartum period present a diagnostic challenge. Though most can be diagnosed with unipolar depression, at least 14% of these women go on to be diagnosed with bipolar I disorder.[18] Some women previously diagnosed with major depressive disorder convert to bipolar II disorder in the postpartum period.[19] Other factors that may signal a latent bipolar disorder include early age of onset, psychosis, atypical features, and an abrupt onset.[20] Thus, care should be taken when diagnosing and prescribing for women with PPD symptoms, as patients who have an undiagnosed bipolar depression can become manic if antidepressants are prescribed. Chapter 12: Treating Depression and Bipolar Disorder in Integrated Care Settings provides additional information.

Perimenopausal Depression

Studies suggest that a past history of PMDD or PPD, related to hormonal fluctuations, is a significant risk factor for perimenopausal depression.[21] However, depression during perimenopause may present as qualitatively different than depression at other phases. Women with perimenopausal depression may present as more irritable, labile, tense, and nervous[21] than sad and anhedonic. Women going through perimenopause may also struggle psychologically with a loss of their reproductive ability (even if they don't plan on becoming pregnant) or loss of youth, or may experience a "midlife crisis."

Anxiety Spectrum Disorders in Women

Peripartum Anxiety

Anxiety may be more prominent than depression during the peripartum period. Though more common during this period, anxiety disorders have similar presentations compared to other times in a woman's life and often meet DSM-5 criteria for unspecified anxiety disorder.

Postpartum Anxiety Disorders

The three most commonly occurring anxiety disorders in the postpartum period are generalized anxiety disorder, panic disorder, and obsessive-compulsive disorder (OCD). Generalized anxiety disorder and panic disorders in the postpartum phase present as they do in all phases in the reproductive life cycle. For OCD, some common intrusive thoughts or obsessions include letting go of the baby, dropping the baby down the stairs or out of a window, or stabbing the baby. Women may deal with these thoughts by avoiding the baby.[22] A nonjudgmental inquiry by a sensitive nurse or primary care provider (PCP), explaining that violent/aggressive thoughts are common, can facilitate open sharing of a mother's anxieties. Postpartum OCD symptoms need to be distinguished from psychosis. OCD symptoms are ego-dystonic, and judgment and reality testing are typically intact. Obsessive thoughts often involve fears of contamination, fears about hurting the baby, or feeling terrified that she will do so. In these cases, with good support from the behavioral health specialist (BHS) and their family, these patients often can be treated as outpatients since the baby is unlikely to be harmed. See Chapter 11: Integrated Care for Anxiety Disorders for additional information about the subtypes of anxiety disorders.

Bipolar Disorder

Hormonal fluctuations, including those around childbirth, place women with existing bipolar disorder at risk for affective dysregulation. Of all women with bipolar disorder, 60% to 70% experience a mood episode during pregnancy or the postpartum phase;[23] primarily they experience depression, though manic episodes may also emerge.

The majority of bipolar relapses occur within four weeks after delivery. Mania or hypomania may begin in the first 72 hours after delivery, while depressive symptoms may occur later. The number of previous hospitalizations, the duration of the most recent illness, and the time proximity of hospitalization to the pregnancy all increase the risk of experiencing a bipolar episode after birth. Family history is just as important as taking a personal history, as it has been shown that there is a much higher prevalence of bipolar or postpartum depression if a first-degree relative has experienced these disorders.[24] It is imperative to identify women at risk for initial onset or relapse before they give birth, as detailed in Table 20.1, and to observe them

TABLE 20.1 POSTPARTUM DETECTION OF BIPOLAR DISORDER AND ACTIONS[a]

Warning Signs for Initial Onset	Risk Factors for Relapse
• Bipolar history in immediate family member	• Bipolar history in immediate family member
• Sleep loss can trigger mania.	• Sleep loss can trigger mania.
• Euphoria that is more intense than expected, increased goal-directed activity, increased speech, racing thoughts, decreased need for sleep, and irritability, especially in first 72 hours	• History of bipolar disorder • Younger age at delivery • Unplanned pregnancy • Unwell at referral
• Depressive symptoms	• Number of previous hospitalizations • Duration of the most recent illness • Time proximity of hospitalization to the pregnancy • Severity of mental illness prior to pregnancy

Actions

- Consult with a psychiatrist immediately.
- If this is an initial depressive episode and the woman is taking an antidepressant, discontinue this immediately.
- Choose medication specific to treatment of bipolar depression, as antidepressants do not work for bipolar depression.
- Consider lithium, antipsychotics. Consider mood stabilizers for management of manic symptoms. Avoid valproate.
- Institute frequent monitoring if the woman has a history of depression or bipolar, or "new" depression.
- If the woman is not getting better quickly, consider hospitalization. If left untreated, women may harm themselves, and in rare cases harm their children.
- Call child protection services when appropriate.
- Include family in treatment planning and safety measures.
- Manage sleep regimen.
- Provide frequent psychotherapy in addition to medication management.

[a]Relapse rate is higher during the postpartum phase for patients with a diagnosis of bipolar disorder than for any other form of mental illness.

for symptoms after delivery so that actions can be taken to decrease risk and provide appropriate support and treatment.[22]

Postpartum Psychosis

Postpartum psychosis can present with psychotic symptoms such as suspiciousness, paranoia, thought disorder, hallucinations, delusions, and suicidality or as a delirium with common symptoms such as extreme confusion, hopelessness, insomnia, exhaustion, agitation, refusal to eat, or overeating. Delusions are present about half the time and tend to be about harm to the infant or feeling controlled by an outside force. In contrast to OCD symptoms, delusions may be ego-syntonic, reality testing is impaired, and there may be a compulsion to act. The worst cases can result in infanticide or homicide. Postpartum psychosis is exceedingly rare but potentially dangerous. In contrast to other disorders, it develops rapidly, usually 48 hours to two weeks after delivery. It can be difficult to diagnose and is considered a psychiatric emergency. Risk factors for postpartum psychosis include bipolar disorder, history of PPD, and family history of bipolar disorder.

INTEGRATED CARE TEAM: FUNCTIONS AND ROLES

When a woman presents to an integrated practice, she should initially be interviewed and screened by a nurse or medical assistant. Depending on her reproductive life stage, she may be screened for PMDD, peripartum or postpartum depression, anxiety, bipolar illness, psychosis, and perimenopausal depression (a list of screening tests may be found below in the "Nurses and Medical Assistants" section). The interview should include a personal history and a family history component since women with a first-degree relative with bipolar illness are more prone to develop postpartum bipolar disease. The PCP should review the results of the mental health screening tests and questionnaires. If the registry alerts the team to a history of PMDD, the medical assistants or nurses should screen extensively for depression and bipolar disorder during the postpartum and perimenopausal phases of the woman's reproductive life cycle. A positive history of PPD, major depressive disorder, and/or bipolar depression should also be added to the patient registry. A prior history of any depression has been shown to be a risk factor for developing PPD and other depressive variants in the future. Should the PCP suggest referral to a BHS, health coach, and/or psychiatrist, we recommend collaborative team meetings to address all facets of the woman's care. This means including obstetricians/gynecologists (OB/GYNs), case managers, health coaches, and other members of the health care team. As pregnancy and the postpartum phase are times of extreme hormonal, emotional, and social transition, which may need a team management, we recommend holding collaborative meetings at least once per trimester and monthly in the postpartum period should the woman present with mental health struggles during these times.

ROLES OF SPECIFIC TEAM MEMBERS

Nurses and Medical Assistants

For any pregnant woman presenting to the practice, the nurses/medical assistants can obtain part of the patient's personal and family history and can administer questionnaires for each phase of the reproductive life cycle. Nurses and/or medical assistants may need to be trained to administer screening tests specifically for women, which include the Calendar of Premenstrual Experiences diary (COPE)[25] and the Edinburgh Postnatal Depression Scale (EPDS).[26] COPE asks women to rate the severity of the most commonly reported physical and behavioral symptoms over the menstrual cycle. These symptoms include anxiety, depression, fatigue, and pain, and are rated daily and scored. A score of less than 40 in days three through nine of the menstrual cycle and greater than 42 in the last seven days is diagnostic for PMDD. EPDS screens for depression, focusing more on anxious and anhedonic symptoms without the inclusion of somatic symptoms that may be present as a part of a normal pregnancy and postpartum period.[26] For example, questions about weight change or change in sleep patterns are not included. Alternative prompts that are part of the EPDS include "I have been able to laugh and see the funny side of things," "I have been anxious or worried for no good reason," and "things have been getting on top of me." It is also recommended to administer the PHQ-9, GAD-7, and the Mood Disorder Questionnaire (MDQ)[27] (which screens for bipolar disorder) and to screen for smoking, alcohol, and other substances of abuse.

Nurses or medical assistants should also routinely ask about PMS symptoms at regular medical checkups. This applies especially to screening adolescents and young adults who may not have been educated about their menstrual cycles or who have not had enough experience to know what to expect about possible PMS symptoms and/or PMDD. Some women may feel shame discussing their symptoms with their support persons or physicians. It is therefore important that team members educate women and normalize PMS symptoms. If PMDD is suspected, the patient can be added to the registry and followed by using the COPE.[25] Patients can record their daily symptoms for one to three months with monthly results added to the registry. Three months are required for accurate diagnosis, but patients may not want to wait this long. Often, mild to moderate PMDD can be managed without medications. Some women may experience relief of symptoms from following recommendations by nurses, health coaches, or specifically trained medical assistants for lifestyle changes such as eating a healthy diet, weight management, exercise, sleep, harm reduction (e.g., reducing or stopping cigarettes, alcohol, or other substance use), and stress management. See Chapter 22: Wellness An Integrated Care Approach to review an approach to lifestyle modifications.

Because of societal expectations that a new mother is joyful and at peace, both patients and team members may be reluctant to discuss the patient's mental health symptoms even when they are not pathologic. The new mother's feelings are of paramount importance; nurses/medical assistants should first ask how she is feeling, and follow with general questions about mood and anxiety. For new mothers, an important aspect for prevention of postpartum mood episodes is sleep management. The nurse or specifically trained medical assistant can educate the mother and partner about basic sleep hygiene recommendations, including suggesting that the partner wake up with the baby as often as possible. Women can schedule their nights to sleep through (in a guest room) and some may hire a night nurse. In these discussions, a concern about breastfeeding is often raised. Nurses can be helpful by not framing this as an all-or-nothing proposition. A child can be nursed or fed expressed milk or formula by a husband or other caregiver. Emphasizing that the mother's well-being is the most important factor in the child's well-being, will be helpful. Sometimes permission from a nurse or other professional to get sufficient sleep, rely on others, not breastfeed, or not breastfeed 100% of the time, can be enormously supportive for a struggling new mother. When a nurse/medical assistant suspects the mother is having difficulty bonding with her child, the PCP and BHS should immediate consult and intervene, as needed.

For some women, perimenopause may be a confusing time. They might experience mood swings, sleep disturbances, hot flashes, irritability, and/or decreased libido that they may initially not associate with hormonal factors. In addition, perimenopause may present its own challenges such as experiencing a "midlife crisis," an empty-nest syndrome, and/or the care of elderly parents. Nurses/medical assistants should screen all women with perimenopausal symptoms for depression, paying particular attention to symptoms such as irritability, worsened premenstrual symptoms, and sleep disturbances. This is especially true for women who may have an individual risk for developing a perimenopausal mood disorder if they had a history of past depression, in particular during hormonal transitions, or a history of bipolar disorder.

Nurses or medical assistants may also discuss with women approaching their 40s what to expect from perimenopause. The care team should be prepared to help these women identify symptoms early on and discuss treatment plans that may reduce or prevent symptom escalation. Nurses may recommend and educate patients about mindfulness, relaxation skills, exercise, and diet, or discuss the possible need for medications. These suggestions may alleviate or prevent symptoms.

Primary Care Providers

Often the PCP in an integrated care practice may be the first or only provider a woman chooses to see. Therefore, when treating a female patient, the PCP should identify the chief complaint that led to the visit and inquire about obstetrical/gynecological issues, other physical symptoms, substance use, and behavioral, psychological, and familial needs.

Psychotropic Medications

When prescribing psychotropic medication for any woman, the PCP needs to understand, explore, and adjust the treatment based on the hormonal phase within her life cycle. Medications may affect a woman's sexual and reproductive functions, reproductive choices, and a potential fetus. When prescribing psychotropics for a woman in her childbearing years, the PCP must recognize and manage the risks of fetal exposure to psychiatric medications, weigh benefits versus risks, and not reflexively default to rapid discontinuation of medication. The patient should be counseled about what she should do if she becomes pregnant unexpectedly. It is also important to examine the interactions of psychotropic medication with oral contraceptives. Valproate should be vigorously avoided in all women of childbearing age due to the risk of birth defects[28] and polycystic ovarian syndrome.[29] Up to half of women who were positive for PMS or PMDD and for whom lifestyle education is not sufficient will respond to 1,200 mg of calcium daily.[30]

During pregnancy and the postpartum phase, the PCP must also consider the psychotropic effects on the newborn from in utero exposure, as well as medication effects on lactation. When prescribing for pregnant women, providers may be tempted to "protect" the fetus by withholding psychotropic medications, but a risk–benefit analysis requires that the PCP and the patient weigh the potential harm caused by medications against the potential harm caused by untreated or worsened maternal mental illness. A consensus paper by both the American College of Obstetrics and Gynecology and the American Psychiatric Association[31] recommends medications be used during pregnancy in the following situations: psychosis, suicidality, moderate to severe symptoms of the psychiatric disorder, less than 6 months of stability, poor response to psychotherapy, history of relapse, patient preference, and/or bipolar disorder.

Though it is popular to use U.S. Food and Drug Administration (FDA) warnings in advising women about medications in pregnancy, these are outdated and overly simplistic. They do not take the mother's illness into account and do not provide a distinction for the severity, type, or timing of harm.[32] Very few good studies have been performed on pregnant women. When available, it is far better to review the information available in Micromedex[33] or Reprotox[34] than to rely on the FDA.

The risks with each medication differ depending on the timing of exposure. Teratogenic risks are incurred in the first trimester, whereas neurocognitive effects and potential for withdrawal are associated with third-trimester exposure. The use of psychiatric medications in the peripartum period is reviewed in Table 20.2.

Antidepressant Use During Pregnancy

For patients who are already taking an antidepressant, reducing the dosage or not increasing it according to the clinical picture can exacerbate the maternal illness during pregnancy. Medication changes can also expose the fetus to potentially harmful drug effects. With antidepressants, the pregnant patient's response to medications is similar to the response of non-perinatal depression. Switching to a medication thought to be "safer" in pregnancy is not recommended. Absolute risks for teratogenicity in the first trimester are very small, including those for cardiac malformations.[35] Risks related to third-trimester exposure include preterm birth,[35] although depression may confer the same risk. The dosage of antidepressants may need to be increased after 20 weeks for agents metabolized by CYP2D6 or CYP3A4.

Selective serotonin reuptake inhibitors (SSRIs) are commonly used and considered to be safe. Tricyclic antidepressants and serotonin–norepinephrine reuptake inhibitors (SNRIs) are also considered relatively safe, although they are less well studied.

Patients experiencing pregnancy loss/miscarriage should be allowed to grieve and do not necessarily progress to a diagnosable mood or anxiety disorder. Thoughts of wanting to die to be with the child are common and do not necessarily represent active suicidal ideation. For these patients, the PCP should resist the urge to provide an antidepressant, as this sends a message that the patient's grieving is pathologic. Brief, symptomatic treatment (benzodiazepines or sleep aids) may be appropriate, and a referral for brief supportive grief/loss-focused treatment with the team's BHS is indicated.

Benzodiazepine Use During Pregnancy

Studies show that judicious and brief use of benzodiazepines are associated with little to no risk of teratogenicity and may be reasonable prescribed for intense anxiety, including panic disorder.[36] Referral to a behavioral therapist for relaxation training and short-term cognitive-behavioral therapy may also be considered.

Bipolar Medication Use During Pregnancy

In most cases of known bipolar disorder, women should be generally advised to continue their medication, with special consideration given to the use of anticonvulsants and avoidance of valproate because of the risk of birth defects and polycystic ovarian syndrome. Review Table 20.2 for medication options and doses for bipolar patients.

There is also an increased risk of postpartum psychosis in women with bipolar disorder. A PCP

TABLE 20.2 USE OF PSYCHIATRIC MEDICATIONS DURING PREGNANCY AND THE PERIPARTUM AND POSTPARTUM PERIODS

Medication Classes	Disorders	Teratogenicity	Maternal Considerations	Neonatal Considerations	Lactation	Medication Options	Notes
Antidepressants (SSRIs, SNRIs, tricyclics, bupropion)	Major depression, anxiety disorders	None confirmed, except avoid paroxetine due to the risk of cardiac malformation	May need to increase dose due to increased metabolism	Potential withdrawal syndrome	Compatible	Sertraline 50–200 mg Fluoxetine 20–60 mg Escitalopram 10–20 mg Citalopram 20–40 mg Paroxetine 20–60 mg Venlafaxine XL 75–225 mg Duloxetine 40–120 mg Nortriptyline 50–150 mg Bupropion XL 150–300 mg	Do not change pregnant woman from antidepressant that is working.
Benzodiazepines and sleep medications	Anxiety disorders, insomnia	Possible small increase in cleft lip or palate with first-trimester exposure	Watch for dependence; ultrasound for facial morphology	Withdrawal syndrome up to 3 months postpartum	Compatible; watch for sedation of baby	Lorazepam 1–4 mg/day divided Clonazepam 0.5–4 mg/day divided Diazepam, alprazolam not recommended Zolpidem 5–10 mg QHS	Advise against co-sleeping given increased risk to the child of injury or smothering.
Lithium	Bipolar disorders	Low absolute increased risk of cardiac defect	High-resolution ultrasound of heart at 16–18 weeks. Check blood level every 2 weeks; likely need to increase dose. Return to prepregnancy dose at delivery.	Risk of floppy baby	Thyroid-stimulating hormone, creatinine, complete blood count, lithium levels monitored	Lithium or lithium CR 300–1,200 mg/day, to level of 0.7–1.1	

(continued)

TABLE 20.2 CONTINUED

Medication Classes	Disorders	Teratogenicity	Maternal Considerations	Neonatal Considerations	Lactation	Medication Options	Notes
Antipsychotic medications	Bipolar disorders, schizophrenia, other psychotic disorders	None confirmed	Weight gain and metabolic syndrome. Check triglyceride levels each trimester.	Extrapyramidal symptoms and withdrawal	No known complications	Haloperidol 0.5–20 mg Quetiapine 25–800 mg Risperidone 0.5–4 mg Olanzapine 2.5–20 mg Lurasidone 20–120 mg	
Anticonvulsant medications	Bipolar disorders	Increased risk of neural tube defect, other structural abnormalities	Dose likely needs to be increased during pregnancy. Supplementation with 4 mg folate may help prevent defects.	None known	Check liver function tests in baby.	Lamotrigine 25–300 mg Carbamazepine 400–1,200 mg (recommended after first trimester) Do not use valproic acid because of risks of birth defects and polycystic ovarian syndrome.	Valproic acid with high rate of major malformations and later cognitive effects in baby

treating a patient with known bipolar disorder should do so in conjunction with a psychiatrist, as psychological and medication treatments can be complex. Most mood-stabilizing medications have some potential teratogenic effects, as described in Table 20.2. Women with bipolar disorder are unlikely to be stabilized with psychotherapy or behavioral measures alone. Postpartum mood episodes are likely to be depressive, though manic and mixed states may emerge, which are associated with high morbidity and may require psychiatric hospitalization. Patients presenting with mania or hypomania may be referred to the emergency department for further evaluation.

Even with treatment, patients with bipolar disorder are at a high risk for relapse. In one study, patients with bipolar disorder had an 85.5% recurrence of mood episode with discontinuation of their mood stabilizer versus 37% in those who maintained treatment.[37] Even if a woman desires to discontinue her medication, she should be advised to taper it slowly to reduce her time to relapse.[38] Chapter 12: Treating Depression and Bipolar Disorder in Integrated Care Settings offers additional information on the use of mood stabilizers.

Thyroid Disorders

The PCP should consider primary thyroid disorders or exacerbation of preexisting thyroid disorders in the differential diagnosis for all women presenting with PMS symptoms, PMDD, depression, bipolar disorder, or postpartum mood or anxiety symptoms.

In the presence of any menstrual change, the PCP should screen for hypothyroidism, which can present as mood disturbances or depression, by ordering a serum thyroid-stimulating hormone level. If elevated, repeating the test with the addition of a free thyroxine (free T4) level[39] can confirm the diagnosis. Providers may begin thyroid replacement treatment as necessary or refer the patient to an endocrinologist for management.

Postpartum thyroiditis is a syndrome of thyroid dysfunction typically occurring in the first year after delivery. Symptoms of postpartum thyroiditis may be transient or permanent and occur in 5% to 7% of postpartum women.[40] Most commonly, there is a thyrotoxic phase followed by a hypothyroid phase, though some cases are exclusively hyperthyroid or hypothyroid. During the thyrotoxic phase, symptoms may include fatigue, irritability, nervousness, insomnia, weight loss, and other somatic disturbances. Hypothyroid states are well known to mimic depression. Symptoms can include fatigue, poor concentration, weight gain, and depressed mood. Clinical management of these conditions requires accurate diagnosis.

Use of Other Medications

For perimenopausal women, should lifestyle changes not suffice, low-dose oral contraceptive pills can help to regulate periods, regulate moods, and treat acne. Providers should use the lowest possible dose due to potential cardiovascular risks. SNRIs may be particularly effective for treatment of both mood and vasomotor symptoms in this group. There is also data for successful symptomatic treatment using gabapentin, pregabalin, and clonidine.[41]

Obstetrician/Gynecologist

The PCP may refer a woman to an OB/GYN when lifestyle and calcium recommendations to treat PMDD do not suffice in order to explore whether she might benefit from the use of a combined oral contraceptive, a vaginal ring, a levonorgestrel intrauterine device, or depot medroxyprogesterone acetate (DMPA).[9] These medications help to maintain steady hormone levels throughout the month. An oral contraceptive, drospirenone/ethinyl estradiol (Yaz), has been approved for PMDD, though most other estrogen or combination oral contraceptives may improve symptoms as well. Triphasic oral contraceptives should be avoided as they can exacerbate symptoms. In extreme cases a woman may elect to undergo a "medical oophorectomy" (using exogenous hormones to completely suppress ovarian hormone production) to manage these symptoms.

Behavioral Health Specialist

When a woman's PMDD is not alleviated by lifestyle education, or when the medical team suspects that psychological, substance use, or cultural issues are contributing to PMDD, a referral to a BHS or health coach should be considered. The PCP or nurse may introduce the BHS/health coach in a "warm handoff." The therapist can explain and educate the woman about treatment of PMDD, validating that her symptoms are real and reassuring her that she is not being referred because of major mental health concerns. A qualitative study by Ussher and Perz[11] found that normalization and offering anticipatory awareness of uncomfortable premenstrual symptoms allows women to better accept the symptoms and reduce the perceived stress that accompanies PMS for some women. The study found that women who did not have anticipatory awareness of PMS were more likely to self-pathologize, describing themselves as "crazy," "psycho," or a "nutcase" in the days before their periods. Women who did not self-pathologize used more effective coping strategies and self-care, such as avoiding situations that may provoke anger or distress during this phase or allowing more time for rest. Psychosocial treatment for PMDD may also be done in a group setting, given the common recommendations for behavioral modification for this disorder and the camaraderie these women may share in a group. More on setting up groups in an integrated care setting can be found in Chapter 28: Group Interventions in Integrated Care Settings.

Infertility treatments, miscarriage and stillbirth, abortion, and unwanted pregnancies are events that should immediately signal the medical care team to consider involving a BHS. These situations may take their toll on a woman's self-worth and control. She may present with difficulty dealing with loss or issues with her partner, and/or she may experience an exacerbation of a depression, OCD, or other mental health condition. For pregnancies that go full term, it is important to monitor the woman's attitude toward the pregnancy and screen for any previous mental health conditions. If feasible, we recommend scheduling routine meetings with a BHS once per trimester to monitor the mother's well-being and provide a sense of emotional support so the pregnancy is not overly "medicalized."

Pregnancy, or pregnancy loss, is a time of heightened emotionality. The entire care team's attitude and communication with the patient around these events is crucial. A study by Kelley and Trinidad[42] found that the doctor's management of stillbirth made a huge difference in how women felt. They found that it is easier for doctors to focus on the medical aspects than to deal with the woman's emotional needs. Most women reported that the most meaningful interactions with the care team were when they experienced members of the team as human and when team members sat with them, expressed empathy, and even cried with them. The BHS may encourage the team to provide this nurturing and also conduct educational seminars for the other team members on how to approach women around these sensitive issues.

Women often have a specific birth plan in mind, but it is important for the BHS to prepare them to be flexible with this plan. For example, an unexpected cesarean section, a child born with a health concern, or an extremely long labor can be detrimental to a mother's mood if she was not fully prepared to "change plans," as needed. Attitudes toward breastfeeding, much like the birth plan, should also be somewhat flexible. For some women, breastfeeding can be quite different from what they expected; it can be painful or the baby may not thrive on the mother's milk. Some women will report having "baby blues," which is contrary to what they fantasized about when considering giving birth and becoming a mother. It important for the BHS to educate, prepare, and help a mother to be flexible at this most significant transitional phase.

Problematic thoughts that should indicate to the care team that the woman may require therapy include (1) the woman questioning her ability to be a parent, feeling resentment toward the unborn child, or admitting that she is afraid she will hurt her child; (2) resurfacing of prior traumas; (3) severe impact on self-worth (e.g., "What good am I if I can't get pregnant?" or "A life without children is not worth living"); (4) severe anxiety, mood symptoms, or substance use during pregnancy or after a miscarriage or stillbirth; or (5) depression around a loss. There is increasing evidence that interpersonal psychotherapy efficaciously treats depression during pregnancy and the postpartum phase.[43]

The team should keep in mind that a mother is born long before she actually gives birth. Her attachment to the idea of a baby may begin in childhood or adolescence; for others, it begins when she is trying to get pregnant or is pregnant. Attachment studies[44] have shown that a mother's sense of her own attachment as a child to her parents will determine the attachment she has with her children, even before they are born. If there are concerns about a mother's inability to attach to her unborn child or unresolved issues affecting the mother's parenting or well-being, a BHS should meet frequently with the woman to conduct a thorough assessment and develop a behavioral treatment plan. If the BHS is concerned about attachment difficulties, the Parenting Stress Index Short Form[45] may be administered. This test is a 36-item form that yields three scales (parental distress, parent–child dysfunctional interaction, and difficult child) as well as a validity scale.

Mother–child dyadic therapy is highly recommended in the postpartum phase for women struggling to bond with their child. In their classic paper "Ghosts in the Nursery," Fraiberg, Adelson, and Shapiro[46] show the positive effects of treating mother–child dyads even in very disturbed and traumatized mothers. In fact, family therapy should be considered in all constellations while the mother is in treatment to allow greater systemic support. Mother–child dyadic therapy can be used to educate the mother about the baby's needs and her impact on the baby's well-being and development. Individual therapy with the mother is also useful to allow her to manage her symptoms and reframe her relationship with herself and consequently with the child and her partner. Parental/couples therapy can be used to help the couple adjust to family life, to educate the partner on how to best support the mother, and/or to decrease marital discord, if it is present. Family therapy can be used to help the whole family adapt to the tasks of a growing family. More information about treating families can be found in Chapter 27: Best Practice for Family-Centered Health Care: A Three-Step Model. If the integrated care practice serves many postpartum women, the practice would benefit from hiring a BHS with specific training in family therapy. Alternatively, families can be referred to community family therapists who can consult with the integrated care team.

All team members need to be aware of just how much women with a history of severe PPD, bipolar exacerbation, or psychotic disorders are terrified about relapse with subsequent pregnancies. Women with preexisting mental illnesses may also be wary of the stresses of new motherhood. Thus, patients can preemptively complete a "care plan" to be implemented should they become ill, in addition to active medication management, as needed. Excellent resources are detailed in Table 20.3, including templates for such care plans, which can be found at the website for children of parents with a mental illness.[47]

BHSs who are trained to do so may also offer couples therapy when appropriate. Common issues for partners of pregnant women are not having control over the pregnancy or confusion about what the partner needs or is experiencing. For couples with infertility, partners may feel shame or guilt if they believe the infertility is "my fault" or anger directed toward the woman trying to get pregnant if they feel the infertility is "her fault." Some couples may not agree about wanting a pregnancy or how they approach loss in cases of miscarriage, stillbirth, or wishes for an abortion. Many couples whose

TABLE 20.3 COMMUNITY AND INTERNET RESOURCES FOR WOMEN'S ISSUES

Name of Organization	Website	Website overview
Office on Women's Health (OWH), U.S. Department of Health and Human Services	Womenshealth.gov	Reliable, commercial-free information on the health of women. Wide variety of health topics, ranging from adolescent health, to reproductive health, to healthy aging. OWH also offers free assistance by phone through an information referral center.
Massachusetts General Hospital Center for Women's Mental Health	womensmentalhealth.org	A perinatal and reproductive psychiatry information center. Presents new research findings in women's mental health and how such investigations inform day-to-day clinical practice.
Postpartum Support International	postpartum.net	Offers support, education, and local resource information such as a guide for each state with information about coordinators and support groups for postpartum issues
Children of Parents with a Mental Illness	copmi.net.au/parents/helping-my-child-and-family/care-plans	Offers templates for care plans a mother can fill out should she become mentally ill
North American Menopause Society	menopause.org	A commercial-free resource offering information about all aspects of menopause for patients and health care providers

pregnancy goes full term report that, after a "honeymoon" phase, having a new child presents a strain on the couple. Differences in childrearing practices, less time together as a couple, and a constant balancing act of personal/couple/familial needs may present a challenge. Partners of women who recently gave birth may also report feeling left out. They may feel unable to soothe the baby as well as the mother. If the mother is breastfeeding, the partner may feel left out of feeding/nurturing experiences. If the mother is experiencing PPD or other mental illness, the partner may feel alone and overwhelmed by the double responsibility of taking care of the baby and the mother. The BHS should help the couple openly communicate their emotions, identify their struggles, and negotiate the gentle balance of each of the partner's needs.

How a woman approaches menopause is of paramount importance. If the woman has difficulty dealing with aging or experiences a significant loss or stressors during this phase (e.g., divorce or the empty-nest syndrome), group therapy may be a great treatment alternative. Meeting like-minded women, in a similar life phase, can offer tremendous support. An integrated care team can offer yearlong or time-limited groups led by a nurse, health coach, and/or BHS. These groups can offer support, camaraderie, and psychoeducation, as these women often find they share many of the same symptoms and struggles. For more on setting up groups, see Chapter 28: Group Interventions in Integrated Care Settings.

Psychiatrist

Prescribing psychotropic medications throughout the women's lifespan can be complex. Both the PCP and the patient may benefit from a psychiatric consultation to assess complex diagnoses, complex medication needs, and assessment and treatment of high-risk or complicated comorbid psychiatric and addiction issues.

For PMDD, there is some evidence for intermittent dosing of antidepressants[48] (only taking medication 14 days before expected menstruation, then stopping with menses each cycle). However, most psychiatrists will recommend consistent dosing to foster adherence and avoid unnecessary complications. Nonetheless, intermittent dosing may be reasonable for cases of troublesome side effects and patient preference. It is imperative to screen for bipolar disorder (using the MDQ)[27] as part of the differential diagnosis of PMDD. Women with PMS can be identified in the patient registry and reviewed with the psychiatrist, since they can be up to twice as likely to experience PPD.[15]

For any comorbid psychiatric disorders, substance use, or addictive disorders during pregnancy, the postpartum phase, or lactation, collaboration with a psychiatrist who specializes in women's mental health issues is warranted, either by a live consultation or via telehealth. Psychiatrists experienced with women's mental health can help weigh the benefits of continuing medication versus the risks of discontinuing or changing a medication or dosage while a woman is pregnant or breastfeeding. Psychiatrists may also consult and educate the PCP, the OB/GYN, the patient, and/or her partner about the maternal and fetal risks and implications for the support system of treatment versus nontreatment. The psychiatrist may also work with the practice, using the registry, to develop population approaches and algorithms for groups of women with specific diagnoses.

Depression with a postpartum onset can generally be approached similarly to an episode of major depression during any other time of life. However, a woman presenting with depression during this period is at increased risk for suicide and having a bipolar disorder, so she will likely need further psychiatric evaluation and management. Patients with an unknown bipolar diathesis, who present with depression, can inadvertently be activated into mania by use of antidepressants. Symptoms suggestive of possible hypomania induced by an antidepressant include increased energy, anxiety, agitation, increased irritability, and decreased need for sleep. A patient with these symptoms should stop taking antidepressant medications and be seen immediately by a psychiatrist. If a psychiatric consultation is not readily available, the team should consider referral to an emergency department. Psychiatrists are in the best position to develop the treatment plan for bipolar patients and especially for prescribing and managing antipsychotic and mood stabilizers in women with a bipolar depression. (See Chapter 12: Treating Depression and Bipolar Disorder in Integrated Care Settings.) Because of these issues, we recommend frequent and early follow-up (one week) with a psychiatrist, with strict return precautions, education for the patient about suicide and bipolar risk, and involvement of family members for additional support.

Use of Mood Stabilizers

Lithium may be considered the medication of choice for pregnant women. However, it can be difficult to manage, given the small therapeutic window and the patient's changing, fluid status. There are risks to the fetus, including Ebstein anomaly (septal and posterior leaflets of the tricuspid valve are displaced toward the apex of the right ventricle of the heart), but these risks are now considered to be very low. Nonetheless, a psychiatrist, in coordination with the PCP, OB/GYN, or perinatologist, should prescribe lithium. Lithium is a viable option during breastfeeding if the mother is stable, the infant is healthy, and the medication regimen is simple. Monitoring in the baby should include monthly measurement of lithium, thyroid-stimulating hormone, blood urea nitrogen, creatinine, and a complete blood count.

Use of Anticonvulsants

Anticonvulsants are commonly prescribed in bipolar disorder but can present significant risks to the fetus, including a twofold increase in neural tube defects, craniofacial anomalies, growth retardation, microcephaly, or heart defects and a threefold increased risk of miscarriage or stillbirth. Valproate, in particular, is very dangerous and carries a black box warning. This medication should be avoided in women of childbearing age and a pregnant woman should discontinue this medication. Some experts recommend 4 to 5 mg of folate for patients taking carbamazepine and lamotrigine during the first trimester as this reduces the risk of neural tube defects. Postpartum, there are no known withdrawal symptoms in infants. For infants exposed to anticonvulsants through breast milk, liver function tests should be monitored.

Use of Antipsychotics

Antipsychotics rather than anticonvulsants are preferred in the treatment of acute mania in a pregnant woman. They may also be used for the initial treatment of postpartum psychosis and for maintenance bipolar treatment. Mid- or high-potency typical antipsychotics (haloperidol or perphenazine) may carry less risk of fetal malformation. There are few studies involving atypical antipsychotics, but they are nonetheless commonly prescribed. Most of the risks of using atypicals during pregnancy have to do with metabolic side effects and weight gain. While the patient is taking an antipsychotic, a lipid profile should be checked each trimester since there is a risk for increased triglyceride levels.

For women who were taking antipsychotics during pregnancy, the psychiatrist or PCP should collaborate with a pediatrician immediately after birth to monitor the baby for extrapyramidal symptoms and withdrawal. Extrapyramidal symptoms could include agitation, abnormally increased or decreased muscle tone, tremor, sleepiness, difficulty breathing, or difficulty feeding. There is little known about the use of antipsychotics during lactation, though few adverse events have been reported.

Use of SSRIs

If a mother is already taking antidepressants, the PCP or psychiatrist should inform her and the infant's pediatrician to observe the child for SSRI-related side effects or a withdrawal syndrome characterized by restlessness, rigidity, and/or tremor. This is not dangerous and usually resolves in one to four days. The link between SSRIs and an increased risk for autism[49] has been largely disproven with improved methodology of subsequent studies. Despite previous concern, the absolute risk of persistent pulmonary hypertension of the newborn is very low.[50] Antidepressants are generally considered to be compatible with breastfeeding.

Use of Benzodiazepines

Clinically, benzodiazepines are not a problem when used at usual doses. A baby exposed to higher doses in utero may experience a withdrawal syndrome after delivery, which includes restlessness, hypertonia, hyperreflexia, tremor, apnea, diarrhea, and/or vomiting up to 3 months after delivery. Very few studies have been done with lactation. When prescribing, the psychiatrist should consider the patient's need to get up with the child and ask if the patient is co-sleeping with the child. A medication with a shorter half-life, such as lorazepam (1–2 mg), should be considered for new mothers who need to wake up frequently. For sleep, trazodone (25–150 mg at bedtime) may also be effective and safe but may be too sedating.

Zolpidem is popular, though we recommend against it due to a patient's likely need to wake up and the increased risk for sleep-related behaviors such as amnestic nocturnal eating, sleepwalking, sleep driving, and so forth.

Health Coaches

Health coaches can be "certified health coaches" (a new national credential). Other health professionals with other degrees (e.g., medical assistants, community case workers, nurses, social workers, psychologists, or others with specialized behavioral health skills) may also be health coaches. Health coaches share a common philosophy that health behavior change comes from the individual. Coaches focus on the patient's values, beliefs, and goals for managing his or her health. They are typically trained in motivational interviewing and have five roles:[51] (1) acting as a bridge between doctors and patients; (2) providing emotional support for patients; (3) assisting patients as they develop self-management skills, based on patients' values and preferences; (4) helping patients navigate the health care system; and (5) providing follow-up continuity of care. Coaches have been shown to increase patients' trust in their physicians.[52] Most are also trained to foster wellness behaviors, working with nutrition/weight, exercise, stress management, harm reduction (e.g., smoking cessation), and adherence to medical recommendations, and providing assistance to patients who need help managing chronic health and mental health conditions. Based on these roles and abilities, coaches can track wellness activities and other health outcomes for the team in the registry, can remind and teach the team about wellness strategies useful for women, and can offer emotional support and education for patients who want to make lifestyle changes to help them with PMS, PMDD, menopausal symptoms, depression, and anxiety. Coaches can also facilitate smoking cessation, help pregnant women adjust to new diets, monitor weight, suggest safe exercise regimens, and assist with sleep hygiene. They can also help women navigate the world of specialists and may function as care managers for women with PPD, bipolar disorder, or other mental health issues, addictions, or chronic medical conditions associated with pregnancy such as diabetes and hypertension. See Chapter 25; Health Coaching in Integrated Care for an extensive overview of the roles and functioning of this new health professional.

Case Manager

Case managers coordinate and assist women with referrals to other specialists, community self-help support groups, hospitals or emergency departments, addiction treatment services, and community mental health support services. A care coordinator or case manager can assist single mothers, new immigrants, and women with a sparse support system, along with women struggling with housing, food, and/or financial issues. This supportive team member can provide community resources or offer assistance such as applying for health insurance (e.g., Medicaid, Children's Health Insurance Program), finding low-cost child care programs (e.g., Head Start), help paying for food (e.g., Women, Infants and Children [WIC] food program, food stamps, the U.S. Department of Agriculture's National Hunger Clearinghouse), and/or connecting patients with local support groups. Establishing these supports early during pregnancy will support a smoother transition into the postpartum period.

CONCLUSION

Each woman has unique needs depending upon her personality, where she is in her life cycle, her response to hormonal changes, her familial, social, and financial contexts, and more. It is important for all team members in an integrated practice to be aware of the woman's hormonal life cycle and its potential interaction with biological, psychological, and social factors. Beyond the global recommendations made in this chapter, the team should remember that every woman responds differently to her own hormonal fluctuations and to hormonal treatments and has her own unique cultural and personality makeup. Thus, the care of women may need to be highly individualized. Team members should allow the time to find the best medical and psychosocial treatments. Integrated care practices seeing many women will benefit from consulting with psychiatrists specializing in women's mental health. All practices need education and training to manage and respond in sensitive ways to women's unique needs. Box 20.2 summarizes the evidence for treatment approaches for women's mental health issues across the reproductive lifespan.

BOX 20.2

SUMMARY OF RECOMMENDED TREATMENT APPROACHES AND RELEVANT EVIDENCE

Strength of recommendation taxonomy (SOR A, B, or C)

PREMENSTRUAL SYMPTOMS/PREMENSTRUAL DYSPHORIC DISORDER

- **Exercise, diet, and stress management are indicated for the initial treatment of premenstrual syndrome and premenstrual dysphoric disorder (SOR B).[5]**
- **Up to 50% of women can reduce symptoms associated with premenstrual syndrome and premenstrual dysphoric disorder by taking 1,200 mg of calcium per day (SOR B).[30]**
- **Oral contraceptives and serotonin selective reuptake inhibitors are efficacious in the management of symptoms associated with premenstrual syndrome and premenstrual dysphoric disorder (SOR A).[9,48,53]**
- **Psychoeducation is important to help women cope with menstrual symptoms (SOR B).[11]**
- **Psychosocial treatment for premenstrual dysphoric disorder may be done in a group setting, given the recommendations for behavioral modification for this disorder and the sense of camaraderie these women may share (SOR B).[54,55]**

PREGNANCY

- **The American College of Obstetrics and Gynecology and the American Psychiatric Association recommend that psychotropic medications be used during pregnancy in the following situations: psychosis, suicidality, moderate to severe symptoms of a psychiatric disorder, less than 6 months of stability, poor response to psychotherapy, history of relapse, patient preference, and/or bipolar disorder (SOR C).[31]**
- **Psychotropic medications can be used with relative safety during pregnancy to treat depression, anxiety, and bipolar illness (SOR C).[13,56]**
- **Valproate should be avoided during pregnancy because of the risk of birth defects (SOR A)[28] and polycystic ovarian syndrome (SOR B).[29]**
- **There is increasing evidence that interpersonal psychotherapy is efficacious for the treatment of depression during pregnancy and the postpartum period (SOR B).[43]**
- **Other forms of psychotherapy, including cognitive-behavioral therapy, relaxation skills, psychodynamic therapy, and couples therapy, can be helpful for women dealing with issues related to pregnancy (SOR C).[55]**

POSTPARTUM PERIOD

- **Educating about a proper sleep regimen and sleep hygiene is important (SOR B).[57,58]**
- **Psychotropic medications are efficacious in the treatment of depression, anxiety, and bipolar illness in the postpartum period (SOR B).[56]**
- **Attachment studies have shown that a mother's sense of her own attachment as a child to her parents will determine the attachment she has with her children. The Parenting Stress Index Short Form may be used to help with an attachment assessment (SOR A).[44,45]**
- **Interpersonal therapy can be used to treat postpartum depression (SOR B).[43]**
- **Other forms of psychotherapy (e.g., cognitive-behavioral, psychodynamic, family) may also be useful treatment approaches during the postpartum period (SOR C).[55]**

MENOPAUSE

- **Exercise, diet, and stress management can help relieve perimenopausal and menopausal symptoms (SOR C).[21]**
- **Low-dose oral contraceptive pills and serotonin–norepinephrine reuptake inhibitors may be particularly effective for the treatment of both mood and vasomotor symptoms in this group (SOR B).[7,21] There are also data for successful symptomatic treatment using gabapentin, pregabalin, and clonidine (SOR B).[41]**
- **Group therapy can be a helpful adjunctive treatment for women experiencing difficulty dealing with menopause (SOR B).[54,59]**

REFERENCES

1. Dossett EC. The role of reproductive psychiatry in women's mental health. In: Barnes DL, ed. Women's Reproductive Mental Health Across the Lifespan. New York: Springer International Publishing; 2014:301–327.
2. World Health Organization. Gender and women's mental health. http://www.who.int/mental_health/prevention/genderwomen/en/. Accessed September 22, 2015.
3. Spitzer RL, Kroenke K, Williams JB. Validation and utility of a self-report version of PRIME-MD: The PHQ primary care study. JAMA. 1999;282(18):1737–1744.
4. Spitzer RL, Kroenke K, Williams JBW, Löwe B. A brief measure for assessing generalized anxiety disorder: The GAD-7. Arch Intern Med. 2006;166(10):1092–1097.
5. Epperson NC, Hantsoo L. Menstruation and premenstrual dysphoric disorder: Its impact on mood. In: Barnes DL, ed. Women's Reproductive Mental Health Across the Lifespan. New York: Springer International Publishing; 2014:49–72.
6. Hendrick V, Altshuler LL, Suri R. Hormonal changes in the postpartum and implications for postpartum depression. Psychosomatics.1998;39(2):93–101.
7. Schuiling KD, Likis FE. Women's Gynecological Health. 2nd ed. Burlington, MA: Jones and Bartlett Learning LLC; 2006.
8. American Psychiatric Association. Diagnostic and Statistical Manual of Mental Disorders. 5th ed. Washington, DC: American Psychiatric Association; 2013.
9. Hatcher RA, Trussell, J, Nelson AL, Cates W, Kowal D, Policar MS. Contraceptive Technology. 20th Rev. ed. New York: Ardent. Media Inc; 2011.
10. Johnson TM. Premenstrual syndrome as a Western culture-specific disorder. Cult Med Psychiatry. 1987;11(3):337–356.
11. Ussher J, Perz J. PMS as a process of negotiation: Women's experience and management of premenstrual distress. Psychol Health. 2013;28(8):909–927.
12. Weissman MM, Wickramaratne P, Nomura Y, Warner V, Pilowsky D, Verdelil H. Offspring of depressed parents: 20 years later. Am J Psychiatry. 2006;163(6):1001–1008.
13. Cohen LS, Altshuler LL, Harlow BL, et al. Relapse of major depression during pregnancy in women who maintain or discontinue antidepressant treatment. JAMA. 2006;295(5):499–507.
14. Sit DK, Perel JM, Helsel JC, Wisner K. Changes in antidepressant metabolism and dosing across pregnancy and early postpartum. J Clin Psychiatry. 2008;69(4):652–658.
15. Buttner MM, Mott SL, Pearlstein T, Stuart S, Zlotnick C, O'Hara MW. Examination of premenstrual symptoms as a risk factor for depression in postpartum women. Arch Womens Ment Health. 2013;16(3):219–225.
16. Wisner KL, Sit DKY, Hanusa BH, et al. Major depression and antidepressant treatment: impact on pregnancy and neonatal outcomes. Am J Psychiatry. 2009;166(5)557–566.
17. Jennings KD, Ross S, Popper S, Marquita E. Thoughts of harming infants in depressed and nondepressed mothers. J Affect Disorders. 1999;54(1):21–28.
18. Munk-Olsen T, Laursen TM, Meltzer-Brody S, Mortensen PB, Jones I. Psychiatric disorders with postpartum onset: Possible early manifestations of bipolar affective disorders. Arch Gen Psychiatry. 2012;69(4):428–434.
19. Sharma V, Xie B, Campbell MK, et al. A prospective study of diagnostic conversion of major depressive disorder to bipolar disorder in pregnancy and postpartum. Bipolar Disord. 2014;16(1):16–21.
20. Forty L, Smith D, Jones L, et al. Clinical differences between bipolar and unipolar depression. Br J Psychiatry. 2008;192(5):388–389.
21. Gibbs Z, Kulkarni J. Risk factors for depression during perimenopause. In: Barnes DL, ed. Women's Reproductive Mental Health Across the Lifespan. New York: Springer International Publishing; 2014:215–233.
22. Puryear LC. Postpartum adjustment: What is normal and what is not. In: Barnes DL, ed. Women's Reproductive Mental Health Across the Lifespan. New York: Springer International Publishing; 2014:109–122.
23. Freeman MP, Smith KW, Freeman SA, et al. The impact of reproductive events on the course of bipolar disorder in women. J Clin Psychiatry. 2002;63(4):284–287.
24. Henshaw C. Screening and risk assessment for perinatal mood disorders. In: Barnes DL, ed. Women's Reproductive Mental Health Across the Lifespan. New York: Springer International Publishing; 2014:91–108.
25. Mortola JF, Girton L, Beck L, Yen SS. Diagnosis of premenstrual syndrome by a simple, prospective, and reliable instrument: The Calendar of Premenstrual Experiences. Obstet Gynecol. 1990;76(2):302–307.
26. Cox JL, Holden JM, Sagovsky R. Detection of postnatal depression. Development of the 10-item Edinburgh Postnatal Depression Scale. Br J Psychiatry.1987;150(6):782–786.
27. Hirschfeld RM, Williams JB, Spitzer RL, et al. Development and validation of a screening instrument for bipolar spectrum disorder: The Mood Disorder Questionnaire. Am J Psychiatry 2000:157(11);1873–1875.
28. Walker SP, Permezel M, Berkovic SF. The management of epilepsy in pregnancy. Br J Obstet Gynaecol. 2009;116(6):758–767.

29. Joffe H, Cohen LS, Suppes T, et al. Valproate is associated with new-onset oligoamenorrhea with hyperandrogenism in women with bipolar disorder. Biol Psychiatry. 2006;59(11):1078–1086.
30. Thys-Jacobs S, Starkey S, Bernstein D, Tian J. Calcium carbonate and the premenstrual syndrome: Effects on premenstrual and menstrual symptoms. Am J Obstet Gynecol. 1998;179(2):444–452.
31. Yonkers KA, Wisner KL, Stewart DE, et al. The management of depression during pregnancy: A report from the American Psychiatric Association and the American College of Obstetricians and Gynecologists. Obstet Gynecol. 2009;114:703–713.
32. Wood W. FDA pregnancy categories: Help or hindrance? Ment Health Clin. 2013;3(2):78–80.
33. Micromedex Solutions. http://micromedex.com. Accessed April 18, 2016.
34. Reprotox. https://reprotox.org. Accessed April 18, 2016.
35. Wisner KL, Bogen DL, Sit DK, et al. Does fetal exposure to SSRIs or maternal depression impact infant growth? Am J Psychiatry. 2013;170(5):485–493.
36. Ornoy A, Arnon J, Shechtman S, Moerman L, Lukashova I. Is benzodiazepine use during pregnancy really teratogenic? Reprod Toxicol. 1998;12(5):511–515.
37. Viguera AC, Tondo L, Koukopoulos AE, Reginaldi D, Lepri B, Baldessarini RJ. Episodes of mood disorders in 2,252 pregnancies and postpartum periods. Am J Psychiatry. 2011;168(11):1179–1185.
38. Viguera AC, Whitfield T, Baldessarini RJ, et al. Risk of recurrence in women with bipolar disorder during pregnancy: Prospective study of mood stabilizer discontinuation. Am J Psychiatry. 2007;164(12):1817–1824.
39. Gaitonde DY, Rowley KD, Sweeney LB. Hypothyroidism: An update. Am Fam Physician. 2012;86(3):244–251.
40. Muller AF, Drexhage HA, Berghout A. Postpartum thyroiditis and autoimmune thyroiditis in women of childbearing age: Recent insights and consequences for antenatal and postnatal care. Endocr Rev. 2001;22(5):605–630.
41. Reddy SY, Warner H, Guttuso Jr. T, et al. Gabapentin, estrogen, and placebo for treating hot flushes: A randomized controlled trial. Obstet Gynecol. 2006;108(1):41–48.
42. Kelley MC, Trinidad SB. Silent loss and the clinical encounter: Parents' and physicians' experiences of stillbirth—a qualitative analysis. BMC Pregnancy Childbirth. 2012;12(1):1.
43. Cuijpers P, Geraedts AS, van Oppen P, Andersson G, Markowitz JC, van Straten A. Interpersonal psychotherapy for depression: A meta-analysis. Am J Psychiatry. 2011;168(6):581–592.
44. Fonagy P, Steele H, Steele M. Maternal representations of attachment during pregnancy predict the organization of infant-mother attachment at one year of age. Child Dev. 1991;62(5):891–905.
45. Abidin RR. Parenting Stress Index, 3rd ed.: Professional Manual. Odessa, FL: Psychological Assessment Resources, Inc.; 1995.
46. Fraiberg S, Adelson E, Shapiro V. Ghosts in the nursery. A psychoanalytic approach to the problems of impaired infant–mother relationships. J Am Acad Child Psychiatry. 1975;14(3):387–421.
47. About "care plans." Children of Parents with a Mental Illness. http://www.copmi.net.au. Accessed September 20, 2015.
48. Steiner M, Pearlstein T, Cohen LS, et al. Expert guidelines for the treatment of severe PMS, PMDD, and comorbidities: The role of SSRIs. J Womens Health. 2006;15(1):57–69.
49. Hviid A, Melbye M, Pasternak B. Use of selective serotonin reuptake inhibitors during pregnancy and risk of autism. N Engl J Med. 2013;369(25):2406–2415.
50. Huybrechts KF, Bateman BT, Palmsten K, et al. Antidepressant use late in pregnancy and risk of persistent pulmonary hypertension of the newborn. JAMA. 2015;313(21):2142–2151.
51. Bennett HD, Coleman EA, Parry C, et al. Health coaching for patients with chronic illness. Fam Pract Manag. 2010;17(5):24–29
52. Thom DH, Hessler D, Willard-Grace R, et al. Does health coaching change patients trust in their primary care provider? Patient Educ Couns. 2014;96(1):135–138.
53. Pearlstein T, Steiner M. Premenstrual dysphoric disorder: Burden of illness and treatment update. J Psychiatry Neurosci. 2008;33(4):291–301.
54. Burlingame GM, Fuhriman A, Mosier J. The differential effectiveness of group psychotherapy: A meta-analytic perspective. Group Dyn. 2003;7(1):3–12.
55. American Psychological Association. Recognition of psychotherapy effectiveness. http://www.apa.org/about/policy/resolution-psychotherapy.aspx. Accessed November 1, 2015.
56. Doyle K, Heron J, Berrisford G, Whitmore J, Jones L, Wainscott G, Oyebode F. The management of bipolar disorder in the perinatal period and risk factors for postpartum relapse. Eur Psychiatry. 2012;27(8):563–569.
57. Armstrong KL, van Haeringen AR, Dadds MR, Cash R. Sleep deprivation or postnatal depression in later infancy: Separating the chicken from the egg. J Paediatr Child Health. 1998;34(3):260–262.
58. Dennis CL, Ross L. Relationships among infant sleep patterns, maternal fatigue, and development of depressive symptomatology. Birth. 2005;32(3):187–193.
59. McRoberts C, Burlingame GM, Hoag M. Comparative efficacy of individual and group psychotherapy: A meta-analytic perspective. Group Dyn. 1998;2(2):101–117.

21

Assessing and Treating Sexual Problems in an Integrated Care Environment

KENNETH M. POLLOCK AND ALAN M. ALTMAN

BOX 21.1

KEY POINTS

- **Many sexual problems go undetected and untreated in primary care settings.**
- **Patients want doctors to ask about sexual problems.**
- **There are four major sexual problem areas: desire, arousal, orgasm, and pain.**
- **Sexual problems are multifactorial, with combined biological, psychological, and relationship etiologies. The clinician needs to think like Sherlock Holmes when determining etiologies.**
- **A small, incremental increase in sexual health knowledge among the members of an integrated care team can have a major effect on helping patients with their sexual functioning.**
- **Understanding partner functioning is crucial when assessing and treating a patient's problem.**
- **Primary care physicians functioning in integrated care teams can do time-efficient assessments, collaboratively treat some sexual problems, and make well-informed referrals within and outside of their practices to appropriate specialists.**
- **Treatment usually requires concurrent, *not* sequential, interventions on multiple levels, such as the biological, psychological, and relationship level.**
- **Estrogen and testosterone are effective and safe hormonal treatments that can be used to treat some sexual problems.**

INTRODUCTION

Sex plays an important and transcending role in most people's lives. See Box 21.1 for an overview of the key points discussed in the chapter. Sexual functioning is directly affected by a combination of medical/physical, psychological, and relationship factors. Few if any areas in health have a greater mind–body connection than sex. Problems existing in the mind or body impair and often preclude sexual functioning, as well as play a major role in decreasing quality of life. Simply thinking about sex can lead to physical arousal, yet without a functional neurohormonal system, arousal cannot occur. For example, in the absence of bioavailable testosterone, arousal for either sex is impossible. Hence, effective detection, assessment, and treatment require practitioner knowledge in both arenas.

This chapter is written for the primary care physician (PCP) and all members of the integrated care team. The aim is to provide a framework that will enable the team to increase their level of expertise in assessing, diagnosing, and treating common sexual problems. It directly addresses sexual problems encountered by couples as well as unpartnered individuals who are or who want to be sexual. It does not address other sex-related topics, such as birth control, sexually transmitted diseases, sexual abuse detection, and adolescence. In this chapter, the word *physical* encompasses other terms such as "biological," "physiologic," or "neurologic." Similarly, the title "clinician" may refer to any treating practitioner: the PCP, psychologist, behavioral health specialist (BHS), clinical social worker, health coach, urologist, gynecologist, nurse practitioner, or care manager.

In the majority of primary health care practices, relatively few sexual complaints are presented by patients. At the same time, proactive physician screening for sexual concerns is limited by a number of barriers, including: (1) time-limited visits; (2) insurance reimbursement limitations; (3) physician discomfort in talking about sex; (4) a natural tendency of physicians to think along medical rather than psychological dimensions; and (5) physician training about sexual problems that does not always include approaches to multifactorial diagnosis and assessment.

Many of these same barriers exist in urology and gynecology practices, which often function as the primary providers for sexual problems. While these specialists are frequently presented with sexual problems by patients, they too have time-limited visits, as well as a predisposition toward medical and away from psychological and relationship dimensions. Another structural barrier to integrated, within-practice team functioning is that current insurance reimbursement in medical practices is largely limited to covering the medical-surgical aspects of care and rarely reimburses for the critical-to-success psychological and relationship components of treatment. This results in the need to refer out of the practice in order to obtain behavioral health expertise in treating patients. This may change if value-based incentives, team-based billing, and global budgeting are widely implemented.

In an equally problematic way, nonmedical clinicians such as psychologists, social workers, and other mental health counselors are generally not well versed in understanding the medical aspects of sexual problems, limiting their ability to effectively assess and treat the large number of patients with sexual problems that have medical causes. Too often, this results in psychotherapeutic and sex therapy interventions that fail as a consequence of not including causal physical factors either diagnostically or in the treatment.

To compound the problem, only a tiny percentage of all mental health practitioners are trained in the specifics of how to assess and treat sexual problems. Therefore, while physicians face one set of barriers in being able to provide care, nonmedical practitioners are equally impeded by another set. Psychiatrists stand somewhere in the middle, as they have general medical training as well as skill in assessing psychological problems. Yet, like most other mental health professionals, those with specialized training in sexual health are rare.

As a result of these barriers and knowledge deficits, many sexual problems remain undetected, inadequately treated, or untreated. Increased integration of sexual health care within a practice team, along with a new insurance environment, and accompanied by a small but nevertheless significant increase in sexual health knowledge in all of the professions mentioned, has the potential to profoundly improve what is currently done for the sexual health of patients. This includes becoming increasingly adept at making informed referrals to another team member or to a specialist outside of the practice.

To be specific, increasingly well-informed and targeted referrals will put the referred-to specialist in a better position to therapeutically exploit the diagnostic formulations and treatment recommendations proffered by the team. Improving the PCP's understanding of sexual problems will put him or her in a better position to target a referral to a specialist with the appropriate skillset. For example, after asking some core questions about loss of arousal in a patient, the PCP determines that the couple's relationship is harmonious, but the problems are limited to sexual interaction and communication. In this case, the PCP may want to refer them to a nonmedical sex therapist rather than a gynecologist, or someone who treats depression or troubled marriages. Specialists will not only appreciate the preliminary work done by the PCP, but will have an increased likelihood of being more collegial and communicative when handing the patient back to the PCP, increasing the *effective* integration of care.

For some practitioners, their increase in knowledge, diagnostically and interventionally, will potentially result in a small but nevertheless intriguing and possibly enjoyable widening of their *effective* scope of practice.

YOUR PATIENTS WANT YOU TO ASK THEM ABOUT SEX

A number of systematic studies of primary care physicians support the conclusion that 85% of patients believe their physician *should* inquire about sexual problems, with 75% of these same patients reportedly being "under satisfied" by their physician's queries about sexual matters.[1] The vast majority of patients reported feeling uncomfortable about mentioning sexual problems and expressed the wish that their physician bring up the subject.[1] In another study, patients were reluctant to raise sexual issues with their physician, stating that they were worried no treatment would be available, the physician would dismiss the problem as being psychological, and the physician would be uncomfortable discussing sexual topics.[2] It appears that inhibitions increase when topics are potentially more embarrassing (e.g., masturbation, unusual ways of having sex, and when patients are elderly). The importance of physicians and other clinicians asking about and discussing sex cannot be overemphasized. Sometimes, simply talking about a problem can be therapeutic in itself. As physicians go through the process of assessing, diagnosing, and treating sexual problems, they must be sensitive to and respectful of the cultural, religious, and spiritual context in which their patients live.

THE MAJOR SEXUAL PROBLEMS

The four major problem areas in sexual functioning are desire, arousal, orgasm, and pain. Each has variations and they frequently co-occur, as shown in detail in Table 21.1. For each of these specific problem areas, patient or partner distress is a requirement. For example, low desire without distress in either partner is not a problem, since there would be no motivation to change it. However, a person without distress who has low desire, but whose partner is distressed, has a *relationship problem*, not necessarily one that is sexual.

Unlike the *Diagnostic and Statistical Manual of Mental Disorders*, fifth edition (DSM-5),[3] which defines almost all sexual difficulties as "disorders," this chapter emphasizes that many sexual problems are not necessarily disorders. For example, the loss of desire is normal and common in long-term relationships.

OVERVIEW OF SEXUAL ASSESSMENT, DIAGNOSIS, AND TREATMENT PLANNING

Table 21.2 represents the core conceptual model that can and should be used in three ways: (1) as an overview for understanding the multifactorial and complex nature of sexual problems; (2) as a guide, framework, and checklist for conducting an assessment interview; and (3) as a guide and checklist for determining a treatment plan.

The first column to the left delineates the four major areas of sexual problems (desire, arousal, orgasm, and pain). The next three columns list the three etiologic categories, suggesting to the clinician that it is important to *always* consider etiologies that are biological (B), psychological (P), and relationship-based (R) in origin. The next column "reminds" the clinician to consider interactions between [B-P-R] (all of the possible identified etiologies). Caution is indicated, as there is a natural tendency, once a significant causal factor is located, to proceed to treatment rather than to keep searching the etiologic horizon. The identification of the first of several potential etiologies is often a treatment as well as a diagnostic "fork in the road." It is an opportunity to integrate care while also incrementally expanding the scope of one's practice. A common example would be the determination that low desire in a woman is secondary to pain associated with an atrophic vagina, a condition that often engenders negative relationship effects. The PCP might choose to continue as the direct care provider by prescribing a topical estradiol cream (Estrace), or ospemifene (Osphena), which is a selective estrogen receptor modulator (SERM), while simultaneously referring the patient to a BHS who would provide counseling aimed at addressing the secondary relationship problems.

Numerous etiologic subcategories exist within each of these three categories. For instance, "biological" can include a wide range of causes, including, but not limited to, hormonal deficits, birth injuries, medication side effects, diabetes, traumatic injuries, and neurologic damage from bicycle seats. "Psychological" can include depression, anxiety, anti-sexual attitudes from childhood, posttraumatic stress disorder, or other psychiatric disorders. "Relationship" can include marital discord, changes in life priorities, boredom, and extramarital relationships. Sub-categories can, and frequently are, both additive and interactive.

Problems	Women	Men	Comments
Desire	Discrepant levels between partners. Two major kinds of desire: (1) sexual hunger/innate desire, lust versus (2) receptive desire, which involves the wish to become aroused without lust/hunger being initially present.	Similar to women, although most men frequently experience loss of innate desire.	For women: Important to distinguish between *receptive* desire and *innate* desire. For both genders: a loss of desire can feel distressing even when not partnered, i.e., people like to feel desire, even if they do not masturbate.
Arousal	Desire for sex may exist but arousal does not occur or is negligible. Often involves both subjective non-arousal as well as physical, e.g., not lubricating.	The most common form is inability to attain or maintain a satisfying (hard) erection: erectile dysfunction (ED). Often co-occurs with high as well as low desire.	For women: Some may experience subjective or mental arousal, but no corresponding physical excitement (e.g., engorgement of the genitals, lubrication) and vice versa. Often, this results in loss of arousal. Diagnosis: genital arousal disorder.
Orgasm	Inability to achieve orgasm even when aroused; frequently coexists with low arousal.	Two major forms: (1) Early/premature ejaculation (PE) is defined as ejaculation occurring prior to the man's wishes. (2) Inhibited or delayed ejaculation in which the man is unable to ejaculate or has extreme difficulty doing so inside his partner.	For women: There are two major types: 1) *Primary*: a life-long condition. 2) *Secondary:* previously experienced orgasms but no longer does. Many women cannot experience orgasm solely with penile penetration and are distressed by this, when in fact it is a normal variation. For men: Premature ejaculation does not occur during masturbation but with penetration. *Delayed ejaculation* is often, but not always, associated with overuse of pornography. A rarer form tends to be lifelong, which does not happen when the man is masturbating.
Pain	Different types: (a) introital/vestibulitis (b) vulvovaginal atrophy (c) vulvodynia (d) poor lubrication (e) endometrial (f) pelvic inflammatory disease (g) vaginismus	Peyronie disease (chronic fibrous inflammation of the penis): not a sexual problem but pain is often experienced during sexual activity.	For women: Often but not always associated with menopausal transition as well as relationship issues; can engender problems in the partner (e.g., ED). Caution is required when assuming pain is psychogenic.

TABLE 21.1 MAJOR SEXUAL PROBLEM AREAS*

* This table is based on the most clinically useful description of the major sexual problems. It does not necessarily follow DSM-5.[3]

TABLE 21.2 TEMPLATE FOR MULTIFACTORIAL ASSESSMENT AND TREATMENT

Sexual Problems	Causes				Treatments			
	Biological (B)	Psychological (P)	Relationship (R)	Interactions between B-P-R	Biological Interventions	Psychological Interventions	Relationship Interventions	Multifactorial Interventions
Desire								
Arousal								
Orgasm								
Pain								

Focus on Interactions Between Causes

Interactions typically occur within and between one or more of these major causes of sexual problems. For example, in women, dyslipidemia is associated with increases in sex hormone binding globulin (SHBG) and causes low bioavailable testosterone levels. Consequently, there is a lowering of desire and arousability, often leading to nonarousal (including both vaginal dryness and an absence of subjective excitement). Chronic sexual pain can easily lead to negative emotional reactions and then to relationship distress. Another example of interactions between causes would be biologically induced erectile dysfunction (ED), which might easily trigger feelings of rejection and unattractiveness in the partner. These reactions could manifest with the partner withdrawing emotionally, becoming defensively angry, or feeling unloved, resulting in patients blaming themselves or their partners. In this case, the original vascular insufficiency could lead to an essentially incorrect conclusion by the clinician or BHS that there is a relationship "cause" of the problem. Always keep in mind that as you subsequently develop a treatment plan, eliminating a primary symptom may not cure the problem unless the secondary relationship dysfunction is also treated, as it can easily take on a life of its own.

Using the ED example, a man who has been prescribed sildenafil (Viagra) may be anxious about resuming sex with his partner. His anxiety could result in avoidance of sex, premature ejaculation secondary to fear of erection loss, and/or the inability to attain and maintain the erection. He might also feel hurt and criticized, resulting in a loss of sexual self-confidence.

These examples lead to several suggestions regarding assessment that may prevent treatment failures:

1. It is critical to determine whether the identified complaint is primary or secondary to another problem.
2. When conducting the assessment, automatically assume that there are multiple causes that may be additive as well as interactive.
3. Be aware that the existing skillset gaps between all practitioners could easily result in missing a significant etiologic element.

The chain of one problem leading to another (including physical leading to psychological and vice versa) is complex but nevertheless comprehensible. Problems are often additive and interactive within an individual as well as within a relationship. Biology affects the relationship, the relationship affects individual psychology, and a cascade of interacting phenomena cycle into a spiral of sexual and relationship difficulties. Many of the links in this chain can be identified through a careful interview, plus a consideration of the patient's medical history and the partner relationship.

At first glance, doing this may appear to be beyond the time availability and technical knowledge of the PCP, but a few good questions along with an existing medical history can produce the needed clinical information (see the next section, "Detection and Screening").

In summary, both critical thinking and the potential value of collaboration between specialties on the team (all of them thinking like Sherlock Holmes) can have a positive impact on accurate assessments and impactful treatment.

Detection and Screening

While both clinician and patient willingness to discuss sexual concerns are important aspects of treatment, the primary care team, just as with hypertension, diabetes, and gastrointestinal problems, should *proactively screen for sexual problems.*

Approaches to detection and screening include (1) active, direct questioning; (2) pre-consultation screening questionnaires (see Boxes 21.2 and 21.3); and (3) clinician-initiated discussions. PCPs should look for propitious moments to ask questions that will lead to discussion. For example: "Women can often have vaginal dryness which may affect their sex life. Are you having any difficulties with this?" Or, "People in your situation (e.g., new baby, perimenopausal, partner recently was ill, elderly, status post an illness or surgery) often encounter problems with sexual functioning (e.g., ED, dryness, low desire). How about you?"

Assessment and Diagnosis

Here are four core questions integrative care clinicians should ask their patients:

1. "Are you sexually active?"
2. If Yes, "Are you having any problems or concerns with your sexual activity or lack of it?"
3. If Yes, "Is this distressing to you? Is this distressing to your partner (if partnered)? Would you like to become sexually active

BOX 21.2
BRIEF SEXUAL SYMPTOM CHECKLIST FOR WOMEN*

The brief questionnaire can be incorporated into a patient intake form and used as a pre-consultation screening tool or administered clinically.

Please answer the following questions about your overall sexual function in the past 3 months or more.

1. **Are you satisfied with your sexual function?**
   Yes____ No____ If No, please continue.
2. **How long have you been dissatisfied with your sexual function? __________________**
3. **The problem(s) with your sexual function is/are: (Mark one or more)**
   a. **Problems with little or no interest in sex**
   b. **Problems with decreased genital sensation (feeling)**
   c. **Problems with decreased vaginal lubrication (dryness)**
   d. **Problems reaching orgasm**
   e. **Problems with pain during sex**
   f. **Other____________________**
4. **Which problem in question 3 is most bothersome to you?____________**
5. **Would you like to talk about it with your health care provider?**
   Yes_____ No_____

* This instrument is in the public domain.

BOX 21.3
SEXUAL HEALTH CHECKLIST FOR MEN*

Please answer the following questions about your overall sexual function in the past 3 months or more.

1. **Are you satisfied with your sexual functioning?**
   Yes____ No____ If No, please continue.
2. **How long have you been dissatisfied with you sexual functioning?**
   ____
3. **The problem with your sexual functioning is (mark one or more):**
   a. **Problems with little or no interest in sex**
   b. **Problems with getting or keeping an erection**
   c. **Problems with ejaculating *before* you want to**
   d. **Problems with being able to ejaculate or reach an orgasm**
   e. **Other problems__________________________**
   f. **If you have a sexual partner, is your partner bothered by your problem? Yes____ No___**
4. **Which problem in question 3 is most bothersome to you?____________**
5. **Would you like to talk about it with your health care provider?**
   Yes______ No______
6. **Would you like to talk to another health care provider with whom you might be more comfortable? Yes______ No______**

* Authors: Kenneth M. Pollock, Ph.D. (kmpollock@aol.com) and Alan M. Altman, M.D., FACOG. IF. Permission is granted to all practitioners: (alanaltmanmd.com) who wish to reproduce and employ this checklist as a screening instrument for sexual problems in men providing that they give credit to the authors.

again?" Note: if patient is unpartnered and/or elderly, ask about self-stimulation in a nonjudgmental way that normalizes it: "Many people in your situation masturbate. Does that work well for you or are you having any difficulties that get in the way?"
4. "Perhaps I can be of help. Would you be willing to tell me more about it?"

Once the patient has indicated willingness to discuss the problem, follow-up questions can be useful in developing a clearer clinical picture (asked by PCP or sexual health–trained nurse practitioner or BHS if patient has been referred). In the following list, questions 1 through 3 are relevant to both genders, while questions 4 through 9 focus directly upon the assessment of ED:

1. "Does the problem occur in specific situations or all the time? For example, with your regular partner, but not with others? When you are with your partner but not when you are masturbating? Does it occur when you are with the opposite sex but not the same sex?"
2. "Is the problem lifelong or acquired?" If the problem is acquired, "When was it acquired? Gradually or over a certain amount of time? Was it around a specific event? (e.g., after childbirth, an illness, loss of a loved one)"
3. "What is your partner's reaction to this problem? Are you comfortable discussing it with your partner? Does your partner have any sexual problems?" (This is a mandatory question if the patient is partnered.)
4. "Do you have difficulty acquiring or maintaining an erection?"
5. "Is it different during masturbation?"
6. "Using a hardness scale of 1 to 10, at what number would you stay in or pop out of your partner during penetrative sex?"

7. "Are there occasions that ED does or does not happen either solo or partnered, (e.g., during an illicit affair, while using drugs, drinking, with same sex, during a fantasy, etc.?)"
8. "Do you experience morning erections? How hard?"
9. "Approximately when was the last time you had an erection?"

The answers to these questions are usually informative enough to suggest which of three major treatment options may be indicated: (1) medication alone (e.g., a phosphodiesterase type 5 inhibitor [PDE-5] or a phosphodiesterase type 11 inhibitor [PDE-11]); (2) medication in combination with couple sex therapy; or (3) couple sex therapy alone. Details on these options are described in the section on treating ED. Figure 21.1 presents a treatment algorithm for ED.

Interviewing the partner alone may create an opportunity for the PCP to hand off part or all of the treatment to an in-practice BHS. Additionally, there are several clinically important facts or feelings that people are frequently unwilling to express candidly in front of their partners. These include negative feelings about unappealing aspects of their partner that they are reluctant to say out of a wish to not hurt him or her. A partner's unspoken experiential truths frequently preclude the understanding needed by the clinician in order to intervene successfully. Obtaining both sides of the story is diagnostically useful, not only in treating troubled relationships, but also in assessing the interpersonal intricacies and nuances of sexual problems even when a relationship is untroubled.

For example, possible responses to the clinician's question about whether the sexual problem is situational or general might be:

> "I only experience the problem (low desire, pain, ED, etc.), when my children are home."
>
> "When I masturbate, I do not have any problem keeping my erection, but when I'm with my partner I lose it." "I have a lot of sexual desire, but not for my partner."
>
> "I have desire and arousal but lose arousal during sex with my partner."

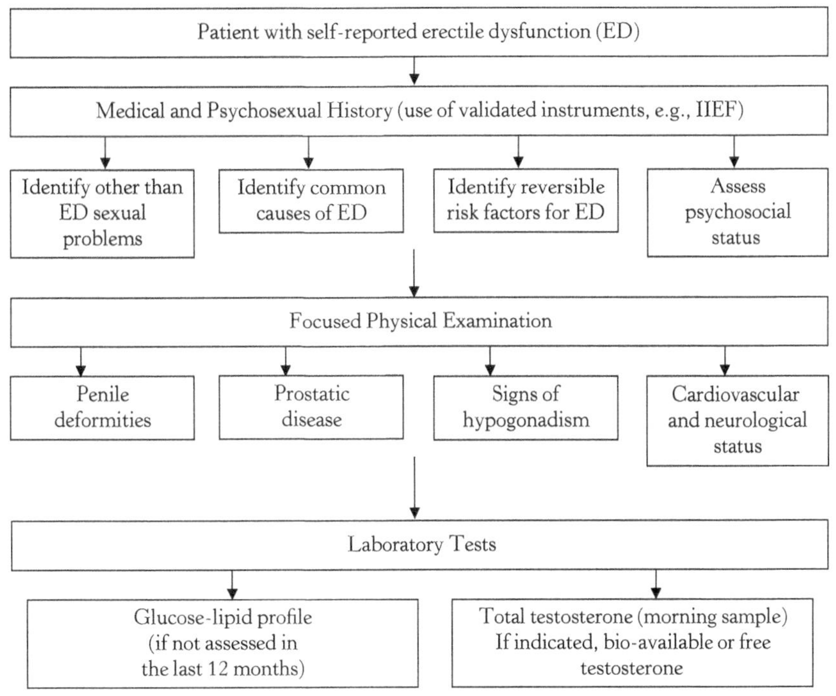

FIGURE 21.1 Treatment Algorithm for Erectile Dysfunction.[4]

All of these responses illustrate situational differences and mitigate toward relationship causes and away from biological etiologies. On the other hand, if these same responses were to be generalized (e.g., "I experience erection problems in all contexts"), then the clinician should consider biological/physical etiologies.

In another example, the clinician asks if the problem is lifelong or acquired. Possible responses are:

> "My sexual desire went downhill after the birth of my baby." (This should trigger the clinician to consider multiple possibilities, such as pelvic floor injury, postpartum depression, changes in priority from spouse to baby, hormonal deficits, etc.)
>
> "My low interest started when I began to have vaginal dryness." (In this case, the clinician might consider estrogen deficiency leading to vaginal atrophy and/or depression.)
>
> A response from a man: "My desire went down after I lost my job, got depressed, and started to take medication for it." (The clinician might consider medication side effects, loss of self-esteem, low testosterone, reduced energy, or marital conflict associated with anxiety.)

BRIDGING THE GAP FROM ASSESSMENT TO TREATMENT

After reaching basic diagnostic conclusions and some indication of the nature and direction of treatment or specialist referrals, some problems will necessitate a deeper understanding of psychological and relationship processes, often involving questions about how symptoms are specifically experienced. *The essence of treatment success is inextricably linked to assisting the patient in describing both their psychological and physical experience to the clinician as well as to their partner.* This is especially the case regarding sexual pain. For those reasons, a few assessment comments and questions are included in the "Treatment Intervention" section of this chapter.

The primary care team determines appropriate roles for assessment and treatment follow-through. The PCP is at the center of care with an ever-increasing role for the BHS, along with a health coach and any required external specialists; all are concurrently involved or at least informed, as the process unfolds.

From Biology and Culture to Relationships

Sexual problems are a function of the biological, cultural, and psychological differences between men and women. These differences are the source of both attraction and trouble. Sexual situations become exciting when there is a certain tension and distance between the partners. For some, the most intense sexual relationships are between partners who cannot instantly take each other for granted, where there exists some anxiety, and where there is an element of the unknown and unconquered.

For thousands of years, women, as conceptualized by men, have been seen as possessing a curious combination of traits ranging from overdependency to secret powers that mystify and are magnetic but also dangerous. In this context, men have nevertheless continually and explicitly attempted to define themselves as more powerful, while acknowledging in a host of ways that women are ultimately more powerful and need to be controlled. There is an age-old struggle around aggression and submission not only based on physical and temperamental differences but from the symbolic connotations of sexual intercourse, involving penetration and receptivity, and an acute awareness of *who is on top*. Attraction and the troubles that inevitably follow, even in satisfied couples, rest on the ever-changing, almost unconscious awareness that in virtually every sexual interaction, there is a *doer* and a *done-to*, and a built-in instability that in its existence is associated with pleasure, and in its absence, with acquired neutrality and loss of excitement. What may begin with interpersonal sexual electricity and magnetism often, over time, emerges into a sense of interpersonal blandness. Out of this eternal, ever-shifting matrix, sexual desire and excitement, including the ultimate excitement of orgasm, serve as both the fuel and glue for the creation and recreation of relationships and continuity of the species. A delicate balance exists between the sexes. When it is disrupted, problems with desire, arousal, and orgasm emerge. The disruption itself, while uncomfortable, presents an opportunity for relationship renewal or, if not taken, a long pathway toward neutrality and chronic, resigned acceptance of a less-than-exciting relationship.

Prior to addressing specific treatment interventions, the psychological/relationship phenomena discussed below need to be considered. Combined, they play a major role in the creation of sexual difficulty. Hence, diminishing their power constitutes the essence of sexual repair and growth.

From Acquired Sexual Neutrality to Desire

Desire problems are the most common sexual difficulties encountered by sexual health professionals. They frequently co-occur with other sexual troubles and also typically affect both arousal and orgasm (with pain being the handmaiden of low arousal in women). However, this is not always the case; a person can have low desire but still experience high arousal or, conversely, have high desire but problems with arousal. Desire problems typically manifest within couples as a *distressing* discrepancy between the partners. In unpartnered individuals, lost or lower desire is experienced as a wish to recover desire and to resume sex with a "hoped-for" new partner or for masturbatory pleasure.

The clinician's understanding of the profound difference between *innate* and *receptive* desire in women is of critical importance. *Innate* desire is best understood as primary sexual hunger and lusting. *Receptive* desire is characterized by the wish to become aroused as well as receptivity to stimulation and a wish for the arousal that follows—while *not* actually feeling lust or innate desire. Receptive desire is often misinterpreted by both clinicians and patients as a problematic loss of desire, but in fact it is simply a *different* kind of desire. The clinician should keep in mind that the wish to be close is the "mother" of *receptive desire* and typically involves the absence of erotic lusting. It is a predecessor to both lust and subsequent arousal.[5]

While keeping in mind possible physical and biological etiologies, the clinician needs to be perpetually mindful of the common, but normal and problematic, sexual interaction difficulties that exist between the sexes. As described in the following paragraphs, some of them can be misinterpreted as blaming men for many desire-reducing phenomena that commonly occur. For the most part, however, they are a manifestation of complex biological, psychological, evolutionary, and cultural differences between men and women. Through sex therapy, counseling, education, and treatment, sexual problem-inducing phenomena are amenable to alteration and change in a positive and pro-sexual direction.

Sexual Problem-Inducing Phenomena

There are at least eight phenomena that take place between men and women that can induce sexual problems.

1. In long-term relationships, it is normal for both partners to experience a *loss of desire*. Loss of desire is a common and expectable outcome associated with increased complementarity and closeness, and not necessarily a sign of a disorder. In well-balanced, enduring relationships, interpersonal compatibility improves while erotic energy often declines.[6] This distressing phenomenon implies more of a need for psychoeducation, couple creativity, and the possible use of a health coach knowledgeable about sex.
2. *Loss of desire for a specific partner* is different than generalized loss of desire for all partners or potential partners. Part of any treatment intervention involves helping couples confront an uncomfortable experiential reality by being truthful. It is virtually impossible to address individual or specific desire loss without such an acknowledgment.
3. Many women complain that their male partner is *too predictable*. Many women feel they always know what he is going to do next. Predictability can be boring, while surprise and differences can be exciting. Despite constant feedback from women, many men continue to be repetitive and stereotyped in their sexual behavior.
4. Many happily partnered women experience their male partner as trying to *turn every affectionate encounter into a sexual one*. This experience by women is a major factor in creating interpersonal distance and lowered desire. This often has a negative impact on women's desire and an unintended secondary and reciprocal effect on her male partner, who feels unwanted.
5. Low desire in women can be an indirect result of men being penile-centric and expecting women to be *genitally focused* as well. Women are more globally responsive, and prefer global stimulation both physically and verbally. Also, many men tend to focus on the women's genitals and breasts, often with more force and vigor than is comfortable for the woman. Despite being presented with this complaint by women, as well as having good intentions, some men have difficulty altering this behavior.

6. A significant number of women complain that men *do not pay sufficient attention to how they react both* before and during sex. As a result, women may feel that men are nonresponsive to their needs. This behavior is experienced as interpersonally insensitive, frequently results in low desire, and also impairs arousal. It triggers a belief that the man is not making love to the woman but instead is overly focused on her body and sex organs in a way that is objectifying and degrading and renders them personally invisible. Women say things like: "It feels as though he is masturbating on my body, and that I am unimportant." These experiences frequently exist in relationships that are, in an overall sense, satisfying to both partners, but are even more common in troubled relationships.
7. Women often do not understand that many men *access their real feelings of love and affection mostly when they are sexually aroused.*
8. Women may mistakenly conclude that they are only desired for what they can offer sexually. This is exemplified by women hearing "I love you" immediately before and during sex, and only then, and not in other non-erotic, affectionate contexts. In long-term relationships, women's interest in sex with their partner is usually associated with the man's nonsexual psychological expressed affection, presence, attentiveness, helpfulness, and the degree to which he demonstrates a caring attitude. Such is the case both prior to and after explicit sexual interaction is on the table.

In summary, the integrated care team needs to consider the responses to all of the core questions presented in the section on assessment, plus the presence of any of these eight phenomena, as well as medications, and medical history. Together, these factors will be suggestive of the next steps needed in order to arrive at a conclusive diagnosis or, alternatively, to direct the team toward a well-targeted referral and/or treatment(s).

TREATMENT SPECIFICS FOR SEXUAL PROBLEMS

The focus of the chapter to this point has been to present a foundation for understanding sexual problems from a multifactorial/multidisciplinary perspective, with an eye on assessment and diagnosis. From here on, the emphasis is upon treatment, with the clinician always being mindful that interventions along biological, psychological, and relationship dimensions may be required, even in cases where the primary etiology rests in only one of the three causal areas.

Psychosocial Interventions: All Major Problems in Couples and Individuals

Depending upon the assessment, different types of interventions include: (1) individual counseling/psychotherapy; (2) patient and partner coaching/sex education; (3) couples' therapy for relationship difficulties that cause sexual problems; and (4) exercise-based sex therapy for a relationship that works satisfactorily except for sex. One or more of these interventions should take place *concurrently* with any needed medical intervention conducted by the PCP, the BHS, or an external specialist. Most experienced BHSs are familiar with these approaches, except for exercise-based sex therapy, which will be described next.

Traditional exercise-based sex therapy was originally developed in an organized form by Masters and Johnson as a set of mutual touching exercises for couples to use. It was aimed at reducing anxiety and then expanded to include a psychodynamic perspective by Helen Singer Kaplan.[7–9] Depending upon the state of the couple's relationship, it can often be used in a straightforward, almost protocol-driven manner by psychotherapists without having to endlessly analyze resistances and deeper issues. Kaplan, in her landmark volumes,[7,8] which include illustrations, provides specific steps for treating low desire, arousal, orgasm problems, and premature ejaculation. All clinicians who choose to work in this area are strongly encouraged to familiarize themselves with her work.

The first two steps in the sex therapy treatment process are referred to as *sensate focus* exercises, in that they remove all demands for sexual excitement, arousal, and performance. In Sensate Focus I, the partners are asked to touch each other sensually (staying away from genitals and breasts), without the expectation of becoming aroused or orgasmic, but simply to *focus upon giving and receiving sensual (not erotic) pleasure.* In Sensate Focus II, mutual pleasuring is expanded to include breasts and genitals, but without any attempt to bring about high levels of arousal and/or orgasm. During these first two early but crucial steps, the couple is asked to agree *not to turn or convert unplanned arousal into a full-scale erotic encounter.* This agreement cannot be overemphasized, as violation of it usually results in an unwitting sabotage of the treatment. Following Sensate Focus I and II, and over a series of visits with intermittent homework, the partners are helped to gradually progress to incrementally higher levels of erotic pleasure. Between homework sessions, and during visits to the therapist's office, the couple discusses how each session felt, what worked, what did not work, and what can be learned from the problems that emerged during the homework. Further steps include highly specific exercises targeting the identified problem.[7,8]

A word of caution: Assigning a couple the exercises without parallel and intermittent office consultations is inevitably a formula for treatment failure. In even the best treatments, things often go wrong during homework. These may include physical discomfort, interpersonal tension, a reluctance to tell one's partner that something does not feel good, etc. It is the explicit exploration of such problems, along with the therapist's help, that is often the key to treatment success.

Desire, Arousal, Orgasm, and Pain Problems (Women)—Medical Interventions

The overriding primary medical approach to the major sexual problem areas is to add agonists and remove antagonists (Table 21.3). Agonists are typically pharmaceutical, hormonal, or moisturizing agents that are pro-sexual. They facilitate and/or increase desire, arousal, and orgasm while lessening pain. Antagonists are essentially antisexual in that they serve to decrease desire, arousal, orgasm and/or to increase pain.

Overall, major antagonists are oral estrogens when used for hormone replacement therapy, including birth control pills, as well as the adverse effects associated with common medications such as selective serotonin reuptake inhibitors (SSRIs), selective norepinephrine reuptake inhibitors (SNRIs), antipsychotics, antihypertensives, and antifungals. Most major agonists fall into a few basic categories: hormonal (e.g., transdermal estrogens, testosterone), dopaminergics, lubricants, and moisturizers.

Some medical interventions involve approaches that do not by definition easily fall into either of these categories. For example, some women may need to consult with a pelvic floor physical therapist experienced in dealing with sexual problems associated with childbirth-induced trauma, loss of pelvic tone associated with the perimenopausal transition, bicycle seat–induced damage, and so on. While the reader may be familiar with the Kegel exercise, there are a range of other pelvic floor interventions that have proven efficacious in the treatment of arousal, orgasm, and pain (e.g., myofascial release). Every primary care team should locate a pelvic floor physical therapist in its area.[30]

While Table 21.3 presents a multiplicity of ways to administer estrogen and testosterone for women, a few key points need to be reemphasized:

1. While testosterone is the hormone of desire, a woman requires sufficient estrogenization as a precondition for the effective circulation of bioavailable testosterone.
2. Exogenous, transdermal estrogen should almost always be the first medical intervention prior to employing transdermal testosterone.[13,23,24]
3. Before prescribing testosterone, the clinician should seek endogenous approaches to increasing the patient's own bioavailable levels, such as reducing medications and changing poor lifestyle choices that increase sex hormone-binding globulin (SHBG).

Desire Problems (Men)—Medical Interventions

As with women, the primary medical approach for men is to remove antagonists, such as antisexual medications, particularly SSRIs and antihypertensives, as well as other agents that reduce bioavailable testosterone (e.g., beer and chronic moderate alcohol use), while adding agonists, such as testosterone and phosphodiesterase inhibitors.[31–33] Notably, many testosterone antagonists are linked with a resistant-to-change unhealthy lifestyle (e.g., poor diet and insufficient exercise). Positive lifestyle changes, which increase bioavailable testosterone by lowering SHBG and hemoglobin A1C, can play a major role in increasing desire. The clinician can easily overlook chronic, moderate alcohol use because it is socially acceptable. Simply asking a patient to evaluate and consider reducing alcohol consumption may prove helpful. Many physicians report that decreasing alcohol use increases bioavailable testosterone.[33]

TABLE 21.3 WOMEN: HORMONAL, PHARMACOLOGIC, MECHANICAL, PHYSICAL INTERVENTIONS TO ADDRESS PROBLEMS WITH DESIRE, AROUSAL, AND PAIN

Targeted Symptom/ Problem	Treatment Intervention	Generic Name (Brand Name)	Dosing	Comments
		Non-Systemic Treatments		
Vaginal dryness/ Dyspareunia	Water-based lubricants	Glycerol (Astroglide), Glycerol (KY)	Apply topically to genitals.	Used to reduce friction; effects can diminish during sex. Reapplication might be necessary. Episodic use.
Dyspareunia—Mild/ moderate vaginal dryness, not responsive to emollients (topical)	Moisturizers	Vitamin E gel (Replens)	Apply topically to genitals.	Coats the vaginal lining. Used daily to reduce vaginal discomfort. Not for episodic use.
Vaginal dryness, atrophy, dyspareunia; not responsive to treatments above.	Topical and internal estradiol and other estrogens. Note: Many patients with atrophic vaginas benefit greatly from progressive self-dilation over several weeks.[10] See comments.	Topical estradiol cream (Estrace), Conjugated Equine Estrogen (Premarin cream), local estradiol tablets (Vagifem)	Apply topically or internally.	Dyspareunia causes low desire (ospemifene and testosterone cream, via different pharmacologic mechanisms, also can be used to treat dyspareunia). Dilator sets can easily be purchased through the Internet, or are available by prescription.
		Systemic Estrogen (with the Exception of Estring)		
Vaginal atrophy, dyspareunia, vasomotor symptoms (e.g., hot flashes), depression, hormonally related low sexual desire.	Oral estrogen, conjugated equine estrogen (often used in conjunction with medroxyprogesterone acetate [MPA]). See comments.[11,12]	Example: Premarin	Once daily	Oral and transdermal estrogens address vaginal atrophy over the long term. A topical, vaginally applied estrogen cream and/or progressive dilation accelerates the curative process dramatically. (Oral estrogen increases SHBG, decreases bioavailable testosterone and estrogen. Do not use oral as first-choice estrogen therapy.)
		Patches and Transvaginal Approaches to Systemic Estradiol		
Vaginal atrophy, dyspareunia, vasomotor symptoms (e.g., hot flashes, insomnia), depression, hormonally related low sexual desire	Transdermal estrogen patches (bio-identical 17β estradiol) (most popular route of administration)[13,14]	Examples: Climara and Vivelle Dot	Once or twice weekly (five dose levels available)	See comment above. For women with a uterus, authors, as supported by research, suggest bio-identical progesterone (e.g., micronized progesterone [Prometrium]). MPA has been associated with adverse reactions.[15]

Vaginal atrophy, dyspareunia, vasomotor symptoms (e.g., hot flashes), hormonally related low sexual desire and depression	Transdermal estradiol gels or mist (bio-identical 17β estradiol). Some patients do not like transdermal patch and prefer these routes.	Examples: Elestrin, Divigel, Estrogel, Evamist	Apply once daily to the skin:	Alternative to patches: non-oral, non-transdermal patches, as route of administration. Precise control of dose levels is challenging with mist and gel products, often resulting in chronic lower-than-prescribed amounts being applied by the patient.
Vaginal atrophy, dyspareunia, vasomotor symptoms (e.g., hot flashes), depression, hormonally related low sexual desire	Transvaginal estradiol rings	Estradiol (Femring and Estring)	Insert vaginally for 3 months. First time inserted by physician, thereafter by patient.	Femring targets both vaginal atrophy and vasomotor symptoms, while Estring is local and non-systemic and targets only vaginal atrophy.
Vaginal atrophy, dyspareunia, vasomotor symptoms (e.g., hot flashes), depression, hormonally related low sexual desire	Topical compounded estradiol advertised as "bio-identical," containing estrogen, progesterone, and testosterone[15]	No brand name, provided by compounding pharmacies	Varies: applied to skin or in tablet form sublingual	Caution: Not approved by the U.S. Food and Drug Administration (FDA). What is on the label is not necessarily in the container; what the patient actually gets may vary from day to day. It is *unnecessary* to employ commercially promoted so-called bio-identical compounds as all are available in FDA-approved, pharmaceutically produced formulations.[16] Exception is compounded testosterone/E2 for vestibulitis.
		Non-Estrogen Approach		
Dyspareunia with vaginal atrophy	Oral selective estrogen reuptake modulators (SERMs)[17]	Ospemifene (Osphena)	60 mg/day with food	FDA-approved oral SERM that effectively and safely treats dyspareunia. May be beneficial for bones and similar to tamoxifen in breasts.
Dyspareunia: pain and erythema located at the vestibule. Also commonly referred to as vulvar vestibulitis, vestibulodynia, and VVS.	Topical compounded testosterone/estrogen cream[18]	Compounding pharmacy	Estradiol 0.03%, testosterone 0.01% twice daily to the erythematous vestibule. Discontinue oral birth control pills.	Usually responds within a few weeks. Goldstein now suggests dose as estradiol 0.01% and testosterone 0.1% (A. Goldstein in email 3/11/16 to A. Altman).
		Electro-Mechanical Devices		
Vaginal atrophy	Intravaginal CO_2 laser treatment[19,20]	Mona Lisa Touch	Not applicable	FDA approved, with early studies indicating high patient satisfaction. Claims to work by enhancing vaginal epithelium and blood supply.

(continued)

TABLE 21.3 CONTINUED

Targeted Symptom/ Problem	Treatment Intervention	Generic Name (Brand Name)	Dosing	Comments
		Testosterone		
Desire and arousal	Dehydroepiandrosterone (DHEA)[21,22]	Prasterone (Intra-Rosa)	0.5% Vaginal suppository daily	DHEA is a precursor to testosterone and is an indirect way to elevate levels; slow in action and more efficacious in older women. Caution: Purchase from reputable manufacturers.
Desire and arousal/orgasm problems	Transdermal testosterone[23,24]	Testosterone (Androgel, Testim, Axiron)	Use of male products off-label for women in much lower doses	Not FDA approved for women but used off-label. Beware of side effects, including hair growth, acne, hair loss, voice lowering, and clitoromegaly. Aromatized to estradiol: use caution with breast cancer patients. See methyltestosterone and ospemifene (Osphena) as alternatives.
Low desire	Flibanserin[25]	Flibanserin (Addyi)	100 mg/daily at bedtime	Modulates serotonin and dopamine in frontal cortex and can be used concurrently with sex therapy. FDA approved for premenopausal women.
Low desire and as antidote to SSRI side effects	Buproprion,[26] buspirone[27]	Bupropion (Wellbutrin XL), buspirone (Buspar)	Doses vary.	Bupropion is a desire agonist. Buspirone is effective for side effect reduction *only* in women.[26]
Low desire, arousal, orgasm problems	Discontinue and/or reduce oral estrogen, SSRIs, and other antisexual medications.[26–28]	All hormone replacement therapy oral hormones, SSRIs, SNRIs, oral contraceptive pills, antihypertensives, and antipsychotics	Most adverse effects are dose-related. Reduce to minimum effective dosing.	Side effects of SSRIs vary but appear to be strongest in inhibiting orgasm.[26]
Genital arousal problems	Phosphodiesterase inhibitors (PDE-5s or PDE-11s)	Tadalafil (Cialis), Sildenafil (Viagra), Vardenafil (Levitra), Sildenafil	Doses vary.	PDE-5s have some reported efficacy for many women but especially for genital arousal disorder (always rule out other medical etiology).[28,29]

Similarly, the clinician should consider the role of chronic masturbation and concomitant use of internet pornography when the patient is reporting low desire.[4] Stopping or radically reducing compulsive masturbation can both increase desire and improve the ability to achieve and maintain a lasting erection. Table 21.4 gives details on medical and behavioral interventions for men.

Arousal Problems (Men, Women, and Couples)

Psychosocial Interventions

The core of nonmedical psychosocial intervention for arousal problems is couple sex therapy. It involves dialogue-rich counseling, interspersed with exercises and supplemented by relevant educational information from the clinician.

TABLE 21.4 MEN: HORMONAL, PHARMACOLOGIC, MECHANICAL, SURGICAL, PHYSICAL, AND BEHAVIORAL INTERVENTIONS FOR PROBLEMS WITH DESIRE, AROUSAL, AND ORGASM

Symptom/ Problem	Treatment Intervention	Generic Name/Brand Name and Dosing	Comments
Desire	Transdermal testosterone[32]	Testosterone (Androgel, Testim, Axiron, Testopel); dosing varies as per manufacturer and patient response.	Axiron applied to the armpits. Testopel injectable, subdermal tablet form. Employed when transdermals do not absorb.
Desire	Injectable testosterone[32]	Testosterone enanthate (Delastryl), testosterone cypionate (Depo-testosterone); 50 mg twice a week by injection	Possible long-term negative effects on bioavailable testosterone as a result of increased estrogen[33]
Desire, erectile dysfunction inhibited, delayed/ impaired ejaculation	Discontinue/reduce SSRIs/SNRIs, antihypertensives, benzodiazepines, and other antisexual medications.[32,34,35]	Multiple generic names, including hydrochlorothiazide, metoprolol, atenolol, and many others	Review all medications and interactions. SSRIs/SNRIs inhibit ejaculation.
Desire, erectile dysfunction inhibited, delayed/ impaired ejaculation	Stop/dramatically decrease masturbation for several months. Includes elimination of compulsive pornography.[4,36,37]	Not applicable	A virtual epidemic of delayed/inhibited ejaculation exists among younger men in conjunction with compulsive use of pornography.[36]
Premature ejaculation	Add SSRIs/SNRIs.[38,39]	Multiple generics (e.g., fluoxetine, sertraline). Begin with low dose (e.g., 50 mg of sertraline) and increase if needed.	Often unnecessary as exercise-based sex therapy is usually effective, but can be useful as adjunct
Premature ejaculation	Topical lidocaine	Many brands (e.g., Promescent); one pump from spray container	Applied to the glans penis. Mixed efficacy, but appears to help some men.

(continued)

TABLE 21.4 CONTINUED

Symptom/ Problem	Treatment Intervention	Generic Name/Brand Name and Dosing	Comments
Desire, erectile dysfunction	Discontinue/reduce alcohol use.	Not applicable	Negative impact of chronic and even short-term use of ethyl alcohol (ETOH) on desire and performance. The problem is often ignored by clinicians.
Erectile dysfunction	PDE-5 and 11	Sildenafil (Viagra), 25–100 mg Vardenafil (Levitra), 2.5–20 mg Vardenafil (Staxyn), 10–20 mg Tadalafil (Cialis), 2.5–20 mg; 5 mg/day or 20 mg prior to sex	Approved by U.S. Food and Drug Administration (FDA). Staxyn dissolves on tongue. Tadalafil lasts for up to 36 hours, not influenced by food intake (see text).
Erectile dysfunction	Intercavernosal injections of Alprostadil	Alprostadil = Prostaglandin (Caverject, Edex); doses vary and are determined by physician	FDA approved. Patient learns to self-inject at home. Often effective when other approaches fail.
Erectile dysfunction	Vacuum erection device	Not applicable	FDA approved. Vacuum suction device mechanically engorges the penis.
Erectile dysfunction	Surgically inserted prosthesis; nonreversible	A variety of inflatable and non-inflatable devices exist.	Generally, high patient satisfaction despite anxiety associated with procedure

Arousal is defined as becoming sexually excited, both physically and subjectively (mentally). In men, it is manifested by an erection, in women by both a subjective sense of excitement and genital vascularization, lubrication, swelling, and usually an increase in erotic breast sensation. Women, in contrast to most men, have a more global sense of excitement throughout much of their bodies while men experience arousal more locally in the penis.

Arousal or sexual excitement is the experience of desire immediately before or during sex. *The essence of arousal is the desire to become even more aroused* and ultimately experience orgasm. Desire feeds on itself. Aside from physiology, it is a product, during coupled sex, of reciprocal physical and psychological stimulation. In many long-term relationships, partners struggle to maintain excitement during sex. This phenomenon is often, but not always, directly related to loss of desire. In men, the loss of excitement is associated with loss of an erection, while in women it is experienced both physically and subjectively.

Therapeutically, it is essential for the clinician to promote interpersonal risk taking, often based upon information garnered earlier during individual meetings with each of the partners. Although partners may be worried about offending and hurting their counterpart, candor is a requirement for treatment success. During such dialogues, which are often uneasy and anxiety-laden, explicit acknowledgment by each partner of his or her experiential *truths* can serve as a springboard for helping the couple reinvent and revitalize their sexual enjoyment.

Some typical "truths" or comments people make include: "He (or she) is a lousy lover," "I hate it when he touches me the way he does," "He (she) never washes his (her) hands and face and then jumps into bed with me," "His (her) smell bothers me," and "The way he (she) makes love to me is boring and predictable."

Finally, many couples benefit from a variety of attempts to "spice things up" through the use of sensate focus, sex games, role playing, erotic films, and having sex in unconventional locations. There is a plethora of books available, not to mention magazine articles, on how couples can enhance their sexual pleasure.[6–8]

Combined Medical and Psychosocial Interventions for Arousal (Women)

A small but significant percentage of women experience subjective arousal without physiologic correlates (vascularization/lubrication), as well as the converse (physical arousal/lubrication without subjective pleasure). Also, physiologic arousal can occur with or without pain. During subjective arousal, if pain is present, possible structural and/or hormonal intervention may be required. Often, examination and treatment by a pelvic floor physical therapist can be useful. However, in the presence of "working physiology" and a healthy pelvic floor, questions arise about what may be transpiring psychologically or in the relationship. When chronic, subjective arousal is unaccompanied by physiologic arousal, the condition is known as genital arousal disorder. A few major causal possibilities should be considered. These include genital atrophy and physical trauma (e.g., childbirth injuries, playground accidents, bike seat injuries). Often, and regardless of etiology, genital arousal disorder can frequently be treated successfully with a PDE-5 inhibitor.[29]

Among the most widely employed and efficacious approaches to arousal and orgasm problems is directed masturbation.[7,8,40–42] It is described in detail by Kaplan in her classic handbook, *The Illustrated Manual of Sex Therapy*.[8] It is employed for both partnered and unpartnered women.

The clinician advises and instructs the woman on how to masturbate, using a sex toy, often a vibrator, along with erotic stimuli of her choice (visual, literature, fantasy). For some naïve or inhibited patients, it may be necessary to provide them with assistance in purchasing a device. Instructional videotapes are widely available. Showing patients the illustrations in the manual can be helpful for both instructional and normalizing purposes.

The clinician always needs to be sensitive to cultural, religious, and/or deeply held values in patients that forbid self-stimulation. Often, this objection disappears if the patient masturbates in the presence of her partner rather than alone. (Also see the section on "Orgasm in Women").

Combined Medical and Psychosocial Interventions for Arousal (Men)

ED is the most common male complaint heard by primary care clinicians.[1] All male arousal problems are characterized by ED, the inability of a man to attain and/or maintain an erection. While usually discussed in the literature with respect to penetrative sexual intercourse, it also a frequent and distressing problem for couples and individuals who engage in nonpenetrative sex.

Pharmaceutical companies tend to present ED as due to vascular insufficiency or performance anxiety, but there are many other causes. Common examples include fear about causing pain to a partner secondary to vaginal atrophy, fears of hurting his recently ill partner, and anxiety in a man with cardiovascular disease due to fear of overexertion. Bicycle seats are a cause of ED, as well as many medications, especially SSRIs and antihypertensives.[34] Other major culprits include diabetes and nerve damage secondary to prostatectomies.

The primary psychosocial treatment of ED is exercise-based couple sex therapy, employing Sensate Focus I and II plus specific steps during which the man's partner stimulates him to purposely gain and lose, and then regain, an erection, followed by "non-demand intercourse."[7] In one variation of this approach, the couple is instructed to have the man intentionally lose his erection, withdraw, and then regain it (with stimulation from the partner), and then restart intercourse. The relationship and individual psychological dimensions of ED or premature ejaculation are almost impossible to treat without couple sessions.

The most common medical treatments for ED are phosphodiesterase inhibitors.[4,7] While it is traditional in medicine to start a patient with the lowest possible effective dose, there may be some advantage to starting with a moderately higher dose and then lowering it once the patient has success in achieving a workable erection. Specifically, performance anxiety can often trump a PDE-5, even at higher doses. Hence, it is suggested to start higher, achieve success, then lower the dose, as an initial failure due to a low dose is likely to stimulate anxiety and possibly reduce probability of success.

The clinician has a range of other medical options, some of which include the removal or decrease of antisexual medications, surgical prostheses, vacuum erection devices, intracavernosal injections, and lifestyle changes. Table 21.4 gives details on these and other medical interventions.

Often psychosocial interventions, in conjunction with medication, can be efficacious. The combination of the two modalities has proven clinically advantageous, especially when the man's anxiety is high.

Orgasm Problems (Men)

Premature ejaculation and inhibited/delayed ejaculation are the two major male orgasm problems. Inhibited ejaculation typically occurs with non-penetrative couple sex as well as intercourse, except when a man is stimulating himself in or out of the presence of his partner.

Premature ejaculation ranges from unwanted ejaculation prior to penile insertion into a vagina, to the most common form in which ejaculation occurs within a minute or less after insertion and/or prior to when the man would choose to ejaculate. Ultimately, the definition is subjective. Men *never* complain about ejaculating prematurely when masturbating, indicating that the problem typically has psychological and/or relationship causation and consequences. When chronic, it is a frustrating experience for both partners and typically results in mutual avoidance of partnered sex.

Inhibited or delayed ejaculation (historically referred to as retarded ejaculation) is categorized by the authors into Type I and Type II. Type I is usually lifelong and associated with extreme difficulty in ejaculating during penetrative sex (not during masturbation). Due to low prevalence, as well as disagreement between practitioners over causes and treatment, it will not be addressed here. Type II inhibited/delayed ejaculation is often secondary to compulsive masturbation and/or overuse of pornography and is treated by the man dramatically reducing or stopping masturbation. In some cases, it presents as a symptom of guilt—for example, when having sex with a new partner following the death of a lifelong partner. It is most effectively treated with brief psychodynamic individual psychotherapy.[7,43]

Sex therapy, employing Sensate Focus I and II plus Stop, Start, Squeeze (SSS) techniques in the context of couple counseling, is the first choice for treating premature ejaculation, although it is often supplemented by the use of an SSRI (Table 21.4).[7,38] Essentially, SSS helps the man to focus his attention on when he reaches an arousal level just prior to ejaculatory inevitability; he then immediately asks his partner to stop stimulating him until his arousal level reduces, then restart stimulation, repeating this same SSS cycle up to about four times during the same session. On the last cycle, the man and his partner are given "permission" for him to reach orgasm without any attempt to stop. This intervention has a high rate of success.[7,8]

Another less frequently employed but nevertheless effective approach is *directed repetitive sex* occurring within a two-day time span. It may be used in conjunction with sensate focus/stop-start interventions. It typically begins on a Friday evening and continues over a weekend. The couple first has an initial session with the therapist. The partners are directed to engage in penetrative sex after the visit, using Sensate Focus I and II plus SSS when they subsequently have sex. They are asked to repeat penetrative sex in the morning when they arise, return to a midmorning therapy session, engage in sex again in the afternoon, return to the therapist in the evening, after which they will be directed to have sex again, and then again the next morning, always following the same sequence described above. It is common for men to have erectile difficulties due to diminished physiologic reserve associated with having sex so frequently. A PDE-5 can be useful in this circumstance as the couple continues to have repeated sex over the weekend. Parallel, intermittent couple counseling during the two days is an essential element in this intervention.

Lidocaine spray also appears to be helpful for some men. It dulls sensations on the penis, but also can induce loss of erection and/or transfer to the woman's genitals. A recent, as yet unpublished study indicates that one particular over-the-counter lidocaine spray (Promescent) has demonstrated high patient satisfaction with no transfer of anesthesia effects to the partner.

Orgasm Problems (Women)

The lifelong inability of a woman to achieve orgasm, despite the arousal level, has been classified as *primary anorgasmia*. If she experienced orgasms in the past but no longer does, the problem is classified as *secondary anorgasmia*. The clinician must distinguish whether the problem exists generally or only in certain situations. If she is able to achieve an orgasm with masturbation but not with a partner, the treatment implications are different: Anorgasmia occurring only with a partner suggests the need for sex therapy. *Primary anorgasmia* is considered to be easily treatable with brief couple sex therapy or through directed masturbation. Again, if consistent with the patient's values, permission and encouragement should be given by the clinician to explore self-stimulation in private, using erotica of her choice, and various sex toys including a vibrator and/or a genital suction device.[7,8,40–42]

Many women believe there is something wrong with them if they are anorgasmic during penetrative sex. In fact, it is a very common experience, and the clinician should normalize this with both the patient and her partner. Many men experience distress in reaction to female anorgasmia and often blame themselves or the woman.

For a number of reasons, including possible feelings of shame or lack of awareness, some women are uncomfortable simultaneously stimulating themselves during intercourse or asking the partner to do it for them. This should be suggested by the clinician, who might also encourage the patient and partner to obtain educational materials that illustrate and normalize these techniques. A mixture of couple counseling along with Sensate Focus, followed by exercises aimed at having the partner unselfishly please the woman, is the treatment of choice. For orgasm-relevant medical interventions, see Table 21.3, since most of the listed interventions address problems in the sexual arousal cycle that ultimately lead to orgasm.

Sexual Pain (Women)

The following overview of pain treatment contains information and concepts pertinent to assessment and diagnosis rather than direct intervention. *However, in the case of treating the nuanced complexity of sexual pain, the assessment/interview is an integral element of the treatment itself.* It is, therefore, presented at this juncture rather than earlier in the chapter.

Sexual pain or *dyspareunia* is often, but not always, reported to clinicians, especially gynecologists. Pain can be experienced in many different places and contexts: at the introitus, deep in the vagina, only with motion, when a tampon or finger is inserted, and so forth. For some women, it may hurt in all contexts, while in others only during sex, and for others in some, but not all, sexual positions.

Many women consider sexual pain to be normal, choose to ignore it, and then do not report the problem to their physician. Sometimes, pain leads to an inability to allow, let alone enjoy, even wished-for penile entry (vaginismus). Painful sex has a wide variety of psychological and biological etiologies. It should always be treated as a *pain* problem, not necessarily as one that is psychological in origin. Although it often has psychological causes and negative relationship sequelae, the treatment team needs to be acutely aware of the possibility that disorders such as pelvic inflammatory disease and endometriosis may play a causal role. The clinician should keep in mind that vulvovaginal pain can exist with and without penetration, in both sexual and nonsexual contexts.

The physical, psychological, and relationship factors that can cause dyspareunia are complex, with no particular health care specialty necessarily trained to sort them out. The integrated care team, including a BHS collaborating with a gynecologist, offers the best choice for effective care. If possible, it is helpful for the partner to be present during the discussion of these issues.

Aside from being attentive to medical/physical factors as outlined and detailed in Table 21.3, the centerpiece for treating pain in women should be couple counseling integrated with exercise-based sex therapy, including Sensate Focus exercises and the use of progressive dilation, when indicated. Nondemand intercourse, with the woman in control of penetration and motion, is often a crucial element in this enterprise.[7,8] On occasion, individual psychodynamic therapy as well as cognitive-behavioral therapy can be useful.[43] Finally, encouraging results of the newly approved laser therapy for atrophic vaginas may be worth considering as another option.[19,20]

HORMONE TREATMENT: SUGGESTIONS AND PRECAUTIONS

Laboratory assays should not be the sole determinant for making conclusions about hormonal treatments. Laboratory results can be misleading, and many individuals with "normal" levels are often quickly responsive to exogenous testosterone or estrogen.[16] For example, it is common for clinicians to obtain an estradiol or follicle-stimulating hormone (FSH) level that falls within normal assay parameters. The clinician then sends the patient away, despite her experiencing florid hot flashes and night sweats, without prescribing transdermal estrogen. No one knows what the "right" levels are. *Symptoms should determine treatment.*

Exogenous estrogen received negative publicity as a result of the misleading interpretation of the findings from the Women's Health Initiative study, as well as its inappropriate choice of subjects. Both clinicians and patients subsequently became reluctant to employ it, despite many outstanding re-analyses of the data, as well as other excellent studies and meta-analyses, all of which have demonstrated that when properly used, *estrogen is both efficacious and safe.*[7,11,12]

The evidence that transdermal estrogen can restore sexual desire in a patient using oral estrogen is both logical and strong. The increase in SHBG, due to oral estrogen's first pass through the liver, is avoided with transdermal products, which will ultimately correct the unfavorable decrease in both bioavailable testosterone and estrogen. Transdermal use will also avoid the first-pass increase in C-reactive protein and clotting factors associated with oral estrogen, and their negative impact on cardiovascular health.[13,14]

Testosterone in men and women is efficacious and safe. There are numerous studies indicating that exogenous testosterone, either by injection or patches, increases sexual desire in both genders.[23,24,31,33] With respect to safety in men, the U.S. Food and Drug Administration in 2014 suggested that physicians exercise caution in employing previously approved testosterone, citing two recent studies that suggested an increase in cardiovascular events.[44] However, in a compelling analysis reviewing all the published findings on testosterone efficacy and safety in men, other investigators concluded: "There is no convincing evidence of increased cardiovascular (CV) risks with testosterone (T) therapy. On the contrary, there appears to be a strong beneficial relationship between normal T and CV health that has not yet been widely appreciated."[45] Similar findings on its safety in women have been published. Especially notable is the work of Davis at Monash University in Australia.[24] Finally, very recent evidence on Addyi, a non-hormonal, FDA approved pill for low desire in premenopausal women, also has beneficial impact on sexual pain, arousal and satisfaction.[46,47] Furthermore, at least one other investigation indicates it is equally efficacious for post-menopausal women.[25]

CONCLUSION

We hope that this chapter stimulates the interest of the integrated care team to engage in a discussion of sexual problems and functioning with their patients, thus opening the door to an important aspect of people's lives that is rarely addressed. See Box 21.4 for the summary of the evidence supporting our approach for this chapter.

BOX 21.4

SUMMARY OF RECOMMENDED TREATMENT APPROACHES AND RELEVANT EVIDENCE

Strength of recommendation taxonomy (SOR A, B, or C)

- **Exogenous estrogen is efficacious and safe for the treatment of vasomotor symptoms associated with the menopausal transition within 10 years of a woman's last period (SOR A).[11,12]**
- **Transdermal estrogen, as contrasted with oral, is even safer with respect to cardiovascular events such as venous thromboembolism (SOR A).[13,14]**
- **Exogenous testosterone is efficacious and safe for the treatment of low sexual desire in hypogonadal men who do not have a diagnosis of prostate cancer and women (SOR A).[23,24,31,45]**
- **Flibanserin is efficacious and safe for treating low sexual desire in premenopausal women (SOR B).[25]**
- **Osphemipene is a safe and efficacious treatment for vaginal dyspareunia causing low sexual desire in postmenopausal women (SOR B).[17]**
- **Testosterone is efficacious and safe for the treatment of low sexual desire in postmenopausal women (SOR B).[23,24]**
- **Sex therapy techniques are a primary form of treatment for most sexual problems (SOR C).[6,7]**
- **Compounded testosterone cream is highly successful in treating vestibulitis (SOR C).[18]**

A small but incremental increase in knowledge of sexual health by PCPs in collaboration with their integrated team colleagues, accompanied by the proactive use of simple screening instruments and a few basic questions asked to patients, can lead to effective treatment of sexual problems. The positive impact on the lives of patients, partners, and their families will be appreciated by all.

The authors wish to express their deepest gratitude to Jannet Gaesser for her wonderful editorial skills, persistence, patience and thoughtful contributions to this chapter.

REFERENCES

1. Metz ME, Seifert MH. Men's expectations of physicians in sexual health concerns. J Sex Marital Ther. 1990;16(2):79–88.
2. Marwick C. Survey says patients expect little physician help on sex. JAMA. 1999;281(23):2173–2174.
3. American Psychiatric Association. Diagnostic and Statistical Manual of Mental Disorders, 5th ed. Washington, DC: American Psychiatric Publishing; 2013.
4. Hatzimouratidis K, Amar E, Eardley I, et al. Guidelines on male sexual dysfunction: Erectile dysfunction and premature ejaculation. Eur Urol. 2010;57(5):804–814.
5. Basson R. The female sexual response: A different model. J Sex Marital Ther. 2000;26(1):51–65.
6. Schnarch DM. Sexual desire: A systemic prescriptive. In: Leiblum SR, Rosen RC, eds. Principles and Practices of Sex Therapy. 3rd ed. New York: Guilford Press; 2000:17–56.
7. Kaplan HS. The New Sex Therapy. New York: Brunner/Mazel; 1974.
8. Kaplan HS. The Illustrated Manual of Sex Therapy. New York: Quadrangle/New York Times Book Co.; 1975.
9. Masters WH, Johnson VE. Human Sexual Response. Toronto, Canada: Bantam Books; 1966.
10. Lindahl SH. Reviewing the options for local estrogen treatment of vaginal atrophy. Int J Womens Health. 2014;6(1):307–312.
11. Hodis HN, Mack WJ. The timing hypothesis and hormone replacement therapy: A paradigm shift in the primary prevention of coronary heart disease in women. Part 1: Comparison of therapeutic efficacy. J Am Geriatr Soc. 2013;61(6):1005–1010.
12. Hodis HN, Mack WJ. The timing hypothesis and hormone replacement therapy: A paradigm shift in the primary prevention of coronary heart disease in women. Part 2: Comparative risks. J Am Geriatr Soc.2013;61(6):1011–1018.
13. Canonico M, Oger E, Plu-Bureau G, Conrad J, Meyer G, Levesque H, et al. Hormone therapy and venous thromboembolism among postmenopausal women: Impact of the route of estrogen administration and progestogens: The ESTHER study. Circulation. 2007;115(7):840–845.
14. Postmenopausal estrogen therapy: Route of administration and risk of venous thromboembolism. Committee Opinion No. 556. American College of Obstetricians and Gynecologists. Obstet Gynecol. 2013;121:887–890.
15. Ghatge RP, Jacobsen BM, Schittone SA, Horwitz KB. The progestational and androgenic properties of medroxyprogesterone acetate: Gene regulatory overlap with dihydrotestosterone in breast cancer cells. Breast Cancer Res. 2005;7(6):R1036–R1050.
16. What are bioidentical hormones? Harvard Medical School. http://www.health.harvard.edu/womens-health/what-are-bioidentical-hormones. Published August 1, 2006. Updated December 4, 2015. Accessed June 6, 2016.
17. Ciu Y, Zong H, Yan H, Li N, Zhang Y. The efficacy and safety of ospemifene in treating dyspareunia associated with postmenopausal vulvar and vaginal atrophy: A systematic review and meta-analysis. J Sex Med. 2014;11(2):487–497.
18. Burrows LJ, Goldstein AT. The treatment of vestibulodynia with topical estradiol and testosterone. J Sex Med. 2013;1(1):30–33.
19. Perino A, Calligaro A, Forlani F, et al. Vulvovaginal atrophy: A new treatment modality using thermos-ablative fractional CO_2 laser. Maturitas. 2015;80(3):296–301.
20. Salvatore S, Nappi RE, Parma M, et al. Sexual function after fractional microablative CO_2 laser in women with vulvovaginal atrophy. Climacteric. 2015;18(2):219–225.
21. Labrie F. Intracrinology in action: Importance of extragonadal sex steroid biosynthesis and inactivation in peripheral tissues in both women and men. J Steroid Biochem Mol Biol. 2015;145:131–132.
22. Davis SR, Panjar M, Stanczyk FZ. Clinical review: DHEA replacement for postmenopausal women. J Clin Endocrinol Metab. 2011;96(6):1642–1653.
23. Bonfim Reis SL, Abdo CHN. Benefits and risks of testosterone treatment for hypoactive sexual desire disorder in women: A critical review of studies published in the decades preceding and succeeding the advent of phosphodiesterase type 5 inhibitors. Clinics (Sao Paulo). 2014;69(4):294–303.
24. Davis SR, Davison SL. Current perspectives on testosterone therapy for women. Menopausal Med. 2012;20(2):S1–S4.
25. Simon JA, Kingsberg SA, Shumel B, Hanes V, Garcia M, Sand M. Efficacy and safety of flibanserin in postmenopausal women with hypoactive sexual desire disorder: Results of the SNOWDROP trial. Menopause. 2014;21(6):633–640.
26. Primary Psychiatry. In Session with Anita H. Clayton, MD: An Update on the Sexual Side

Effects of Medication. http://primarypsychiatry.com/issue/march-2008-primary-psychiatry. Accessed June 6, 2016.
27. Clayton AH, Warnock JK, Kornstein SG, Pinkerton R, Sheldon-Keller A, McGarvey EL. A placebo-controlled trial of bupropion SR as an antidote for selective serotonin reuptake inhibitor-induced sexual dysfunction. J Clin Psychiatry. 2004;65(1):62–67.
28. Kennedy SH, Rizvi S. Sexual dysfunction, depression, and the impact of antidepressants. J Clin Psychopharmacol. 2009;29(2):157–164.
29. Lo Monte G, Graziano A, Piva I, Marci R. Women taking the "blue pill" (sildenafil citrate): Such a big deal? Drug Design, Development and Therapy. 2014;(8:)2251–2254. doi:https://dx.doi.org/10.2147/DDDT.S71227
30. Rosenbaum TY. Managing postmenopausal dyspareunia: Beyond hormone therapy. The Female Patient. 2006;31:1–5.
31. Morgentaler A. Testosterone for Life. New York: McGraw Hill; 2009.
32. Dean JD, McMahon CG, Guay AT, et al. The International Society for Sexual Medicine's process of care for the assessment and management of testosterone deficiency in adult men. J Sex Med. 2015;12(8):1660–1686.
33. Shippen E, Fryer W. The Testosterone Syndrome: The Critical Factor for Energy, Health and Sexuality Reversing the Male Menopause. New York: M. Evans and Company, Inc.; 1998.
34. Seagraves RT, Balon R. Sexual Pharmacology: Fast Facts. New York: WW Norton; 2003.
35. Seagraves RT. Effects of psychotropic drugs on human erection and ejaculation. Arch Gen Psychiatry. 1989;46(3):275–284.
36. Bergner RM, Bridges AJ. The significance of heavy pornography involvement for romantic partners: Research and clinical implications. J Sex Marital Ther. 2002;28(3):193–206.
37. O'Donohue WT, Geer JH. The habituation of sexual arousal. Arch Sex Behav. 1985;14(3):233–246.
38. Giuliano F. Hellstrom WJ. The pharmacological treatment of premature ejaculation. BJU Int. 2008;102(6):668–675.
39. Corona G, Ricca V, Bandini E, Mannucci E, Lotti F, Boddi V, et al. Selective serotonin reuptake inhibitor–induced sexual dysfunction. J Sex Med. 2009;6(5):1259–1269.
40. Phillips NA. Female sexual dysfunction: Evaluation and treatment. Am Fam Physician. 2000;62(1):127–136.
41. Goldstein I, Meston CM, Davis SR, Traish AM. Women's Sexual Function and Dysfunction. Study, Diagnosis and Treatment. London: Taylor and Francis; 2006.
42. Meston C. Sexual Psychophysiology Laboratory, University of Texas at Austin. http://labs.la.utexas.edu/mestonlab/. Accessed June 6, 2016.
43. Shedler J. The efficacy of psychodynamic psychotherapy. Am Psychol. 2010;65(2):98–109.
44. Vigen R, O'Donnell CI, Baron AE, Grunwald GK, Maddox TM, Bradley SM, et al. Association of testosterone therapy with mortality, myocardial infarction, and stroke in men with low testosterone levels. JAMA. 2013;310(17): 1829–1836.
45. Morgentaler A, Miner MM. Testosterone therapy and cardiovascular risk: Advances and controversies. Mayo Clin Proc. 2015;90(2): 224–251.
46. Goldstein S, Goldstein I. Sexual and non-sexual improvements in women with HSDD: Personal experiences with Flibanserin treatment of women with and without resolved sexual pain and post-traumatic stress disorder. Paper presented at: 2016 IPPS Annual Fall Meeting on Chronic Pelvic Pain; October 13-16, 2016; Chicago, Illinois.
47. Simon JA, Goldstein I, Kim NN, Freedman MA, Parish SJ. Flibanserin Approval: Facts or Feelings? ISSM. 2016;4(2):e69-e70. doi: http://dx.doi.org/10.1016/j.esxm.2016.03.025.

22

Wellness

An Integrated Care Approach

MEEGAN LIPMAN, JACQUELINE CALDERONE, JOEL YAGER, AND MARYANN WAUGH

BOX 22.1

KEY POINTS

EXERCISE

- **An exercise prescription is important for both the prevention and treatment of cardiovascular disease, diabetes, obesity, metabolic syndrome, depression, anxiety, bipolar disorder, attention-deficit/hyperactivity disorder, Parkinson disease, and dementia.**

NUTRITION

- **Nutritional factors affect the risk of developing diabetes, cardiovascular disease, depression, and anxiety, and impact the quality of life and the severity of symptoms from autism, Alzheimer disease, and Parkinson disease.**
- **Dietary factors that may broadly affect wellness include omega-3 fatty acids, food-based antioxidants, vitamin D, sugar and sweeteners, and the intestinal microbiota.**

WEIGHT

- **Weight management is critical for the prevention of chronic diseases and the reduction of health care costs.**
- **Obesity increases many cardiovascular disease risk factors, is harmful to the brain, and increases the risk for depression, anxiety, and dementia.**

SLEEP

- **Between 35% and 40% of the U.S. adult population experience some form of sleep disturbance.**
- **Sleep disorders are independent risk factors for both mental and physical disorders.**
- **A full sleep evaluation includes a complete medical and psychiatric history and physical examination in addition to specific evaluations of daytime and nocturnal symptoms related to the sleep disturbance.**
- **Most people with insomnia have coexisting psychiatric illness and/or medical illness; they often have another sleep disorder as well.**
- **Cognitive-behavioral therapy for insomnia (CBT-I) is the first-line, gold-standard treatment for long-term and sustained improvement in insomnia.**

- **Medications might be indicated for short-term treatment of insomnia, but some have significant adverse effects, and long-term use is often problematic.**

STRESS REDUCTION

- **Mortality rates are more than double for persons with high psychological distress versus low distress.**
- **National surveys show that stress received inadequate attention in primary care settings, with only 3% of primary care visits including some kind of stress-reduction counseling.**
- **Research suggests that mindfulness-based stress reduction, cognitive-behavioral stress management, autogenic training, relaxation-response training, and other meditation and mind–body practices may effectively mitigate stress-related symptoms.**

INTRODUCTION

Wellness encompasses a broad range of health, lifestyle, and emotional factors that impact overall well-being and influence the prevention and treatment of many physical and mental disorders.[1] Lifestyle factors such as exercise, nutrition, weight management, sleep, and stress reduction (see Box 22.1 for a summary of key points related to wellness) affect numerous psychological symptoms and disorders, including mood, anxiety, psychosis, dementia, and attention-deficit/hyperactivity disorder. Chronic diseases caused by lifestyle factors are leading causes of death and health care costs worldwide.[2] The National Prevention Council estimates that overall medical costs decrease by approximately $3.27 for every dollar spent on wellness programs.[3] Unfortunately, only half of patients report discussing lifestyle choices with their health care providers.[2] Since studies demonstrate that behavioral counseling by primary care physicians (PCPs) effectively promotes behavior change,[4] wellness considerations are foundational for effective integrated care and deserve attention in every preventive care visit and in chronic disease management.

DESIGNING A WELLNESS PLAN

This chapter focuses on five aspects of wellness: exercise, nutrition, weight management, sleep, and stress management. Following the 5A's Behavior Change Model,[5,6] we consider how integrated primary care teams can address the following functions for each aspect of wellness: **A**ssess, **A**dvise, **A**gree, **A**ssist, and **A**rrange. Sleep issues are addressed in terms of overall sleep hygiene as well as diagnosis and treatment of defined sleep disorders. We assume an integrated care team model likely to consist of front desk administrative staff, medical assistant, PCP, behavioral health specialist (BHS), health coach, psychiatrist, and clinical care coordinator (CCC). Practices will also variably include or refer to registered dietitians, pharmacists, or other ancillary professionals and paraprofessionals. The roles and functioning of an integrated care team are outlined in Table 22.1.

Assessing Priorities to Create Lifestyle Change

For patients with multiple barriers to wellness, clinicians and patients should prioritize which lifestyle issues to address first, considering cardiometabolic risk factors, patient preference, patient motivation and confidence regarding achieving behavioral change, and the patient's likelihood of success with related interventions.[7,8] For example, successful quit rates for smoking cessation are low, while physician-designed interventions for increasing exercise are generally more effective. The literature suggests that rather than starting with smoking cessation, getting an early success with exercise may increase the patient's motivation and confidence, subsequently increasing the likelihood that smoking cessation will also be successful.[7] Once physicians and patients establish behavioral health change priorities, primary care teams can provide patients with lists of community providers and resources for specific needs that the team cannot adequately address.

Biopsychosocial-Cultural Evaluation

It is important to fully assess a patient, in multiple areas, before moving toward a lifestyle change plan. Medical assessment should include physical

TABLE 22.1 LIFESTYLE AND WELLNESS CRITICAL CARE PATHWAY

Personnel	Initial Visit	Follow-up Visits
Front office staff	Distribute screening questionnaires: PHQ-2/GAD-7, health history questionnaire, exercise screening questionnaire, food diary, sleep quality scale	• Distribute repeat screening questionnaires for tracking as indicated
Medical assistant/ nursing staff	• Vital signs and BMI • Chief complaint • Administer/distribute follow-up screening questions: Epworth Sleepiness Scale, questions #3 and #4 on PHQ-9; mental health: PHQ-9, GAD-7 • Document pertinent acute psychosocial issues for PCP • Alert PCP to any core issues identified • Document in registry	• Vital signs and BMI • Chief complaint • Administer/distribute and update responses to follow-up screening questions: Epworth Sleepiness Scale, questions #3 and #4 on PHQ-9; mental health: PHQ-9 GAD-7 • Document pertinent acute psychosocial issues for PCP • Alert PCP to any core issues identified • Document in registry
Primary care provider/ Advance practice nurse	• Establish the working alliance • Attend to medical evaluation and illnesses through physical exam, labs, specialized testing, and referral • Review screeners • Ask appropriate follow-up questions • Assess priorities for lifestyle change and assign to appropriate registries • Sleep: consider medical and medications causes and determine differential diagnosis for sleep disorders with appropriate referrals (BH, psychiatry, neurology, sleep specialist) prior to initiating medications • Assist in team-based development and achievement of short- and long- term goals • Medication management as indicated • Warm handoff to BHS or psychiatrist as needed and coordination of care with all team members	• Update prescriptions for lifestyle change, monitor progress, review priorities • Adjust duration and intensity of exercise • Clarify/adjust nutritional plan • Adjust prescription for calorie intake as needed to achieve weight loss goals • Consider addition of meal replacement and/or weight loss medications • Review stress-reduction efforts • Follow-up on labs, studies and consult recommendations • Warm handoff to BHS, health coach, or psychiatrist as needed and coordination of care with all team members • Coach, or psychiatrist as needed and coordination of care with all team members
Behavioral health specialist	Initial wellness or mental health consultation, if needed	• Wellness groups • Psychotherapy and behavioral interventions for patients with identified mental health barriers to lifestyle change

(*continued*)

TABLE 22.1 CONTINUED

Personnel	Initial Visit	Follow-up Visits
Health coach	• Do complete wellness assessment for exercise, nutrition/weight, sleep, stress, and harm-reduction plan (tobacco, alcohol, etc.) • Develop initial wellness plan with PCP and/or other integrated care team members (as available) • Refer outside the practice for stress test, complex nutritional counseling, or other wellness counseling prn • Add wellness plan and set up tracking in patient registry	• Implement individual exercise program (FITT prescription) and monitor progress • Provide basic health nutritional counseling • Track food diaries • Offer basic sleep hygiene counseling • Track sleep diaries • Offer basic stress-management techniques • Track stress levels • Start harm reduction (decrease smoking and alcohol, etc.) • Track progress in registry • Revise wellness plan • Refer out, prn • Develop wellness groups and work as a teamlet with BHS
Psychiatrist	Assess (as needed) all comorbid psychiatric and substance abuse conditions that are inhibiting lifestyle change	• Consult on and/or treat co-occurring disorders or refer for assessment and treatment to BHS or community resources
Clinical care coordinator	Add patients to appropriate registries	• Manage and update patient registries • Coordinate referrals

examination, relevant laboratory testing, specialized testing or consults (such as stress test, cardiopulmonary testing, and orthopedic evaluations as needed) as a prelude to wellness interventions. As comorbid psychiatric problems can be significant barriers to lifestyle change, patients should also be screened for mood, anxiety, eating disorders, substance use (e.g., tobacco, alcohol), and sexual disorders (which can be barriers to weight loss). Also, social factors can impact wellness planning; for example, living in a dangerous neighborhood may influence exercise plans, just as living in crowded conditions may affect sleep, increase stress, and influence efforts at smoking cessation. Socioeconomic factors may affect nutrition, weight, sleep, and stress wellness planning. Cultural factors inevitably interact with biology to impact all wellness efforts. Sociocultural factors can determine a person's experience and definition of health and illness, access to wellness care, and response to wellness interventions, and can influence treatment expectations and wellness outcomes.

EXERCISE

Benefits of Exercise

All wellness treatment plans, after medical clearance for exercise, should include regular physical activity. Exercise is necessary to maintain cardiovascular fitness, healthy metabolism, and bone density, and provides both immediate and long-term physical, emotional, and cognitive benefits.[9] Exercise can help with weight loss and weight maintenance, reduce the risk of type 2 diabetes, and improve lipid levels.[10] Exercise can also help with behavioral health symptom management, substance use disorder symptoms, and attention-deficit/hyperactivity disorder symptoms.[11,12] Cognitive benefits may come from exercise-induced stimulation of brain-derived neurotrophic factor and associated neurogenesis.[13,14]

Moderate exercise can be as effective as medications and psychotherapy for treatment of unipolar and bipolar depression.[11,15] It also mitigates symptoms for patients with treatment-resistant depression, comorbid personality disorders, comorbid medical problems, or a history of significant substance abuse. Exercise is recommended and offered as a treatment for depression in Scotland and the United Kingdom.[12]

Structured, supervised group exercise or fitness training helps with exercise regimen adherence.[10] Physical activity can be offered as an individual plan for each patient or programmatically, in an integrated practice, by a health coach or via a practice that chooses to develop group wellness offerings. Exercise or fitness training groups are most effective for treating depression, suggesting that this effect might result from increased social contact and distraction from negative thoughts.[12]

Assess Exercise Ability

Integrated care practices should briefly assess patients' activity levels and fitness at initial and follow-up visits. An exercise history begins by asking whether patients exercise recreationally, participate in structured fitness routines, feel satisfied with current fitness levels, or experience barriers preventing exercise. A practice may obtain a more formal exercise history, asking about the patient's current exercise regimen in terms of the frequency, intensity, type, and time for exercise (called a FITT history), and can offer a new FITT prescription as part of the exercise recommendation.

Common barriers to exercise include low self-esteem, not understanding the importance of exercise, not knowing how to exercise, lack of access, cost, lack of social-cultural support, poor health, and mental illness. Medical assistants, nursing professionals, health coaches, or BHSs may help identify patient barriers. Validated questionnaires include; the Exercise Benefits/Barriers Scale[16] and the Motivators and Barriers of Healthy Lifestyle Behaviors Scale,[17] which is specifically validated for black adults.

Advise on Exercise

Primary care providers should educate patients about the benefits of exercise at initial visits. Health coaches alone or BHSs with health coaching experience can provide ongoing education at follow-ups. Optimally, studies recommend 45 to 60 minutes of moderate aerobic exercise three times per week, although benefits have been demonstrated with as little as 20 minutes at target aerobic heart rate three times per week. Dose–response relationships exist, with largest effects seen going from sedentary to walking and with greater frequency, intensity, and duration of exercise, as well as with combinations of exercise and strength training.[18] Patients new to exercise or those with chronic illness or cardiovascular risks should be medically cleared first and then, with the help of a knowledgeable care coordinator, referred to experienced fitness professionals. The American College of Sports Medicine further recommends that men over 40, women over 50, and young people with two or more coronary risk factors be classified at increased risk, suggesting complete medical examinations and diagnostic exercise tests before participation in vigorous exercise.[18] Detailed recommendations for these American College of Sports Medicine exercise guidelines have been published and are readily available.[19]

Agree on an Exercise Plan

Through informed shared decision making based on a strong working alliance, patients and providers or health coaches should develop realistic goals for a fitness plan. PCPs or trained health coaches should develop the initial FITT prescriptions for every patient, starting with current abilities and gradually increasing the intensity and frequency of exercise until patients reach their goals.

Assist in Implementing an Exercise Plan

Patients often need assistance to overcome barriers to exercise. Minimally, patients should receive written exercise recommendations as a FITT prescription. Some patients require more intense interventions such as educational groups conducted by nurses, health coaches, or other trained staff. Including friends and family in educational sessions increases support. CCCs should offer information about low-cost accessible community resources (e.g., at recreation centers, exercise meet-up groups, or classes in local parks). If co-occurring mental health or substance use issues are barriers to exercising, the patient may best be treated in a "teamlet" made up of a health coach, a BHS, and a psychiatrist or referred out of the practice for mental health care if these resources are not available

Arrange for Exercise Action Plans

Based on patients' interests and goals, PCPs, health coache or BHS can create basic action plans, obtain agreement on regular daily exercise plans, ask patients to keep exercise diaries, assess progress at follow-up visits, or even develop a wellness group program. They can help patients adhere to their exercise plans by listing specific goals and encouraging patients to share their plans with friends and family. At follow-up visits health coaches, nurses, or other trained ancillary staff can measure fitness indicators such as blood pressure, weight, and body mass index (BMI); assess the plan's effectiveness; and adjust plans as needed. As the patient's fitness improves, PCPs and the practice team members should encourage the patient to increase the frequency, intensity, and duration of his or her activities, and/or try new activities. PCPs can decide what information to include in a patient registry, managed by the nurse, CCC, or BHS, so that patients' plans and progress can be monitored and updated. The registry can also be used so that patients can receive reminders, educational information, and/or letters of encouragement at regular intervals.

When to Refer

PCPs should consider internal and/or external referrals when significant exercise barriers or risks exist. Patients with severe depression, anxiety, or other mental health barriers will likely benefit from referral to a BHS or psychiatrist, as needed. Patients with specific physical health risks may benefit from evaluation by a specialist. CCCs can ensure that referrals are aligned with wellness goals and economic needs.

NUTRITION

Nutrition and weight management are closely related areas in integrated primary care practices. Depending on staffing patterns, each integrated care practice should designate staff members (medical assistant, health coach, BHS, or registered dietitian) to oversee nutrition and weight management programs and to determine when patients need referral outside the practice. For brevity and consistency, in the following sections we will refer to individuals designated by the practice to manage nutrition and weight-related issues as "nutrition managers" (NMs).

Benefits of Healthy Eating

Dietary choices have a tremendous impact on risks for obesity, diabetes, hyperlipidemia, and cardiovascular disease. They also impact mood, cognition, and sleep.[20,21] Counseling patients about their nutrition is an important part of wellness care. Many dietary factors, such as calories, fat, sodium, and fiber, that affect weight and cardiovascular risk also affect mental health.[22] Studies have demonstrated a link between nutritional status and sleep quality,[20] and between dietary patterns and the long-term risk for depression.[21] Factors that influence the microbiome are also important to consider, as evidence exists that the microbiome might influence body and brain health.[23] Other dietary factors such as omega-3 fatty acids, vitamin D, antioxidants, and gluten may also have important effects, although much controversy exists about whether and how much this is true.

Most Americans consume more calories, sugar, refined grains, saturated fatty acids, and trans-fatty acids (which confer greater cardiovascular risks than saturated fats) and less fiber, whole fruits, and whole vegetables than recommended by dietary guidelines.[24] The overabundance of unhealthy foods in the modern Western diet has been associated with pro-inflammatory and immunosuppressing effects.[25] Plant-based diets beneficially affect blood lipid levels and cardiovascular risk and are associated with a decreased risk of depression, stroke, dementia, and all-cause mortality.[26]

Unfortunately, 2010 data shows that only 13.8% of physician visits made by youth or adult patients included nutritional counseling and only 19.1% of physician visits made by patients with cardiovascular disease, diabetes, or hyperlipidemia included counseling or education related to nutrition.[27] Since physician counseling can effectively change patients' dietary practices,[28] PCPs, nurse practitioners, health coaches, and mental health providers may be optimally positioned to provide such counseling.

Increasingly recognized as important in human physiology, the gut microbiome influences resistance to pathogenic bacteria and affects immune functioning, inflammation, pain sensitivity, obesity, diabetes, bone density, and cancer risk.[29] The microbiome is postulated to play a role in well-established correlations between obesity and depression and between unhealthy diets and depression.[30] Probiotics and prebiotics that positively impact healthy microbiota, available in natural food sources and in supplement form,[31] have shown preliminary promise for microbiota-related disorders but are not yet evidence-based treatments.

Assess Nutritional Status

Several reliable and effective dietary assessment tools enable clinicians to quickly assess dietary patterns and guide patient counseling.[32] Dietary assessment tools generally focus on the intake of calories, fat, fruits, vegetables, proteins, and fiber but do not address specific nutrients such as calcium, vitamin D, or omega-3 fatty acids. NMs must ask patients about those directly. The Diet History Questionnaire is generally considered to provide the most valid energy and nutrient intake assessment in diverse patient populations,[33] but the Dietary Intervention in Primary Care (DINE) questionnaire might most pragmatically assess overall "healthy" or "unhealthy" dietary behaviors.[34] A descriptive summary of tools developed by the National Obesity Observatory to measure dietary intake and behaviors is also available online.[35] NMs should also assess patients' understanding of nutritional issues and identify barriers to eating well, such as cultural or family influences, resource limitations, lack of access/skills, or mental health issues that challenge healthy choices.

Advise on Nutrition and Healthy Eating

Every patient should receive basic education about healthy diets and the recommended intake of calories, fat, fiber, fruits, vegetables, protein, grain, calcium, vitamin D, and omega-3 fatty acids, as detailed in Table 22.2. PCPs or NMs should create initial dietary prescriptions and NMs should conduct follow-up assessments and ongoing education. The U.S. Department of Agriculture and the U.S. Department of Health and Human Services,[36] as well as the American Heart Association,[37] have the most recently published dietary guidelines for cardiovascular, metabolic, and mental health.

Agree on Nutritional Goals

At initial wellness visits, PCPs or NMs should help patients identify nutritional goals (based on individual needs/motivation for change), and create action

TABLE 22.2 DIETARY FACTORS

Dietary Supplement	Effects	Recommendations	Natural Sources
Omega-3 fatty acids	• Decreased incidence of cardiovascular disease • Beneficial to intestinal microbiota • May be protective against depression, anxiety, Alzheimer disease, autism, and attention-deficit/hyperactivity disorder • Stabilize neuronal membranes and intracellular enzymatic pathways • Involved in catecholamine regulation • Effective treatment for mood disorders	• 1–2 g fish oil daily or • One fish meal per week (8–12 oz high omega-3 fish) • Flaxseed is not recommended for supplementation due to a lack of studies demonstrating clinical efficacy	• Salmon, halibut, herring, tuna (limit to 6 oz/week due to high mercury content), walnuts, flaxseeds
Vitamin D	• Important for bone health • Involved in blood glucose regulation • Affects intestinal microbiota • Involved in catecholamine regulation • Protective against type 2 diabetes, cardiovascular disease, autoimmune disorders, and certain cancers • Protective against depression, anxiety, insomnia, fatigue, and dementia	• 2,000 IU daily • 5,000 IU daily or prescription ergocalciferol if verified deficiency	• Sunlight, soy milk, orange juice, vitamin D supplement

(continued)

TABLE 22.2 CONTINUED

Dietary Supplement	Effects	Recommendations	Natural Sources
Dietary antioxidants	• Protective against neuronal injury and neuroinflammation • Protective against atherosclerosis	• Diets rich in vegetables, fruits, legumes, sprouts, seeds and antioxidant-containing spices • Supplements are not recommended and have been found to be harmful in many cases.	• Citrus fruits, red grapes, blueberries, green and yellow vegetables, soybeans, cocoa beans, red wine, peanuts, turmeric
Gluten	• Increasing incidence of celiac disease, wheat allergy, non-celiac gluten sensitivity, and gluten ataxia • Exposure in gluten-sensitive individuals may cause gastrointestinal complaints, chronic pain, fatigue, paresthesias, ataxia and skin rashes • Gluten-related disorders may exacerbate some neuropsychiatric conditions, including attention-deficit/hyperactivity disorder, depression, autism, schizophrenia, and dementia	• Refer for testing if sensitivity is suspected • Avoidance is the treatment for both celiac disease and non-celiac sensitivity	• Wheat, wheatberries, durum, emmer wheat, semolina, spelt, farina, farro, graham, rye, barley, triticale, malt, brewer's yeast, wheat starch
Sugar and sweeteners	• Both sugar and non-calorie sweeteners contribute to obesity • Sweetened beverages are considered to be one of the largest contributors to the obesity epidemic and increase the risk of developing type 2 diabetes	• Water is the perfect source of hydration, even during moderate exercise • Water should be recommended in place of juices and sweetened beverages for optimal hydration and weight management • Patients should be advised to limit their intake of added sugars and non-nutritive sweeteners in foods	

plans. For example, a patient may decide to add one fruit or vegetable to each meal in place of a starch, or drink water in place of soda. NMs should advise patients to keep simple food diaries so that they can record types and quantities of everything they eat for purposes of self-awareness and ongoing monitoring with professional staff. Sample food diaries are available online at the National Institute for Health website[38] and WebMD.[39]

Assist with Dietary Change

Dietary changes can be challenging, and many patients will require extensive education and support. NMs should provide all patients with written educational materials about diet and nutrition. Although the U.S. Department of Agriculture's Dietary Guidelines for Americans are excellent, they may be overwhelming for many. Educational groups and classes, conducted by registered dietitians or other trained NMs, can effectively educate and support multiple patients and their families. CCCs should provide information about free/low-cost cooking classes, food co-ops, and other cost-effective grocery options, as for many patients the cost of fresh foods is prohibitive.

Arrange for Support to Meet Nutritional Goals

NMs can conduct follow-up visits to assess and support progress on a monthly basis, along with quarterly PCP visits, until patients meet their goals. Patient registries, managed by CCCs, can help clinics track the efficacy of programming and help target patient communication and support by email, text, or social media.

When to Refer

Consider referral to a nutritionist outside the practice if the practice does not have a skilled NM. NMs, nutritionists, or registered dietitians within the practice should develop individualized initial nutrition prescriptions and can be vital team members within a wellness group program. Also consider having the CCC refer patients to a gastrointestinal specialist in cases of specific nutritional deficiencies or dietary sensitivities. The CCC can also assist patients who may benefit from purchasing monthly meal replacement programs (e.g., Blue Apron, Nutrisystem).

WEIGHT MANAGEMENT

The prevalence of obesity in the United States has reached 35% among adults and 17% among children and adolescents.[40] Obesity increases the risk for many health problems, including type 2 diabetes, hypertension, hyperlipidemia, cardiovascular disease, and even some cancers.[24] Obesity is also associated with increased rates of depression and anxiety, poorer cognitive performance among otherwise healthy children and adults, and increased cognitive decline associated with aging.[41,42] Weight gain is driven by overall calorie consumption compared to energy expenditure. Individual food choices affect weight gain, as certain food items are more calorically dense or are easy to overconsume. The U.S. Preventive Services Task Force recommends that PCPs screen all adults for obesity and offer treatment for all obese patients.[43]

Assess Weight Issues

Weight management needs assessments should begin with the medical assistant's measurement of the patient's height and weight, and BMI calculation. BMI tables are available on the Centers for Disease Control and Prevention[44] and National Institute of Health[45] websites. There is evidence from the World Health Organization that the waist-to-hip ratio is a better indicator or measure of health, and better at predicting the risk of developing serious health conditions.[46] Research shows that people with "apple-shaped" bodies (with more weight around the waist), face more health risks than those with "pear-shaped" bodies who carry more weight around the hips. The World Health Organization defines abdominal obesity as a waist–hip ratio of more than 0.90 for males and more than 0.85 for females, or a BMI of more than 30.[46]

Patients needing to lose weight should schedule detailed assessments and planning sessions with either the PCP or NM. They should keep food diaries that are evaluated by NMs using dietary assessment tools that focus on intake of total calories, fats, protein, and fiber. PCPs or NMs should assess how patients understand the impact of body weight on metabolic functioning, cardiovascular risk, and mental health, and work with patients to reduce barriers preventing weight loss.

Advise on Weight Loss Plan

Weight loss coaching should include dietary prescriptions and instructions to increase physical activity as tolerated, until patients reach FITT goals described earlier. Dietary prescriptions should include appropriate daily caloric intakes for age and level of physical activity and appropriate proportions of fat, protein, and carbohydrates. The U.S.

Department of Agriculture publishes online tables to estimate daily caloric needs based on age, gender, and level of activity.[47]

Weight loss prescriptions should include dietary changes, dietary restrictions, exercise, stress management, and adequate sleep. Calorie reduction is the single most effective weight loss strategy, accounting for 80% of weight loss. Exercise is much less effective than calorie restriction in producing weight loss, but programs that combine weight loss first, followed by exercise afterwards, are even more effective. Exercise is also essential for maintaining a stable weight. Increased consumption of water and whole fruits and vegetables aids in weight loss and can also help prevent weight gain.[48,49] Increased protein intake improves satiety, stimulates endocrine responses associated with lipolysis, increases loss of body fat, and maintains muscle mass during weight loss.[50] Contrary to common belief, rapid weight loss does not predict weight regain in the long term; thus, patients do not necessarily need to lose weight slowly.[50]

Weight loss interventions in integrated care settings can effectively produce moderate weight loss among obese patients. The most effective interventions include monthly weight loss coaching, quarterly PCP visits, meal replacement, and weight loss medications.[51,52] NMs or trained ancillary clinic staff may provide weight loss coaching.[51] Bariatric surgery, the most effective treatment for morbid obesity, confers a significant level of risk and requires high levels of patient compliance and commitment to be effective.[53] Potential candidates should seek specialist evaluation.

Weight loss medications can decrease appetite, increase satiety, lead to greater weight loss when combined with weight loss coaching,[43] and can help maintain weight loss.[54] In some cases they may also decrease absorption of nutrients and calories. Pharmacotherapy for weight loss is indicated for patients with a high BMI and comorbid conditions, such as type 2 diabetes, hypertension, hyperlipidemia, or sleep apnea.[55] To supplement calorie restriction and exercise, medications with U.S. Food and Drug Administration (FDA) approval for short-term use (up to 12 weeks) include benzphetamine, diethylpropion, phendimetrazine, and phentermine. Medications approved for long-term use include orlistat, lorcaserin, a combination of phentermine and topiramate, a combination of bupropion and naltrexone, and the subcutaneously injected medication liraglutide. See Table 22.3 for doses, mechanism of drug action, and risks and side effects. While weight loss medications have been shown to improve cardio-metabolic risk factors, none is proven to decrease cardiovascular morbidity or mortality.[56] Further, these medications can be expensive, are not covered by insurance, and potentially have adverse side effects.[43] Meal replacements are as effective and have fewer risks and costs than medications.[43,54]

Agree on Weight Loss Action Plan

Based on patients' individual needs, goals, and motivation for change, the PCP or NM should engage in a shared decision-making process with the patient that creates specific agreed-upon weight loss action plans that include both dietary changes and exercise, all tracked by patient diaries with relevant information also tracked in patient registries. Individualized nutritionist-created diet plans may be appropriate for some patients. Depending on patient preferences and circumstances, PCPs should consider meal replacement and/or weight loss medications as needed.

Assist in Implementation of Weight Loss Plan

Weight loss programs should include education, support, and/or psychotherapy groups delivered by the NM, BHS, or a psychiatrist. Obese patients often struggle with shame and have co-occurring mental illness. Goal setting, recordkeeping, weight loss support and psychoeducation groups, and a higher frequency of counseling visits improve adherence and effectiveness.[43]

Arrange Weight Loss and Follow-up Plans

Even after desired weight has been achieved, weight maintenance is improved by monthly follow-up visits with the NM, in some instances scheduled indefinitely, and quarterly visits with the PCP.[43] At follow-up visits, the NM should track the patient's weight and BMI or waist–hip ratio and, if desired, changes in body composition, provide encouragement, and adjust plans as necessary for unmet goals. The NM or CCC should enter follow-up data into patient registries.

When to Refer

When primary care practices are unable to provide in-house weight loss counseling, the CCC should refer patients to reputable community-based or online weight loss programs, some of which are

TABLE 22.3 WEIGHT LOSS MEDICATIONS

Weight Loss Medications with FDA Approval for Short-Term Use (up to 12 weeks)		
Name/Doses	Mechanism	Risks and Side Effects
Benzphetamine (25 mg/d to 50 mg tid) Diethylpropion (25 mg tid for IR; 75 mg/d for controlled release) Phendimetrazine (35 mg bid or tid for IR; 105 mg/d for ER) Phentermine (15–37.5 mg/d in one or two divided doses)	• Sympathomimetic agents • Inhibit reuptake of norepinephrine	• Xerostomia, headache, insomnia, hypertension, tachycardia • Contraindicated for patients with a history of cardiovascular disease
Weight Loss Medications with FDA Approval for Long-Term Use		
Orlistat (Xenical) (120 mg tid with meals)	• Inhibitor of pancreatic lipase • Prevents absorption of fat in diet	• Decreased absorption of fat-soluble vitamins, flatus, oily discharge, increase defecation, urgency, oily stools • Rare cases of severe liver injury and breast cancer.
Lorcaserin (Belviq) (10 mg bid)	• Serotonin type 2C receptor agonist	• Headache, nausea, dizziness, constipation, xerostomia, serotonin syndrome • Should not be combined with selective serotonin reuptake inhibitor or monoamine oxidase inhibitors
Phentermine/topiramate extended release (Qsymia) (complex advancing regimen; starting dose phentermine 3.75 mg + topiramate 23 mg once daily for 14 days)	• Sympathomimetic and anticonvulsant • Topiramate is thought to decrease appetite via GABA receptor agonism.	• Paresthesias, dizziness, dysgeusia, insomnia, constipation, xerostomia • Contraindicated in pregnancy due to increased risk of fetal malformations
Bupropion ER + naltrexone ER (Contrave) (initial dose naltrexone 8 mg/bupropion 90 mg once daily in am for 1 week, followed by complex advancing regimen. Usual dose ultimately 2 tablets twice daily.)	• Naltrexone is an opioid antagonist, and bupropion is a weak inhibitor of dopamine and norepinephrine reuptake.	• Boxed warning for suicidality and antidepressant drugs, neuropsychiatric reactions • Should not be combined with monoamine oxidase inhibitors
Liraglutide (Saxenda; Victoza) (Initial dose is 0.6 mg subcutaneous injection daily for a week; weekly increase to target of 3 mg/day)	• Long-acting analog of human glucagon-like peptide-1, which increases glucose-dependent insulin secretion	• Boxed warning: thyroid C-cell tumor risk; contraindicated in patients with family or personal history of medullary thyroid cancer

more effective and less costly than PCP-driven programs.[43,57] All patients who are severely obese or have cardio-metabolic risk factors should consult with medical weight loss specialists.

Bariatric surgery is the most effective treatment for morbid obesity, as noted above, however, it confers a significant level of risk and requires a high level of patient compliance and commitment in order to be effective.[53] Indications for bariatric surgery include patient preferences, a BMI of 40 or greater (or a BMI of 35 with associated medical or psychological comorbidities, such as type 2 diabetes, obstructive sleep apnea, or severe joint disease[53]), or when obesity is conferring other significant mortality risk. Patients seeking bariatric surgery should be referred to a specialist for evaluation.

INSOMNIA AND OTHER SLEEP–WAKE DISORDERS

Average American adults sleep 6.9 hours, while experts recommend seven to nine hours of sleep per night.[58] Individuals who sleep four to five hours per night show impaired neurocognitive, behavioral, metabolic, and autonomic functioning as well as mood disturbances.[59] Approximately 35% to 50% of U.S. adults have problems falling asleep or staying asleep, experience daytime sleepiness, or have combinations of these three, resulting in up to 60 different International Classification of Sleep Disorders diagnoses. Sleep disorders are associated with increased mortality and are independent risk factors for mood disorders and cardiovascular disease; both chronic insomnia and sleep apnea may increase the risk of depression.[60] Sleep disorders have varied and complex precipitating and perpetuating causes. Sufferers commonly have more than one type of sleep disorder. These disturbances are symptomatic of many psychiatric and medical illnesses, and in addition can constitute independent disorders. Although several schemes have been proposed, for the purpose of this chapter, we use the American Psychiatric Association's *Diagnostic and Statistical Manual of Mental Disorders*, Fifth Edition (DSM-5) terminology and categorization of sleep–wake disorders.[61]

The most prevalent disorders in the U.S. population include insomnia (10–20%), obstructive sleep apnea (3–7%), restless leg syndrome (2.5–5%), narcolepsy (0.02%),[62] and circadian rhythm disorders (the delayed sleep phase type is most prevalent, at 0.17%).[63] This section provides guidance for integrated care teams to identify and begin managing the most common sleep problems. Given the high prevalence of sleep–wake disorders, we recommend that all patients be questioned about their sleep.

Assess Sleep Problems/Disorders

Medical assistants or front desk staff can administer general health screening questionnaires that include at least one question concerning sleep quality. The validated single-item self-report Sleep Quality Scale or questions #3 and #4 on the Patient Health Questionnaire-9 Item (PHQ-9) are useful.[64] The Epworth Sleepiness Scale (ESS)[65] is also a useful follow-up screen for patients reporting daytime sleepiness, snoring, or suspected sleep apnea. An elevated BMI or waist–hip ratio or patient reports of fatigue and low energy should also alert staff to a probable sleep disturbance.

When a patient has a positive screen for sleep disturbance, the PCP and the integrated team can follow up with detailed sleep questions to determine sleep duration and quality as well as precipitating and perpetuating factors. PCPs, primarily responsible for assessing medical and psychiatric factors as they develop a differential diagnosis, should consider current medications, general medical illnesses, and psychiatric conditions that might contribute to sleep disturbances. Medications that can affect sleep include antidepressants (e.g., bupropion, selective serotonin receptor inhibitors), antihypertensive medications, corticosteroids, stimulants, second-generation H1 antagonists, weight-management medications, over-the-counter herbal preparations, and many substances of abuse. Queries regarding sleep-related habits should assess basic sleep hygiene practices (sleep and wake times, sleep habits, bed and bedroom partners, sleep environment), and use of sleep aids, alcohol, caffeine, and other substances. Review of symptoms should include nocturnal pain, nocturia, and undiagnosed or undertreated psychiatric illnesses. For example, nightmares might signify trauma or posttraumatic stress disorder (PTSD), early morning rising might indicate depression, and difficulty falling asleep or staying asleep might indicate an anxiety disorder. It's helpful to differentiate daytime sleepiness from fatigue (feeling tired but unlikely to fall asleep even when given the chance). Patients with fatigue but low excessive daytime sleepiness (low ESS score) often show chronic hyperarousal due to anxiety, depression, or sleep worry. Elevated ESS scores (normal < 9) suggest sleep apnea, insufficient sleep opportunity, narcolepsy, and/or restless leg syndrome. This will help PCPs differentiate between a primary sleep disorder and a secondary sleep disorder (resulting from an underlying physical or mental condition). Since many mental health disorders produce coexisting insomnia, we recommend diagnosing these conditions first, before pursuing a diagnosis of a primary sleep disorder.

Insomnia, the most common sleep disorder, is defined as subjective dissatisfaction with sleep despite having the opportunity to sleep, causing evidence of distress or impairments, occurring at least three times per week for 3 months.[66] Patients with insomnia are much more likely to report daytime fatigue and inability to fall asleep than excessive daytime sleepiness. Common contributing medical and psychiatric causes of insomnia include gastroesophageal reflux disease, chronic pain, hyperthyroidism, heart failure, stroke, fibromyalgia, mood and anxiety disorders, PTSD, alcohol and substance use disorders, Alzheimer disease, and Parkinson disease.

Advise About Sleep Problems

For patients with insomnia, the PCP must first attend to contributing medical and psychiatric conditions. Cognitive-behavioral therapy for insomnia (CBT-I) is the recommended first-line evidence-based treatment.[66] Since chronic insomnia is commonly conceptualized as a disorder of hyperarousal that appears to override sleep drive, CBT-I is specifically designed to decrease arousal, increase sleep drive, and stabilize circadian rhythm.[67,68] CBT-I consists of five components: sleep hygiene, stimulus control, relaxation therapy, cognitive therapy, and sleep restriction. PCPs will ordinarily assign this treatment to the BHS or a health coach with specialized training. When CBT-I is insufficient, PCPs might consider medication management for insomnia, even though hypnotic medications are often ineffective in the long term. Medications alone are less effective than medications plus CBT-I.

The "gold standard" treatment for obstructive sleep apnea is positive airway pressure delivered via a continuous positive airway pressure (CPAP) machine. Other treatments include weight loss or mandibular advancement performed by oral surgeons or dentists. CPAP adherence is often challenging; patients may need a trial of multiple masks for comfort since masks induce anxiety or panic in some patients. Follow-up by a BHS or a health coach to provide motivational interviewing and cognitive-behavioral therapies can increase adherence.

For restless leg syndrome, effective treatments include: iron replacement for a ferritin level less than 75 mcg/L, pramipexole (0.125–0.75 mg/day), ropinirole (0.25–4 mg/day), rotigotine patch (0.5–4 mg/day), levodopa (200–300 mg/day), gabapentin enacarbil (600–1,800 mg/day), and pregabalin (300 mg/day).[69] Massage, warm baths, relaxation, and exercise may also help. Referral to a sleep clinic, a neurologist, or a psychiatrist is indicated if initial treatments fail.

For circadian rhythm disorders, treatment requires estimating the individual's spontaneous wake time (generally two hours after the lowest core body temperature occurs) and then gradually shifting the endogenous alerting system through the use of bright-light treatments and melatonin.[70] Morning bright light advances sleep to earlier times and evening bright light pushes sleep to later times. Referral to a sleep specialist is recommended.

For narcolepsy, medication treatments include modafinil (200–400 mg/day). Second-line agents include methylphenidate (initial dose 10 mg bid), dextroamphetamine (initial dose 10 mg bid), and the supplement gamma hydroxybutyric acid (GHB). Patients who do not respond should be referred to a sleep clinic.

Agree on Sleep Problem Diagnosis and Plan

PCPs and patients should collaboratively explore the details of sleep complaints, agree on diagnoses, and collaboratively formulate treatment plans. Patients often have long standing insomnia histories and strong preferences regarding treatments. PCPs can employ team members to provide education and support for patients and families regarding medical recommendations.

Assist with Sleep Problems

CBT-I

CBT-I is a prescribed treatment usually conducted by BHSs, specifically trained health coaches, or sleep specialists. BHSs, health coaches, and CCCs can initiate basic education and provide printed materials on sleep hygiene and sleep diaries.[71] The American Academy of Sleep Medicine recommends keeping a sleep diary for at least two weeks because individuals commonly misperceive sleep duration. Supplemental actigraphy (the use of a small device [actigraph] that continuously measures activity or movement and can also mark events such as bedtimes or wake times) may assist with accurate sleep accounting. In addition, weekly phone calls by the BHS or coach using motivational interviewing to identify and support stepwise change can increase success.

BHSs or health coaches can review sleep logs to determine whether sleep difficulties are acute or chronic and whether disturbances are with sleep onset, maintenance, and/or early awakening. In addition, they can address specific precipitating and perpetuating factors. While a BHS or health coach can implement the first four strategies of CBT-I, sleep restriction may require more specialized expertise. Sleep restriction is intended to increase sleep drive and stabilize circadian rhythm by increasing sleep efficiency. Sleep efficiency is defined by total sleep time divided by time in bed as a percent. An individual's time in bed is restricted, not less than five hours, until the weekly average sleep efficiency is at least 85%, and then time in bed is gradually increased by 15-minute increments. Evidence for using online CBT-I modules is limited.[72]

Medication

Although clinical guidelines recommend behavioral interventions for first-line treatment, most patients who have insomnia receive sedative-hypnotic medications. Approximately 20% of U.S. adults use hypnotic medications despite their adverse effects, limited efficacy, and risk of dependence.[73]

If medications seem necessary to assist with sleep onset and/or sleep maintenance, prescribing the lowest possible dose for primarily acute episodes will reduce related risks. Many sedative-hypnotics, particularly benzodiazepines, can be habit-forming. Dependence may develop within one to two weeks, after which patients may experience rebound insomnia, reporting an inability to sleep without pills. In these instances, patients often attribute their sleep problems to "chronic insomnia" rather than to the medication-induced rebound insomnia/mild withdrawal symptoms they are most likely experiencing during attempts to discontinue these medications. Alpha-adrenergic blockers such as prazosin used to specifically treat nightmares and associated nocturnal hyperarousal states in patients with PTSD might require prolonged administration. Many medications prescribed for insomnia cause daytime somnolence or sedation, and some have been associated with parasomnias, memory impairment, and occasional cases of transient global amnesia. Patients differ widely in how much difficulty they experience when discontinuing various medications. A discussion of these related risks is an important component of medication consent. Therefore, in addition to considering patient preferences, PCPs must exert considerable judgment in how they prescribe hypnotics. Table 22.4 lists medications currently used to treat symptoms of insomnia; some are used off-label for their sedative side effects, and not all have FDA indications.

Registry and Tracking

The CCC, health coach, or BHS can enter information into integrated care or depression registries or specific sleep–wake registries. Registries are very useful for tracking sleep screening results (e.g., PHQ-9 questions, ESS scores), documentation from sleep diaries, treatment recommendations, outcomes, and as aid for development of population approaches to improve sleep.

Arrange for Treatment and Referrals for Sleep Problems

Four different types of referrals might be necessary for patients with sleep–wake disorders. These will be ordered by the PCP and arranged by the CCC. These include: (1) Half of patients with insomnia have psychiatric and/or substance use disorders with behavioral difficulties (e.g., refractory illness, suicidality, psychotic symptoms) exceeding the capacities of a BHS and requiring referral to psychiatrists for best care. (2) Patients with obstructive sleep apnea and unusual sleep–wake complaints not responding to first-line interventions need a referral to specialty sleep-disorder clinics to obtain polysomnography for a specific diagnosis. (3) Treatment-resistant patients with restless leg syndrome, and (4) Patients with rapid-eye-movement sleep disorders thought to manifest because of Parkinson disease, Lewy body dementia, or multiple-systems atrophy should have a neurologic consultation.

STRESS ASSESSMENT AND STRESS MANAGEMENT

Nearly 15% of the population reports significant levels of psychological distress,[74,75] and nearly 60% of primary care patients report significant distress,[76] while 60% to 80% are thought to have a stress-related component to other physical or mental problems.[77] Mortality rates are more than double for individuals with high psychological distress versus low distress.[78] Despite these findings, PCPs give little attention to stress-related concerns. A national study showed that only 3.0% of office visits from 2006 to 2009 included

TABLE 22.4 MEDICATIONS FREQUENTLY USED TO TREAT INSOMNIA[a]

Benzodiazepine Receptor Agonists	Adult Dose (mg/hs)	Half-life in hours	Comments (Use lower doses for patients age ≥ 65)
Clonazepam (Klonopin)	0.25–1	18–50	Used to treat parasomnias
Eszopiclone (Lunesta)	2–3	6–9	
Lorazepam (Ativan)	0.05–2	8–12	
Temazepam (Restoril)	7.5–30	8–10	
Triazolam (Halcion)	0.125–0.5	2–5	
Zaleplon (Sonata)	5–20	1	
Zolpidem (Ambien)	5–10	2.5	
	Antidepressants		
Amitriptyline (Elavil)	10–50	17–40	Used in low doses, as for migraine, neuropathic pain
Doxepin (Sinequan)	10–50	12–18	
Mirtazapine (Remeron)	7.5–30	20–30	May lose sedative effects at higher doses
Trazadone (Oleptro)	25–300	7	Caution if cardiac disease; can rarely cause priapism
	Antihistamines		
Hydroxyzine (Vistaril)	25–100	20	
Diphenhydramine (Benadryl)	25–50	8.5	
	Orexin Receptor Antagonist		
Suvorexant (Belsomra)	10–20	9–13	Contraindicated in patients with narcolepsy
	Melatonin Agonist		
Melatonin	5	0.5–2	Less expensive, over the counter
Ramelteon (Rozerem)	8	1	
Atypical Antipsychotic/Mood Stabilizer (e.g., quetiapine, olanzapine)			NOT indicated for insomnia per se (but sedative effects may benefit anxious patients)

[a] Not all have FDA indications.

stress management counseling by the PCP. Stress management was the least common type of PCP counseling, following rates of counseling about nutrition (16.8%), physical activity (12.3%), weight reduction (6.3%), and tobacco cessation (3.7%).[79] Furthermore, in one study of primary care visits, an average discussion between a PCP and patient included 3.6 different lifestyle issues during a total discussion length of 2.9 minutes. Weight, diet, and nutrition, physical activity, and tobacco use were the topics most frequently covered. Discussions were more likely to occur with female physicians and when PCPs perceived poorer patient mental health status.[80]

Since many psychologically distressed individuals qualify for specific mood, anxiety, PTSD, and substance use disorders (diagnoses discussed elsewhere in this book), this section addresses only assessment and interventions for milder forms of distress, those seen in the "worried well," including subclinical forms of mixed depression/anxiety, demoralization, and situational adjustment reactions.

Assess for Stress

Screening by front desk staff or the medical assistant is usually performed via general health questionnaires or specific instruments such as the PHQ-2, PHQ-9, or Generalized Anxiety Disorder 7-Item (GAD-7). These instruments require little time to complete and broadly cover symptoms of depression and anxiety.[81] Screening personnel should bring positive responses to the clinician's attention at the time of the visit.

Clinicians continue assessment by observing patients' body language and voice tones, and by asking additional screening questions in culturally suitable language: How is it going? How are things with the family? How is work? How are your finances? Are you getting around? Are you taking care of business? How are your nerves? How well are you managing and coping? Are you stressed? By these means, clinicians can identify and acknowledge patients presenting with high degrees of distress, and rule in or rule out more clinically concerning psychiatric and substance use disorders that might require more elaborate psychosocial and possibly pharmacologic interventions.

Advise About Stress and Agree on a Plan

Where indicated, PCPs can educate and advise patients regarding the need for stress-reduction interventions, and suggest options. Based on collaboratively identified patient preferences, stress-reduction interventions can include brief individual or group counseling, self-guided readings with stress-reduction activities, mindfulness exercises, yoga, physical activity, lifestyle management to better balance work/family/personal activities, stress-reduction apps, and other activities. High-quality studies suggest benefits for mindfulness-based stress reduction, cognitive-behavioral stress management, autogenic training (a form of relaxation therapy that involves training the body to respond to verbal suggestions),[82] relaxation-response training, and other meditation and mind–body skills practices. See Chapter 25 Health Coaching in Integrated Care for additional discussion of approaches to stress reduction.

Assist with Stress Reduction

Assistance tasks are generally assumed by the BHS, health coach, and CCC, who can schedule one or more sessions for individuals or groups of patients offering stress counseling, detailed education about stress reduction, and classes in specific stress-reduction methods. They might opt to organize and offer multifaceted stress-reduction programs modeled on activities promulgated by employee assistance programs, insurance companies, and some health care agencies, including the U.S. Department of Veterans Affairs (the VA). For example, an excellent, no cost stress-reduction program (promoted by the VA) combines problem solving, relaxation training, improved personal expression, time-management skills, positive thinking, and pleasant activities.[83]

Arrange for Stress-Reduction Activities

The CCC, health coach, or BHS may provide internal "warm handoffs" within the integrated practice or may help patients access outside resources, providing pamphlets, reading lists (including self-help workbooks), websites, and referrals to activities and services not available within the practice. Designed for the use of veterans but equally useful for non-veterans, links to many free resources are available at the Center for Integrated Care website.[83] A valuable stress-reduction self-help workbook that includes stress trackers and activity/progress worksheets aligned with the various stress-reduction undertakings can be downloaded from their website.[84] The National Center for Telehealth and Technology website also offers excellent free self-help stress-reduction apps including Breath2Relax and Mindfulness Coach, among many others.[85] Registry tracking can be initiated by the BHS or CCC, using the rating scales mentioned above.

CONCLUSIONS

Integrated care practices, by attending to exercise, nutrition, weight management, sleep/wake difficulties, and stress management, can help patients stay well or become healthier, prevent disease, and potentially reduce the deleterious effects of diseases that already exist. Many activities, supported by a

BOX 22.2
SUMMARY OF RECOMMENDED TREATMENT APPROACHES AND RELEVANT EVIDENCE

Strength of recommendation taxonomy (SOR A, B, or C)

- **Most if not all patients are likely to benefit from behavioral counseling by PCPs directed to nutrition and exercise-related behaviors, including screening, counseling/education, and regular phone/in-person visits to monitor progress. (SOR B)[2,4,28]**
- **The 5A's distributed among primary care staff (Assess, Advise, Agree, Assist, and Arrange) can be used as a platform for addressing behavior change. (SOR A)[5]**
- **Each patient's treatment plan should include an exercise program, which may help improve cardiovascular fitness, metabolism, bone density, blood sugar control (SOR A),[9,10,79] mood and substance-use disorder symptoms, attention-deficit/hyperactivity disorder (ADHD) symptoms (SOR A),[11,12,15,80] and cognition (SOR A).[13,14] Exercise programs aligned with the patient's current risks, needs, and abilities should include goals that move (in some cases gradually) toward nationally endorsed fitness standards (SOR A).[18]**
- **Patients should undergo primary care–based nutrition assessment (SOR A)[19,22,24] based on quick self-report instruments that can be delivered by front desk or other clinic staff members to efficiently gather a reliable picture of their nutritional intake (SOR B).[32]**
- **Primary care facilities should offer weight loss interventions that include monthly weight loss coaching, quarterly PCP visits, meal replacement, and weight loss medications (SOR C)[51,52] augmented by specialist support (SOR C).[51]**
- **Primary care practices should advocate and/or offer cognitive-behavioral therapy for insomnia (CBT-I), since its demonstrated efficacy regardless of insomnia etiology is considered the gold-standard intervention. (SOR A)[66]**
- **Promising interventions that primary care practices may initiate to help patients reduce stress include mindfulness-based stress reduction, cognitive-behavioral stress management, autogenic training, relaxation response training, and other meditation and mind-body practices. (SOR C)[82]**

team approach involved in addressing these lifestyle areas, empower patients and challenging them to take responsibility for improving their health and functioning, thereby improving both their physical and emotional well-being. See Box 22.2 for a summary of the evidence supporting various wellness approaches.

REFERENCES

1. World Health Organization. Definition of health. http://www.who.int/about/definition/en/print.html. Accessed December 15, 2015.
2. Sagner M, Katz D, Egger G, et al. Lifestyle medicine potential for reversing a world of chronic disease epidemics: From cell to community. Int J Clin Pract. 2014;68(11):1289–1292. doi:10.1111/ijcp.12509.
3. The role of primary care and wellness in reshaping healthcare economics. Medical Economics. http://medicaleconomics.modernmedicine.com/medical-economics/news/role-primary-care-and-wellness-reshaping-healthcare-economics. Updated 2016. Accessed January 5, 2016.
4. Lin JS, O'Connor E, Whitlock EP, Bell TL. Behavioral counseling to promote physical activity and a healthful diet to prevent cardiovascular disease in adults: A systematic review for the U.S. Preventive Services Task Force. Ann Intern Med. 2010;153:736–750.
5. Riekert KA, Ockene JK, Pbert L. Handbook of Health Behavior Health. 4th ed. New York: Springer Publications; 2013.
6. Whitlock EP, Orleans CT, Pender N, Allan J. Evaluating primary care behavioral counseling interventions: An evidence-based approach. Am J Prev Med. 2002;22(4):267–284.

7. Feinstein RE. Prevention-oriented primary care: A collaborative model for office-based cardiovascular risk reduction. Heart Dis.1999; 1(5):264–271.
8. Rabinowitz PM, Cullen MR, Feinstein RE. Host/environment medicine: A family practice model for the future. Fam Med. 1998;30(4):297–300.
9. Penedo FJ, Dahn JR. Exercise and well-being: A review of mental and physical health benefits associated with physical activity. Curr Opin Psychiat. 2005;18(2):189–193.
10. Garber CE, Blissmer B, Deschenes MR, et al. Position Stand. Appropriate physical activity intervention strategies for weight loss and prevention of weight regain for adults. Med Sci Sports Exerc. 2011;43(7):1334–1359. doi:10.1249/MSS.0b013e318213fefb.459–471.
11. de Sá Filho AS, de Souza Moura AM, Lamego MK, et al. Potential therapeutic effects of physical exercise for bipolar disorder. CNS Neurol Disord Drug Targets. 2015;14(10):1255–1259.
12. Cooney GM, Dwan K, Greig CA, et al. Exercise for depression. Cochrane Database Syst Rev. 2013;12:9. doi:10.1002/14651858.CD004366.pub6.
13. Cotman CW, Berchtold NC, Christie LA. Exercise builds brain health: Key roles of growth factor cascades and inflammation. Trends Neurosci. 2007;30(9):464–472.
14. Wrann CD, White JP, Salogiannnis J, et al. Exercise induces hippocampal BDNF through a PGC-1α/FNDC5 pathway. Cell Metab. 2013;5:18(5):649–659. doi:10.1016/j.cmet.2013.09.008.
15. Hogan CL, Mata J, Carstensen LL. Exercise holds immediate benefits for affect and cognition in younger and older adults. Psychol Aging. 2013;28(2):587–594. doi:L10.1037/a0032634.
16. Sechrist KR, Walker SN, Pender NJ. Development and psychometric evaluation of the Exercise Benefits/Barriers Scale. Res Nursing Health. 1987;10(6):357–365.
17. Downes LS. Further validation of the motivators and barriers of a healthy lifestyle scale. South J Nurs Res. 2010;10(4):1–21.
18. American College of Sports Medicine. ACSM's Guidelines for Exercise Testing and Prescription. 5th ed. Baltimore: Williams & Wilkins; 1995:18–25.
19. Nelson ME, Rejeski J, Blair SN, et al Physical activity and public health in older adults: Recommendation from the American College of Sports Medicine and the American Heart Association. Med Sci Sports Exerc. 2007;39(8):1435–1445.
20. Beydoun MA. The interplay of gender, mood, and stress hormones in the association between emotional eating and dietary behavior. J Nutr. 2014;144(8):1139–1141. doi:10.3945/jn.114.196717.
21. Grosso G, Pajak A, Marventano S, et al. Role of omega-3 fatty acids in the treatment of depression. PLoS One. 9(5):e96905. doi:10.1371/journal.pone.0096905.
22. Jacka FN, Sacks G, Berk M, Allender S. Food policies for physical and mental health. BMC Psychiat. 2014;14:132. doi:10.1186/1471-244X-14-132.
23. Selhub EM, Logan AC, Bested AC. Fermented foods, microbiota, and mental health: Ancient practice meets nutritional psychiatry. J Physiol Anthropol. 2014;33(2):1–12.
24. U.S. Department of Agriculture and U.S. Department of Health and Human Services. Dietary Guidelines for Americans, 2010, 7th ed. Washington, DC: U.S. Government Printing Office, December 2010. http://health.gov/dietaryguidelines/dga2010/DietaryGuidelines2010.pdf. Accessed December 28, 2015.
25. Myles IA. Fast food fever: Reviewing the impacts of the Western diet on immunity. Nutr J. 2014;13(1):61. doi:10.1186/1475-2891-13-61.
26. Psaltopoulou T, Sergentanis TN, Panagiotakos DB, et al. Mediterranean diet, stroke, cognitive impairment, and depression: A meta-analysis. Ann Neurol. 2013;74(4):580–591. doi:10.1002/ana.23944.
27. Ambulatory Medical Care Survey (NAMCS), CDC/NCHS. http://www.healthypeople.gov/2020/data-search/Search-theData?&f[0]=field_topic_area%3A3502. Updated 2010. Accessed December 28, 2015.
28. Holtrop JS, Dosh SA, Torres T, et al. Nurse consultation support to primary care practices to increase delivery of health behavior services. Appl Nurs Res. 2009;22(4):243–249.
29. Bruce-Keller AJ, Salbaum JM, Luo M, et al. Obese-type gut microbiota induce neurobehavioral changes in the absence of obesity. Biol Psychiat. 2015;77(7):607–615. doi:10.1016/j.biopsych.2014.07.012.
30. Dash S, Clarke G, Berk M, et al. The gut microbiome and diet in psychiatry: Focus on depression. Curr Opin Psychiatr. 2015;28(1):1–6. doi:10.1097/YCO.0000000000000117.
31. Bhawana D, Nettu S. Availability of prebiotic and probiotic foods at household and commercial level: Constraints ahead for health. Int J Sci Res. 2015;4(9):1095–1098.
32. Calfas KJ, Zabinski MF, Rupp J. Practical nutrition assessment in primary care settings. Am J Prev Med. 2000;18(4):289–299.
33. Beechy L, Galpern J, Petrone A, Das SK. Assessment tools in obesity—psychological measures, diet, activity, and body composition. Physiol Behav. 2012;107(1):154–171. doi:10.1016/j.physbeh.2012.04.013.
34. DINE Tool. American Journal of Preventive Medicine Online Appendix. http://www.

ajpmonline.org/cms/attachment/250589/1594869/mmc1.pdf. Accessed December 28, 2015.

35. Review of dietary assessment methods in public health. National Obesity Observatory: August 2010; 1–30. http://www.noo.org.uk/uploads/doc/vid_7237_Review_new.pdf. Accessed December 28, 2015.
36. Dietary Guidelines. Office of Disease Prevention and Health Promotion. http://health.gov/dietaryguidelines/. Updated February 2, 2016. Accessed February 2, 2016.
37. American Heart Association. Diet and lifestyle recommendations. http://www.heart.org/HEARTORG/HealthyLiving/HealthyEating/Nutrition/The-American-Heart-Associations-Diet-and-Lifestyle-Recommendations_UCM_305855_Article.jsp#.VrI9FbIrKM8. Updated August 2015. Accessed December 28, 2015.
38. US Department of Health and Human Services, National Heart, Lung, and Blood Institute. Daily food and activity diary. https://www.nhlbi.nih.gov/health/educational/lose_wt/BMI/bmi_dis.htm. Accessed December 16, 2015.
39. WebMD. Weight loss and diet plans. Food and fitness journal. http://www.webmd.com/diet/printable/food-fitness-journal. Updated November 26, 2008. Accessed December 28, 2015.
40. Ogden CL, Carroll, MD, Kit, BK, Flegal M. Prevalence of childhood and adult obesity in the United States, 2011–2012. JAMA. 2014;311(8):806–814. doi:10.1001/jama.2014.732.
41. Li Y, Dai Q, Jackson JC, et al. Overweight is associated with decreased cognitive functioning among school-age children and adolescents. Obesity (Silver Spring). 2008;16(8):1809–1815. doi:10.1038/oby.2008.296.
42. Scott KM, Bruffaerts R, Simon GE, et al. Obesity and mental disorders in the general population: Results from the world mental health surveys. Int J Obes (Lond). 2008;32(1):192–200.
43. Wadden TA, Volger S, Tsai AG, at al. Managing obesity in primary care practice: An overview with perspective from the POWER-UP study. POWER-UP Research Group. Int J Obes (Lond). 2013;37(Suppl 1):S3–S11. doi:10.1038/ijo.2013.90.
44. Centers for Disease Control and Prevention, Division of Nutrition, Physical Activity, and Obesity. About adult BMI. http://www.cdc.gov/healthyweight/assessing/bmi/adult_bmi/. Updated May 15, 2015. Accessed December 28, 2015.
45. U.S. Department of Health and Human Services, National Heart, Lung, and Blood Institute. Classification of overweight and obesity by BMI, waist circumference, and associated disease risks. https://www.nhlbi.nih.gov/health/educational/lose_wt/BMI/bmi_dis.htm Accessed December 16, 2015.
46. Waist circumference and waist-hip ratio: Report of a WHO Expert consultation, Geneva, 8–11 December 2008. http://whqlibdoc.who.int/publications/2011/9789241501491_eng.pdf. Accessed February 3, 2016.
47. U.S. Department of Agriculture. Estimated calorie needs per day by age, gender, and physical activity level. http://www.cnpp.usda.gov/sites/default/files/usda_food_patterns/EstimatedCalorieNeedsPerDayTable.pdf. Accessed December 16, 2015.
48. Lafontan M, Visscher TL, Farpour-Lambert N, Yumuk V. Opportunities for intervention strategies for weight management: Global actions on fluid intake patterns. Obes Facts. 2015;8(1):54–76. doi:10.1159/000375103.
49. Bertoia ML, Mukamal KJ, Cahill LE, et al. Changes in intake of fruits and vegetables and weight change in United States, men and women followed for up to 24 years: Analysis from three prospective cohort studies. PLoS Med. 2015;12(9):e1001878.
50. Layman DK, Boileau RA, Erickson DJ, et al. A reduced ratio of dietary carbohydrate to protein improves body composition and blood lipid profiles during weight loss in adult women. J Nutr. 2003;133(2):411–417.
51. Vetter ML, Wadden TA, Chittams J, et al. Effect of lifestyle intervention on cardiometabolic risk factors: Results of the POWER-UP Trial. Int J Obesity (Lond). 2013;37(1):S19–S24. doi:10.1038/ijo.2013.92.
52. Carvajal R, Wadden TA, Tsai AG, Peck K, Moran CH. Managing obesity in primary care practice: a narrative review. Ann NY Acad Sci. 2013;1281(1):191–206. doi:10.1111/nyas.12004
53. Miras AD, le Roux CW. Can medical therapy mimic the clinical efficacy or physiological effects of bariatric surgery? Int J Obes (Lond). 2014;38(3):325–333. doi:10.1038/ijo.2013.205.
54. Johansson K, Neovius M, Hemmingsson E. Effects of anti-obesity drugs, diet, and exercise on weight-loss maintenance after a very-low-calorie diet or low-calorie diet: A systematic review and meta-analysis of randomized controlled trials. Am J Clin Nutr. 2014;99(1):14–23. doi:10.3945/ajcn.113.070052.
55. Apovian CM, Aronne LJ, Bessesen DH, et al. Pharmacological management of obesity: An Endocrine Society clinical practice guideline. J Clin Endocrinol Metab. 2015;100(2):342–346.
56. Yanovski SZ, Yanovski JA. Long-term drug treatment for obesity: A systematic and clinical review. JAMA. 2014;311(1):74–86. doi:10.1001/jama.2013.281361.
57. Dixon KJ, Shcherba S, Kipping RR. Weight loss from three commercial providers of NHS primary care slimming on referral in North Somerset: Service

evaluation. J Public Health. 2012;34(4):555–561. doi:10.1093/pubmed/fds034.
58. National Sleep Foundation. 2005 adult sleep habits and styles. https://sleepfoundation.org/sleep-polls-data/sleep-in-america-poll/2005-adult-sleep-habits-and-styles. Accessed December 16, 2015.
59. Dinges D, Pack F, Williams K, et al. Cumulative sleepiness, mood disturbance, and psychomotor vigilance performance decrements during a week of sleep restricted to 4-5 hours per night. Sleep. 1997;29(4):267–277.
60. Shukla A, Aizer A, Holmes D, et al. Effect of obstructive sleep apnea treatment on atrial fibrillation recurrence: A meta-analysis. J Am Coll Cardiol. 2015;1(1):41–51. doi:10.1016/j.jacep.2015.02.014.
61. American Psychiatric Association. Diagnostic and Statistical Manual of Mental Health Disorders, fifth ed. (DSM-5). Washington, DC: American Psychiatric Publishing; 2013.
62. Arnardottir ES, Bjornsdottir E, Olafsdottir KA, Benediktsdottir Bl, Gislason T. Obstructive sleep apnea in the general population: Highly prevalent but minimal symptoms. Eur Respir J. 2016;47(1):194–202. doi: 10.1183/13993003.01148-2015.
63. Zhu L, Zee PC. Circadian rhythm sleep disorders. Neurol Clin. 2012;30(4):1167–1191. doi:10.1016/j.ncl.2012.08.011
64. Kroenke K, Spitzer R L, Williams J B. The PHQ-9: Validity of a brief depression severity measure. J Gen Int Med. 2001;16(9):606–613.
65. Johns MW. A new method for measuring daytime sleepiness: The Epworth Sleepiness Scale. Sleep. 1991;14(6):540–545.
66. Schutte-Rodin S, Broch L, Buysse D, Dorsey C, Sateia M. Clinical guideline for the evaluation and management of chronic insomnia in adults. J Clin Sleep Med. 2008;4(5):487–504.
67. Morgenthaler TI, Lee-Chiong T, Alessi C, et al. Practice parameters for the clinical evaluation and treatment of circadian rhythm sleep disorders. An American Academy of Sleep Medicine Report. Sleep. 2007;30(11):1445–1459.
68. Winkelman JW. Insomnia disorder. N Engl J Med. 2015;373(15):1437–1444. doi:10.1056/NEJMcp1412740.
69. Garcia-Borreguero D, Kohnen R, Silber MH, et al. The long-term treatment of restless legs syndrome/Willis–Ekbom disease: Evidence-based guidelines and clinical consensus best practice guidance: a report from the International Restless Legs Syndrome Study Group. Sleep Med. 2013;14(7):675–684. doi:10.1016/j.sleep.2013.05.016.
70. Dodson ER, Zee PC. Therapeutics for circadian rhythm sleep disorders. Sleep Med Clin. 2010;5(4):701–715. doi:10.1016/j.jsmc.2010.08.001.
71. National Sleep Foundation. Sleep hygiene. https://sleepfoundation.org/ask-the-expert/sleep-hygiene. Accessed December 28, 2015.
72. Anderson KN, Goldsmith P, Gardiner A. A pilot evaluation of an online cognitive behavioral therapy for insomnia disorder—targeted screening and interactive Web design lead to improved sleep in a community population. Nature Sci Sleep. 2014;6:43–49. doi:10.2147/NSS.S57852.
73. Bertisch SM, Herzig SJ, Winkelman JW, Buettner C. National use of prescription medications for insomnia: NHANES 1999–2010. Sleep. 2014;37(2)343–349.
74. Aldworth J, Colpe LJ, Gfroerer JC, et al. The National Survey on Drug Use and Health Mental Health Surveillance Study: Calibration analysis. Int J Meth Psych Res. 2010;19(Suppl 1):61–87.
75. Golub A, Vazan P, Bennett AS, Liberty HJ. Unmet need for treatment of substance use disorders and serious psychological distress among veterans: A nationwide analysis using the NSDUH. Mil Med. 2013;178(1):107–114.
76. Rosenberg E, Lussier MT, Beaudoin C, Kirmayer LJ, Dufort GG. Determinants of the diagnosis of psychological problems by primary care physicians in patients with normal GHQ-28 scores. Gen Hosp Psychiatry. 2002;24(5):322–327.
77. Avey H, Matheny KB, Robbins A, Jacobson TA. Health care providers' training, perceptions, and practices regarding stress and health outcomes. J Natl Med Assoc. 2003 95(9):836–845.
78. Russ TC, Stamatakis E, Hamer M, Starr JM, Kivimäki M, Batty GD. Association between psychological distress and mortality: Individual participant pooled analysis of 10 prospective cohort studies. Br Med J. 2012;345:e4933. doi:10.1136/bmj.e4933.
79. Nerurkar A, Bitton A, Davis RB, Phillips RS, Yeh G. When physicians counsel about stress: Results of a national study. JAMA Intern Med. 2013;173(1):76–77.
80. Beaudoin C, Lussier MT, Gagnon RJ, Brouillet MI, Lalande R. Discussion of lifestyle-related issues in family practice during visits with general medical examination as the main reason for encounter: An exploratory study of content and determinants. Patient Educ Couns. 2001;45(4):275–284.
81. Crawford C, Wallerstedt DB, Khorsan R, Clausen SS, Jonas WB, Walter JAG. A systematic review of biopsychosocial training programs for the self-management of emotional stress: Potential applications for the military. Evidence-Based Complementary and Alternative Medicine : eCAM. 2013;2013:747694. doi:10.1155/2013/747694.
82. National Center for Health Promotion and Disease Prevention, Office of Patient Care Services, Veterans

Health Administration. Healthy living message: Manage stress. http://www.nyharbor.va.gov/docs/HPDPmanagestress.pdf. Accessed December 28, 2015.

83. Clinical Resources: VISN 2 Center for Integrated Healthcare (CIH). U.S. Department of Veterans Affairs. http://www.mentalhealth.va.gov/coe/cih-visn2/clinical_resources.asp. Updated June 3, 2015. Accessed February 15, 2016.

84. U.S. Department of Veterans Affairs, Veterans Health Administration, Patient Care Services. Manage Stress Workbook. http://www.prevention.va.gov/mpt/2013/docs/managestressworkbook_dec2013.pdf. Accessed February 15, 2016.

85. National Center for Telehealth and Technology. Mobile Applications. http://t2health.dcoe.mil/products/mobile-apps. Updated 2016. Accessed February 15, 2016.

23

Integrated Chronic Pain and Psychiatric Management

ROBERT M. MCCARRON, AMIR RAMEZANI, IAN KOEBNER, SAMIR J. SHETH, AND JESSICA PALKA

BOX 23.1

KEY POINTS

- **Chronic pain and psychiatric conditions are highly comorbid.**
- **Early screening and use of a team approach optimizes the treatment of chronic pain.**
- **An integrated, multidisciplinary treatment approach is recommended for patient who have both chronic physical pain and psychiatric illness.**
- **Treatments for chronic pain include pharmacologic consultations, cognitive-behavioral therapy, trauma-focused therapies, biofeedback and mindfulness-based therapies, acupuncture, community engagement, nutrition consultation and behavioral weight management, and behavioral sleep management.**

CHRONIC PAIN: AN OVERVIEW

Pain is the number-one reason individuals seek medical attention. According to the Institute of Medicine, nearly 100 million Americans suffer from chronic pain,[1] more than the number of Americans suffering from heart disease, cancer, and diabetes combined.[2] Twenty-five million adults (11.2%) report experiencing pain every day for the last 3 months; those with more severe pain have worse overall health, use more health care, and have more disability than those with less severe pain.[3]

The International Association for the Study of Pain defines pain as "an unpleasant sensory and emotional experience associated with actual or potential tissue damage, or is described in terms of such damage."[4] Implicit in this definition is recognition that pain is never purely a physiologic phenomenon. While chronic pain is widely acknowledged as a biopsychosocial phenomenon, its psychological and social dimensions are often inadequately addressed clinically,[5–7] despite an established body of literature demonstrating the relationship of chronic pain to numerous psychosocial factors including but not limited to depression, stress, anxiety, posttraumatic stress disorder (PTSD), and perceived social connection.[8–11] Therefore, there is a need to develop integrative pain medicine models that both acknowledge and address chronic pain as a biopsychosocial phenomenon. See Box 23.1 for key points to consider when developing a integrated chronic pain program.

Unfortunately, usual care for some chronic pain conditions increasingly relies on diagnostic tests and treatment options that have not been well validated in terms of safety or effectiveness, and abuse of pain medication has become a major public health concern.[12] Since 2003, more overdose deaths have involved opioid analgesics than heroin and cocaine combined.[13] For every unintentional overdose death related to an opioid analgesic, nine persons are admitted for substance abuse treatment, 35 people visit emergency departments, 161 people report drug abuse or dependence, and 461 people report nonmedical uses of opioid analgesics. The Institute of Medicine estimates the annual economic burden of chronic pain in terms of medical costs and lost productivity in the United States to be over $600 billion, which exceeds the cost of each of the nation's priority health conditions.[1,2] See Chapter14: Treating Substance Use Disorders in Integrated Care Settings for a discussion about treatments for opiate abuse.

Complementary health approaches to chronic pain management are prevalent in the United States, with 33.2% of adults with pain acknowledging the use of at least one complementary modality.[15] American adults who use complementary health approaches to treat or manage pain spent out of pocket an estimated $14.9 billion on them, according to the 2007 National Health Interview Survey (NHIS). This accounts for 20% to 25% of all out-of-pocket spending to treat or manage pain, including complementary and conventional care. Back pain was the number-one condition by far in terms of cost, with $8.7 billion spent out of pocket on complementary approaches. This was more than a quarter the amount spent on all conventional health care for back pain ($30.5 billion, according to Medical Expenditures Panel Survey data). Most of the $4.7 billion complementary-approach spending for back pain was for practitioner visits rather than dietary supplements.[15]

Chronic pain is a complex biopsychosocial phenomenon with significant costs to society in terms of both personal suffering and economic burden. The need for integrated evidence-based care that incorporates the psychosocial components of chronic pain is essential and timely given the dual epidemics of chronic pain and abuse of certain pain medications that our country faces.

CHRONIC PAIN AND PSYCHIATRIC COMORBIDITY

Patients with chronic pain conditions disproportionately have comorbid psychiatric conditions. An estimated 40% to 50% of patients with chronic pain conditions have a comorbid mood disorder and an estimated 35% have a comorbid anxiety disorder.[16,17] Major depressive disorder, dysthymia, generalized anxiety disorder, agoraphobia, panic disorder, social phobia, PTSD, and substance use disorders each have a greater prevalence among patients receiving treatment for chronic pain conditions.[18] Table 23.1 includes a listing of select psychiatric disorders and the odds ratio of comorbid psychopathology among patients with low back or neck pain compared to those without such pain.

Comorbid psychiatric conditions complicate the management of chronic pain conditions. For example, depression and anxiety are associated with poorer treatment outcomes, more pain complaints, greater pain intensity, longer duration of pain, and greater likelihood of nonrecovery.[19,20]

Another group of disorders frequently comorbid with chronic pain are the somatic symptom and related disorders. See Chapter 16: Somatic Symptom Disorders and Illness Anxiety in Integrated Care Settings. However, due to frequently changing diagnostic categorization of these disorders and disagreement over diagnostic validity, reliable estimates of the prevalence of these disorders are not available.[21] With the advent of "somatic symptom disorder, with predominant pain" in the most recent edition of the *Diagnostic and Statistical Manual of Mental Disorders*, Fifth Edition (DSM-5),[22] the diagnosis has become more inclusive and would likely

TABLE 23.1 LIKELIHOOD OF COMORBID PSYCHOPATHOLOGY AMONG PATIENTS WITH NECK OR LOW BACK PAIN[a]

DSM-5 Diagnosis	Comorbidity, Odds Ratio (Confidence Interval)
Major depressive episode	2.8 (2.3, 3.5)
Dysthymia	3.7 (2.8, 5.0)
Generalized anxiety disorder	3.0 (2.3, 3.9)
Agoraphobia or panic disorder	2.1 (1.6, 2.7)
Social phobia	1.9 (1.5, 2.3)
Posttraumatic stress disorder	2.8 (2.3, 3.5)
Alcohol abuse/ dependence	1.8 (1.4, 2.5)

[a] Odds ratio of each psychiatric diagnosis being found in an individual with low back or neck pain compared to individuals without such pain. Based on the World Mental Health Surveys.[18]

include a significant percentage of chronic pain patients.[23]

Personality disorders are present in an estimated 31% to 81% of chronic pain patients, while only 15% of the general U.S. population is felt to have a personality disorder.[24,25] See Chapter 17: Working with Personality Disorders in an Integrated Care Setting. Patients with borderline, paranoid, histrionic, and dependent personality disorders commonly experience comorbid pain.

Patients with both personality disorders and multiple somatic complaints are often labeled as "difficult" by their providers.[26,27] Such difficult encounters are estimated to make up 10% to 20% of primary care visits.[26,28] Lack of training in the management of patients with personality disorders and multiple somatic complaints can lead to provider burnout and worse patient outcomes.

From a theoretical standpoint, the "diathesis-stress model" is most often used to explain the development of comorbid chronic pain disorders and mental illness.[29] This model proposes that a given patient has preexisting, semidormant psychological characteristics that are activated by the stress of chronic pain and eventually result in psychopathology; for example, the patient sustains an injury, experiences functional impairment leading to loss of employment, and subsequently develops depression. Consistent with this model, most studies suggest that mental disorders, in particular depressive disorders, occur after chronic pain begins.[30] Personality disorders also appear to fit the diathesis-stress model for development in chronic pain patients. This raises concern that what is diagnosed as a personality disorder may in reality be an overrepresentation of maladaptive coping mechanisms in a patient experiencing chronic pain.[31]

Among patients with chronic pain and psychiatric comorbidity, suicide is a devastating potential outcome. Mental disorders have long been considered independent risk factors for suicide, suicide attempt, and suicidal ideation.[32] Among the psychiatric diagnoses, major depressive disorder is the most common single diagnosis and anxiety disorders are the most common group of diagnoses associated with suicide, suicide attempt, and suicidal ideation.[32,33] A growing body of literature has also established chronic pain conditions as independent risk factors for suicidal ideation and suicide attempt. Migraines, "back problems," and abdominal pain have been the most frequently researched chronic pain conditions associated with suicidal ideation and suicide attempts. A large epidemiologic study using the Canadian Community Health Survey found migraine and "back problems" to be independently associated with suicidal ideation and suicide attempts.[34] Comorbidity with multiple psychiatric diagnoses and chronic pain conditions only strengthens the association. However, not all chronic pain conditions (e.g., fibromyalgia, arthritis) are associated with suicidal ideation and suicide attempts.

THE INTEGRATED BEHAVIORAL PAIN MEDICINE TREATMENT MODEL

The Integrated Behavioral Pain Medicine (IBPM) treatment model is a multidisciplinary, team-based treatment approach designed to address the complexity and increasing prevalence of chronic pain and related opioid use in the primary care setting. The main goals of IBPM are as follows:

1. Early recognition of those who have chronic pain and comorbid psychiatric illness
2. Early recognition of those who are at increased overall risk from taking opioid medications
3. Alleviation of the inherent stress to the patient and health system associated with treating complex chronic pain conditions in the primary care setting
4. Provision of evidence-based and wellness-based therapies to those who have chronic pain and comorbid psychiatric illness
5. Reduction of morbidity and mortality associated with poorly treated chronic pain and opioid medication use.

IBPM consists of a four-stage system that begins in the primary care setting and, depending on the severity of illness, may evolve into treatment within a pain medicine clinic. Close collaboration between the primary care provider and IBPM staff is critical to the success of this care model.

IBPM Triage Process

Figure 23.1 provides a broad overview of the IBPM process, with specific inclusion and exclusion criteria detailed for each assessment.

The four-stage process starts with Stage 1, when a primary care provider (PCP) treats uncomplicated pain that is present for less than 3 months. For patients who have had pain for longer than 3 months

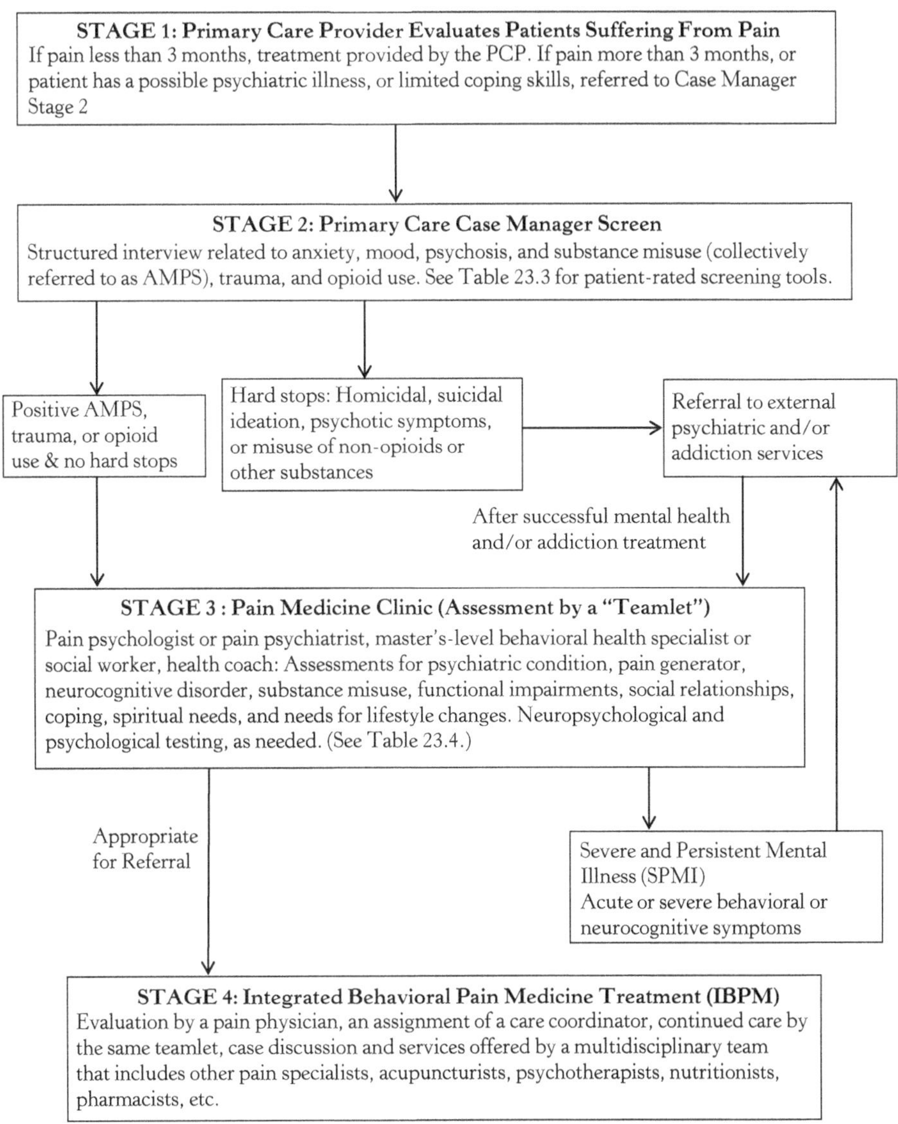

FIGURE 23.1 Overview of the four stages of the Integrated Behavioral Pain Medicine (IBPM) model.

and have possible psychiatric illness or limited coping skills, a referral is placed to the primary care manager (Stage 2). The case manager is located in the primary care setting and, as a nonlicensed person with a minimum of a bachelor's degree, will follow a structured interview and provide the patient with self-rated screening tools (Stage 2). The results of the structured interview and screening tools will determine whether the patient moves forward to the pain medicine clinic (Stage 3) for more extensive clinical assessment with a doctoral-level mental health provider and an IBPM health coach and/or a social worker, collectively forming a clinical "teamlet."

Before enrollment into the Stage 4 IBPM treatment program, the patient will meet with the pain management teamlet for further assessment and more extensive clinical screening tools. After this assessment, most patients will join the IBPM program (Stage 4), which includes treatment by a pain medicine physician as well as other nonphysician providers (e.g., acupuncturists, psychotherapists, nutritionists, pharmacists).

Our model is unique for two main reasons. First, the patient receives a comprehensive "pain psychiatric" assessment before seeing the pain medicine physician. Second, the treatment is largely based on a multidisciplinary approach, which is individually tailored and strongly focused on addressing psychosocial stressors, which often amplify or even generate the perception of pain.

The Four Stages of the IBPM

Stage 1: Primary Care Provider

In the initial triage stage, the PCP initiates a referral by way of the electronic medical record or through other technology. This referral is initiated if the patient has treatment-refractory chronic pain (greater than 3 months in duration) and possible comorbid psychiatric illness, including somatization or "psychiatric pain generators/amplifiers." The referral criteria are meant to be broad so that the majority of patients can move forward to access IBPM services. Patients are referred to the primary care case manager.

Stage 2: Primary Care Case Manager

In Stage 2, the primary care case manager determines whether the patient meets criteria for a broader pain management assessment by using structured interviews and brief screening measures. Since the case manager may not be an independent and licensed clinical provider, there are explicit criteria for the case manager to follow. Review Figure 23.1, which illustrates the IBPM Stage 2 criteria.

The case manager's manualized interview consists of questions related to anxiety, mood, psychosis, and substance misuse (collectively referred to as AMPS). (See Chapter 11: Integrated Care for Anxiety Disorders and Chapter 12: Treating Depression and Bipolar Disorder in Integrated Care Settings.) Patients are also routinely asked about use of opioid medications. Patients who report current use of opioids or significant psychosocial stressors or disclose symptoms of anxiety or depression will likely be seen in the pain medicine clinic (Stage 3) for further assessment and eventual IBPM treatment (Stage 4). Patients who exhibit homicidal/suicidal ideation, psychotic symptoms, or misuse of nonopioid substances (referred to as "hard stops" in the IBPM triage process) will need to be referred externally and/or treated for these conditions before moving forward in the process.

The primary care case manager's criteria for brief screening measures include the presence of any of the following:

1. Elevated depression scores ranging between 5 (mild depression) and 19 (moderately severe depression) on the Patient Health Questionnaire-9[35]
2. Elevated trauma scores of 1 or more on the Primary Care-Posttraumatic Stress Disorder questionnaire[36]
3. Elevated functional impairment scores of 7 or more on any item of the Pain Disability Index[37]
4. Positive substance use/opioid use on any items of the modified CAGE questions[38]

Table 23.2 lists case manager screening tools and domains assessed with respect to chronic pain patients. Table 23.3 provides a more extensive list that PCP and pain medicine providers can use when assessing patients who have chronic pain.

See Chapter 10: Automated Mental Health Assessment for Integrated Care: The Quick

TABLE 23.2 PRIMARY CARE CASE MANAGER SCREENING TOOLS

Tools	Psychological Functioning	Pain and Sleep Functioning	Substance/ Opioid Use
Anxiety, Mood, Psychosis and Substance Abuse (AMPS)	√		
Patient Health Questionnaire-9 (PHQ-9)[35]	√		
Primary Care-Posttraumatic Stress Disorder (PC-PTSD)[36]	√		
Pain Disability Index (PDI)[37]		√	
CAGE[38] for problem drinking			√

TABLE 23.3 OVERVIEW OF BRIEF SCREENING TOOLS

Tools	Psychological Functioning	Pain and Sleep Functioning	Opioid Use
Anxiety, Mood, Psychosis and Substance Abuse (AMPS)[a]	√		
Patient Health Questionnaire-9 (PHQ-9)[35]	√		
Generalized Anxiety Disorder-7 (GAD-7)[39]	√		
Primary Care-Posttraumatic Stress Disorder (PC-PTSD)[36]	√		
Brief Pain Inventory (BPI)[40]	√	√	
Multidimensional Pain Inventory (MPI)[41]	√	√	
Pain Disability Index (PDI)[37]		√	
Provokes, Quality, Radiates, Severity, Time (PQRST) [42,a]		√	
McGill Pain Questionnaire (MPQ)[43]		√	
STOP-BANG[44] for obstructive sleep apnea		√	
CAGE[38] for problem drinking			√
Prescription Drug Monitoring Program[45,b]			√
Screener and Opioid Assessment for Patients in Pain (SOAPP)[46]			√
Current Opioid Misuse Measure[47]			√
Urine drug test			√
4 A's Opioid Assessment[48,a]			√

[a]Interview tool that provider can use with the patient
[b]Tool available for provider to order or obtain

PsychoDiagnostics (QPD Panel) for an additional diagnostic screening instrument.

Based on the manualized interview and brief screening measures, the primary care case manager may refer the patient to Stage 3 care. Figure 23.1 shows the referral criteria.

Stage 3: Pain Medicine Clinic

Once patients enter the pain medicine service (Stage 3), they undergo a pain medicine assessment by a small behavioral health team, the IBPM teamlet. *Teamlet* is a term used to describe a small team of providers who meet with the patient in a systematic way, which helps to increase access, improve efficient delivery of clinical services, and reduces the burden on the patient and provider.[49] The teamlet is composed of a doctoral-level behavioral health specialist (BHS) (e.g., pain psychologist or pain psychiatrist), a master's-level BHS (e.g., social worker), and a health coach. The PCP will not routinely be a part of the teamlet meetings unless he or she would like to attend. This general teamlet format is used for the pain management assessment, the pain physician assessment, and other clinical visits in the IBPM program. An integral part of this teamlet is the IBPM health coach. In our program, this unlicensed team member works closely with IBPM patients and will be available to address and triage questions. See Chapter 25: Health Coaching in Integrated Care for more details on the roles and functioning of health coaches.

The primary purpose of the Stage 3 pain management assessment is to determine whether the patient meets entrance criteria to Stage 4 IBPM treatment services and to develop an integrated treatment plan. Figure 23.1 shows the referral criteria that the behavioral teamlet uses to determine entrance into the Stage 4 program.

Doctoral-level BHSs and psychiatrists are best qualified in the assessment, diagnosis, and treatment of mental health conditions. They both can play a major role in assessing (1) the presence of a psychiatric condition, psychiatric pain generator, neurocognitive disorder, substance misuse, suicide risk, and functional status; (2) the severity and functional impairments of the aforementioned conditions; and (3) the patient's appropriateness for IBPM services.[50] Unlike the brief screening tools used by the case manager in Stage 2, the BHS or psychiatrist determines whether a comprehensive assessment or battery of tests would be psychiatrically or medically indicated. For example, the team may see a 64-year-old man who is filing for a disability claim; has no history of psychiatric illness; and reports inconsistent physical, cognitive, and psychiatric symptoms in the context of generalized, whole-body pain and a history of traumatic brain injury. In this case, the Stage 3 team provider may wish to obtain objective neuropsychological and psychological tests that help diagnose cognitive functioning, somatization processes, personality disorder, and symptom magnification. The Stage 3 team provider would make a referral for a comprehensive neuropsychological and psychological testing by a neuropsychologist. The results may provide a clear direction for referral to the IBPM treatment (e.g., in the case of somatization) or may identify an inappropriate candidate for IBPM (e.g., a case of malingering, factitious disorder, or dementia). The results can assist not only in ruling out neurocognitive disorders (e.g., mild or major neurocognitive disorders) but also in assessing core brain functioning abilities that underlie activities of daily living (e.g., memory, executive functioning, motor function). This further assists the PCP and integrated team in understanding the level of assistance the patient requires. Several comprehensive standardized psychological tests are listed in Table 23.4.

Social workers are highly qualified in assessing psychosocial, family, cultural, and societal aspects of mental health and medical conditions.[53,54] The social worker can function as a case manager and coordinates closely with other health care professionals. The role of the social worker as an integral part of the IBPM teamlet is to assess the impact of medical and psychological conditions with regard to the patient's (1) social, family, and community relationships; (2) ability to cope with such conditions and distress; (3) spiritual or religious beliefs and practices; and (4) need for lifestyle changes (e.g., exercise and healthy eating).

In the context of the IBPM team, social work specialists also help track patient outcome data in a unified registry. The registry is used to determine treatment algorithms and the effectiveness of the program. For example, the registry can be used to discover which patients respond best to

TABLE 23.4 COMPREHENSIVE STANDARDIZED PSYCHOLOGICAL AND NEUROPSYCHOLOGICAL TOOLS

Tools	Psychiatric Conditions	Pain and Somatization	Minimization/ Exaggeration of Symptoms	Habits Affecting Medical Condition
Personality Assessment Inventory (PAI)[51]	√	√	√	
Minnesota Multiphasic Personality Inventory-II RF (MMPI-II RF)[52]	√	√	√	
Millon Behavioral Medicine Diagnostic (MBMD)[53]	√	√		√

opioids, antidepressant medications, biofeedback, or cognitive-behavioral therapy (CBT); which patients are good candidates for the IBPM program; and for which patients the program is efficacious.

Health coaches often focus on exercise, stress management, nutrition, and harm reductions, and most are well trained in motivational interviewing and some form of problem solving. The health coach plays an essential role in facilitating efficient behavioral pain medicine services and serves as a support to the rest of the clinical team. See Chapter 25: Health Coaching in Integrated Care.

Stage 4: IBPM Treatment

The overall goal of IBPM services is to help patients receive comprehensive biopsychosocial care that squarely addresses physical, behavioral, cognitive, and social aspects of their chronic pain condition. IBPM treatment service provides an evaluation by a pain physician, the assignment of a care coordinator, continued care by the same health coach, teamlet case discussion, and participation in the multidisciplinary management plan.[49]

Once patients start IBPM treatment services, they meet with their pain physician and part of the IBPM teamlet. At a minimum, the health coach will be present during most visits with the pain medicine physician. The IBPM teamlet includes the following:

1. Providers who are typically medical, such as a physician who is a pain specialist (e.g., anesthesiologist, neurologist, psychiatrist)
2. Health coaches, who can have various degrees and often serve multiple roles. Some of the bachelor's-level individuals are trained in how to best support patients within their established treatment plans. Health coaches help the patient and providers to seamlessly navigate the IBPM program and organize patient care activities.
3. Care coordinators, who are typically master's-level clinicians, such as social workers, marriage and family therapists, nurses, or nurse practitioners. The care coordinator may supervise and mentor the IBPM health coaches, monitor the delivery of IBPM services, and update the patient and providers when there is a deviation from the treatment plan.

IBPM treatment also includes a wide range of pharmacologic and nonpharmacologic treatments and services that address multiple aspects of chronic pain. These services are aimed toward the primary goal of enhancing behavioral, physical, emotional, and social/community functioning.

TREATMENTS FOR CHRONIC PAIN

Examples of evidence-based treatments for various forms of chronic pain include pharmacologic consultations, CBT, trauma-focused therapies, biofeedback and mindfulness-based therapies, acupuncture, community engagement (e.g., Art Rx, which is a pilot program at University of California, Davis), physical therapy, nutrition consultation and behavioral weight management, and behavioral sleep management.

Pharmacologic Consultation

Pharmacologic consultation meetings are conducted with a psychiatrist who specializes in pain medicine; the purpose is to assess and monitor pain and use of psychotropic medications. The IBPM teamlet works with the PCP or other prescriber and patient to monitor adherence to treatment, while providing written information about prescribed medications and side effects to patients and their families.

Cognitive-Behavioral Therapy

CBT is an evidence-based psychotherapy that improves psychiatric conditions and chronic pain.[55,56] CBT includes a broad spectrum of clinical interventions that aim to change thoughts, beliefs, and behaviors that commonly interfere with the management of pain. CBT helps the patient learn cognitive and behavioral strategies that expand coping strategies for emotional distress, functional impairment, and severe pain. CBT can be used for those who have fibromyalgia, irritable bowel syndrome, somatic symptoms disorder, depression, anxiety, and other disorders. Some examples of cognitive strategies that help patients manage pain include the following:

1. Recognition of the effects of irrational thinking on emotion and pain sensation
2. Identification of unrealistic thinking patterns, such as "all-or-none" thinking and overgeneralization (see Table 25.3 in Chapter 25: Health Coaching in Integrated Care)
3. A change from unrealistic thinking to helpful and goal-directed thinking (see

Table 25.4 in Chapter 25: Health Coaching in Integrated Care)
4. Completion of dysfunctional thought records (see Fig. 25.1 in Chapter 25: Health Coaching in Integrated Care)

Some additional examples of behavioral strategies for pain management include the following:

1. Recognition and change of pain behaviors that reinforce inactivity, decreased functioning, and increased emotional distress
2. Recognition and change in sick role or pain-mediated interpersonal relationships that solicit people to assist with functional activities, which ultimately reinforce pain behaviors
3. Management of daily activity levels via activity–rest cycle/timed pacing
4. Medication management and adherence training

Trauma-Focused Therapies

Trauma-focused therapies are psychotherapy modalities that help to decrease symptoms associated with PTSD and related conditions. A wide range of psychotherapy systems have been empirically validated to treat posttraumatic stress and related trauma symptoms. Trauma-focused therapies include CBT, cognitive processing, exposure therapy, and eye movement desensitization and reprocessing (EMDR).[57,58] See Chapter 11: Integrated Care for Anxiety Disorders for additional information on PTSD and trauma-related treatments.

Psychophysiologic and Biofeedback Interventions

Psychophysiologic treatments, such as biofeedback interventions, are evidence-based treatments that have a long history of being applied to musculoskeletal, neurologic, pain, neurocognitive, and psychiatric conditions.[59] Psychophysiologic treatment teaches the individual how to self-regulate a physiologic system (e.g., cerebral blood flow, electrophysiologic activity of the brain, muscle tension, galvanic skin response, heart rate variability) via cognitive and attention processes with the goal, in a pain patient, of reducing pain.

Mindfulness-Based Therapies

Mindfulness is the purposeful act of bringing attention to "moment-to-moment" experience in an accepting, nonjudgmental, and curious manner.[49] Mindfulness and acceptance-based psychotherapies have been shown to improve psychiatric conditions and chronic pain conditions.[60] Patients can participate in mindfulness-based interventions by participating in a traditional mindfulness-based stress reduction course and/or in newer but well-established forms, such as mindfulness-based cognitive therapy or mindfulness-based self-compassion. The majority of mindfulness-based interventions include an eight-week class that includes sitting meditation, walking meditation, body scans, breathing meditation, silent one-day meditation retreats, mindful eating, moving meditation, yoga, and tracking pleasant activities.

Acupuncture

According to the 2007 NHIS, approximately 3 million Americans used acupuncture within the past year, a 50% increase from 5 years earlier.[61] The 2002 NHIS demonstrated that roughly 80% of acupuncture treatments were directed at pain conditions and 72% of respondents reported receiving "some" or "a great deal" of help for their first condition.[62] The largest systematic review and meta-analysis of acupuncture for chronic pain to date, by Vickers et al,[63] analyzed data from 17,922 individuals to determine the effect size of acupuncture for several chronic pain conditions, including back and neck pain, osteoarthritis, chronic headache, and shoulder pain. Acupuncture was superior to both sham and no-acupuncture control for each pain condition ($p < .001$ for all comparisons).[55] In practical terms the effect sizes in this study demonstrate that half of patients receiving acupuncture would have had a 50% or more reduction in pain compared to 30% in the no-treatment group and about 43% percent receiving sham acupuncture. This study of high-quality randomized controlled trials, using individual patient data meta-analyses of nearly 18,000 randomized patients, represents the most robust evidence to date that acupuncture is both effective and efficacious for chronic pain.

Community Interventions: Art Rx

An appreciation for the social determinants of health[64–67] has reframed "where health happens" and has opened up new opportunities for organizations outside of the clinical enterprise, such as museums,

BOX 23.2

SUMMARY OF RECOMMENDED TREATMENT APPROACHES AND RELEVANT EVIDENCE

Strength of recommendation taxonomy (SOR A, B, or C)

- **Cognitive-behavioral therapy (CBT) is an evidence-based psychotherapy that improves psychiatric conditions and chronic pain. (SOR B)[4,5]**
- **Trauma-focused therapies, which include CBT, cognitive processing, exposure therapy, and eye movement desensitization and reprocessing (EMDR), help to decrease symptoms associated with posttraumatic stress and related conditions. (SOR B)[57,58]**
- **Biofeedback interventions have been successfully used to treat musculoskeletal, neurologic, pain, neurocognitive, and psychiatric conditions. (SOR C)[59]**
- **Mindfulness and acceptance-based psychotherapies have been shown to improve psychiatric conditions and chronic pain conditions. (SOR B)[6]**
- **The National Health Interview Survey (NHIS) 2002 demonstrated that roughly 80% of acupuncture treatments were directed at pain conditions and 72% of respondents reported receiving "some" or "a great deal" of help for their first condition. (SOR A)[62]**
- **Vickers et al[63] analyzed high-quality randomized controlled trials, using individual patient data meta-analyses of nearly 18,000 randomized patients. This represents the most robust evidence to date that acupuncture is both effective and efficacious for chronic pain. (SOR A)[62]**
- **Art Rx encourages positive social experiences in a museum setting that reduce chronic pain. (SOR C)[72]**
- **Dietitian counseling helps patients change unhealthy eating habits, thereby reducing comorbid medical and psychiatric conditions that contribute to pain. (SOR C)[73]**
- **Behavioral weight management and behavioral sleep management can reduce some of the comorbid conditions that occur with chronic pain, such as obesity, eating disorders, and sleep disorders. (SOR C)[74,75]**

to become public health partners. Art museums can be restorative environments[68,69] that foster a sense of social inclusion,[70,71] and group tours led by docents may create a sense of community among participants that facilitates the experience of social connection. The Integrative Pain Management Program at UC Davis has initiated an innovative program for individuals with pain, as well as their families, called Art Rx. Based on the understanding that social connection may be analgesic,[11] Art Rx seeks to encourage positive experiences that reduce the burden of chronic pain[72] through specialized tours of the museum and facilitated discussion. The program is free and open to any individual with chronic pain. In addition, participants are encouraged to invite family members and caregivers to attend free of charge.

Nutrition/Dietitian Intervention

Nutritional counseling, offered by dietitians, helps patients to address maladaptive eating patterns and reduces comorbid medical and psychiatric conditions that contribute to pain.[73] For example, nutritional interventions help to improve meal planning and healthy eating to reduce diabetes and obesity, which can indirectly reduce pain sensitivity. Intervention offered by dietitians also helps to improve eating habits associated with binge eating, which frequently contribute to obesity and diabetes. See Chapter 22: Wellness; An Integrated Approach for discussion about delivering wellness interventions in integrated care settings.

Behavioral Weight and Sleep Management

Cognitive, behavioral, and mindfulness strategies are also applied to comorbid medical conditions that often accompany chronic pain. CBT and mindfulness interventions also encompass behavioral weight management and behavioral sleep management. These interventions aim to reduce obesity, disordered eating, and the effects of sleep disorders, which often are comorbid with chronic pain.[74,75] Behavioral weight management interventions help address emotional eating, overeating, night eating, grazing, and loss of control while eating. These interventions also include managing urges to eat, managing relationships that sabotage healthy eating, and managing body image dissatisfaction. See Chapter 15: Integrated Care for Binge Eating Disorder and Other Eating Disorders for additional information. Sleep management interventions include planning a sleep–wake schedule, sleep hygiene prior to sleep and upon awakening from sleep, controlling environmental sounds and light, and management of arousal/stimulating thoughts, emotions, and behavior. See Chapter 22 Wellness: An Integrated Care Approach for additional information about sleep interventions.

CONCLUSION

PCPs are at the forefront of pain management, but they are often limited by time constraints and a paucity of pain medicine referral resources. The authors suggest incorporating the IBPM treatment model into integrated care practices and pain medicine clinics, with the hope that this multidisciplinary approach to care will supply much-needed services to those with chronic pain. If these models are not readily available in your environment, we recommend using parts of this model (e.g., nutritionist, psychotherapist, acupuncturist). In addition, clinicians must recognize the critical importance of addressing frequently comorbid psychiatric conditions in those who have chronic pain; this should be a routine part of its treatment. See Box 23.2 for an overview of evidence based treatment approaches for treating chronic pain.

REFERENCES

1. Institute of Medicine. Committee on Advancing Pain Research C, Education. Relieving Pain in America: A Blueprint for Transforming Prevention, Care, Education, and Research.Washington, DC: National Academies Press; 2011.
2. Gaskin DJ, Richard P. The economic costs of pain in the United States. J Pain. 2012;13(8):715–724.
3. Nahin RL. Estimates of pain prevalence and severity in adults: United States, 2012. J Pain. 2015;16(8):769–780.
4. Task force on taxonomy of the International Association for the Study of Pain. Classification of Chronic Pain: Description of Chronic Pain Syndromes and Definitions of Pain Terms. 2nd ed. Seattle, WA: IASP Press; 1994.
5. Turk DC, Monarch ES. Biopsychosocial perspective on chronic pain. In: Turk GC, Gatchel RJ, eds. Psychological Approaches to Pain Management: A Practitioner's Handbook. 2nd ed. New York: Guilford Press; 1996:3–32.
6. Gatchel RJ, Peng YB, Peters ML, Fuchs PN, Turk DC. The biopsychosocial approach to chronic pain: Scientific advances and future directions. Psychol Bull. 2007;133(4):581–624.
7. Blyth FM, Macfarlane GJ, Nicholas MK. The contribution of psychosocial factors to the development of chronic pain: The key to better outcomes for patients? J Pain. 2007;129(1):8–11.
8. Kroenke K, Wu J, Bair MJ, Krebs EE, Damush TM, Tu W. Reciprocal relationship between pain and depression: A 12-month longitudinal analysis in primary care. J Pain. 2011;12(9):964–973.
9. Van Uum S, Sauve B, Fraser L, Morley-Forster P, Paul T, Koren G. Elevated content of cortisol in hair of patients with severe chronic pain: A novel biomarker for stress: Short communication. Stress Med. 2008;11(6):483–488.
10. McWilliams LA, Cox BJ, Enns MW. Mood and anxiety disorders associated with chronic pain: An examination in a nationally representative sample. J Pain. 2003;106(1):127–133.
11. Eisenberger NI. The pain of social disconnection: Examining the shared neural underpinnings of physical and social pain. Nat Rev Neurosci. 2012;13(6):421–434.
12. Deyo RA, Mirza SK, Turner JA, Martin BI. Overtreating chronic back pain: Time to back off? J Am Board Fam Med. 2009;22(1):62–68.
13. Dowell D, Haegerich TM, Chou R. CDC Guideline for prescribing opioids for chronic pain—United States, 2016. JAMA. 2016;315(15):1624–1645. doi:10.1001/jama.2016.1464.
14. Centers for Disease Control Prevention. CDC grand rounds: Prescription drug overdoses—a US epidemic. MMWR. 2012;61(1):10–13.
15. Nahin RL, Stussman BJ, Herman PM. Out-of-pocket expenditures on complementary health approaches associated with painful health conditions in a nationally representative adult sample. J Pain. 2015;16(11):1147–1162.
16. McWilliams LA, Cox BJ, Enns MW. Mood and anxiety disorders associated with chronic pain: An examination in a nationally representative sample. J Pain. 2003;106(1–2):127–133.
17. Relieving pain in America: A blueprint for transforming prevention, care, education, and research. Choice. 2012;49(11):2098–2098.
18. Demyttenaere K, Bruffaerts R, Lee S, et al. Mental disorders among persons with chronic back or neck pain: Results from the World Mental Health Surveys. J Pain. 2007;129(3):332–342.
19. Bair MJ, Robinson RL, Katon W, Kroenke K. Depression and pain comorbidity: A literature review. Arch Intern Med. 2003;163(20):2433–2445.
20. Bair MJ, Wu J, Damush TM, Sutherland JM, Kroenke K. Association of depression and anxiety

alone and in combination with chronic musculoskeletal pain in primary care patients. Psychosom Med. 2008;70(8):890–897.
21. Dersh J, Gatchel RJ, Polatin P, Mayer T. Prevalence of psychiatric disorders in patients with chronic work-related musculoskeletal pain disability. J Occup Environ Med. 2002;44(5):459–468.
22. American Psychiatric Association. DSM-5 basics. In: American Psychiatric Association, ed. Diagnostic and Statistical Manual of Mental Disorders. 5th ed. Arlington, VA: American Psychiatric Association; 2013.
23. American Psychiatric Association. Diagnostic and Statistical Manual of Mental Disorders. 5th ed. Arlington, VA. American Psychiatric Association; 2013.
24. Grant BF, Hasin DS, Stinson FS, et al. Prevalence, correlates, and disability of personality disorders in the United States: Results from the National Epidemiologic Survey on Alcohol and Related Conditions. J Clin Psychiatry. 2004;65(7):948–958.
25. Davis JL. Personality disorders affect 15% of Americans. Web MD. http://www.webmd.com/mental-health/news/20040804/personaity-disorders-affect-15-of-americans August 3, 2004. Accessed June 10, 2016.
26. Hahn SR, Thompson KS, Wills TA, Stern V, Budner NS. The difficult doctor-patient relationship: Somatization, personality and psychopathology. J Clin Epidemiol. 1994;47(6):647–657.
27. Hahn SR. Physical symptoms and physician-experienced difficulty in the physician-patient relationship. Ann Intern Med. 2001;134(9 Pt 2):897–904.
28. Jackson JL, Kroenke K. Difficult patient encounters in the ambulatory clinic: Clinical predictors and outcomes. Arch Intern Med. 1999;159(10):1069–1075.
29. Dersh J, Polatin PB, Gatchel RJ. Chronic pain and psychopathology: Research findings and theoretical considerations. Psychosom Med. 2002;64(5):773–786.
30. Fishbain DA, Cutler BR, Rosomoff HL. Comorbidity between psychiatric disorders and chronic pain. Curr Rev Pain. 1998;2(1):1–10.
31. Monti DA, Herring CL, Schwartzman RJ, Marchese M. Personality assessment of patients with complex regional pain syndrome type I. Clin J Pain. 1998;14(4):295–302.
32. Kessler RC, Berglund P, Borges G, Nock M, Wang PS. Trends in suicide ideation, plans, gestures, and attempts in the United States, 1990–1992 to 2001–2003. JAMA. 2005;293(20):2487–2495.
33. Kessler RC, Borges G, Walters EE. Prevalence of and risk factors for lifetime suicide attempts in the National Comorbidity Survey. Arch Gen Psychiatry. 1999;56(7):617–626.
34. Ratcliffe GE, Enns MW, Belik SL, Sareen J. Chronic pain conditions and suicidal ideation and suicide attempts: An epidemiologic perspective. Clin J Pain. 2008;24(3):204–210.
35. Kroenke K, Spitzer RL. The PHQ-9: A new depression diagnostic and severity measure. Psychiatr Ann. 2002;32(9):509–515.
36. Cameron RP, Gusman D. The Primary Care PTSD Screen (PC-PTSD): Development and operating characteristics. Prim Care Psychiatr. 2003;9(1):9–14.
37. Chibnall JT, Raymond C. The Pain Disability Index: Factor structure and normative. Arch Phys Med Rehabil. 1994;75(10):1082–1086.
38. Ewing JA. Detecting alcoholism: The CAGE questionnaire. JAMA. 1984;252(14):1905–1907.
39. Spitzer RL, Kroenke K, Williams JB, et al. A brief measure for assessing generalized anxiety disorder: The GAD-7. Arch Intern Med. 2007;166(10):1092–1097.
40. Shahid A, Wilkinson K, Marcu S, Shapiro CM. Brief Pain Inventory (BPI). In: Shahid A, Wilkinson K, Marcu S, Shapiro CM, eds. STOP, THAT and One Hundred Other Sleep Scales. New York: Springer; 2011:81–88.
41. Okifuji A, Turk DC, Eveleigh DJ. Improving the rate of classification of patients with the Multidimensional Pain Inventory (MPI): Clarifying the meaning of "significant other." J Pain. 1999;15(4):290–296.
42. Blainey S. Consultation and clinical historytaking skills. In: Abbott H, Braithwaite W, Ranson M, eds. Clinical Examination Skills for Health Professionals. Keswick, UK: M & K Publishing; 2014:1–19.
43. Burckhardt CS, Jones KD. Adult measures of pain: The McGill Pain Questionnaire (MPQ), Rheumatoid Arthritis Pain Scale (RAPS), Short Form McGill Pain Questionnaire (SF MPQ), Verbal Descriptive Scale (VDS), Visual Analog Scale (VAS), and West Haven Yale Multidisciplinary Pain Inventory (WHYMPI). Arthrit Care Res. 2003;49(5):96–104.
44. Vasu TS, Doghramji K, Cavallazzi R, et al. Obstructive sleep apnea syndrome and post-operative complications: Clinical use of the STOP-BANG questionnaire. Arch Otolaryngol. 2010;136(10):1020–1024.
45. Prescription Drug Monitoring Programs. Office of National Drug Control Policy. https://www.whitehouse.gov/sites/default/files/ondcp/Fact_Sheets/pdmp_fact_sheet_4-8-11.pdf. Published April 2011. Accessed June 30, 2016.
46. Akbik H, Butler SF, Budman SH, Fernandez K, Katz, NP, Jamison RN. Validation and clinical application of the Screener and Opioid Assessment for Patients with Pain (SOAPP). J Pain Symptom Manag. 2006;32(3):287–293.
47. Meltzer EC, Rybin D, Saitz R, et al. Identifying prescription opioid use disorder in primary care: Diagnostic characteristics of the Current Opioid Misuse Measure (COMM). J Pain. 2011;152(2):397–402.
48. Fine PG, Mahajan G, McPherson ML. Long-acting opioids and short-acting opioids: Appropriate use

in chronic pain management. Pain Med. 2009; 10(2):79–88.
49. Bodenheimer T, Laing BY. The teamlet model of primary care. Ann Fam Med. 2007;5(5):457–461.
50. McDaniel GC, Cubic BA, Hunter CL, et al. Competencies for psychology practice in primary care. Am Psychol. 2014;69:409–429.
51. Cashel ML, Rogers R, Sewell K, Martin-Cannici, C. The Personality Assessment Inventory (PAI) and the detection of defensiveness. Psychol Assessment. 1995;2(4):333–342.
52. Wygant DB, Sellbom M, Gervais RO, et al. Further validation of the MMPI-2 and MMPI-2-RF Response Bias Scale: Findings from disability and criminal forensic settings. Psychol Assessment. 2010;22(4):745–756.
53. Antoni M. Millon Behavioral Medicine Diagnostic (MBMD). In: Gellman MD, Turner JR, eds. Encyclopedia of Behavioral Medicine. New York: Springer; 2013:1243–1244.
54. Edmond T, Megivern D, Williams C, Rochman E, Howard M. Integrating evidence-based practice and social work field education. J Soc Work Educ. 2006;42(2):377–396.
55. Beck AT, Rush AJ, Shaw BF, Emery G. Cognitive Therapy of Depression. New York: Guilford Press; 1979.
56. Jensen MP, Turk DC. Contributions of psychology to the understanding and treatment of people with chronic pain: Why it matters to ALL psychologists. Am Psychol. 2014;69(2):105–118.
57. Ehring T, Welboren R, Morina N, Wicherts JM, Freitag J, Emmelkamp PM. Meta-analysis of psychological treatments for post-traumatic stress disorder in adult survivors of childhood abuse. Clin Psychol Rev. 2014;34(8):648–657.
58. Silver SM, Rogers S, Russell M. Eye movement desensitization and reprocessing (EMDR) in the treatment of war veterans. J Clin Psychiat. 2008;64(8):947–957.
59. Yucha C, Gilbert C. Evidence-Based Practice in Biofeedback and Neurofeedback. Wheat Ridge, CO: Association for Applied Psychophysiology & Biofeedback; 2008.
60. Kabat-Zinn J. Full Catastrophe Living: Using the Wisdom of Your Body and Mind to Face Stress, Pain and Illness. New York: Delacorte; 1990.
61. Zhang Y, Lao LX, Chen HY, Ceballos R. Acupuncture use among American adults: What acupuncture practitioners can learn from National Health Interview Survey 2007. Evid Based Complement Alternat Med. 2012;2012:1–8. doi:10.1155/2012/710750
62. Burke A, Upchurch DM, Dye C, Chyu L. Acupuncture use in the United States: Findings from the National Health Interview Survey. J Altern Complem Med. 2006;12(7):639–648.
63. Vickers AJ, Cronin AM, Maschino AC, et al. Acupuncture for chronic pain: Individual patient data meta-analysis. Arch Intern Med. 2012172(19):1444–1453.
64. Marmot M, Allen J, Goldblatt P, et al. Fair society, healthy lives: Strategic review of health inequalities in England Post 2010. London: Marmot Review; 2010.
65. Marmot M. Social determinants of health inequalities. Lancet. 2005;365(9464):1099–1104.
66. Koh HK, Piotrowski JJ, Kumanyika S, Fielding JE. Healthy people: A 2020 vision for the social determinants approach. Health Educ Behav. 2011;38(6):551–557.
67. Commission on Social Determinants of Health. Closing the Gap in a Generation: Health Equity Through Action on the Social Determinants of Health: Commission on Social Determinants of Health Final Report. Geneva, Switzerland: World Health Organization; 2008.
68. Packer J, Bond N. Museums as restorative environments. Curator. 2010;53(4):421–436.
69. Reynolds F, Prior S. "A lifestyle coat-hanger": A phenomenological study of the meanings of artwork for women coping with chronic illness and disability. Disabil Rehab. 2003;25(14):785–794.
70. Silverman LH. The Social Work of Museums. New York: Routledge; 2009.
71. Silverman LH. The therapeutic potential of museums as pathways to inclusion. In: R. Sandell, ed. Museums, Society, Inequality. London: Psychology Press; 2002:69–83.
72. Malchiodi C. Defining art therapy in the 21st century: Seeking a picture of health for art therapy. Psychology Today, April 2, 2013. https://www.psychologytoday.com/blog/arts-and-health/201304/defining-art-therapy-in-the-21st-century Accessed June 10, 2016.
73. Wadden TA, Volger S, Tsai AG, et al. Managing obesity in primary care practice: An overview and perspective from the POWER-UP Study. Int J Obese. 2013;37(1):S3–S11. doi:10.1038/ijo.2013.90.
74. Zachariae R, Lyby MS, Ritterband LM, O'Toole MS. Efficacy of Internet-delivered cognitive-behavioral therapy for insomnia—A systematic review and meta-analysis of randomized controlled trials. Sleep Med Rev. 2015;30:1–10.
75. Jungquist CR, O'Brien C, Matteson-Rusby S, et al. The efficacy of cognitive-behavioral therapy for insomnia in patients with chronic pain. Sleep Med. 2010;11(3):302–309.

24

Death and Dying

Integrated Teams

ANNE A. BREWER AND JOSEPH V. CONNELLY

> **BOX 24.1**
> KEY POINTS
>
> - **Dealing with dying patients is a common challenge for primary care practices. A team approach can facilitate this care.**
> - **Advance care planning is best executed in a primary care setting in advance of serious medical challenges and is facilitated by a team approach.**
> - **Breaking bad news to patients is an important communication skill often shared by the team.**
> - **Palliative care addresses all domains of suffering and is best delivered by teams.**
> - **Hospice care from multidisciplinary teams is appropriate for patients in the last 6 months of life.**
> - **Bereavement is the response to loss and has physical, emotional, and spiritual components. Each patient may benefit from discussion of these issues, which are tailored to each patient and the immediate circumstance.**

INTRODUCTION

Death and bereavement are universal experiences. However, working with the bereaved and dying challenges the innate denial of mortality that most people, including health care professionals, maintain. Further, the very essence of a health care professional's work is healing to prevent suffering and death. For this reason, health care professionals, especially primary care providers (PCPs), may view the death of a patient as a personal failure and may distance themselves from the dying patient. Nonetheless, PCPs are in a unique position to accompany their patients through these final, very painful experiences. The PCP who has been the dying patient's principal health care provider often has known the patient and family members for many years. PCPs can lead in developing protocols to assist patients and communities in discussing goals of care and end-of-life issues.

Dealing with the dying and the bereaved is emotionally and professionally challenging for everyone involved with the patient and family. Because of the influential role the PCP plays in the patient's life, he or she is in a unique position to bring comfort, understanding, and emotional support to the patient and the patient's family during this most difficult and painful period. This chapter will provide resources for primary care practices or integrated care teams to deal compassionately and competently with persons facing life-limiting illness, death, and bereavement. It provides an overview of attitudes and techniques that may be helpful in this challenging part of medical practice. Because some situations will warrant special psychosocial support, the chapter will offer guidelines to assist in determining when a referral to a mental health professional may be appropriate. Box 24.1

summarizes some of the key issues that will be discussed in this chapter.

INTEGRATED CARE FOR DYING AND DEATH

The modern model of caring for those going through the dying process began in the 1970s and 1980s with the growth and development of the hospice and palliative care movements. This model developed in response to the deficiencies of the technologically and biologically predominant care that patients at the end of life were receiving. As articulated in the World Health Organization definition, key components of palliative care are integration of psychological and spiritual aspects of patient care and use of a team approach to address the needs of patients and families.[1] This biopsychosocial-spiritual orientation to caring for dying patients within the context of their family unit, when used by a trained multidisciplinary team, has revolutionized the experience of those going through this universal process.

Proper care of the dying patient and their family requires a team approach.[2] See Table 24.1 for a description of how team members participate in the care of these patients.

In larger integrated practices, many team members may be members of the practice itself. In most situations, however, the team will also include those with expertise from the local or regional community. The PCP functions as the team leader and addresses the primary medical problems. In some practices, much of primary care may be delegated to advanced practice nurses or physician assistants. Medical assistants and registered nurses can administer screeners for depression, anxiety, or posttraumatic stress disorder. (For screeners that may be used, see Chapter 12: Treating Depression and Bipolar Disorder in Integrated Care Settings, Chapter 11: Integrated Care for Anxiety Disorders, and Chapter 10: Automated Mental Health Assessment for Integrated Care: The Quick PsychoDiagnostics Panel Meets Real-World Clinical Needs.) Medical assistants and nurses can also help to identify signs or symptoms of caregiver distress that families may try to hide from the PCP. Behavioral health specialists (BHSs) may provide counseling and support to patients and families who are experiencing significant distress. They also provide bereavement services, another key component of palliative care, to surviving family members. Psychiatrists may be called in (for face-to-face, telepsychiatry, or "curbside" consultation) when there are signs or symptoms of psychosis, suicidal ideation, previous history of psychiatric disease, or questions about psychotropic medication management. Social workers and case managers help patients and families negotiate the complex issues that arise with housing, insurance, financial, placement, and support services. Health coaches can help patients with important issues such as proper nutrition, exercise, and activity (see Chapter 25: Health Coaching in Integrated Care). The team may also be able to help patients continue to find meaning in this last period of their lives. Specialists in palliative medicine, who may be physicians or advanced practice nurses, may be consulted when there are questions about managing complicated or intractable symptoms, such as pain, nausea, delirium, and insomnia. Chaplains with experience in dealing with patients at the end of life can be invaluable in helping patients deal with the existential questions and distress that arise. Depending upon patient needs, other team members may include dietitians, pharmacists, art therapists, music therapists, physical therapists, recreational therapists, occupational therapists, and others as appropriate.[3] The care manager plays an important role in coordinating the care of the various team members.

Many, if not most, communities in the United States have access to formal hospice programs that incorporate many of these team members. Patients can usually be referred to these programs when they have a life expectancy of 6 months or less.

An important part of team functioning is the team meeting. These meetings occur on a regular basis and are attended by as many team members as possible. Patient status and upcoming plans are discussed. An electronic health record that is shared among team members can facilitate communication and care. Ideally, the electronic record would also have the ability to create a registry to better track these patients.

ADVANCE CARE PLANNING

The shift from treating acute illness to caring for persons with chronic illness brought new challenges to the medical profession. Aggressive treatment of all conditions may impose burdens on patients and families and may adversely affect quality of life. Recent attention to advance care planning has begun to address these issues. Some communities have adopted a community-wide approach to this process, notably LaCrosse, Wisconsin, where the Respecting Choices program[4] has enabled nearly

TABLE 24.1 DEATH AND DYING: AN INTEGRATIVE APPROACH

	Age 65 or at Onset of Chronic Disease	Follow-up Visits	At Diagnosis of Terminal Illness or Significant Deterioration
Primary Care Provider/ Advanced Practice Nurse	1. History and physical exam 2. Social history 3. Assess safety risk factors. 4. Assess functional status. 5. Depression screen 6. Check labs. 7. Diagnostic/preventive tests as indicated (electrocardiogram, cancer and heart screens, diabetes, etc.)	1. Review results from last visit. 2. Agree on shared priorities. 3. Assess functional status. 4. Assess for new symptoms or problems. 5. Refer as indicated. 6. Review advance directives.	1. Assess goals of care. 2. Shared decision making regarding treatment plan 3. Review advance directives. 4. Assess for new symptoms.
Medical Assistant, Nurse, and Staff	1. Screen for substance abuse, mood, stress. 2. Provide advance directive form if not yet completed.	1. Screen for mood, substance use, and stress. 2. Distribute appropriate patient education material.	Screen for mood, substance use, stress, grief.
Behavioral Health Specialist/ Psychiatrist	Mental health referral or consultation, if needed	1. Assess for mood and psychiatric disorders. 2. Treat associated psychiatric disorders as needed.	1. Assess for mood and psychiatric disorders. 2. Treat associated psychiatric disorders as needed.
Social Work	1. Assess financial and insurance needs. 2. Assess home and housing needs. 3. Assess spiritual resources and needs.	1. Assess financial needs 2. Assess home and housing needs. 3. Assess spiritual resources and needs.	1. Assess financial needs. 2. Assess home needs. 3. Assess need for other services such as art, music, physical, occupational, recreational therapies. 4. Assess spiritual resources and needs.
Care Coordinator/ Case Manager	Coordinate any needed follow-up and referrals.	Arrange for indicated referrals.	Arrange for indicated referrals.
Palliative Medicine Specialist		Evaluate complex or intractable symptoms.	1. Evaluate complex or intractable symptoms. 2. Refer to hospice if indicated.

90% of adults to create advance care documents.[5] Proper advance care planning has been demonstrated to positively impact care at the end of life.[6]

The team approach facilitates discussion of care goals and decision making for patients. This process should be routine and the topics addressed in a matter-of-fact way. Front office staff can begin by inquiring whether patients have completed an advance directive. Medical assistants and nurses can provide advance directive forms and answer basic questions when getting patients set up to see the PCP. The PCP reinforces the importance of advance care planning and answers other questions not addressed so far. The PCP, BHS, and/or social worker can help the patient and family explore their values and goals so the advance care directive accurately reflects their wishes.

Advance care planning should take place across the lifespan of adults and target likely causes of mortality. For healthy younger adults, for whom accidents and sudden catastrophic illness are the major causes of mortality, designation of a health care proxy is the primary aim. Adults should be encouraged to discuss their views on organ donation and desired care in the event of catastrophic illness. As adults age and may develop chronic illnesses, more detailed advance care planning becomes appropriate and should be addressed regularly during comprehensive visits. Designation of a health care proxy should be reviewed and open discussions with the proxy encouraged. Patients' thoughts and fears about aging and mortality can be explored, as many older adults have experienced serious illness and death among family or friends.

After the diagnosis of a life-limiting disease, advance care planning should be reemphasized and goals of care addressed. Sometimes it is necessary to change the advance directives, as illustrated in the case example in Box 24.2.

As the illness progresses, the patient's wishes about pursuing aggressive care, which may adversely affect quality of life, should be explored. Further progression of the disease is signaled by repeated hospitalizations, poor response to treatment, and a prognosis of less than 6 months. Knowing the trajectories of the most common conditions can be helpful to physicians and the care team. As illness progresses, the focus of care appropriately shifts from seeking a cure to quality of life, relief of symptoms, and maintenance of function.

At this time, patients should be offered formal palliative care and hospice services, which focus on symptom relief and quality of life rather than life-prolonging care, which often comes at the expense of severe symptoms and side effects. Some families may benefit from audiovisual and other tools that give concrete information about end-of-life care and certain procedures and treatment options. At each stage of the process, patients should be screened for depression, anxiety, substance use, and other psychiatric comorbidities and should be referred as needed to a BHS, psychiatrist, or other mental health resources in the community.

COMMUNICATING BAD NEWS

One of the more difficult tasks for a PCP is communicating bad news[7]: the death of a loved one, the diagnosis of a life-threatening illness, or a grave prognosis. The way in which the PCP handles this demanding task may influence how a family copes and adapts to grave news or grief or how a person copes with a life-threatening or terminal illness. The PCP is often the best person to convey this news because of the continuity and closeness of the PCP–patient relationship. Even if the patient learns of the bad news from another source, the PCP may need to provide education, care, and support.

The PCP must be adequately prepared to deliver bad news. Also, the PCP must be attentive to the setting in which the news in conveyed, how the news is to be delivered, and the necessary follow-up care for the patient and/or family members. For example,

BOX 24.2

CASE EXAMPLE: CHANGING ADVANCE DIRECTIVES

An 87-year-old man was admitted to a nursing home with a primary diagnosis of Alzheimer's dementia. He had discussed advance directives with his daughter early in the course of his illness, so "Do Not Resuscitate" orders were written when he was admitted. Six months later, he had an episode of pneumonia for which he was hospitalized and treated with intravenous antibiotics. One month later, he was again hospitalized and treated for pneumonia after having aspirated food. After this hospitalization, the PCP discussed with his daughter the change in his condition. She decided to modify the advance directive so that no feeding tube would be inserted and not to hospitalize him again. A few weeks later, he developed recurrent aspiration pneumonia and died peacefully in the nursing home.

conveying a diagnosis of a terminal or grave illness requires an approach that may be somewhat different from that used to communicate with a family after a sudden or unexpected death. The manner in which bad news is conveyed is extremely important. It is not unusual for patients or families to recount, years later, bitter tales of how a PCP delivered bad news "badly," in an off-handed or callous manner. The SPIKE protocol (Setting, Perception, Invitation, Knowledge, Emotion) provides a format for the delivery of bad news with accuracy and compassion.[8]

Setting Up the Interview

PCPs need to prepare for conveying bad news in several ways. First the PCP needs to gather all the available facts. In the case of a sudden death, data collection includes review of prehospital and hospital care, assembling diagnostic information, and being prepared to answer the family's questions about the patient's care and the last moments prior to death. In cases in which a terminal or grave illness is suspected or diagnosed, the PCP should review available data on the patient's condition and research treatment options.

PCPs should also be prepared for the various ways in which patients and family members respond emotionally to bad news. There may be numbness, stoicism, hostility, or hysterics. By allowing patients and families time to express strong feelings, the PCP may facilitate their assimilation of the bad news and their coping. On some occasions, the individual or family's emotional responses may be so strong as to constitute a crisis, and the PCP will need to employ techniques described in Chapter 26: Crisis Intervention in Integrated Care. Patients or families with a history of substance abuse or other personality disorders may be particularly volatile. The PCP should be prepared for the rare occasion when a severe emotional reaction or physical violence is a possibility. If such reactions are anticipated, the PCP should arrange in advance for assistance from a BHS, psychiatrist, other staff members, or even police or security officers. See Chapter 18: Violence and Suicide for strategies for managing these rare violent encounters.

The PCP may also have to prepare psychologically to deliver bad news in the most effective way. When possible, PCPs should plan to deliver bad news when they are rested and not pressured for time. PCPs have to decide what their own comfort level of personal emotional expression is, and should mentally rehearse what, where, when, and how they will convey the bad news.

The setting in which bad news is conveyed is important. A location that is quiet, private, and comfortable is preferable, one in which the PCP, patient, and/or family are seated at the same level with no barriers, such as a desk, between them. Delivering bad news in a hallway or in the middle of a crowded, busy emergency department adds stress to an already difficult situation. It is essential to allow adequate time and to schedule the discussion for a time convenient for the patient and family. In an office setting, it may be best to see the patient or family prior to a lunch break or at the end of the day to allow more time for discussion and care. In many situations, having the family accompany a patient or drawing together the family's support network (extended family, close friends, or clergy) may facilitate the discussion and provide support. If the PCP is not fluent in the language of the patient or family, the PCP should arrange to have an interpreter present.

Perception

The discussion of bad news, except in an emergency situation, should begin with what the patient and/or family members already know and fear. The PCP may ask questions such as "What have you been told so far?" "What is your understanding about the reason for doing this test?" "What are you fearful about?" This allows the PCP to assess the patient's knowledge and level of understanding about medical conditions, as well as determining whether there is denial or unrealistic expectations.

Invitation

The PCP should obtain the patient's invitation to convey information and assess how much information the patient wishes to receive and how he or she wishes to receive it. A possible format would be asking "Would you like me to discuss the results of your tests?" or "Would you prefer me to talk with your family?" Some patients prefer not to receive complete information (as partial denial, which may help them) or wish for their families to receive the information instead.

Knowledge

The PCP then conveys the information to the patient. It is helpful to soften the bad news by revealing information in stages. The PCP can express concern about how the patient has been feeling and/or concern about the results of a diagnostic test. For example, a verbal "warning shot" such as "I'm concerned about your biopsy report ... it suggests a tumor" is preferable to the bluntness of "You have cancer." Information should be provided in an honest, straightforward, and realistically hopeful manner, including acknowledgment of uncertainties that may exist. The PCP should convey empathy and warmth while reassuring the patient and family that he or she will not abandon them in this grave situation. Where it is appropriate, the PCP can provide hope to the patient and family in terms of possibilities for further diagnostic workup or other treatment options. In this case, the PCP needs to maintain hope while discussing the uncertainty about the diagnosis and the plans for further evaluation. When there is little hope for survival, the PCP can offer continued care and support and reassurance that death will be as painless as is possible.

Emotion

Patients react to bad news in a variety of ways: stoicism, anger, sadness, disbelief. The PCP needs to respond to the emotions with empathy and allow time for expression. This can be disconcerting to PCPs who are not comfortable with negative feelings, but any further discussion (e.g., about treatment options) will not be assimilated by patients in the midst of strong feelings.

Follow-up After Discussing Bad News

During the initial discussion of bad news, the PCP should encourage questions and answer them honestly. The PCP should anticipate that patients will not retain much of the information they receive at the first discussion. Having the family present for the first discussion of bad news may improve comprehension somewhat, but the emotional reaction to bad news may lessen everyone's ability to absorb information. PCPs may need to schedule follow-up visits or phone calls to deal with questions that arise as people gradually assimilate the diagnosis and prognosis.

Near the end of the follow-up meeting, the PCP should attempt to assess the understanding of the patient and family and should review the information and plans for additional follow-up. For some patients and families, providing written information and instructions may be necessary. Patients and their families may require additional support, and the PCP should make arrangements for necessary follow-up care or referrals. In most situations, particularly when the patient or family is distraught, PCPs should assume responsibility for arranging care using the multidisciplinary team. Otherwise, the patient's or family's denial or strong emotional reactions may delay necessary ongoing medical care.

Where there is hope, the PCP should reinforce that message. Where death is the likely outcome, the PCP should reassure the patient and family of his or her ongoing support and involvement and offer the hope of death with dignity.

Conveying the news of the death of a family member or loved one encompasses many of the same elements as giving news of a terminal illness to a patient, although some factors are different. Death may be sudden or it may be expected. In America, it is most likely to occur in a hospital or nursing home. Whenever possible, news of a death in the family should be conveyed in person by the PCP who has cared for the patient. If the covering PCP, other physicians, emergency department staff, or other members of the care team have been directly involved in the patient's care, delivering the news of a death may become their responsibility. In all these situations, attention to the setting and method of delivery is just as important as in the case of advising about terminal illness.

STAGES OF COPING WITH TERMINAL ILLNESS

Elisabeth Kübler-Ross, in her seminal work *On Death and Dying*,[9] outlines five stages of dealing with terminal illness and death: denial, anger, bargaining, depression, and acceptance. She describes these stages based on her interviews with many terminally ill patients at a time when physicians generally regarded death as the ultimate enemy to be combated. Kübler-Ross characterizes the movement of patients through these stages not as a linear progression, but as a process in which patients may move back and forth between stages or experience several stages simultaneously during their illnesses. Moreover, not all patients experience all five stages; some may remain in one stage until death.

Denial

Denial is often the first reaction of people when they are confronted with the news of a terminal illness: "This cannot be happening to me." Denial is usually present to some degree and can be adaptive or damaging. Denial may serve an important coping function as it temporarily protects the person from a reality that may be overwhelming, allowing additional time for other defenses to be mobilized. If denial prevents reasonable medical care or pursuit of potentially beneficial treatment options, or causes the patient isolation from his or her social supports, it may be necessary to attempt to help a patient work through this maladaptive behavior. This can be done by scheduling follow-up appointments to continue the discussion or by enlisting the assistance of family or other support persons to encourage a patient to pursue medical care or reconnect with social supports. In cases of severe denial that prevents ongoing care, referral to a BHS or requesting a psychiatric consultation may be warranted.

Anger

Anger usually surfaces as denial lessens, is no longer necessary, or cannot be maintained any longer. Anger is characterized by the statement, "Why me? Why not someone else?" Anger can be very intense and difficult for families and health care providers to deal with. Anger or blame may be directed toward the self, the family, staff, clergy, or God. A patient's expression of rage and resentment can alienate those close to him or her at the very time they are most needed. If family members or the PCP reacts to anger defensively or returns the anger, the patient may become angrier or more isolated. If, however, the patient can express the anger to a receptive listener, the anger may dissipate over time. The BHS may be able to help patients and families with angry feelings and families who are blaming each other.

Bargaining

Bargaining often follows anger. Bargaining is characterized by the statement, "What can I do, how can I behave, or what can I trade that will give me back my life?" Bargaining is often directed toward God. It is an attempt to postpone death, either as a reward for good behavior or to achieve a specific goal. Bargaining may progress to guilt or even depression if terminally ill patients feel they did not keep promises or if they regret past actions. For example, patients may feel that if they had loved their children more or expressed that love more readily, they would not have become sick or be facing death.

Depression

Depressive symptoms are common in people facing terminal illness. These symptoms may involve grieving for losses caused by the disease (e.g., loss of vitality, physical beauty, energy, finances, activities). Depressive symptoms also may involve anticipatory grief for the losses that the disease will cause for loved ones and loss of life itself. Both these forms of grieving may be alleviated by receptive listening and psychological work with letting go and accepting the inevitability of death.

In some cases, normal depressive symptoms grow to become a major depressive disorder. This form of clinical depression is not uncommon in the terminally ill; however, it should not be considered a normal part of the death and dying process. If a major depressive disorder occurs, it should be treated aggressively (see Chapter 12: Treating Depression and Bipolar Disorder in Integrated Care Settings). Otherwise, it has the potential to adversely affect medical treatment, prognosis, and the ultimate course of many terminal illnesses, including terminal heart disease, HIV infection, and many cancers. Referral to a BHS or psychiatrist, depending on the degree of symptoms or treatments needed, may be indicated.

Acceptance

Acceptance is the final stage of dealing with terminal illness. It is characterized by the statement, "I am prepared to die and accept dying and death as a part of the natural order of living." Acceptance is typically gradual, and it may wax and wane. Full acceptance of death may be accompanied by a reaching out to loved ones, a heightened sense of spirituality, and peace and contentment that comes from a life well lived. Acceptance may also come about from a combination of exhaustion and/or a delirium that appears as a resignation to death. This resignation may be characterized as "Leave me alone. I can't fight any more." Resignation to death may occur when a patient has worsening weakness, chronic pain, overwhelming exhaustion, or withdrawal from interest in activities or people. However, it is important not to mistake the signs of resignation, untreated depression, and a total loss of hope for acceptance.

These five stages are descriptive rather than prescriptive. Every person who deals with terminal illness is an individual with a unique history and web of relationships. Most people with terminal illnesses move in and out of the various stages over the course of the illness and only some patients will ever attain true acceptance of death.

PALLIATIVE CARE FOR THE DYING PATIENT

Care of the dying patient and the suffering associated with terminal illness can be very difficult for both patients and families. Effective care of the dying seeks to relieve suffering, ameliorate symptoms, preserve the best quality of life possible, and ease the transition for dying persons and their families.[10] The suffering of a dying person can be physical, emotional, social, and spiritual, and care for the dying must address all these realms. A multidisciplinary approach, using the team members described above, is essential to provide holistic care to the dying patient and their family.

The hallmark of palliative and hospice care is a focus on care and relief of symptoms, maintaining the quality of life as best as possible, instead of on cure. One of the most difficult aspects of caring for the dying, particularly with the powerful medical technology now available, is discerning when it is appropriate to shift from an emphasis on cure to an emphasis on quality of life and relief of symptoms. PCPs, patients, and families struggle with this discernment, and conflicts often arise when different parties to the decision have different views of the situation.

Since Kübler-Ross published her seminal book in 1969, there has been a resurgence of interest in palliative care. Hospice programs, mostly outpatient but some inpatient, have been organized in many communities. Laws have been passed to allow people to execute advance directives for their care in a terminal situation. However, it is still common to see deaths in the intensive care unit where the patient's pain and suffering was not optimally managed and medical interventions prolonged dying without providing clear benefit.

Physical Aspects of Palliative Care

The physical suffering that accompanies terminal illness is often the most feared aspect of dying. Yet many PCPs, concerned about addiction or audits from agencies that regulate controlled drugs, undermedicate pain in terminal illness. Concerns about addiction should not deter PCPs from treating pain. See Chapter 23: Integrated Chronic Pain and Psychiatric Management. The development of concentrated oral opioids, extended-release opioids, transdermal narcotic patches, and narcotic infusions that can be delivered in the outpatient setting have allowed many patients with severe pain to be cared for outside of hospitals. Visiting nurses or hospice nurses can assist physicians in managing pain by monitoring symptoms and relaying concerns to the PCP. Aggressive treatment of nausea, dyspnea, anorexia, itching, skin breakdown, and constipation can improve the quality of life of dying patients. Specialists in palliative medicine may be consulted to help manage multiple or intractable symptoms.[11]

Psychological Aspects of Palliative Care

Attention to emotional and psychiatric issues is central to care for the dying patient. Although depressive symptoms are a common experience as people journey toward death, treatment of major depressive disorders often improves the quality of life for dying patients.[12] It is not always easy to distinguish between depression that is one of the stages of moving toward death, and major depressive disorder that warrants treatment. However, depression that is accompanied by vegetative signs such as insomnia or anorexia or by atypical signs such as hypersomnia and weight gain or by suicidal ideation often responds to treatment with antidepressants and/or psychotherapy.[13] See Chapter 12: Treating Depression and Bipolar Disorder in Integrated Care Settings for a fuller discussion. PCPs sometimes do not treat depression in terminally ill patients, believing that the patient has good reason to be depressed.[14] They thus miss the opportunity to improve the quality of life for the dying person and in some cases miss opportunities to extend life.

Other psychiatric conditions that occur frequently during the dying process are panic attacks, generalized anxiety disorder, and insomnia. Nurses and medical assistants can assist in screening for these disorders. These should also be treated aggressively with no concern about possible habituation (e.g., to anxiolytics). Prompt referral to the BHS, or psychiatrist when indicated, is important in properly managing these conditions. Stress reduction and relaxation techniques provided by the BHS or health coach may provide additional benefit. See Chapter 25: Health Coaching in Integrated Care for additional interventions.

Delirium may occur during the course of terminal illness, and this may be distressing for the patient and family alike. As in any other situation in which delirium occurs, the PCP should undertake a vigorous search for underlying medical causes. An exception to this is during the final phase of a terminal illness, when psychotropic medications can be used without an exhaustive medical evaluation.

Social Aspects of Palliative Care

Care of the dying patient also must address the needs of the family or social unit in which the person lives.[3] Terminal illness places a great deal of stress on those who are caring for the dying patient.

If this stress exceeds the capacity of the family, the caregiving system will break down. Many caregivers feel guilty if they take time for themselves, and some terminally ill persons resist receiving care from outsiders. However, if a terminal illness is lengthy, caregivers may not be able to sustain the care that is needed, and a crisis may arise as a result. Care managers and social workers have expertise in helping families access helpful support services. Respite care, whether through home nursing agencies, hospice volunteers, or short-term hospital or nursing home placement, may allow families to continue to care for the ill family member. PCPs need to discuss self-care with families openly, especially the primary caregivers, and offer family support and counseling when indicted. See Chapter 27: Best Practice for Family-Centered Health Care: A Three-Step Model.

END-OF-LIFE CARE

Advance Directives

Early in the course of a terminal illness, after the patient and family have assimilated the diagnosis and before physical and psychological deterioration are far advanced, it is appropriate to address the issue of end-of-life care. Advance directives offer patients a way to make their wishes known and to facilitate their care at the end of life or if a crisis arises. Patients may execute documents giving family members durable power of attorney for health care decisions as well as for financial affairs. These discussions, though often difficult for patients, families, and PCPs, can prevent inappropriate interventions that are contrary to the person's values and wishes and prevent future family disagreements about end-of-life care. It is not uncommon for families to panic if the dying person becomes severely dyspneic, for example. If clear do-not-resuscitate (DNR) orders are not in place, which may include special bracelets for persons who request DNR, the emergency medical system is obliged to transport the person to a hospital and apply advanced life-support measures. Instead of a peaceful death, the patient and family are subjected to a chaotic transfer and emergency department experience.

The issue of advance directives may need to be discussed with the person and the family repeatedly during the course of an illness. When there is a major change in the person's condition, the type of care and a revised advance directive may be appropriate. Box 24.2 gives a case example.

Setting for Dying and Death

The setting in which death occurs has changed over the course of the past century. Early in the last century, many deaths occurred at home. After World War II, most deaths occurred in hospitals, particularly with the advent of more powerful medical technology.[15] In the past 20 years, there has been a shift back to the home or nursing home as the setting for dying and death. The palliative care and hospice movement has strongly influenced this shift by providing programs and support that make it possible for families to care for dying persons at home. Hospice also provides respite care in a nursing home or hospitals to assist families. The hospice approach also provides the option for hospitalization for terminal care if the patient's symptoms become unmanageable at home. Care managers and social workers are knowledgeable about community resources and can aid families is choosing the appropriate setting for end-of-life care.

Hospice care, whether in the home, the nursing home, or the hospital, focuses on comfort and relief of symptoms. Medical and nursing interventions, even those that are routine, are often omitted when they do not directly contribute to the person's comfort. The focus of care is shifted to relief of symptoms such as pain, nausea, dyspnea, insomnia, anxiety, and depression. If a person has been cared for in a nursing home, it is often appropriate for the patient to be cared for in a familiar environment during the terminal phase of an illness. Many nursing homes have developed expertise in terminal care. There are also freestanding hospice facilities that may be options for some patients.

Spiritual Aspects of Terminal Care

From the beginning, the palliative care and hospice movement, with its focus on the care of the whole person, has included spiritual care. Assessment for spiritual needs is part of initial and ongoing care, and chaplains are an integral part of palliative care and hospice teams.[3] Recent interest in spirituality within the medical profession has widened this focus. Some terminally ill patients have a strong connection with a spiritual community, which may provide support and participation in religious rituals. Dying persons can be encouraged to maintain their spiritual practices, reconnect with their religious leaders or community, or develop new spiritual practices or connections. Additional support from team chaplains may also be helpful. Other patients may have no particular religious or spiritual

BOX 24.3
CASE EXAMPLE: RECONNECTING TO THE SPIRITUAL LIFE

A man with terminal cancer was receiving care from a hospice team in his home. He had been estranged from his church for many years. The hospice nurse noted that he was extremely anxious and seemed to feel guilty about events in his past. He was encouraged to contact the priest in his parish, and the hospice nurse spoke with the priest before he visited the patient. After the priest's visit, the man was much less anxious and died peacefully a few weeks later.

connection and may prefer a psychological approach to dying. They may be offered a referral to the BHS if they wish to discuss these issues. Terminal illness raises profound questions about the meaning of life and death, what happens after death, and the purpose and accomplishments of one's life. These spiritual issues often affect a patient, and reconnection with the spiritual aspects of living can be a source of great comfort. A case example is given in Box 24.3.

HOSPICE CARE

Hospice care has offered benefit to many terminally ill patients. Although hospice care is usually associated with cancer, the same principles can be applied to most terminal illnesses. Hospice care addresses the physical, emotional, behavioral, social, and spiritual needs of terminally ill persons.[16] Most hospice programs have an interdisciplinary team as described in the section earlier in the chapter.

Most hospice programs offer care to persons with severe or terminal illnesses whose life expectancy is limited (usually less than 6 months). The Medicare hospice benefit requires a PCP's statement that the prognosis is less than 6 months, although patients may remain on the hospice benefit if they survive longer.[17] Most hospice programs require that patients have chosen not to pursue aggressive therapies for their disease, although therapy for symptom relief is considered part of hospice care. Therapy for symptom relief may include radiation and chemotherapy for some oncology patients, pain management, or the use of psychotropic drugs for depression or anxiety.

Referral to a hospice program is appropriate for any patient with an illness that is expected to cause death within a limited time. Diagnoses for which hospice care may be indicated include cancer; acquired immunodeficiency syndrome (AIDS); cardiac, pulmonary, cerebrovascular, renal, and liver diseases; and dementia. Hospice care can be most helpful to patients and families if it is begun early in the terminal phase of a patient's illness. Early referral allows the hospice team to assess needs, develop plans of care, and build relationships with the patient and family.

For many patients and families, hospice allows a better quality of life during the dying process. Not only does this relieve the suffering of the patient, but it also aids the family in caring for the patient and in the bereavement process, which may prevent pathologic grief reactions.

BEREAVEMENT

Bereavement, the loss of a loved one, is one of the most powerful stressors that people experience. Although its expression is very much culturally determined, it is a universal phenomenon that for most people affects all aspects of functioning: physical, emotional, behavioral, spiritual, and social. The emotions produced by bereavement are among the most painful known to human beings.

Normal Grief

Although bereavement has been experienced and described from biblical times, the systematic study of grief began with the work of Lindemann.[18] Uncomplicated grief, or "normal" grief, begins with shock, numbness, and disbelief at the news of a death.[19] These normal grief responses occur whether a death was expected or unexpected. At this point, the reality of the loss has not yet set in, and the bereaved person may appear to be functioning well. As the reality of the loss is felt, numbness often gives way to intense waves of painful emotions of sadness, loss, or anger. The bereaved person may experience somatic distress including fatigue, exhaustion, insomnia, changes in appetite, gastrointestinal symptoms, somatic pain, and involuntary sighing. Bereaved persons frequently present to a PCP with illnesses such as bronchitis or gastric pain that may be slow to resolve. They may experience an altered mental state described as numbness, shock, derealization, or depersonalization. Behavioral symptoms may include sobbing, screaming, and/or periods of intense sadness and yearning that are often experienced in waves of great intensity. These mood swings are often accompanied by anger, irritability, anxiety, and guilt. Some patients experience intense dreams or sensations of seeing the deceased, which may represent the attempt to find or reconnect with the lost person. In most patients, the physical manifestations of grief are resolved in approximately six weeks.[18] Psychological symptoms with or without depressive mood swings may last from several months to more than a year.

Except in cases of complicated grief, bereaved persons resume normal daily behavioral functioning quickly and incorporates more gradually the loss into their lives. Many survivors describe a "hole" in their lives that never goes away, although the acute pain of the loss abates.

The process of grief, like the process of dying, is not linear. Bereaved persons move in and out of the various stages of the process for many months, even years. The time course of normal grief is variable, from a few months to years, depending upon the circumstances of the loss, ambivalence in the relationship, and/or the closeness of the relationship.

Bereavement in children and adolescents differs in some ways from bereavement in adults. Young children, who do not understand the finality of death, may not express grief verbally but may demonstrate somatic or behavioral manifestations such as sleep or eating disturbance, enuresis, and aggressive or withdrawn behavior. School-age children and adolescents may react with school problems, depression, aggression, or withdrawal. The presence of a reliable caregiver and social supports may assist children and adolescents in coping with their grief.

Complicated Grief

It is not always easy to distinguish between normal and complicated grief. The time course of grief is variable, and the intensity of the feelings that surface may be intense.[20] However, if any of the stages of grief remain unresolved over a period of time and there is persistent social or occupational dysfunction, the grief reaction may be considered complicated. For example, depressed mood, tearfulness, difficulties with concentration, and sleep disturbances occur in normal grief. If these symptoms do not lessen over time, or if suicidal ideation, psychosis, intense somatic preoccupation, or progressive withdrawal and loss of function occur, a major depressive disorder or complicated grief may be present. Note that this is an area of some controversy, as illustrated in the *Diagnostic and Statistical Manual of Mental Disorders*, fifth edition (DSM-5) by the explanation of the difference between grief and depression in the section on "major depressive disorder" and the inclusion of a condition referred to as "persistent complex bereavement disorder" in the section on "conditions for further study."[21]

Management of Grief

PCPs who care for many or all members of a family may provide assistance to families experiencing grief. Members of the care team (nurses and medical assistants) can help identify patients who may be struggling with grief. PCPs can explain that the patient's physical symptoms are related to grief and can provide reassurance that experiencing an acute grief reaction is not "going crazy." Other sources of support for bereaved persons are friends, family, clergy, support groups, and a BHS. A referral for psychiatric consultation is warranted if the patient requests it, if the PCP suspects pathologic grief or a major depression, or if there is evidence of suicidal ideation or psychosis.

PCPs are often asked to provide medication for bereaved persons, especially those in the midst of acute grief. Often the request is made by other people who are distressed by the acute distress of the bereaved. Sleep medications, such as zolpidem tartrate 5 to 10 mg at bedtime may be judiciously used.[22] Overmedication with other sedative-hypnotic medications may blunt the acute grief reaction or may interfere with grief resolution. If symptoms persist and/or the patient is dysfunctional and headed toward a depression, antidepressant medication may be used to ameliorate symptoms or prevent severe social or occupational dysfunction.

For many bereaved people, referral to a peer bereavement support group can be very helpful, particularly in the later stages of the grief process when the bereaved person is facing the task of reconstructing his or her life. Access to others who have "been there" may provide reassurance, emotional support, and practical advice in dealing with bereavement. Most hospice programs and other agencies, hospitals, or mental health professionals offer bereavement support groups. Some bereaved persons also benefit from books that describe experiences of grief. Books that many recommend highly include *A Grief Observed*,[23] *Tear Soup*,[24] *The Grief Recovery Handbook*,[25] and *Good Grief*.[26]

DEATH OF A CHILD

The death of a baby or child raises all the issues of grief described above, as well as particular issues for bereaved parents. Pregnancy loss, whether through abortion, miscarriage, or stillbirth, can result in profound grief. The grief is usually proportional to the duration of the pregnancy and/or the amount of bonding that has already taken place, and conflicted feelings about abortion. Parents may experience a traumatic loss from voluntary abortions or early miscarriages (particularly of desired pregnancies). It is often helpful to caution women who have sought an abortion or miscarried to ignore the acute advice often given by well-meaning friends or relatives: "You can always have another child." The effects of losing a child may affect parents for years after the loss.[27] Referral to a BHS or social worker experienced in bereavement counseling should be considered.

The death of a baby or child from sudden infant death syndrome (SIDS) or by other means represents an acute trauma for parents and may also represent the potential loss of the future of being a parent. SIDS deaths are particularly distressing as SIDS parents are often under suspicion or investigation for the child's death and have done no wrong. Referral to support groups, a SIDS support group, or a BHS may assist parents in coping with their grief. This is particularly important if the parents are temporarily dysfunctional or if there are other children in the family whose needs may be overlooked during the parents' grief.

UNNATURAL DEATH

Compared with natural death, "unnatural" death often produces more prolonged and complicated bereavement. Unnatural deaths are caused by violence, violation, or volition.[28] An unnatural death can be the result of accident, natural disaster, or violence as a human action. Violation involves disfigurement or other severe damage to the human being. Volition can be directed toward self (suicide) or other (homicide) or may be the result of human error or negligence. These unnatural deaths are usually sudden and involve a disproportionate number of young people.

PCPs who care for survivors of unnatural death should be alert to the likelihood of complicated bereavement, posttraumatic stress disorder, major depression, or other anxiety disorders. When appropriate, referrals should be made to a BHS or a psychiatrist for consultation and treatment. Support groups may also provide benefit for survivors. Many survivors also become involved in political or social action to prevent future deaths (e.g., advocating gun control after a loved one has been killed by a firearm

BOX 24.4
SUMMARY OF RECOMMENDED TREATMENT APPROACHES AND RELEVANT EVIDENCE

Strength of Recommendation Taxonomy (SOR A, B, C)

- **Palliative care teams have been shown to improve the outcomes of patients with advanced cancer. (SOR A)[2]**
- **Pain management: Recommended medications for neuropathic pain are tricyclic antidepressants, selective serotonin–norepinephrine reuptake inhibitors, and gabapentinoids (first line). Opioids also may be effective. (SOR A)[30]**
- **Grief and depression at the end of life: Antidepressants can relieve depressive symptoms, even in patients with advanced illness. (SOR A)[31]**
- **Early palliative care in patients with newly diagnosed non-small cell lung cancer reduces depression, improves quality of life, and extends survival. (SOR A)[32]**
- **Advance care planning: Discussion with patients and families about advance directives that involve goals of care can improve end-of-life care, increase patient satisfaction, and reduce stress. (SOR A)[6,33]**
- **Grief and depression at the end of life: Psychotherapy may be considered for patients with depressive symptoms, even with advanced illness. (SOR B)[34,35]**
- **Home palliative care improves the symptom burden and the likelihood patients will die in their own home. (SOR A)[36]**

or working against drunk driving after a child has been killed by a drunk driver).

PCP'S REACTION TO DEATH AND BEREAVEMENT

Medical education generally focuses on mastery of medical and technical information, with less attention paid to psychological reactions to illness, death, and bereavement. Detachment, which is a necessary part of clinical decision making, may be misinterpreted by patients as impassiveness or uncaring. Excessive detachment on the part of the PCP may serve as a defense against the fear of death that most people experience, medically trained or not. PCPs risk burnout or being perceived as cold or uncaring if they do not recognize their own grief, touch the emotional experience of their patients, and find appropriate ways to deal with their own emotions.

Few PCPs can care for a patient, particularly for long periods of time, without feeling a sense of connection with the patient. When a patient dies, the PCP experiences a loss and should expect to feel some grief.[29] Attending wakes or funerals of patients who have died is one way of expressing that grief. Most families feel honored when a PCP attends a funeral or wake. Writing sympathy letters or sending cards can also express the PCP's grief and help families in their bereavement. A BHS and/or a psychiatrist, as part of the multidisciplinary team, can be used to support the PCP. In addition, a well-functioning interdisciplinary team can serve as an important source of support for all members of the team in dealing with challenging situations.

CONCLUSION

The universal experiences of dying, death, and bereavement challenge PCPs and their multidisciplinary teams to care for patients and families in an empathic manner and to appreciate our common humanity. As team members accept their own mortality, they have the opportunity to form close ties with patients and families at pivotal times in their lives. Box 24.4 summarizes some of the evidence based topics discussed in this chapter.

REFERENCES

1. WHO. Definition of palliative care. http://www.who.int/cancer/palliative/definition/en/. Accessed July 7, 2016.
2. Higginson IJ, Evans CJ. What is the evidence that palliative care teams improve outcomes for cancer patients and their families? Cancer J. 2010;16(5):423–435. doi:10.1097/PPO.0b013e3181f684e5.
3. National Consensus Project for Quality Palliative Care. Clinical Practice Guidelines for Quality Palliative Care, 3rd ed. 2013. http://www.nationalconsensusproject.org/Guidelines_Download2.aspx. Accessed July 7, 2016.
4. Respecting Choices Advanced Care Planning. http://www.gundersenhealth.org/respecting-choices. Accessed July 7, 2016.
5. Hammes BJ, Rooney BL, Gundrum JD. A comparative observational study of the prevalence, availability, and specificity of advance care plans in a county that implemented an advance care planning microsystem. J Am Geriatr Soc. 2010;58(7):1249–1255. doi:10.1111/j.1532-5415.2010.02956.x.
6. Brinkman-Stoppelenburg A, Rietjens JA, van der Heide A. The effects of advance care planning on end-of-life care: A systematic review. Palliat Med. 2014;28(8):1000–1025. doi:10.1177/0269216314526272.
7. Buckman R. How to Break Bad News. Baltimore, MD: Johns Hopkins University Press; 1992.
8. BaileW, BuckmanR, LenziR, GloberG, BealeE, Kudalko A. Breaking bad news. Oncologist. 2000;5(4):302–311. doi:10.1634/theoncologist.5-4-302.
9. Kubler-Ross, E. On Death and Dying. New York: Macmillan Publishing Company; 1969.
10. Sepulveda C, Marlin A, Yoshida T, Ullrich A. Palliative care: The World Health Organization's global perspective. J Pain Symptom Manage. 2002;24(2):91–96.
11. Gomez-Batiste X, Porta-Sales J, Paz S, Stjernsward J. Palliative medicine: Models of organization. In: Walsh D, ed. Palliative Medicine. Philadelphia: Saunders; 2009:23–29.
12. Laoutidis Z, Mathiak K. Antidepressants in the treatment of depression/depressive symptoms in cancer patients: A systematic review and meta-analysis. BMC Psychiatry. 2013;16(13):1–21. doi:10.1186/1471-244X-13-140.
13. Rayner L, Evans A, Valsraj K, Hetoph M, Higganum I. Antidepressants for the treatment of depression in palliative care: Systematic review and meta-analysis. Palliat Med. 2011;25(1):36–51.
14. Widera E, Block S. Managing grief and depression at the end of life. Am Fam Physician. 2012;86(3):259–264.
15. Wilson D, Cable-Williams B. Death in modern society. In: Walsh D, ed. Palliative Medicine. Philadelphia: Saunders; 2009:8–13.
16. National Hospice and Palliative Care Organization. http://www.nhpco.org/about/hospice-care. Accessed July 7, 2016.
17. Centers for Medicare and Medicaid Services. Medicare benefit policy manual. https://www.cms.gov/Regulations-and-Guidance/Guidance/Manuals/downloads/bp102c09.pdf. Accessed July 7, 2016.
18. Lindemann E. Symptomatology and management of acute grief. Am J Psychiatry. 1944;101(2):141–148.

19. Osterweiss M, Solomon F, Green M. Bereavement reactions, consequences, and care. In: Zisook S. Biopsychosocial Aspects of Bereavement. Washington, DC: American Psychiatric Press; 1987:3–18.
20. Shear M, Simon N, Wall N, et al. Complicated grief and related bereavement issues for DSM-5. Depress Anxiety. 2011;28(2):102–117. doi:10.1002/da.20780.
21. American Psychiatric Association. Diagnostic and Statistical Manual of Mental Disorders, 5th ed. Arlington, VA: American Psychiatric Association; 2013.
22. Ramakrishnan K, Scheid D. Treatment options for insomnia. Am Fam Physician. 2007;76(4):517–526.
23. Lewis CS. A Grief Observed [1961]. The Complete CS Lewis Signature Classics. ed. Joseph Rutt. San Francisco: Harper SanFrancisco; 2002:435–462.
24. Schweibert P. Tear Soup, 5th ed. Portland, OR; Grief Watch; 2005.
25. James J, Friedman R. The Grief Recovery Handbook, 20th Anniversary Expanded Ed: The Action Program for Moving Beyond Death, Divorce, and Other Losses including Health, Career, and Faith. New York: William Morrow Paperback; 2009.
26. Westberg G. Good Grief: 50th Anniversary Edition. Minneapolis, MN; Fortress Press; 2010.
27. Rogers C, Floyd F, Seltzer M, Greenberg J, Hong J. Long-term effects of the death of a child on parents adjustment in midlife. J Fam Psychol 2008;22(2):203–211. doi:10.1037/0893-3200.22.2.203.
28. Rynearson E. Psychological adjustment to unnatural dying. In: Zisook S, ed. Biopsychosocial Aspects of Bereavement. Washington, DC: American Psychiatric Press; 1987.
29. Sansone R, Sansone L. Physician grief with patient death. Innov Clin Neurosci 2012;9(4):22–26.
30. Chaparro L, Wiffen P, Moore R, Gilron I. Combination pharmacotherapy for treatment of neuropathic pain in adults. Cochrane Database Syst Rev.11(7);CD008943. doi:10.1002/14651858.CD008943.pub2.
31. Rayner L, Price A, Evans A, Valsraj K, Higginson IJ, Hotopf M. Antidepressants for depression in physically ill people (protocol). Cochrane Database of Systematic Reviews 2008:(4);Art. No.: CD007503. doi:10.1002/14651858.CD007503.
32. Temel J, Greer J, Muzansky A, et al. Early palliative care for patients with metastatic non-small cell lung cancer. N Engl J Med. 2010;363(8):733–742.
33. Detering K, Hancock A, Reade M, Silvester W. The impact of advance care planning on end of life in elderly patients: Randomized control trial. BMJ. 2010;340:c1345. doi:http://dx.doi.org/10.1136/bmj.c1345.
34. Akechi T, Okuyama T, Onishi J, Morita T, Furukawa TA. Psychotherapy for depression among incurable cancer patients. Cochrane Database of Systematic Reviews 2008;(2) Art. No.: CD005537. doi:10.1002/14651858.CD005537.pub2.
35. Li M, Fitzgerald P, Rodin G. Evidence-based treatment of depression in patients with cancer. J Clin Oncol. 2012;30(11):1187–1196.
36. Gomes B, Calanzani N, Curiale V, McCrone P, Higginson IJ, Brito MD. Effectiveness and cost-effectiveness of home palliative care services for adults with advanced illness and their caregivers. Sao Paulo Med J. 2016;134(1):93–94.

PART IV

Psychosocial Treatments in Primary Care and Medical Specialty Clinics

25

Health Coaching in Integrated Care

MARILYN S. FEINSTEIN AND ROBERT E. FEINSTEIN

BOX 25.1

KEY POINTS

- **U.S. health care has moved toward patient-centered, patient-empowered, team-based care, facilitating patient activation for behavioral change, thereby reducing chronic illness.**
- **Prevention, population management, reimbursement reforms, a strong physican-patient working alliance has created fertile soil for the emergence of health coaching within our health care system.**
- **Health coaches have emerged from two professional groups: (1) existing medical professionals (e.g., nurses, nurse practitioners, physician assistants, psychologists, social workers), trained as coaches, or using health coaching approaches, and (2) non-medical, trained coaches, who may or may not be accredited by a major national coaching credentialing body, such as the International Coaching Federation.**
- **The National Consortium for Credentialing Health and Wellness Coaches' defines health and wellness coaches as professionals from diverse backgrounds and education who work with individuals and groups in a client-centered process to facilitate and empower the client to achieve self-determined goals related to health and wellness.[1]**
- **Health coaching roles include: (1) *thinking partner* versus *expert*; (2) facilitates patient discovery of strengths, core values and life goals, healthier choices; facilitates patient recognition of discrepancies between unhealthy lifestyles and patient core values and goals; (3) moves between the roles of non-directive health coach and health educator; (4) supports shared decision making; (5) co-designer of behavioral change goal(s); collaboratively addresses barriers to change; (6) facilitates an accountability plan; (7) champions patient successes; refines contingency plans; works through relapses; (8) As a team member; screenings; tracks outcomes, using a registry; and develops population-based wellness programing.**
- **Health coaches do not engage patients in psychotherapy. If mental illness or addictions emerge during the coaching process, coaches must refer the patient to behavioral health professionals.**
- **Health coaching draws from a wide range of models and theories, including: (1) human needs fulfillment; (2) theories of self-determination and self-efficacy; (3) humanism; (4) adult learning; and (5) positive psychology.**
- **Four predominant models of behavioral change are significantly woven into the fabric of health coaching: (1) the transtheoretical model or stages of change; (2) motivational interviewing; (3) solution-focused coaching; and (4) cognitive-behavioral coaching.**

INTRODUCTION

Health care in the United States is in transition. Facilitating individual patient and population-based lifestyle change is critical for creating a healthier country. Fostering prevention, facilitating lifestyle change, and dealing with the high incidence and prevalence of chronic disease are all within the purview of health coaching, a new health discipline. The Centers for Disease Control and Prevention (CDC) considers chronic disease "the public health challenge of the 21st century."[2] In 2010, chronic disease accounted for seven of the top 10 causes of death, of which heart disease and cancer accounted for nearly 48% of all deaths.[3] As of 2012, about half of all U.S. adults (117 million people) had one or more chronic health diseases, while one of four adults had two or more chronic conditions.[4] According to the World Health Organization (WHO), by 2020, chronic conditions will be not only the leading cause of disability throughout the world, but the most expensive to manage for both high and low income countries.[5] The substantial increase in chronic disease rates has cost the United States $2 trillion[6] in health care costs and an additional $1 trillion[7] in the annual cost of absenteeism and productivity loss. At least one or more chronic medical conditions accounted for eighty-six percent of all U.S. health care spending.[8]

Chronic diseases (e.g., cardiovascular disease, diabetes, obesity) are often exacerbated or caused by lifestyle choices and behaviors. The CDC has characterized American society as *obesogenic* due to the prevalence of environments that promote high sodium and sugar intake, excessive calories through super-sized food portions, high-fat processed food (junk food), and sedentary living.[9] Smoking and stress are additional lifestyle factors contributing to morbidity and mortality.[10]

The current health system not only has been largely focused on treating or managing emergencies and acute diseases, but has inadequately addressed lifestyle factors, as well as prevention. The Patient Protection and Affordable Care Act passed in 2010, and upheld by the U.S. Supreme Court in June 2012, has begun to help turn this around.[11] New national goals have emerged from Title IV, Prevention of Chronic Disease and Improving Public Health, aimed at "increasing the number of Americans who are healthy at every stage of life."[12] Prevention in Title IV focuses on a healthy lifestyle with seven priorities: (1) tobacco-free living; (2) prevention of drug and alcohol abuse; (3) healthy eating; (4) active living; (5) mental and emotional health; (6) sexual and reproductive health; and (7) public safety from injury and violence.[11,12]

This chapter, which provides an introduction to the world of health coaching, describes the emergence, theories and methodologies, and efficacy of this new health discipline. See Box 25.1 to review key points about health coaching. In addition, we describe health coaching in practice, as primary care and integrated care environments incorporate health coaching within their multidisciplinary health care teams. Five major coaching approaches are discussed: (1) the transtheoretical model (stages of change); 2) motivational interviewing; (3) solution-focused coaching; (4) cognitive-behavioral coaching; and (5) mindfulness-based stress reduction. An example of a brief coaching session is presented.

DEVELOPMENTS IN HEALTH CARE

Medical schools were formed in the first half of the 20th century, and physicians were viewed as the "experts," by virtue of their medical training and experience, providing treatment in the form of support, medicine, and surgery. Physicians expected that patients would comply with their recommendations so as to regain or improve their health. In turn, patients expected these "magical" physicians to cure them, with little sense of personal accountability.

In the 1940s and the 1950s, the solo family doctor made house calls and, by developing a relationship (working alliance) with patients, had time to better understand them in their environment. The doctor was better able to understand obstacles preventing them from making lifestyle change. In the 1960s and 1970s, while health care began to move from homes and solo practices to hospitals and outpatient medical groups, medical paternalism continued.

The traditional medical office visit supported what Glaser[13] would call *transactional* and *positional* levels of dialog between physician and patient. The physician directed the patient toward health, by providing advice (*positional*) without first having gained a level of trust with the patient. Without trust, the patient was less likely to comfortably share the undercurrents of his or her current unhealthy behavior, which could provide the physician with a better understanding of the patient's social context from which to work.[13]

The physician-directed communication style, described as *biomedical or paternalistic*,[14] is also known as the *righting reflex*—"the desire to fix what seems *wrong* (medically) with the person."[15] This style of communication is not conducive to biopsychosocial conversations, in which patients express their preference.[14] The "one style fits all" medical/biological visit left many patients feeling that the physician did not really understand them in their own *psychosocial-cultural* context. Discussions of their chief medical complaints with a disease focus, while helpful in a diagnostic and biomedical way, does not readily foster a psychological "safe space" for patients to disclose the individual stories behind their lifestyle choices and at-risk behaviors. Without this safe space, it is difficult to engage the patient in lifestyle changes and self-managed health care, essential for the 21st century.[16]

The Influence of Managed Care

During the age of managed care (1970s–2000s), health care focused on cost cutting, which was disguised as cost savings. As resources for patients were reduced, demands were placed on physicians for greater productivity and "appropriate" medical utilization. The health insurance industry fostered and solidified a dichotomy between physical and mental health care, by developing two totally separate systems of care and reimbursement procedures. Mental health services were predominantly offered by solo practitioners. Medical physicians were asked to manage or treat multiple problems in a 15-minute visit.

Managed care requirements, as well as time constraints imposed on physicians, had profoundly deleterious effects on patient experience: (1) patients felt rushed and unwelcomed; (2) patients reported little eye contact with their physicians; (3) focused visits were limited to chief complaints and diseases; (4) there was little time for physicians to explain test results to their patients; (5) there was no time for physicians to "teach back," ensuring that patients understood their treatment plans; and (6) there was no time to even explore whether the treatment plan was feasible for the patient.[17] While prevention and lifestyle changes were perceived as worthy goals, the managed care demands for physician productivity and time made achieving these goals impractical for a population of patients.

The results of the managed care era remain profound and linger, in that 50% of patients leave primary care visits not understanding what their doctor told them.[18] Patients may not really understand the potential medical repercussions of their at-risk behaviors. Though shared decision making is associated with improved outcomes, only 9% of patients participate in medical decisions.[18] Average adherence rates for prescribed medications are about 50%; rates are below 10% for lifestyle changes.[19]

The Transformation of Health Care

Since 2000, health care has been undergoing a transformation. The Institute of Medicine[20] published *To Err is Human*, and Baker[21] published *Crossing the Quality Chasm*, initiating the quality and safety movement. Don Berwick, MD, formed the Institute for Health Care Improvement (IHI).[22] In 2007, the American Academy of Family Physicians, the American Academy of Pediatrics, the American College of Physicians, and the American Osteopathic Association developed the following seven principles to describe the patient-centered medical home (PCMH):[23,24]

1. Every patient has his or her own physician
2. A team of individuals, directed by the physician, takes care of patients
3. Care is "whole person" oriented
4. Care is coordinated and/or integrated across the system
5. The importance of quality and safety care
6. Enhanced access to care
7. Payment reform (e.g., away from fee-for-service)[23,24]

Furthering the concept of the PCMH, the IHI introduced its "triple aim":

1. Improve the individual care experience
2. Improve population health
3. Reduce the population per capita costs of medical care[25]

Two other developments, crucial to making integrated care possible, were the Mental Health Parity Act of 1996[26] and the Mental Health Parity and Addiction Equity Act of 2008.[26] Mental health parity was mandated in group health plans, while the Affordable Care Act of 2010[11] extended parity to individual insurance plans and advocated for prevention.

Health care transformation has also been greatly facilitated by the rapid development and implementation of the electronic medical record.

Ongoing developments, such as telehealth, promise to improve patient access even further.

HEALTH/WELLNESS AND INTEGRATIVE MEDICINE

The concept of health and wellness has played a critical role in creating a new medical paradigm. The evidence that lifestyle changes reduce risks for chronic disease, facilitate health, increase productivity, boost longevity, and enhance prevention activities (e.g., immunization) is remarkable. See Chapter 22: Wellness: An Integrated Care Approach for additional review.

In the late 1950s, Dunn,[17,27] considered the "father of wellness," advocated for preventive health and the idea of wellness.[17,27] A patient's health and wellness is the flip side of diagnosing and treating the patient with illness or pathology. The National Wellness Institute states that there is consensus from those in the field regarding the following characteristics about wellness:

1. A conscious self-directed and evolving process of achieving full potential
2. Multidimensional and holistic, encompassing lifestyle, mental and spiritual well-being, and the environment
3. Positive and affirming[28]

Wellness includes "health, health promotion, disease prevention, incorporating physical, emotional, social, spiritual, environmental, intellectual, and occupational health."[29]

Health and wellness concepts are fundamental elements of integrative medicine (IM). The inclusive goal of IM is to "focus on health and well-being throughout the health span."[30–32] IM has been offered as a potential solution to the American health care crisis. IM provides health care that is "patient centered, healing oriented, emphasizes the therapeutic relationship, and uses evidence-based therapeutic approaches, originating from either conventional and/or alternative medicine."[32] Overall, the IM initiative aligns with that of the PCMH, as well as that of health coaching.

These changes have been moving current medical practice toward the following:

1. Patient-centered care
2. Patient empowerment
3. A renewed focus, by both patients and physicians, on their working alliance as essential to optimal health care
4. The need to facilitate patient ownership of lifestyle change, to reduce chronic illness
5. Team-based care
6. Prevention
7. Population management
8. Reimbursement reform

These reframed medical perspectives have created fertile soil for health coaches to thrive in new primary care and integrated health care environments.

EVOLUTION OF HEALTH COACHING IN HEALTH CARE

Development of Coaching

In ancient China, coaches were known as 陪導 (*pei dao*), translated as *journeying together, one inch at a time*,[33] while coaches in ancient Greece, *paidotribes*, readied the athletes for sports competition.[34] Socrates's open-ended questions paved the way for the language structure of today's coaching.[35] The word *coach* stems from actual movement. In the 1550s, a carriage maker in the Hungarian village Kocs devised a *kocsi*, the most comfortable carriage known at the time. Over the next century, the *kocsi* became popular all over Europe (*kutsche* in German, *coche* in French, and *coach* in English). The word *coach*, in 18th-century England, was slang for an Oxford University tutor, preparing (carrying) students to their goal of passing examinations. Athletic coaches were known as *coachers* until the late 1880s, when the name was shortened to *coaches*.[36]

The modern coach serves as the metaphorical vehicle, safely carrying the individual from his or her beginning state (point A) to his or her desired state (point B). In the 1950s, business began using executive coaching (based on management consulting, leadership training, and organizational psychology).[35] The 1960s was influenced by sports (performance) coaching, while the 1970s ushered in influence from the personal growth movement, incorporating Eastern philosophy (e.g., Buddhism). Timothy Gallwey's work on the *inner game*[37–39] is a prime example of sports coaching's influence on life coaching. His principles, which permeate the world of life coaching, include the following:

1. Nonjudgmental awareness
2. Trust in oneself
3. Exercise of free and conscious choice

4. Belief that the opponent within is more formidable than the one outside

While others, such as consultants, trainers, directive sports coaches, and mentors, overlap with coaches in helping people move from point A to B, many of these experts still maintain a hierarchal relationship between the practitioner and the consumer. Coaching for health and wellness offers a *partnership* or collegial relationship between coach and individual.[35] Hargrove[40] speaks of the coach as a *"thinking partner."*

Health Coaching as a Discipline

The profession of health coaching is relatively new, inasmuch as national efforts are under way to establish standards. This developmental period is not unusual for a new health discipline; similar dialogs were needed approximately 50 years ago when Duke University established the physician assistant as a new health profession.[10] Definitions of *health coach* originate from various sources, including adaptations of the definition of coaching in general from the International Coaching Federation (ICF),[41] the National Consortium for Credentialing Health and Wellness Coaches (NCCHWC),[1] the National Organization of Nurse Practitioners,[42] the Academy of Integrative Health and Medicine,[43] and individual centers for integrative medicine, such as the one at Duke University.[10] Sample definitions demonstrate similar values, beliefs, and approaches to facilitating change.

The ICF, the leading global organization dedicated to advancing the coaching profession, defines coaching as "a partnership with clients in a thought-provoking and creative process, that inspires and supports them to maximize their personal and professional potential . . . coaches honor the client as the expert in his or her life and work." Coaches believe every client has the potential to be creative and resourceful, in order to become fully self-actualized.[41] The term *client* is preferred by coaches in nonmedical environments, whereas *patient* is more typically used when discussing coaching in a medical setting. Standing on this foundation, the ICF (a nonmedical organization) states that the coach's responsibility is to (1) discover, clarify, and align with what the client wants to achieve; (2) encourage the client's self-discovery; (3) elicit collaborative and client-generated solutions and strategies; and (4) hold clients responsible and accountable for the part of their lives that is under their control.[41]

The NCCHWC has been developing a definition in addition to standards, national certification, and a collaborative research agenda to expand the evidence base for health coaching. The NCCHWC definition is

> Health and wellness coaches partner with patients seeking self-directed, lasting changes, aligned with their values, which promote health and wellness, and thereby, enhance the patient's well-being. In the course of their work, health and wellness coaches display unconditional positive regard for their clients, and a belief in their capacity for change, and honor that each patient is an expert on his or her life, while ensuring that all interactions are respectful and nonjudgmental.[1]

Although the terms *health* coach and *wellness* coach tend to be interchangeable, according to the NCCHWC they are distinguished by the following:

> A certified health coach is a health care professional (e.g., physician, registered nurse, nurse practitioner, licensed mental health provider, social worker) who has studied coaching and has passed the health coaching certification examination.
>
> A certified wellness coach is a professional (e.g., certified personal trainer, registered yoga instructor) who has studied coaching and has passed the wellness coaching certification examination.[42]

The NCCHWC and the National Board of Medical Examiners (NBME) recently signed an agreement for the launch of a national certification for individual health and wellness coaches in the United States. The application period for the first certification examination is expected to open in early 2017. The NBME, which has been responsible for assessing physicians' readiness to practice medicine for 100 years, identified the certification of health and wellness coaches as a vital priority in addressing the national crisis in unhealthy lifestyles. Donald Melnick, MD, the president of NBME, noted:

> NBME has long recognized the need to protect the health of the public through state-of-the-art assessment of health professionals. Moving the spectrum beyond physicians to include health

> and wellness coaches dedicated to helping the public with lifestyle improvement is part of our long-term vision.[1]

Meg Jordan,[29] chair of Integrative Health Studies at the California Institute of Integral Studies, lists the following competencies of a health coach: "specialized training in behavior change, health, nutrition, exercise, stress management, and an expansion of the knowledge base to include integrative and holistic approaches."

A systematic review of articles in the medical literature[44] describes health and wellness coaching as

> a process that is fully or partially patient-centered (86%); includes patient-determined goals (71%); incorporates self-discovery and active learning processes (63%) (versus more passive receipt of advice); encourages accountability for behaviors (86%); and provides some type of education to patients along with using coaching processes (91%). Additionally, 78% of articles indicated that the coaching occurs in the context of a consistent, ongoing relationship with a human coach, trained in specific behavior change, communication, and motivational skills.[44]

ROLES OF THE HEALTH COACH

Using a patient-centered model, the tasks of a health coach include:

1. As a *thinking partner*,[40] establishes a working alliance (partnership) with the patient
2. Uses motivational communication skills, focused primarily on the present/future
3. Facilitates patient identification of strengths, core values, and life goals
4. Facilitates patient identification of discrepancies between current unhealthy lifestyle behaviors, and the patient's values and life goals, and uses those values and goals as a way to elicit the patient's *intrinsic* motivation
5. Facilitates exploration of patient ambivalence about making the change(s)
6. Listens for and supports "change talk"
7. Supports patient decision making (as is medically feasible), for which behavior(s) begin to change
8. Co-designs agreed-upon specific, articulated behavioral change goal(s), with measured, agreed-upon, achievable steps
9. Co-creates ways to deal with anticipated obstacles to the goal
10. Facilitates establishment of a patient accountability plan
11. Fosters the patient's progress
12. Helps the patient work through relapses and refine contingency plans

With the focus on facilitating behavioral lifestyle change for chronic illness, health coaches predominantly work with the 11 most common chronic illnesses. In the United States, in 2010, these chronic illnesses were: hypertension (26.7%); hyperlipidemia (21.9%); allergies, sinusitis, and other upper respiratory conditions (13.5%); arthritis (13%); mood disorders, including depression and bipolar disorder (10.6%); diabetes (9.5%); anxiety disorders (6.7%); asthma (6.2%); coronary heart disease and heart attacks (5.3%); thyroid disorders (4.0%); and chronic obstructive lung disease and bronchiectasis (3.5%).[8]

Within an integrated multidisciplinary medical care team, health coach roles include;

1. Screen patients, using health screen instruments
2. Conduct clinical interviews, focused on assessing the eating/nutrition, weight, exercise, sleep, stress, and harm reduction status of patients (e.g., facilitating smoking cessation, reducing alcohol and drug misuse)
3. Enter data in the patient registries, tracking progress and outcomes toward behavioral change and healthier lifestyles
4. Provide health coaching to patients
5. Provide behavioral health change education, and teach change techniques to other members of the integrated care team
6. Help the team assess population needs, and develop group health and wellness programming for an entire practice, or specified population of patients (e.g., those with diabetes)[10,44–46]

EFFICACY OF HEALTH COACHING

An emerging body of literature demonstrates the general efficacy of health coaching for facilitating behavioral and lifestyle change in primary care environments,[47–50] specifically in patients with chronic disease[51,52] and with specific medical conditions, such as diabetes and cardiovascular disease.[53] Health coaches work in various environments, including in-person one-on-one sessions, with a multidisciplinary medical team or as a *teamlet*[54] (with two or three team members), with groups (within medical environments), and via telecoaching or other promising electronic formats.[55]

Integration of health coaching into integrated medical environments is not without its challenges, including the need to resolve the following:

- Workflow and access issues
- Leadership and culture change
- Definitions of roles/boundaries
- Tracking and use of data to evaluate patients
- Practice-level improvements
- Staff education
- Development of health and wellness population management[49,50]

These kinds of practice issues are common for any new discipline entering a new medical environment, working within an integrated multidisciplinary medical practice.

One other important issue is that a health coach is not currently a licensed medical professional. This may change in the near future. Most current health coaches, working in medical environments, may have additional coaching credentials, but their license to coach comes by virtue of their primary medical state licenses (e.g., as nurses, nurse practitioners, social workers, psychologists, physician assistants, medical assistants).

COMPARISONS OF COACHING AND PSYCHOTHERAPY

The major difference between coaching and psychotherapy is in the frame of reference and focus. Much of psychotherapy was founded on a traditional medical model of evaluation, diagnosing psychiatric or addictive illness (pathology), case formulation, and providing brief or long-term treatment. Psychotherapists often focus on dysfunctional patterns, emanating from the biopsychosocial-cultural past and present, with less focus on the future. Although patients can enter psychotherapy to better understand themselves for personal growth, psychotherapy's main focus has been symptom reduction, improved functioning, and relief from psychiatric conditions and addictions. In contrast, health coaching seeks to facilitate specific health-related behavioral and lifestyle change and to move the patient from point A, his or her present state of health, to point B, his or her desired future state of improved health and well-being.

Most of the coaching literature contrasting coaching with psychotherapy tends to paint these differences in black and white.[56] The following comparisons have been heard at coaching seminars:

> Coaching is for growth, has a whole person perspective, focuses on the present and future, is goal oriented, focuses on behavioral change, with the coach and patient in a collaborative partnership. Psychotherapy, on the other hand, is too focused on psychopathology, for those with mental illness and addictions, unearths the past, is aimless in its goals and time frame, and is delivered by an expert, working in a one-down relationship with a dysfunctional patient.

Perhaps in an effort to distinguish itself as a new discipline/profession, this often skewed differentiation by some coaches misses the beauty of work that both professions share. As evidenced in Table 25.1, coaching has adopted a tremendous amount from psychotherapeutic theories and techniques.

Rather than placing health coaching and psychotherapy professions at odds, an inclusive metaphor might be closer to reality; coaching, which tends to be present, future, and goal-oriented, lies in a compact picture frame, surrounded by a larger frame of the many forms of psychotherapeutic styles it has adopted. Both disciplines use similar techniques, focused within their respective scope of practice. Coaches incorporate therapeutic techniques within the context of coaching, while psychotherapists may use coaching techniques within the context of psychotherapy.

Despite their similarities, it is important to understand that the ICF Code of Ethics[41] mandates that ICF coaches must, in practice, make a clear distinction between coaching and psychotherapy in their contracting with clients. Clients must be referred to a mental health professional if they

1. Exhibit a decline in their ability to experience pleasure and/or an increase in being sad, hopeless and helpless

TABLE 25.1 ELEMENTS OF PSYCHOTHERAPY ADOPTED BY COACHING

Therapy	Influencers	Theory, Skills, or Techniques Adopted by Coaching
Psychoanalysis	Sigmund Freud,[57] Freudian disciples (1890–1960s)	**Talk therapy**: Interactive conversation; predominance of patient talk responding to Socratic questioning **Powerful open-ended questions**: What? How? Tell me more . . . Exploratory questions engage the individual. Discovery questions invite self-reflection by individual. **Individual focus**: patient-centered; patient sets the agenda; individual's autonomy encouraged **Nonjudgmental**: Practitioner's stance of technical neutrality **Nondirective communication**: guided conversations
Psychodynamic Psychotherapy, Psychiatry, Education	Carl Jung[58,59] (1928) Alfred Adler[60] (1964) Rudolf Dreikurs[61] (1974)	**Jung**: Individuation as central process of human development: "individual seeks individuation/self-development"; "individual has innate urge toward wholeness" **Adler**: Holistic view of the individual as a whole person working toward goal; individual's creative power to change for the better **Dreikurs**: Help individuals understand their own power: ability to make decisions; freedom to choose own direction
Adult Education	Malcolm Knowles[62–64] (1973)	Move from dependency toward independence/self-direction, andragogy: successful adult learning
Client-Centered Therapy	Carl Rogers[65] (1940s–1960s)	**Person-centered and first humanistic approach**: Coined the word "client," which is preferred by coaches. "A person cannot teach another person directly; a person can only facilitate another's learning." **Unconditional positive regard for clients**: The client is respected, valued, considered an equal in relationship, rather than one down; client teaches therapist about his/her life and worldview (rather than the client learning from an expert) **Active listening**: Practitioner paraphrases or mirrors what is heard; validates patient's experience
Short-Term Therapy	Milton Erikson[66] (1949–1970s)	**Present-focused, short-term therapy**: "Unconscious mind is creative and solution generating" **Uses metaphor and storytelling** (indirect techniques, i.e., Ericksonian indirect hypnosis): Invites possible lasting change for individual (rather than authoritative commands); often credited as foundational for family systems and neurolinguistic programming communication. **Exception questions**: Client repeats past successes, develops confidence in small steps

Solution-focused Therapy	Steve de Shaser[67] Insoo Kim Berg[67]	**Solution seeking**: Help client create solution for desired outcome; present, future focused; uses client's key words in the sessions **"Miracle Question"**: Imagine desired future is here. What would be the first thing you'd notice; first thing you'd do that is different; how would others notice you have changed for the better? **Measuring questions**: How will client assess success of achieving goal(s)? **Scaling questions**: Client rates level of commitment, confidence, and progress toward goal. **Coping questions**: Elicit information about client's strengths, resources, ways of coping **Time out**: Process check to see how client feels the session is moving **Accolades**: Affirm client on content and process of session **Tasks**: Client sets priorities and specific action steps for goals **Solution talk rather than problem talk** **Resilience**: individual has ability to adapt/recover from challenge
Cognitive-Behavioral therapy (CBT)	Aaron Beck[68]	**Irrational beliefs**; irrational/"hot" thoughts, maladaptive/unhealthy feelings and behaviors **Art of Reframing**; six-column technique for patient/client to reconstruct thoughts/beliefs (see Table 25.3)
Positive Psychology	Martin Seligman[69] Mihalyi Csikszentmihali[70] David Cooperrider[71] Albert Bandura[72]	**Strengths-based**: Personal growth, well-being, what specifically makes person happy **Life of possibilities** rather than problems **Explanatory style**: How person internally perceives situations: Permanent? Pervasive? Personal? **Flow state**: Autotelic state (the zone); holistic sensation created when one is totally engaged **Appreciative inquiry**: apply strengths from peak experiences to current goals **Self-efficacy**: one's belief in own ability to succeed in specific situations or accomplish a task
Transtheoretical Model Stages of Change	James Prochaska[73] Carlo DiClimente	**Begin from person's stage of change**: Pre-contemplation, Contemplation, Preparation, Action, Maintenance, Termination
Motivational Interviewing	Stephen Rollnick[74–76] William Miller	Readiness-to-change rulers (importance/confidence to change) Facilitate/engage individual's intrinsic motivation to change at-risk health behaviors Explore and resolve ambivalence to change Align behavioral change with individual's core values Change Talk (**DARN**): **D**esire; **A**bility; **R**easons; **N**eed; Change Talk (**CAT**): **C**ommitment language; **A**ctivation language; **T**aking action steps Effective approach for guiding patients towards resolution of their ambivalence. OARS communication skills: **O**pen-ended questions; **A**ffirmations; **Reflective listening**; **S**ummarize

2. Have intrusive or illogical thoughts, or cannot concentrate or focus
3. Cannot get to sleep; awaken during the night and cannot get back to sleep; or sleep excessively
4. Have a major change in appetite, whether a decrease or increase
5. Feel guilty because others have suffered or died
6. Have feelings of despair or hopelessness
7. Are hyperalert and/or excessively tired
8. Have increased irritability or outbursts of anger
9. Display impulsive and/or risk-taking behavior
10. Have thoughts of death and/or suicide[41]

According to the ICF Code of Ethics, once entering a coaching agreement with a patient, an ICF-credentialed coach, who may also be trained as a licensed mental health professional, cannot simultaneously do both coaching and psychotherapy with the same patient. Currently, if mental health or addiction issues appear in the coaching, an ICF coach must refer the patient to another psychotherapist, even if he or she may have the training to do both therapy and coaching. However, a mental health professional who is also an ICF-credentialed coach, entering a psychotherapy agreement with a patient, has wide latitude to use coaching techniques within the psychotherapy. This fuller scope of practice is allowed, in as much as many coaching techniques originated from a psychotherapeutic frame. In addition, there is no similar prohibition in the codes of ethics within any of the governing bodies of psychotherapy (e.g., psychiatry, psychology, social work, marriage and family) preventing psychotherapists from using a coaching approach within their work. For this reason, at present, when working with an ICF coach, it is "cleaner" in integrated care settings to have both an ICF health coach (focused on health and wellness) and a mental health professional (focused on mental health issues and addiction) on the same multidisciplinary team.

HEALTH COACHING THEORIES AND METHODOLOGY

An applied field of practice, coaching draws from a wide range of models, theories, and biology of learning, including human needs fulfillment; humanism, reinforced by the personal growth movement; positive psychology; theories of self-determination and self-efficacy; adult learning; and research findings on brain plasticity.

Human Needs Fulfillment and Lifestyle Change

Understanding the individual and his or her worldview, through that person's eyes, includes how he or she satisfies fundamental human needs. Table 25.2 lists various concepts of "human needs."

No matter the model of human needs, patients lean toward satisfying a couple of core needs as their primary motivation. On a daily basis, we set out to satisfy our needs in ways that are either constructive and resourceful, or maladaptive and destructive. The vehicles we use to meet our needs are considered healthy and resourceful when they support the health of the self and of others, and destructive, maladaptive, and unhealthy, when they are at the cost to oneself or others.[82]

For example, while eating is necessary to survive, and healthy eating fosters improved health, many people make unhealthy food choices to meet unfulfilled emotional needs. With such limited time allotted for office visits, primary care doctors may not inquire about emotional eating, with or without purging, as a covert reason why a patient fails to have a healthy diet or to lose weight. Health coaches facilitate exploration of the patient's human needs, as these needs form the basis of every lifestyle choice the patient makes, while also informing his or her actions. Facilitating exploration of one's fundamental needs, and the methods used to satisfy them, and then choosing alternative, healthier methods can be pivotal in helping patients make needed lifestyle and behavioral changes.

Humanism

Health coaching is woven from the fabric of humanism, a philosophy stemming from the Renaissance, in emphasizing human potential. From a macro viewpoint, this perspective was at the core of the human potential movement of the 1960s and is embedded in the following coaching principles:

1. Every person is viewed as a unique being
2. People have a basic striving to reach their full potential and capacity
3. Positive change is a driving ambition
4. Self-actualization means developing or growing into one's full potential[83]

5. The importance of collaborative relationships
6. A belief in the possibility of freedom of choice with accompanying responsibility, rather than "viewing our situations and reactions as inevitable or immutable"[84]

Positive Psychology

Positive psychology, focused on the conditions that allow people to flourish and feel fulfilled in life, has had a tremendous effect on coaching.[85] While there are other pioneers who preceded him (e.g., Alfred Adler, MD),[60] the psychologist Martin Seligman, PhD, is considered the "father of positive psychology."[86–88] Principles of this branch of psychology include the following:

1. One's signature (predominant) strengths often lead to the greatest engagement in life[87]
2. The science of *flow*, the resulting gratifying state of complete engagement[70]
3. The science of happiness, and resilience[89]
4. The understanding that people are often motivated or drawn by the future[90]

Concepts and techniques broadly emerging from within the realm of positive psychology include the following:

1. *Learned optimism*, suggesting that changing one's *explanatory* style (how a person understands events) impacts feelings and subsequent actions[69]
2. *Appreciative inquiry*, gleaning personal strengths from past successes and peak experiences, and using them as internal resources for current and future endeavors[71]
3. *Emotional intelligence*, awareness of self and self with others, as well as self and relationship management[91]

Seligman[88] contends there are five avenues toward attaining a state of *well-being*, described by the acronym PERMA:

1. **P**ositive emotion, subjectively accessed
2. **E**ngagement, in life as a subjective experience, is required to attain the state of *flow*
3. **R**elationships with friends, family, intimacy, or social connection
4. **M**eaning, belonging to and serving something bigger than oneself
5. **A**chievement or accomplishment, pursued for its own sake, without the benefits of positive emotion, meaning, or positive relationships

Positive psychology naturally ties in with coaching, self-determination theory, and adult learning, as the elements of positive psychology can all be learned.

Self-Determination Theory and Self-Efficacy

Self-determination theory (SDT) was conceptualized by Deci and Ryan[92] as a way to explain how an individual's behavior is self-motivated and self-determined. SDT identifies three universal, innate needs—autonomy, competence and relatedness—that, when satisfied, allow for growth, optimal functioning, health, and well-being.[93]

Autonomy

Motivation lies on a continuum of autonomy. *Extrinsic* motivation, at one end of the continuum, involves external motivating factors, such as reward and punishment. In *intrinsic* motivation, which is closer to full autonomy on the continuum, a person initiates an activity because it is interesting and satisfying in itself.[93] Integrated motivation is the most autonomous,[93] as the person is fully invested or committed, whether or not the activity is enjoyable in itself, because the motivation is future oriented and tied in with the person's core values (sense of identity) and life goals. Change arising from integrated, fully autonomous motivation is the most sustainable for maintaining new behaviors.[93]

Health coaches use multiple methods to foster the autonomy of motivation. The degree of autonomous motivation has been directly related to some health care outcomes. For example, long-term weight loss, among morbidly obese individuals, was predicted by more autonomous reasons for treatment participation, which in turn was facilitated by autonomy-supportive counselors.[94,95]

Competence

Competence entails "confidence in one's ability to initiate and sustain a desired behavior." SDT posits that people have an innate need to feel competent,

TABLE 25.2 THEORIES OF FUNDAMENTAL HUMAN NEEDS THAT CAN BE USED IN COACHING

Theoretician	Fundamental Human Needs					Comments
Maslow *Hierarchy of Needs*[77]	**Physiologic:** physical requirements for human survival (food, water, shelter) **Safety and security:** personal and financial security, health and well-being, (having a "safety net") **Love and belonging:** sense of being loved, belonging, and acceptance by others **Esteem:** accepted and valued by self and others **Self-actualization:** desire for self-fulfillment; development of one's potential **Self-transcendence:** giving to some higher goal outside oneself, in altruism and spirituality					Higher needs cannot be satisfied without first satisfying lower needs.
	NEEDS	BEING (*qualities*)	HAVING (*things*)	DOING	RELATING (*settings*)	Comments
Max-Neef *Human Scale Development*[78] *(9 needs fulfilled through Being, Having, Doing, and Relating)*	***1. Subsistence***	Physical and mental health	Food, water, shelter	Feed, clothe, rest, work	Living environment Social setting	Max-Neef agreed with universality of human needs; rejected hierarchy of Maslow's model Max-Neef argued no need is more important than any other (except maybe physical survival [e.g., food and water]) No set order required for self-actualization
	2. Protection	Care Adaptability Autonomy	Social security Health systems Work	Cooperate, plan, help, take care of	Social environment Dwelling	
	3. Affection	Respect Sense of humor Generosity Sensuality	Friendships Family Relationship with nature	Share Take care of Sexual activity Express emotions	Privacy Intimate spaces of togetherness	
	4. Understanding	Critical capacity Curiosity Intuition	Literature Teachers Policies Educational	Analyze Study Mediate Investigate	Schools Families University Communities	
	5. Participation	Receptiveness Dedication Sense of humor	Responsibilities Duties Work Rights	Cooperate Dissent Express opinions	Associations Neighborhoods Churches Parties	

	6. Leisure	Imagination Tranquility Spontaneity	Games Parties Peace of mind	Daydream Remember Relax Have fun	Landscape Intimate spaces Places to be alone	
	7. Creation	Imagination Boldness Inventiveness Curiosity	Abilities Skills Work Techniques	Invent, design Build, compose Work Interpret	Spaces for expression Workshops Audiences	
	8. Identity	Sense of belonging Self-esteem Consistency	Language Religions Values, norms Customs Work	Get to know oneself Grow Commit	Places in which one belongs Everyday settings	
	9. Freedom	Autonomy Passion Self-esteem Open-mindedness	Equal rights	Dissent Choose Run risks Develop awareness	Anywhere	
Deci and Ryan *Self-Determination*[79–81]	***Autonomy:*** self-directed ***Competence:*** self-efficacy, the confidence in one's ability to initiate/sustain a desired behavior ***Relatedness:*** relationship, connection					These needs must be satisfied to achieve psychological growth, integrity, and well-being
Robbins 6 *Universal Needs*[82]	***Certainty:*** safety, stability, security, comfort, order, predictability, control and consistency *(helps anticipate others' behavior and the future)* ***Variety***: adventure, stimulation, challenges, change, novelty, surprise and excitement ***Significance***: to feel as if one matters; has meaning and purpose in one's life ***Love/Connection***: to feel attached, a part of something more than oneself (dyad, group, universe), to feel intimate, to love and be loved ***Growth***: continual intellectual, emotional, and spiritual development ***Contribution***: to give back and generate growth in others					Certainty and variety are complementary (need for balance) Too much focus on significance can preclude healthy love/connection Growth and contribution provide structure for fulfillment

and competence is fostered through affirming positive feedback.[93] This perspective aligns with the coaching tenets that the person is the expert in his or her life and work, and that everyone has the potential to be creative and resourceful in order to become fully self-actualized[41] and has the capacity for change.[1]

Relatedness

Relatedness, the third SDT psychological need,[93] is fostered in coaching. Coaches emphasize the importance of their relationships with patients by establishing an empathic, nonjudgmental *thinking partner*[39] relationship, which supports their patients' wishes to make changes.

Promoting autonomous motivation, the development of competence, and relatedness have all been shown to be particularly helpful in assisting patients in making behavioral change.[93]

Coaches use concepts of self-efficacy as described within Bandura's[96–99] social cognitive model. Self-efficacy develops by achieving goals through positive mastering experiences, perseverance and sustained efforts, overcoming obstacles, and observing how others succeed. Coaches promote self-efficacy by doing the following:

1. Helping the patient set reasonable, attainable behavioral goals to bring desired results; even small successes can set in motion a positive feedback loop for additional behavioral change(s)
2. Affirming successes by the patient, to help the patient build his or her self-esteem
3. Helping the patient improve his or her perception of their ability to achieve a goal
4. Facilitating patient understanding of how others overcome barriers with alternative methods for succeeding

Adult Learning

We cannot teach another person directly; all we can do is facilitate the learning.

Carl Rogers, MD, 1951[65]

In the 1960s and 1970s, Knowles[62–64] developed principles of how adults learn best. He believed his role in education "was not that of a teacher, but rather *a facilitator of learning.*"[64] Five principles from adult learning have informed the practice of coaching:

1. Adult learning is *self-directed*, actively pursued by adults, and need not be dependent on experts or as passive recipients of information
2. Adult learning occurs by accumulating a growing reservoir of experiences.[64]
3. Adults are ready to learn, based on the needs of their social roles.[62]
4. Learning is facilitated by focus and problem solving of an immediate situation, rather than the future
5. Motivation to learn can be sustained when it comes from internal sources (from within)[64]

In the 1970s and 1980s, Tough[100,101] furthered Knowles' work by conceptualizing *self-directed learning* as the ability to teach oneself, and through personal autonomy, to take ownership and control of one's learning. Coaching incorporates Tough's principles:

1. Flexibility, in that coaching is tailored to the patient, his or her personality, learning style, strengths, and values
2. Coaching provides frequent feedback through active and reflective listening
3. Continual affirmation of the learner fosters change
4. Asking patients to reflect on their experiences is crucial for maximizing the learning
5. Coaches initially guide the patient's reflections on his or her learning until the patient internalizes this process and in effect becomes his or her own coach[39]

Coaching is a wonderful learning lab for the patient, in which the coach creates a safe, supporting environment and facilitates self-directed learning by the patient.

COACHING IN PRACTICE

The coach helps the patient prioritize his or her goals without assuming that the health goals recommended by the multidisciplinary integrated health care team are at the top of the patient's list. Because coaches avoid positioning themselves as experts (in an effort to maximize the patient's self-determination and self-efficacy), coaches ask the patient's explicit permission before providing any health education.[17,29]

Five predominant approaches are significantly woven into the fabric of health coaching: (1) the transtheoretical model or stages of change;[73] (2) motivational interviewing;[74–76] (3) solution-focused health coaching (SFHC);[67,102,103] (4) cognitive-behavioral coaching; and (5) mindfulness-based stress reduction.[104] The first four of these approaches were originally developed in a psychotherapy frame and have been adapted for use within a coaching context. Stages of change and motivational interviewing are synergetic and, in working together, present a typical arc for behavioral change. Both approaches suggest ways of facilitating forward movement during each stage. SFHC honors and encourages the patient's innate desire for self-determination and autonomous motivation. Mindfulness, which can be used within any coaching approach, helps clients become centered and more relaxed, as well as work through internal barriers to change.

Transtheoretical Model: Stages of Change

People don't change until they're ready to.

James O. Prochaska[73]

The transtheoretical model, often called *stages of change*, was the first widely used behavioral change model adopted by the medical community to facilitate patient behavioral and lifestyle change.[73] The stages of change model, which is familiar to most health care providers, comprises the following stages: (1) pre-contemplation; (2) contemplation; (3) preparation; (4) action; (5) maintenance; and (6) termination.[73]

In the *pre-contemplation* stage ("I won't, I can't"),[85] the patient is not yet ready for change and does not intend to take action in the next 6 months. The patient might not even be aware of the need to change. In this stage, the coach supports patient self-determination and autonomy, and is empathic to the patient's preference to stay the same, without judgment. The coach asks the patient what concerns he or she may have regarding his or her health, and may (with the patient's permission)[17,29] provide health information.

In the *contemplation* stage ("I might"),[85] the patient considers the positive impact as well as the hard work involved in making the change. The patient may be ambivalent about change, yet intends to take action within the next 6 months. The coach facilitates the patient's exploration of his or her ambivalence to making a change through guidance with the following:

1. Evokes an understanding of the discrepancy between the patient's unhealthy behavior and his or her core values and life goals[76]
2. Explores potential payoff(s) to the patient by maintaining the status quo
3. Reviews the patient's strengths
4. Explores alternative, healthier ways for the patient to meet his or her needs that are currently being met with the unhealthy behavior
5. Reviews ways in which a healthy change aligns with the patient's values and life goals
6. Asks what possibilities open up for the patient as a result of making the change[85]
7. Facilitates patient identification of his or her support system[28]

In the *preparation* stage ("I will"),[85] the patient intends to take action within the next 30 days and has taken steps in this direction. The coach helps the patient do the following:

1. Clarify goal(s) and expectations
2. Discover triggers for the unhealthy behavior
3. Arrive at alternative plans to address obstacles to change
4. Mitigate barriers to change
5. Enlist a support system
6. Set up an accountability process
7. See the change journey as a learning opportunity[29]

In the *action* stage ("I am"), [85] the patient has engaged in a new healthy behavior for less than 6 months. The coach supports the patient by doing the following:

1. Champions the patient's positive actions
2. Reinforces the healthy behavior
3. Acknowledges the commitment and efforts made[17]
4. Helps the patient pull in as much support as possible
5. Reinforces the patient's values, strengths, and support system, connecting them to the goal
6. Helps the patient (if needed) break larger steps into smaller ones
7. Reinforces all successes

8. Supports self-efficacy
9. If there is a relapse, reminds the patient of a contingency plan (reframed as new learning), "like a baby naturally tumbling when learning to walk"[29]

In the *maintenance* stage ("I'm still doing"),[85] the patient has performed the healthy behavior for more than 6 months. The coach supports changes, affirms self-efficacy, discusses coping strategies,[17] and, if a relapse occurs, guides the patient to revisit, revise, and reconnect with his or her strengths, values, resources, visions, goals, and motivators.[85]

Finally, in the *termination* stage ("it's part of me"),[85] the patient adopts the new behavior as a habit. The coach fosters independence and self-sufficiency and supports solution focus, should the patient have a relapse.[17]

Patients do not necessarily move through the stages of change in a linear or sequential progression. Change can occur with jumps over one or two stages, or relapse to earlier stages, before actual change becomes a habit.[73] Prochaska describes 10 processes that can be used to facilitate change:

1. Consciousness raising (raise the patient's awareness) through education and feedback
2. Catharsis (emotional release or expression after a difficult experience)
3. Self re-evaluation (assess if current unhealthy behavior aligns with one's core values and life goals)
4. Environmental re-evaluation (e.g., considering the effects of one's behavior on others, such as noticing the effects that secondhand smoke has on loved ones in the home)
5. Self-liberation (make a commitment, such as a New Year's resolution)
6. Social liberation (make a commitment to a cause, such as healthy foods for school lunches)
7. Counter-conditioning (find alternative healthy behavior, such as knitting or doing puzzles, to quell anxiety)
8. Stimulus control (e.g., manage triggers of unhealthy behaviors, such as eliminating junk food to decrease binge eating)
9. Contingency management (e.g., have a secondary plan as backup in case the original plan fails)
10. The helping relationship (support from others, such as the coach, a therapist, or a self-help group)[73]

Research has shown that some change processes are more effective during certain stages. Consciousness raising (education and feedback) and catharsis (emotional release) work best to help move a patient from pre-contemplation to contemplation. Use of self and environmental re-evaluation can facilitate progression from contemplation to preparation. Use of self-liberation promotes movement to the preparation stage. Counter-conditioning, stimulus control, and contingency management all can be used to facilitate change toward action, maintenance, and termination. Social liberation and helping relationships are useful at any stage.[73]

Motivational Interviewing

People are generally better persuaded by the reasons they have themselves discovered, than by those which have come into the minds of others.

Blaise Pascal, 1623–1662[74]

Motivational interviewing is collaborative and goal-oriented, with particular attention paid to the language of change.[74–76] This person-centered line of inquiry, developed by Miller and Rollnick,[74–76] two clinical psychologists, was first used as a therapeutic approach in the treatment of patients with alcohol addiction. Motivational interviewing is now the most frequently used style by health coaches to facilitate change because it addresses the potential underlying ambivalence while activating the person's own motivation for change. Miller[56] has said that motivational interviewing is "Carl Rogers in new clothes."

Similar to the stages of change model, motivational interviewing recognizes that clients who need to make a change approach coaching at "different levels of readiness to change their behavior."[105] SDT is viewed by many in the field as a good framework for understanding motivational interviewing.[93] Creating sustained behavioral change is predicated on the degree of the patient's ability to develop autonomous motivation for making changes. The four organizing principles of motivational interviewing are the interwoven processes of engaging, focusing, evoking, and planning.[76]

In the first phase, the *engaging* process, the coach develops a partnership with the patient, providing a "safe space" for the patient to feel comfortable, sharing from his or her perspective. Miller and Rollnick credit Jeff Ellison, LCSW,[76] with a beautiful metaphor that the relationship in motivational interviewing is like "dancing, rather than wrestling. Someone is still leading in the dance . . . without tripping or stepping on toes. Without a partnership, there is no dance."[29]

Four core communication skills are used in the opening phase of engaging and continue throughout the coaching. Use of the OARS communication skills, so embedded in psychotherapy, are also basic to coaching:

1. **O**pen-ended questions encourage the patient to elaborate on his or her health situation
2. **A**ffirming or accentuating the positive, particularly one's strengths, sets the stage for future change
3. **R**eflective (active) listening is the process used to develop "accurate empathy,"[65] which helps validate the patient's experience
4. **S**ummarizing or "bottom lining" is used to help synthesize material offered by the patient.

The *righting reflex*, as in advice giving, while offered with the best of intentions, is considered counterproductive. Offering expert opinions elicits *sustain talk* (maintaining the status quo), which can lead to patient disengagement and can derail efforts to create change.

During the engagement phase, coaches often discuss the findings of pre-session self-assessments, which may include the following:

1. Identification of patient values[28]
2. Identification of life goals[29]
3. Identification of the patient's signature (predominant) strengths, which helps the patient mobilize his or her inner resources for creating change[29]
4. A *wheel of health* self-assessment (similar to the wheel of life used in life coaching). This health assessment uses a picture of a wheel with spokes, depicting the relationship of the patient (placed in the wheel's center) to various domains of health, such as nutrition, exercise, rest, spirituality, and relationships.[105] The wheel also depicts the patient's relationship to professional care (traditional medical care, prevention, alternative or complementary medicine). The coach asks the patient to use the wheel to reflect on his or her current state within each of these domains, and explores the patient's vision of optimal health. This process helps the patient uncover his or her core health values and beliefs.[106]

In *focusing*, the second phase of motivational interviewing, the coach helps the patient understand his or her values and goals, which will be used as a way to elicit the patient's autonomous motivation. This phase "shines the light on the gap between a patient's current health behaviors and their values and goals."[85] Facilitated exploration of these discrepancies can be a powerful motivator for change when explored in a safe and supportive atmosphere."[76]

Focusing centers on promoting a collaborative search for direction. Agenda mapping[76] allows a collaborative look at "a menu of behavioral change possibilities" from which to choose when making lifestyle change.[76] Feinstein[107] points out how important it is to continue to support patients' autonomy and to provide them with choices, letting them set their own priorities for change: "What are your priorities for positive change in your health?"[108]

It's important to differentiate between goals (what the patient wants) and outcomes (what is actually achieved).[17] The patient's goal might be to discontinue the need for diabetic medications by losing 25 pounds within 6 months. Even if the desired outcome is not achieved (discontinuing medication), the work done can still be considered positive, in that the client has lost weight. When actual outcomes don't match the original goals, it may be necessary to help the patient renegotiate the goals, providing more time to reach the desired outcome.

In the third phase, *evoking*, the following actions are designed to foster change:

1. Build on the patient's earlier health visioning in the engaging phase
2. Help the patient articulate possibilities for change
3. Elicit the patient's autonomous motivation(s) for change, tied to his or her values and goals
4. Assess the patient's readiness and capacity to make change, using "readiness-to-change rulers"[74]

Motivational interviewing uses two readiness-to-change rulers to examine the patient's strength of motivation for lifestyle and behavioral change.[74,75] The *importance ruler* asks the patient to rate the importance of making a change, on a scale of 1 to 10. The *confidence ruler* asks the patient to rate how confident he or she is in the ability to make a change, on a scale of 1 to 10. For both rulers, it's helpful to evoke the patient's reason for not giving a lower rating (e.g., a 4 instead of a 6 on importance, or a 3 instead of a 5 on confidence to make the change). This line of inquiry invites the patient to clarify how making a change really is important, and how much more confident he or she really feels in making the change. Following up with "What can you do to increase the importance and increase your confidence of making the change?" supports the patient's self-efficacy. Patients with high importance and confidence ratings are most likely to take action, leading to successful change.

Motivational interviewing helps patients give voice to the various sides of their ambivalence, weighing the pros and cons of making the change. This voiced ambivalence is pro/con self-talk and is really just an argument within the person. Ambivalence about change is natural and suggests a discrepancy between the patient's use of unhealthy behavior(s) and his or her core values and health goals. For example, wanting to reduce stress, while feeling obliged to take on more stressful tasks at work, reveals the ambivalence in making a choice. Ambivalence is evident by listening for a mixture of *sustain talk* and *change talk*. Change talk refers to comments related to the reasons to make a change. A predominance of sustain talk, or even an equal mix of sustain and change talk, is associated with maintenance of the status quo, whereas a predominance of change talk predicts subsequent behavioral change. Hearing the patient use a conjunction such as "but" is a tipoff to ambivalence, as in, "I want to stop smoking, *but* if I do I'll gain weight." While patients might talk about wanting to change, their sustain talk focuses on why they cannot or will not change and demonstrates their preference for maintaining the status quo.

Summarized by the acronym **DARN**,[76] change talk occurs when a patient describes his or her **D**esire, **A**bility, **R**eason, or **N**eed to change a behavior:

Desire: Skilled health coaches can evoke change talk with questions that point toward the future and change, such as, "What health behavior(s) do you hope to change?"

Ability questions evoke a patient's skills and confidence. Asking what a patient "can, could, or is able to do" facilitates behavioral change

Reason questions such as, "What do you gain by losing weight?" explore a patient's rationale for wanting to change

Need questions, such as "What makes this change important to you?" highlights the importance and urgency for change

The acronym **CAT**[76] illustrates how to listen for commitment language from the patient:

Commitment language such as "I will," "I promise," or "I give my word" is language preliminarily committed to change.[76]

Activation language such as "I am ready to . . ." or "I am prepared to . . ." is closer to actual movement toward change. The natural coach response to these statements might be to ask for some clarification, such as, "When will you begin to . . .?" "What specifically will you do?"

Taking action steps using action language indicates preparation for change as in, "I went to a support group meeting" or "I bought nicotine patches."

The **DARN CAT** line of inquiry is an effective approach for guiding patients toward resolution of their ambivalence.

Other change strategies include asking the patient to envision the extremes: "What's the worst thing that could happen if you continue to gain weight?" *Appreciative inquiry* explores the patient's past successes, with his or her strengths utilized in those successes, that could be used to elicit positive change. In addition, the process of looking forward and specifically envisioning a happier future can be useful to elicit positive changes.

The final phase of motivational interviewing involves planning and goal setting. The patient's state of readiness for change can be determined by the predominance of change talk (**DARN CAT**) over sustain talk. As change becomes imminent, it is important to help the patient transition to action planning. Drucker's[109] model for planning and goal setting uses the acronym **SMART**. Extending this acronym to **PVCSMART** (as PVC can pave the way to a clear, smart goal), and adapting this to health/behavioral change, the coach helps the patient clarify his or her goal by ensuring the following:

1. **P**ositive statements: Rather than saying, "I don't want to feel so tired," the goal needs a positive frame, as in, "I want to have energy"
2. **V**alues aligned: The goal needs to support the patient's core values and overall life goals
3. **C**ontrol: The goal needs to be within the patient's control
4. **S**pecific: The patient needs to explicitly state the action plan (e.g., lose 25 pounds in 6 months)
5. **M**easurable: The goal needs to be observable, with a way to measure progress
6. **A**ttainable: The goal must be something for which the patient has the skills and/or abilities to achieve
7. **R**ealistic: The goal must be one that the patient is willing and able to achieve, given his or her health
8. **T**ime-sensitive: The goal is pursued within a specific time frame

While the coach guides the patient in the process of clarifying his or her goals, it is the patient who is responsible and ultimately accountable for achieving his or her goals.[17]

Solution-Focused Health Coaching

Every problem is actually a solution in disguise.

Unknown

Solution-focused health coaching a derivative of Solution-Focused Therapy,[66,101] fosters the patient's innate desire for self-determination and autonomy. The SFHC[102] approach emphasizes the following:

1. Inasmuch as the patient, rather than the coach, is the expert in his or her own life, out of curiosity the coach takes the mindset of *the beginner's mind* to learn about the particular patient and his or her worldview
2. Patient strengths
3. Focus is on "solution talk" rather than "problem talk."
4. Exploration of exceptions to the current unhealthy period (periods when the patient was healthy)[67,103]
5. Appreciative inquiry; an exploration of the patient's past that helps focus on how past strengths and skills might again be reawakened to foster health[71]
6. Use of the *Miracle Question* (one of the hallmarks of SFHC): "Imagine when you go to sleep tonight a miracle happens (only you don't know that), and when you wake up tomorrow, you are in your desired healthy state; what's the first thing you'd notice? What's the first thing you'd do that is different? How would others notice you are healthier?"[67,90,103]
7. Reframing the patient's condition, from a different perspective, opening up other possibilities for the patient (e.g., "The minor heart attack you had has allowed you to finally stop smoking")[103]
8. Scaling questions: Ask patients to rate themselves on any number of things, such as identifying their progress on a scale of 1 to 10
9. Set clear and specific health-related tasks and goals[67,90,103]
10. Ask measurement questions, such as, "How will you know you have accomplished the task or goal?"[103]
11. Find existing, but as yet unused, resources available to the patient, rather than what the patient lacks[103]
12. Coping questions: "How have you managed to handle everything that's happened in your life?"[90]
13. Affirming the patient and his or her approach to solutions, as well as celebrating successes[103]

Cognitive Approaches to Coaching

Self-Directed Neuroplasticity

You have brains in your head. You have feet in your shoes.

You can steer yourself any direction you choose.

Dr. Seuss (***Oh, The Places You'll Go***)

To foster behavioral change, the health coach, as *thinking partner*,[40] can facilitate the patient's development of a new healthy behavioral habit (sustained change). Jeffrey Schwartz, MD, a neuroscientist, describes how to create a positive habit in a process he has called *self-directed neuroplasticity* (self-learning, the nature of adult learning).[110] Using a common unhealthy behavior (overeating) as an example, this three-step process comprises the following actions:

1. *Name* the underlying need to satisfy (e.g., the need to calm down or self-soothe). Naming helps the patient become aware and attend to a potential cognitive distortion (e.g., "the purpose of eating is to calm me down").
2. *Reframe* the true purpose of the behavior (e.g., "The true purpose of eating is to refuel and for health, not to relieve my anxiety").
3. *Refocus*, or find a healthy behavioral alternative to satisfy the need (e.g., practice a relaxation exercise to self-soothe). The health coach helps the patient choose an alternative, healthy behavior that aligns with the patient's values and life goals. Should the patient lack knowledge of healthy alternatives, the coach asks the patient's permission to momentarily serve as a consultant/educator and share some information:[29] "May I have your permission to share a behavior that research has found to be very calming for lots of people?" With the patient's agreement, the coach can take the patient through a relaxation exercise such as mindfulness-based stress reduction (MBSR)[111] as a healthy alternative to overeating. After taking on the role of a health educator, the coach returns to the collaborative role of thinking partner.[29]

Once a new behavior is chosen, the coach helps the patient design a plan to incorporate the healthy behavior into his or her life, encouraging the patient to focus and frequently repeat the desired behavior. *Attention density*, the amount of focus and frequency of a behavior, encourages the patient's neurons to "fire together and wire together." These *mirror neurons* allow repetitive health behaviors to become preconscious and more automatic and help create a new healthy habit.[110]

It is also very important to help the patient anticipate and work through barriers/obstacles to practicing the new behavior. This could be done, for example, by guiding the patient to design a ritual (e.g., where and when, to practice and anchor the relaxation technique) and helping the patient create an accountability process. While if asked, the coach can assist, in this accountability process, it's better to invoke the help from the patient's social network (e.g., check in with family or friends prior to going to bed). Ultimately, the patient learns to become self-directed.

Cognitive-Behavioral Coaching

If you think you can do a thing or think you can't do a thing, you're right.

Henry Ford (***Quotations of Henry Ford***, Applewood Books, 2006)

Cognitive-behavioral coaching is based on cognitive-behavioral therapy, which was developed by the psychiatrist Aaron Beck, MD. It is an applied practice of the scientific method.[68,112–114] Cognitive behavioral coaching facilitates the patient's learning in how to use awareness, logic, testing, and practice (altering distorted thoughts and beliefs underlying unhealthy behavior.)[89] Jeff Auerbach, PhD,[104] emphasizes that the coach helps the patient think with "more depth, greater clarity, and less distortion."

The cognitive-behavioral approach is based on the premise that there is a cognitive sequence of events that helps create lifestyle or behavioral dysfunction; when discovered, this sequence can be modified.[113,114] The sequence begins with an environmental trigger (stimulus), leading to negative emotions/feelings, which may cause physical symptoms. These changes in emotions or physical symptoms are really founded on irrational/distorted thoughts, misperceptions, or incorrect interpretations of the event's meaning.[113] Table 25.3[115] gives a list of illogical styles of thinking that affect health-related behaviors, and discusses how patients can more realistically reframe their thinking to facilitate behavioral changes.

Coaches may use a full six-column cognitive behavioral log or diary[113] (see an example of dealing with overeating), depicted in Table 25.4.

Mindfulness-Based Stress Reduction

Mindfulness is not about Buddhism, but about paying attention.

Jon Kabat-Zinn[113]

Neuroscience has validated the positive health effects of Mindfulness-Based Stress Reduction

TABLE 25.3 REFRAMING ILLOGICAL THINKING STYLES TO MORE REALISTIC THINKING[108]

ILLOGICAL (Errors in) THINKING	REALISTIC (Rebalanced) THINKING
1. **Polarized thinking**: All/nothing; good/bad; either/or; black/white; no middle ground *"I ate six pieces of pizza at dinner; I'm a total failure!"*	1. **Assess the whole, not the specific**: What positives am I not considering? *"Overall, I've been moderating my portions."*
2. **Self-reference**: Taking things personally when they have no reference to you *"My doctor missed my appointment; he dislikes me."*	2. **Think of alternative explanations:** What else could have happened? *"Maybe my doctor had an emergency."*
3. **Discounting positives:** Ignoring positive behaviors (they're trivial & don't really count) *"You're just saying that because you're my coach."*	3. **Understand the *value* of the positives:** *"I kept a consistent exercise log; I stayed with the task and I feel good about that."*
4. **Blaming:** **Self**: for problems not within your control *"If I were more attentive, my husband wouldn't drink."* **Others**: for negative outcomes within your control *"He made me so mad! That caused me to overeat."*	4. **Assess realistic locus of control:** **Focus on what is within your control:** *"I'll attend Al-Anon and seek guidance."* **Take responsibility (if warranted):** *"I was so angry at him! I overate."*
5. **Self-labeling/name calling:** Putting oneself down; generalizing about oneself based on a behavior *"I smoke a pack a day; I'm a real loser."*	5. **Separate identity from the behavior**: *"I am a good person and I smoke."* *"This is an addiction; I need some help."*
6. **Negative filter**: Magnify or dwell on negatives. *"When someone sees me, they just see the fat."*	6. **Assess the whole, not the specific:** What positives am I not considering? *"There are many wonderful facets to me."*
7. **Jumping to conclusions:** **Mind reading:** presuming what others think *"They won't like me if I don't drink with them."* **Predicting the future from the past:** *"I fell off the wagon; I'll never stop drinking."*	7. **Stay with the facts in the present:** **Check it out:** *"If drinking is required, do I really want them as friends?"* **The past does not dictate my future destiny:** *"I can stop drinking/learn better ways to cope."*
8. **MOANS**: thinking in absolutes I **M**ust *stay away from soda.* I **O**ught *to do weight training every other day.* I **A**lways *blow my diet.* I **N**ever *feel relaxed.* I **S**hould *quit smoking cold turkey (all at once)*	8. **Linguistic reframe:** *I prefer water or juice over soda.* *I can miss a day of weight training.* *Sometimes I eat unhealthy foods.* *I can practice relaxation techniques.* *I'll smoke fewer cigarettes (harm reduction).*
9. **Catastrophizing, anticipating the worst:** *"My test is positive. I have cancer; I'll die soon."*	9. **Stay in the now, manage uncertainty:** *"There are false positives; I can wait and see."*
10. **Overgeneralization, extrapolating from one experience (e.g., outcome) to that of others:** *"I can't stop smoking, so I'll fail at exercise too."*	10. **Treat each experience as separate:** *"Not yet being able to quit smoking has nothing to do with my engaging in exercise, even just walking."*

TABLE 25.4 COGNITIVE-BEHAVIORAL DIARY

Situation Triggers of Distress	Rate Mood or Feeling	Describe Physical Symptoms	Disturbing Irrational or Hot Thought	Evidence (Pro) Supporting the Hot Thought	Evidence (Con) Opposing the Hot Thought	Revised or Balanced Thought	Revised Rating of Feeling(s) or Mood
1. What happened? 2. When? 3. Where? 4. Who was there?	How were you feeling (mood)? *Rate* your mood Severity: 1 = minimal 5 = severe	List any physical symptoms (e.g., headache, palpitations, heartburn, tightness in stomach, back and neck)	Negative thoughts often contain the "MOANS" **M**ust **O**ught **A**lways **N**ever **S**hould	List evidence that supports (times in the past)	List times you handled the situation differently	Using (con) refuted evidence, write a more realistic thought	How are you feeling now? (including physical) Rate the severity: 1 = minimal 5 = severe
Example: 1. I overate 2. Late at night 3. I was at home 4. I was alone	Example: I felt irritable and cranky Rating = 4	Example: Tightness in neck and back	Example: "I will **N**ever stop binging, or lose weight. I am a total failure"	Example: "I **A**lways pig out late at night; I failed in the past and will fail again; I will never change.	Example: "On vacation, when feeling more relaxed, I ate dinner, read a book, and went to bed; I succeeded that time"	Example: "I can eat moderately without pigging out at night, when relaxed; maybe I *can* succeed" (a self-directed learning moment)	Example: Rating: 2 *Learning:* "I could use some help in choosing a different way to handle my unease at night"

(MBSR)[111] to facilitate behavioral and lifestyle change. With origins arising from Buddhist philosophy, and introduced to America's mainstream by Kabat-Zinn,[116] mindfulness is a state of "full awareness of the present, nonjudgmental attitude toward oneself, and acceptance of what one can or cannot change."[116–118]

Mindfulness practice can facilitate the relaxation response, helping to metabolize stress, and facilitate behavioral and lifestyle change.[111,118] Focused on moment-to-moment awareness and acceptance of "the now," MBSR heightens yet softens the senses, decreases self-judgment, and can help to create a sense of peace and well-being. MBSR triggers shifts in cognition, emotion, biology, and behavior that can synergistically work to reduce a variety of physical and mood symptoms and improve overall health.[111,118,119] Relaxation techniques may be used to bring on a mindfulness state. Deep breathing helps elicit the relaxation response and, used during times of stress, can actually help train one's brain to relax when needed.[111]

A simple way to practice mindfulness throughout the day is to take small breaks or *pit stops*, every 90 to 120 minutes, the amount of time the brain can effectively stay focused, due to ultradian rhythms.[120] Time-out breaks of 15 to 20 minutes from the activity (such as work) are optimal for renewal. Alternatively, 5- or 6-minute mini-pit stops every 1.5 to 2 hours, practicing a short relaxation exercise (e.g., body scan, progressive muscle relaxation, creative visualization, brief meditation), can provide renewal by reducing stress and increasing resilience. This mindful transition from activity to renewal is similar to the peak performance routine for a racecar driver who takes periodic pit stops (e.g., filling tires with air, refueling, recharging) to win the race.

Research has demonstrated that MBSR can facilitate smoking cessation,[121] decrease binge eating,[122] help reduce alcohol and illicit substance use,[123] and improve sleep[124] and is useful for reducing anxiety, depression,[125] and trauma.[126] MBSR has also been shown to help reduce impulsive decision making, or destructive behavior[127] and relieve negative thoughts or a ruminative style of thinking.[111,119] It may help some patients be less judgmental about what they perceive as their own failures.[113]

The practice of mindfulness activities and relaxation techniques,[113] including the use of breathing techniques, body scan, creative visualization, progressive muscle relaxation, and so forth, are not only very popular in peak performance (e.g., sports, performance arts) but are often used alone in therapy and coaching, or in conjunction with therapeutic models, such as motivational interviewing, SFHC, cognitive-behavioral coaching, and so forth. Yoga, tai chi, and meditation can also be used in conjunction with health coaching approaches for their beneficial effects. Mindfulness and relaxation techniques are frequently used as healthy behavioral replacements for unhealthy behaviors such as smoking, drinking, and overeating.

SIX STAGES OF HEALTH COACHING

The six general stages in a health coaching engagement are depicted in Figure 25.1. The following is a brief overview of each stage.

Stage 1. Pre-Engagement Discovery

In pre-engagement discovery, the health coach may be introduced to the patient via a "warm handoff," or may occur via electronic means; the introduction may include recommendations from the multidisciplinary team for behavioral or lifestyle changes. The coach may ask the patient to complete and return an intake package, which often includes a patient profile form, health rating scales used by the team evaluating health symptoms and functioning, and health coaching self-assessment tools, such as the wheel of health,[105] a strengths indicator,[29] or a values assessment.[28]

Stage 2. Establishing the Coaching Agreement: Initial Meeting

The coaching agreement serves as the foundation for the relationship between the coach and the

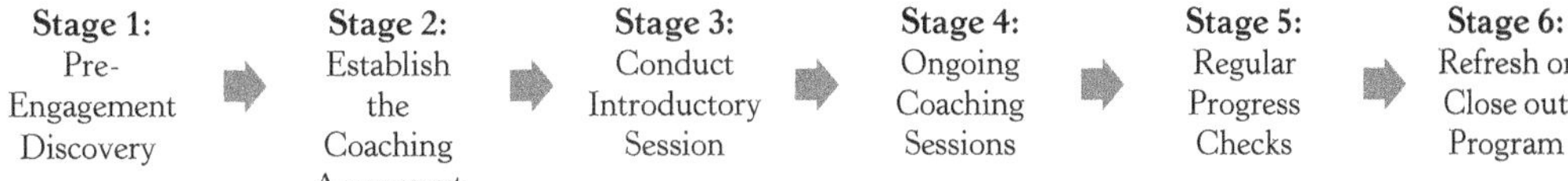

FIGURE 25.1 Coaching session: six stages of engagement.

patient. In a health care setting, Stages 1 and 2 may be combined into one initial meeting, lasting 30 to 60 minutes. The coaching agreement covers roles and responsibilities for both the coach and patient, and clarifies the scope of practice for health coaching with the following understanding:

1. The patient is the expert on his or her life
2. The coach serves as the patient's *thinking partner* to help the patient explore and achieve his or her desired behavioral health goal(s)
3. Together as partners, the health coach and patient will view the patient's health condition within the context of the patient's life
4. Behavioral health goals are ultimately chosen by the patient, taking into account information from the health care team; these choices are the result of alignment with the patient's core values, strengths, personality, life goals, and preferences
5. If symptoms or psychological issues emerge that are better suited for psychotherapy, the patient will be referred to a behavioral health clinician, and the patient may or may not continue health coaching
6. The coach may seek permission (as needed) from the patient to step out of the role of *"thinking partner"* and take on a health educational role, after which the coach returns to the role of thinking partner as soon as feasible[29]

During the initial meeting, the coach provides a brief overview of his or her background and experience, reviews the health summary from the integrated care team with the patient, and may give the patient an intake package (if not previously received in Stage 1), asking for information to be provided prior to the first coaching session. The patient has the opportunity to ask questions about coaching and how they will work together.

As an illustration of a health coaching engagement, we will discuss the case of Joshua (Box 25.2) and demonstrate the arc of the engagement from Stages 3 through 6. For this example, Joshua has already been through Stage 2, during which he has agreed to the parameters of the health coaching engagement and is willing to move forward and consider making some healthy lifestyle changes. He has also agreed that if his mild depressive symptoms do not subside when making lifestyle changes, he will accept a referral to a mental health professional.

BOX 25.2
THE COACHING CASE OF JOSHUA

Joshua is a 36-year-old male, married with two children and one on the way. He was referred to the health coach by his physician, who had diagnosed Joshua with diabetes, obesity, and mild depression. Joshua smokes about a pack of cigarettes a day, goes without breakfast, and eats unhealthy foods throughout the day and evening. Joshua is devoted to his job as an engineer at a major corporation. His job is both sedentary and quite stressful, and he smokes a lot. Joshua does not engage in any regular exercise.

Stage 3. Introductory Coaching Session

The opening full coaching session may last anywhere from 45 to 60 minutes. The session begins with a review and discussion of the patient's wheel of health, which helps the patient assess important domains of his or her health (e.g., nutrition, exercise, rest, spirituality, relationships). This discussion gives the health coach an opportunity to build rapport with the patient and gain an understanding of the patient through his or her eyes, and can help the patient see if each domain currently supports his or her core values and life goals. The coach, employing a *beginner's mind* (rather than making assumptions about how the patient thinks or feels), engages the patient, using reflective (active) listening, empathy, and compassionate curiosity, all of which are important competencies for building rapport.

In Stage 3, Joshua and his coach review his core values (service, contribution, family), strengths (analytic skills, problem solving, applied creativity, humor), personality (empathic, detail-oriented, organized, insightful), and life goals. They look at levels of satisfaction in each of the domains of his completed wheel of health assessment (self-care relationships and communication, physical environment), and use of professional care (preventive, interventional, complementary and alternative). Joshua's vastly uneven levels of satisfaction with many domains, when connected in the diagram, reveal a wobbly wheel of health, one that probably would not smoothly rotate for very long. He envisioned a much healthier future state so he could not only "financially support my family, but have the endurance to engage in all sorts of activities with them, and help each child develop into a healthy adult with life purpose."

Reviewing his health wheel, Joshua laments how far he has fallen from good health. Growing up, he had played many sports, but as a result of current work commitments, has not been exercising and is overeating. "Worst of all," he said, "I'm smoking like a chimney." Joshua's current state of health doesn't align at all with his core values and life goals of financially supporting his family while engaging with them in deep and loving connections. Joshua's coach reflects back his disappointment and adds that his present and past periods of an unhealthy lifestyle do not need to predict the future. The coach suggests that health coaching is an opportunity for him to regain his health.

To ensure a clear agenda, the coach asks Joshua a set of *bookend questions* to help him identify a focused goal and describe the outcome he wants from the session. Joshua says that he wants to "focus on getting my health back," and by the end of the session he wants "to have a game plan of how I can regain my health." These bookend inquiries demonstrate how coaching conversations are very goal-oriented, outcome-driven, and designed to help keep the conversations and agenda on track. At this point, Joshua is in the *contemplation* stage of change.[73]

The health coach and Joshua engage in shared decision making,[108] understanding both Joshua's priorities for making behavioral change and his medical team's recommendations. While his medical team wanted him to first address his smoking, he prefers to focus on his overeating and sedentary living. His coach gains permission to take him through an appreciative inquiry exercise, in which Joshua recalls a specific time growing up when he was active in sports and was healthy. When recalling this healthy period, he remembers that he had abundant energy, was eating healthy meals without binging at night, and felt at peace in his life.

Using the motivational interviewing rulers,[74] Joshua considers healthy eating, and rates himself as a 6 on the importance of eating healthy and a 5 on his confidence in his ability to do so. He rates himself as a 7 on importance for him to exercise and a 4 on his confidence to achieve his exercise goals. When asked, he clarifies that he hasn't rated himself lower because he really feels these things are important for his overarching life goals. He isn't sure that he can do this by himself, but then adds, "but I see that's why I'm in coaching."

The coach agrees with Joshua's priorities and focus, considering that with some healthy new rituals in place, and success with those rituals, they can address smoking cessation at a later date. Guided by the coach's use of PVCSMART (**P**ositively stated, **V**alues aligned, within one's **C**ontrol, **S**pecific, **M**easurable, **A**ttainable, **R**ealistic, and **T**ime sensitive), Joshua decides that his goal is to lose 25 pounds in 6 months, and agrees that he will do this through healthy eating (including portion control) and exercise.

Together, they develop a strategic plan: Joshua *names* the desired behavior (healthy eating), beginning with small, mindful, behavioral steps. He *reframes* the purpose of eating (for health and refueling rather than to control feelings of anxiety or boredom). As Joshua never eats breakfast, he commits to *focus* on doing so every morning. He also agrees to keep a food log (using the cognitive log/diary) depicted in Table 25.4. He will record when, where, and with whom he eats; what he eats; portion size; triggers of his overeating; and what he was feeling and thinking prior to and after eating. He likes this part of the plan because he is detail-oriented and feels this is something he can easily accomplish.

Joshua isn't so sure about the exercise, since he is so out of shape. After considering his busy schedule and brainstorming the types of activity he enjoys, he settles on walking. He commits to walking 20 minutes a day, noting how he feels and what thoughts he has before and again after the walk.

The health coach asks him how he wants to handle accountability for his action plan. He replies that in addition to holding himself accountable, he will ask his wife to be his accountability partner. She has wanted him to do something like this for a long time. Asked about potential obstacles to achieving his action steps, Joshua says his lack of time might preclude achieving his exercise goals, and that his being a "creature of habit" might sabotage his new goals of healthy eating. Using solution-focused coaching, his coach helps him address these obstacles. Joshua commits to getting up a little earlier for breakfast and walking during his lunch break. He adds that with the help of his wife as an accountability partner, he will treat these lifestyle changes (including those around eating) like a scientific experiment.

At the end of this session, the coach asks Joshua what he sees as the takeaways. He says, "Interesting! I was expecting a lecture on nutrition and exercise. While you were guiding me, I felt like I was leading the way. A cool feeling. I was afraid you were going to just put me on some kind of diet. This plan of starting with a food log, and understanding everything around my eating, seems doable. I've never done that before."

Stage 4. Ongoing Coaching Conversations: Middle Phase of the Coaching

The middle phase of a health coaching engagement makes up the bulk of the coaching sessions. These may occur in full sessions, lasting 45 to 60 minutes, or they may be done in parts, over shorter sessions, or even via phone or telecoaching. Health coaching can last up to a year, and occasionally even longer.

In each of these coaching sessions, the coach listens and elicits solution and change talk from the patient. Each coaching conversation is structured in five developing steps and provides a supportive space in which the patient can explore specific behavioral changes within his or her individual context. The five steps are as follows:

1. Checking in with the patient
2. Helping the patient identify his or her agenda
3. Helping the patient become aware of the need to change
4. Action planning, including anticipation of work needed and working through potential obstacles
5. Wrap-up

These steps will be demonstrated through the case of Joshua.

Step 1. Checking In with the Patient

After first welcoming Joshua and asking how things are in general, his coach begins the session by asking about accomplishments made (even the tiniest actions taken) since the last session. The coach checks in on specific, previously agreed-upon actions taken (e.g., eating breakfast, using the food log). The coach affirms Joshua's active participation in making change and his successes, and facilitates his self-directed learning. In addition, the coach invites him to brainstorm how he would handle roadblocks on action steps not yet taken or completed.

COACH: *Joshua, it's nice to see you today! Before we begin, how are you?* (Comment: welcomes the patient and generally checks in, using an open-ended question)

JOSHUA: Well, the good news is that we found out we're going to have a baby boy!

COACH: *Congratulations. How exciting!* (Comment: affirming statement)

JOSHUA: Well, I was so excited that I started to do that food log thing, as promised, and I started to eat breakfast every day.

COACH: *That's great. Just getting started is a success in itself.* (Comment: affirms the patient)

JOSHUA: Well, I started to do that food log, but halfway through, I felt so demoralized that I stopped.

COACH: *Demoralized. Tell me more.* (Comment: using a statement, asks for clarification)

JOSHUA: *Well, the way I overeat at night, it was like holding up a mirror to my lousy behavior.*

COACH: *So, becoming more aware of how you eat was revealing?* (Comment: reflects and checks for accuracy)

JOSHUA: Yes.

COACH: *What did it reveal?* (Comment: open-ended question)

JOSHUA: That sometimes I just lose control.

COACH: *Lose control?* (Comment: asks for clarification)

JOSHUA: You know, I feel like I need to eat something, even though I've already had dinner, and once I get going, I can't stop.

COACH: *So your eating spirals out of control. Is that it?* (Comment: reflects, checks for accuracy)

JOSHUA: Yeah.

Step 2. Helping the Patient Identify the Agenda

COACH: *Joshua, what would you like to discuss, with our time today? Continue with this or something else?* (Comment: (a) asks the first part of the bookend inquiries, on focus; (b) as the agenda is decided by the patient, the coach asks him to choose whether to continue with the eating behavior discussion or something else he might have wanted to discuss prior to coming into the session)

JOSHUA: Yes, let's continue . . . how not to eat again, after dinner . . . that would be helpful.

COACH: *How could you state that in a positive way?* (Comment: asks for a positive reframe, as it's easier to work on a positive than a negative)

JOSHUA: To enjoy dinner as the last meal of the day.

COACH: *So you'd like to focus on how to ensure dinner is your last meal of the day?* (Comment: asks for clarification)

JOSHUA: Yep.

Step 3. Helping the Patient Become Aware of the Need to Change

COACH: *OK. Well, since you've already had dinner, what kind of hunger are you experiencing?* (Comment: asks a discovery question)

JOSHUA: Well, it's really not for food . . .

COACH: *No . . . If it's not for food, what other kind of "hunger" might be triggering your eating?* (Comment: clarifies discovery question)

JOSHUA: I don't know; I feel fidgety, like . . . like I want to do something, but I don't know what. When I eat after dinner, that feeling seems to dissipate.

COACH: *So eating after dinner gives you something to do that calms you down? Is that it?* (Comment: asks for clarification; checks for accuracy)

JOSHUA: Sort of . . . I think. Eating helps me unwind after a day of problem solving at work.

COACH: *. . . helps you unwind.* (Comment: reflects back) *That's an interesting word, "unwind."*

JOSHUA: Well, yeah, by the end of the day, putting out fires, I'm all wound up in a tight ball of knots.

COACH: *A tight ball of knots.* (Comment: echoes the patient's metaphor) *Joshua, you have a gift for painting the scene and your feelings with very clear images.* (Comment: affirms the patient) *Sounds like you come home from work pretty stressed out . . . is that the case?* (Comment: reflects back, asks for accuracy)

JOSHUA: Well, we're understaffed, and I'm the lucky one that gets to pick up all the pieces.

COACH: *You're the go-to problem solver at your job?* (Comment: reflects back with a question, using a paraphrase, checks for accuracy)

JOSHUA: That's me.

COACH: *So after work and dinner, you'd like to unwind.* (Comment: reflects back) *What does unwinding mean to you?* (Comment: asks for clarification)

JOSHUA: Well . . . unwinding means relaxing, I guess.

COACH: *Hmm, relaxing . . . and how does eating after dinner allow you to relax, or "unwind"?* (Comment: stays with the patient's wording, and asks a discovery question)

JOSHUA: Well . . . actually, the more I eat after dinner, the more stuffed and uncomfortable I feel. Hmm . . . I guess it's not exactly relaxing.

COACH: *Good observation.* (Comment: affirms the patient) *Interesting; so you continue to eat throughout the evening to help you unwind after a day of problem solving, yet instead of relaxing, you actually feel stuffed. Is that accurate?* (Comment: summarizes; highlights the discrepancy between action and goal)

JOSHUA: Yup.

COACH: *How does feeling stuffed impact the rest of your evening?* (Comment: asks about potential implications of the patient's stated feeling)

JOSHUA: Well, I feel so stuffed when I go to bed . . . I think this affects my sleep.

COACH: *In what way?* (Comment: asks for clarification)

JOSHUA: I don't sleep very well . . . or feel rested. I wake up tired, like I need to sleep some more . . . and I'm pissed at myself for having lost control of my eating the night before.

COACH: *So not only do you feel stuffed, but you're not getting restful sleep, and the next morning, you're angry with yourself for having overeaten the night before. Am I on target?* (Comment: summarizes; asks for accuracy)

JOSHUA: (Nods yes)

Step 4. Action Planning

COACH: *What specific outcome do you want by the end of our conversation today?* (Comment: asks for the outcome, the second part of the bookend inquiries. The focus and outcome bookend questions are a useful way to streamline the agenda and keep the conversation on track. This is an example of the goal orientation of coaching)

JOSHUA: *I want to find a better way to unwind after work.*

COACH: *What does "better" mean to you?* (Comment: asks for clarification)

JOSHUA: You know . . . healthier.

COACH: *So, by the end of our session today, you'd like to come away with a healthier way to unwind rather than overeating?* (Comment: summarizes; checks for accuracy)

JOSHUA: That's it. I did walk every day, but only for 10 minutes instead of the 20 . . . 'cause, as I started walking, I felt like, "What's the use? Who am I kidding? So I'll walk, but then after dinner, I'll just overeat anyway, so what good is the exercise?"

COACH: *You mean, what's the point?* (Joshua nods yes) *How do you feel about that? (Comment: asks a second-level discovery question that may reveal deeper material)*

JOSHUA: Like a failure; that I've lost control over my eating.

COACH: *Like a failure. So it sounds like you've linked your behaviors: You overeat at night, wake up feeling tired . . . feeling like a failure . . . angry at yourself for overeating. Then, during your lunch break, when you walk, you stop midway, because to exercise while continuing to overeat at night feels like a lost cause. And then you repeat overeating the next evening. Am I capturing the pattern?* (Comment: summarizes, checks for accuracy)

JOSHUA: That's it exactly . . . a "negative feedback loop."

COACH: *"Negative feedback loop"—that's a great way to describe the pattern.* (Comment: affirms the patient) *And how does feeling like a failure play into your overeating?* (Comment: asks for clarification for a potential linked, cognitive triad—linking a thought to a feeling and action)

JOSHUA: I think in a weird way, I punish myself for having lost control of my eating, and I stuff myself; pretty insane, huh?

COACH: *Insane? I don't think so; that negative feedback loop, as you said, around overeating is pretty common . . . if you're human* (Comment: normalizes the behavior; with a little humor)

JOSHUA: (smiles) I'm definitely human.

COACH: *I'm so glad. (They both laugh.)*

JOSHUA: Well, it's pretty stupid . . . I feel "fidgety" before I start eating; kind of irritable; I overeat, then beat myself up for losing self-control by eating more.

COACH: *and then?* (Comment; asks exploration question)

JOSHUA: I start the unhealthy pattern all over again.

COACH: *The pattern repeats. So to create a different, healthier pattern, what could you do instead of overeating?* (Comment: exploration question; asks patient for solution(s)—alternatives to eating after dinner)

JOSHUA: I don't know. Usually, one of us cleans up the kitchen while the other puts the kids to bed. We tend to catch up on the day while watching TV. Of course, there are food commercials, which constantly tempt me.

COACH: *So after dinner, cleanup, and putting the kids to bed, you both sit down, and while watching TV, you catch up on the day. Unfortunately, the food commercials trigger your eating. Yes?* (Comment: summarizes; checks for accuracy) *How would it help if you had a healthier way of unwinding after work and dinner?* (Comment: exploration: asks a needs clarification question, again using Joshua's language)

JOSHUA: Well . . . then I feel I could stay on track with my game plan. Maybe I could have mastery over my eating; then, the walking makes sense, because I can burn off more calories and lose weight, to better manage my diabetes. Right?

COACH: *Absolutely, losing weight will definitely help your diabetes . . . and weight loss is all about more calories burned than ingested.* (Comment: validates the patient)

JOSHUA: So, I can focus on not overeating and not stopping the exercise, and I'll shed the weight.

COACH: *That makes a lot of sense.* (Comment: validates the patient) *How could you rephrase that in a more positive way?* (Comment: asks for a positive reframe)

JOSHUA: Well, when I was my healthiest, I ate okay, and used to work out a lot. I loved to play basketball. In high school, I had a great coach, who drilled me with different kinds of shots . . . different styles of dribbling: hesitation dribbling; the wraparound dribble (Joshua demonstrates the various moves); the ol' behind-the-back dribble; not to mention between-the-legs dribbling. (He and the coach start laughing.)

COACH: *Sounds like you became a great dribbler!* (Comment: affirms the patient)

JOSHUA: Well, he coached me to be a master dribbler, but also fancy layups, bank shots, the turnaround fake jump shot—you name it, I wanted to master it.

COACH: *Joshua, I have noticed a shift in your energy in the last couple of minutes.* (Comment: affirms the patient, picking up on his passion for something healthy—basketball)

JOSHUA: Yeah, well . . . I remember how good it felt as I got so good at so many different shots—and I loved it. I felt powerful . . . like a commander on the court. Aaah . . . so what if I change my goal . . . to master my eating?

COACH: *That's an interesting reframe—so, instead of wanting to lose weight, you want to master your eating?* (Comment: affirms, checks for accuracy, promotes self-efficacy)

JOSHUA: And exercise.

COACH: *And exercise.* (Comment: echoes the patient)

JOSHUA: 'Cause I'm drawn to master things . . . you know, control stuff. I'm an engineer, remember?

COACH: *Yes, you are. Originally your focus was on not overeating and exercise. How might this reframe of wanting to have mastery over your eating and exercise refine your goal?* (Comment: discovery question)

JOSHUA: Well . . . instead of working to lose something, my goal will be to gain more control, have mastery over my eating and exercise. Mastering something seems way easier than wanting to lose something. Huh! (Comment: Aha moment)

COACH: *Sounds like you might have just had a discovery, an "aha" moment.* (Comment: acknowledges his insight)

JOSHUA: I think so.

COACH: *How might your positive reframe align with your core values?* (Comment: discovery question of integration, which could spark more awareness)

JOSHUA: Are you kidding? I enjoy the challenge of mastering new things. I have a workbench in the garage to make things. I've taken some classes; it's something I toy with . . . from time to time.

COACH: *So accepting a challenge and mastering things is part of who you are?* (Comment: interpretation question)

JOSHUA: Definitely.

COACH: *And finding a healthier way to unwind after work and dinner could help you have mastery or get control over your eating? Does that hit the mark?* (Comment: summarizes, checks for accuracy, promotes self-efficacy)

JOSHUA: Got it. Nicely tied up . . . I'll take it.

COACH: *Sounds like we might have found a nicely wrapped gift for you to use?* (Comment: discovery question building on his insight)

JOSHUA: Hopefully.

COACH: *How will you know you're succeeding?*

JOSHUA: I know me; taking one day at a time, feeling like I have more self-control, feeling more competent, and confident . . . gets me really psyched. I look forward to having more energy, like I did when playing B-ball, and taking better care of myself. This could become my positive feedback loop.

COACH: *Wow!* (Comment: affirms the patient) *How could you elaborate on that?* (Comment: exploration question to help create more awareness)

JOSHUA: Well, by eating healthy and exercising, I'll be creating a healthy, positive pattern.

COACH: *Fantastic!* (Comment: affirms the patient) *Since you know yourself better than I do, what other enjoyable things could you do to help you relax and unwind after dinner?* (Comment: asks an exploration question moving the session forward)

JOSHUA: Well, I could go to my workbench and make something, but that's pretty solitary, and I'd rather spend the evenings with my wife. We could turn off TV, maybe listen to music, and read; but we really enjoy vegging out, mindless with the TV . . . Something fun, not too stimulating . . . maybe do some Sudoku puzzles instead.

COACH: *You mentioned several options: using your workbench, spending time with your wife, perhaps putting on some music instead of the TV, maybe read, but you both enjoy the TV "vegging" out while catching up . . . maybe do Sudoku puzzles to relax . . . Have I accurately captured your suggestions?* (Comment: summarizes, checks for accuracy)

JOSHUA: Yeah, not sure any of those would actually do the trick.

COACH: *With your permission, I'd like to share an easy relaxation exercise that has helped other people relax and "unwind."* (Comment: asks for permission, which supports the patient's self-determination and self-efficacy)

JOSHUA: Yeah, that sounds great. Sure.

COACH: *It's called a "**body scan**"; takes just a few minutes, and you can share this or even do it with your wife and maybe unwind together.* (Comment: The coach takes Joshua through a body scan relaxation exercise, guiding him to progressively isolate and relax the muscles throughout his body; body scan is a variation of progressive muscle relaxation without first tensing the muscles).

COACH: *Open your eyes. What do you feel?*

JOSHUA: Oh, wow, so-o-o relaxed . . . something I never feel after stuffing my face with food.

COACH: *You feel relaxed.* (Comment: reflects back) *How long do you think that exercise took?*

JOSHUA: I don't know . . . 20 minutes? Boy, it felt good.

COACH: *Actually, maybe 5 minutes. You can also share this with your kids. It's a great way to help fall asleep. It's something you can do anytime, anywhere, except of course when you're driving.* (Joshua smiles.)

JOSHUA: OK, relaxation . . . the body scan. That's great for after dinner. We do like TV, though.

COACH: *What TV shows can you watch that don't have commercials?* (Comment: exploration question)

JOSHUA: Actually Netflix—we could binge on those—better than binging on food (smiles). I'll practice that relaxation thing and see how that helps.

COACH: *So you'll practice the body scan as a substitute for eating after dinner, watch some Netflix, avoiding those triggering food commercials.* (Comment: summarizes)

JOSHUA: Yeah, I'll start with that—show my wife, my accountability partner. In fact, let's add relaxation to my plan. Maybe I'll give the food log another try . . . it did actually help me understand why I've been overeating.

COACH: *Good point, Joshua. It helped you understand the underlying feelings driving your overeating.* (Comment: affirms the patient, reflects, and summarizes)

JOSHUA: That's right. I'll start adding gold stars to those pages.

COACH: *Why not reward yourself with gold stars? Great idea.* (Comment: affirms the patient and his playfulness)

JOSHUA: OK, so body scan it is . . . after dinner with my wife. And if I can't sleep, I can do it again.

COACH: *That's great, Joshua!* (Comment: affirms the patient) *Practicing relaxation will help instill that healthy pattern you want to develop.* (Comment: elaborates on his statement) *How do you take breaks during the day at work?* (Comment: exploration question)

JOSHUA: I go outside to smoke; they don't allow smoking anymore inside the building.

COACH: *So you take smoking breaks at work?* (Comment: reflects back)

JOSHUA: Yup.

COACH: *How do you feel after you've smoked?* (Comment: asks a second-level discovery question)

JOSHUA: Initially it calms me, but later, when I get back to work, I start craving the nicotine, and I need another smoke. Other than slowly killing me, and the distraction from work, I'm not sure why I still smoke. I wish I didn't. My clothes smell of smoke; I know it's a bad idea, and it's poor role modeling for my kids.

COACH: *Sounds like you have some good reasons to quit smoking.* (Comment: validates patient) *As we agreed, let's pursue that goal a little later. Right now, you have a great game plan: master healthy eating, use the body scan as a substitute for eating, relax, and exercise.* (Coach: affirms the patient and validates their prior agreement to prioritize his focus on eating and exercise, and move toward smoking cessation at a later date.) *As part of your new game plan to relax, how might you use a body scan at work?* (Comment: exploration question, about broadening his action plan)

JOSHUA: Well . . . I guess on a nice day, I could go outside, to a quiet place, where I like to sit and do the scan; or stay in my office, close the door, and take a relaxation break.

COACH: *"Relaxation break:" that has a nice ring to it* (Comment: affirms patient's choice of words)

JOSHUA: Interesting . . . so if I take a couple of 5 minute mini-breaks at work, maybe I will be more relaxed when I get home. I'll explore the mini-breaks with the body scan throughout the day, and walk during my lunch break, every day.

Step 5. Wrap-up

COACH: *Sounds like a plan: getting up earlier to have breakfast, mini-breaks at work, walking for 20 minutes during your lunch hour, food log to stay on track, practicing and sharing the body scan after dinner, maybe watching Netflix . . . no commercials, body scan again before bedtime, as needed. Does that cover your plan?* (Comment: summarizes, checks for accuracy)

JOSHUA: Yup, and if I "fall down" and overeat, I can remember that the walking will still help me. You know, my mother once told me that when I was learning to walk as a toddler, I used to laugh when I fell down; she said I couldn't "wait to get up and begin again with my "wobbly walk"—that's what she called it—my "wobbly walk."

COACH: *What a great way to look at falling down: just a step toward mastering something, then getting up to begin again.* (Comment: reflects back and affirms the patient) *How might you use that reframe of falling down if you find yourself overeating again after dinner?* (Comment: exploration question)

JOSHUA: *I'll go at it again . . . use the food log . . . add some cartoons to it, to remind me of my "wobbly walk."*

COACH: *That's creative — use a fun visual to bring back a memorable learning experience.* (Comment: affirms the patient) *Talking about winding down, we need to wind down the session. Before we close, how would you rate yourself now on the importance of mastering healthy eating and exercise?* (Comment: asks comparative measurement question)

JOSHUA: At a 9, hands down.

COACH: *And how would you rate your confidence in your ability to actually achieve your plan?* (Comment: at the end of the session, asks Joshua about his commitment and readiness to take action)

JOSHUA: My confidence has moved up to an 8. I'm still a creature of habit, although I do feel that with your help and support, I can actually do this.

COACH: *You got it.* (Comment: affirms the support) *So . . . how did we do today, with respect to what you wanted from this session?* (Comment: checks in to see if Joshua felt he had achieved his session outcome)

JOSHUA: Great. I definitely have a game plan to help me with my new goal: to have mastery over my eating and exercise. I have some tools to explore and practice, which I can evaluate as I go. If I fall down . . . it's just feedback, and a natural step in learning how to master my goal . . . so I need to get up, keep practicing, to shape my "wobbly walk" into smooth steps.

COACH: *Joshua, you have so much insight and a wonderful sense of humor. It's a pleasure working with you. I look forward to our next session.* (Comment: affirms the patient; wraps up the session, with a cue for the next session)

JOSHUA: So do I. Thanks.

COACH: *Thank you!*

Stage 5. Conduct Regular Process Checks

During Stage 5, the coach checks in with the patient (weekly, bimonthly, monthly via phone, telecoaching, or in person), and reviews the overall progress made since the last contact. The coach may revisit the patient's baseline health status and health/wellness vision, and affirm and acknowledge successes and accomplishments. Together, they discuss and work through any obstacles the patient might face to making needed changes. The coach assesses the patient's level of commitment to continue with current action plans, and inquires about beginning new behavioral or lifestyle changes, as needed. At the end of each session, the coach asks the patient about session *takeaways* (what he or she has learned).

Stage 6. Recontracting for New Health Goals or Ending the Coaching Engagement

During this last stage, and depending on the outcome of Stage 5, the coach asks Joshua how he would like to proceed with the coaching engagement. Would he like to continue with a new coaching agreement and move forward with the goal of smoking cessation as previously negotiated? Generally, when the partners of coach and client finish the agreed upon goals, they can contract for other desired goals or stop.

BOX 25.3

SUMMARY OF RECOMMENDED TREATMENT APPROACHES AND RELEVANT EVIDENCE

Strength of recommendation taxonomy (SOR A, B, or C)

- **An emerging body of literature demonstrates the general efficacy of health coaching for facilitating behavioral and lifestyle change in primary care environments (SOR B).[47–50]**
- **Health coaching has been shown to be effective in facilitating needed lifestyle changes in patients with chronic disease (SOR B).[51,52]**
- **Health coaching has been a successful approach used to facilitate the lifestyle changes needed for patients with specific medical conditions, such as diabetes and cardiovascular disease (SOR B).[53]**
- **Five evidence-based coaching approaches are effective in facilitating healthy behavioral and lifestyles changes: (1) the transtheoretical model or stages of change; (2) motivational interviewing; (3) solution-focused health coaching; (4) cognitive behavioral coaching and (5) mindfulness-based stress reduction. (SOR A)[52,67,74–76,102,103,112,119,120]**
- **A predominance of "change talk" or "solution talk" predicts subsequent behavior change (SOR B).[67,76]**

In this case, Joshua decides to end the current coaching engagement, at least for the time being. The coach engages Joshua with the following:

1. Asks for clarification as to how to proceed; she supports his decision to stop. They keep open the potential for contracting for smoking cessation after having had several months of successful behavioral change with eating and exercise.
2. Elicits what Josh learned from the coaching, and how he might apply these insights going forward.

3. They celebrate and affirm his progress and successes.
4. Encourages Joshua to continue making progress; offers that he can return anytime and/or check in from time to time, to stay on track.
5. Expresses appreciation for the opportunity to have guided Joshua in his journey to make lifestyle changes.

CONCLUSION

Health coaching is an emerging discipline that will likely make significant contributions toward reducing chronic illness, facilitating health and well-being, and helping foster behavioral and lifestyle change. (See Box 25.3 to review the evidence basis of health coaching.) Medical professionals, such as nurses, nurse practitioners, and other licensed mental health professionals, are the most common professionals using coaching theory and techniques in integrated and primary care practices. Some of these traditionally trained medical professionals are also ICF and NCCHWC certified coaches. ICF and NCCHWC certified coaches do not necessarily have medical training, nor are they currently licensed to practice in medical settings. However, the recent agreement between the NCCHWC and the National Board of Medical Examiners to launch a national certification for individual health and wellness coaches in the United States[1] might help resolve that issue down the road. New standardized medical training and certification standards for standalone coaches will likely qualify them for licensure in the future and permit them to work in a wide array of health care settings. Health coaches have unique perspectives and skills that are needed in the health care system of the 21st century.

REFERENCES

1. National Consortium for Credentialing Health & Wellness Coaches. http://www.ncchwc.org Accessed June 10, 2016.
2. Centers for Disease Control and Prevention. Death and Mortality. NCHS FastStats. http://www.cdc.gov/nchs/fastats/deaths.htm/ Accessed December 20, 2013.
3. Center for Disease Control and Prevention. National Center for Chronic Disease Prevention and Health Promotion. The Power of Prevention; 2009. http://www.cdc.gov/chronicdisease/pdf/2009-Power-of-Prevention.pdf. Accessed June 6, 2016.
4. Ward BW, Schiller JS, Goodman RA. Multiple chronic conditions among US adults: A 2012 update. *Prev Chronic Dis.* 2014;11:130389. doi:http://dx.doi.org/10.5888/pcd11.130389.
5. WHO. Global Statistics 2015. http://www.who.int/gho/publications/world_health_statistics/2015/en/. Accessed June 16, 2016.
6. National Health Expenditure Projections 2010–2020: Forecast Summary. https://www.cms.gov/NationalHealthExpendData/downloads/proj2010.pdf. Accessed March 17, 2013.
7. National Prevention Council, National Prevention Strategy Department of Health and Human Services, Office of the Surgeon General, June 2012. http://www.surgeongeneral.gov/priorities/prevention/about/actionplan.html Accessed June 30, 2016
8. Gerteis J, Izrael D, Deitz D, et al. Multiple Chronic Conditions Chartbook. AHRQ Publications No, Q14-0038. Rockville, MD: Agency for Healthcare Research and Quality. April 2014.
9. Centers for Disease Control and Prevention. Adult Overweight and Obesity: http://www.cdc.gov/obesity/adult/index.html. April 27, 2012 Accessed June 10, 2016.
10. Simmons LA, Wolever RQ. Integrative health coaching and motivational interviewing: synergistic approaches to behavior change in healthcare. Glob Adv Health Med. 2013;2(4):28–35.
11. The Patient Protection and Affordable Care Act of 2010. Pub. L. No. 111-148, 124 Stat 119. Available at: http://www.gpo.gov/fdsys/pkg/PLAW-111publ148/pdf/PLAW-111publ148.pdf. Accessed March 17, 2016.
12. Meeting of the Advisory Group on Prevention, Health Promotion, and Integrative and Public Health, April 12–13, 2011, Washington, DC. http://www.healthcare.gov/prevention/nphpphc/advisorygrp/a-g-meeting-summary-april-12-13.pdf. Accessed March 18, 2016.
13. Glaser JE. Conversational Intelligence; How Great Leaders Build Trust and Get Extraordinary Results. Brookline, MA: Bibliomotion Inc.; 2014.
14. Roter D. The enduring and evolving nature of the patient–physician relationship. Patient Educ Couns. 2000;39(1):5–15.
15. Miller WR, Rollnick S. Motivational Interviewing: Helping People Change. 3rd ed. New York: Guilford Press; 2013.
16. Gruman J, Rovner MH, French ME, et al. From patient education to patient engagement: Implications for the field of patient education. Patient Edu Couns. 2010;78(3):350–356.
17. Miller C, Huffman M. Evidence-Based Health CoachingForHealthCare.3rded.http://www.nshcoa.com/content 2013. Accessed June 16, 2016.
18. Center for Advancing Health. A Snapshot of People's Engagement in Their Health Care. http://www

.cfah.org/file/CFAH_Snapshot_2010_Full.pdf. Accessed June 15, 2016.

19. Bennett HD, Coleman EA, Parry C, Bodenheimer T, Chen EH. Health coaching for patients with chronic illness. J Med Pract Manage. 2010;17(5):24–29.
20. Kohn LT, Corrigan JM, Donaldson MS, eds. Institute of Medicine (IOM). To Err Is Human: Building a Safer Health System. Washington, DC: National Academy Press; 2000.
21. Baker A. Crossing the quality chasm: A new health system for the 21st century. BMJ. 2001;323(7322):1192. doi:http://dx.doi.org/10.1136/bmj.323.7322.1192.
22. Institute for Health Care Improvement. http://www.ihi.org. Accessed June 16, 2016.
23. American Academy of Family Physicians (AAFP), American Academy of Pediatrics (AAP), American College of Physicians (ACP), American Osteopathic Association (AOA). Joint Principles of the Patient-Centered Medical Home; 2007. http://www.aafp.org/dam/AAFP/documents/practice_management/pcmh/initiatives/PCMHJoint.pdf. Accessed June 16, 2016.
24. Agency for Healthcare Research and Quality. Patient-Centered Medical Home Resource Center. https://pcmh.ahrq.gov/. Accessed October 12, 2015.
25. Berwick DM, Nolan TW, Whittington J. The triple aim: Care, health, and cost. *Health Aff (Millwood)*. 2008;27(3):759–769.
26. Centers for Medicare and Medicaid Service. The Center for Consumer Information and Insurance Oversight. The Mental Health Parity and Addiction Equity Act. https://www.cms.gov/CCIIO/Programs-and-Initiatives/Other-Insurance-Protections/mhpaea_factsheet.html. Accessed June 10, 2016.
27. Dunn H. High-Level Wellness. Arlington, VA: Beatty Press; 1961.
28. National Wellness Institute. http://www.nationalwellness.org. Accessed June 16, 2016.
29. Jordon M. How to Be a Health Coach: An Integrative Approach. San Raphael, CA: Global Medicine Enterprises Inc.; 2013.
30. Snyderman R, Dinan MA. Improving health by taking it personally. JAMA. 2010;303(4):363–364.
31. Weisfeld V. Summit on Integrative Medicine & The Health of The Public; Issue Background and Overview 2009. http://www.nationalacademies.org/hmd/~/media/Files/Activity%20Files/Quality/IntegrativeMed/IM20Summit20Background20Paper20Weisfeld2022309.pdf. Accessed June 10, 2016.
32. Maizes V, Rakel D, Niemiec C. Integrative medicine and patient-centered care. *Explore NY*. 2009;5(5):277–289.
33. The Curious Link Between Coaching and the Ancient Chinese. http://www.coachfederation.org/blog. Accessed June 16, 2016.
34. Lehmann CM. Early Greek athletic trainers. J Sports Hist. 2009:36(2):187–204.
35. Edelson M. Values-Based Coaching. A Guide for Social Workers and Other Human Service Professionals. Washington, DC: NASW Press; 2010.
36. Hendrickson R. The Facts on File Encyclopedia of Word and Phrase Origins. Rev. New York: Checkmark Books; 2000:155.
37. Gallwey TW. The Inner Game of Tennis. 1st ed. New York: Random House; 1974.
38. The handbook of knowledge-based coaching: From theory to practice.Wildflower L, Brennan D, eds. San Francisco, CA: John Wiley & Sons; 2011.
39. Whitmore JK. Coaching for Performance: Growing People, Performance and Purpose. London: Nicholas Brealey Publishing; 2002.
40. Hargove R. Masterful Coaching. 3rd ed. San Francisco, CA: Jossey-Bass; 2008.
41. International Coaching Federation. http://coachfederation.org Accessed June 10, 2016.
42. National Organization of Nurse Practitioner Faculties. Nurse Practitioner Core Competencies April 2011. Amended 2012. http://c.ymcdn.com/sites/www.nonpf.org/resource/resmgr/competencies/npcorecompetenciesfinal2012.pdf. Accessed June 16, 2016.
43. Riley DS, Anderson R, William Meeker DC MP, et al. The Academy of Integrative Health and Medicine and the evolution of integrative medicine practice, education, and fellowships. Integr Med. 2016;15(1):38–41.
44. Wolever RQ, Simmons LA, Sforzo GA, et al. A systematic review of the literature on health and wellness coaching: Defining a key behavioral intervention in healthcare. Glob Adv Health Med. 2013;2(4):38–57.
45. Ammentorp J, Uhrenfeldt L, Angel F, Ehrensvärd M, Carlsen EB, Kofoed PE. Can life coaching improve health outcomes? A systematic review of intervention studies. BMC Health Serv Res. 2013;13(1):1–11.
46. Bennett HD, Coleman EA, Parry C, Bodenheimer T, Chen EH. Health coaching for patients with chronic illness. J Med Pract Manage. 2010;17(5):24–29.
47. Olsen JM, Nesbitt BJ. Health coaching to improve healthy lifestyle behaviors: An integrative review. Am J Health Promot. 2010;25(1):e1–e2.
48. Sharma AE, Willard-Grace R, Hessler D, Bodenheimer T, Thom DH. What happens after health coaching? Observational study 1 year following a randomized controlled trial. Ann Fam Med. 2016;14(3):200–207.
49. Davis M, Balasubramanian BA, Waller E, Miller BF, Green LA, Cohen DJ. Integrating behavioral and physical health care in the real world: Early lessons from advancing care together. J Am Board Fam Med. 2013;26(5):588–602.
50. Adelman AM, Graybill M. Integrating a health coach into primary care: Reflections from the Penn State Ambulatory Research Network. Ann Fam Med. 2005;3(suppl 2):S33–S35.

51. Kivelä K, Elo S, Kyngäs H, Kääriäinen M. The effects of health coaching on adult patients with chronic diseases: A systematic review. Patient Educ Couns. 2014;97(2):147–157.
52. Linden A, Butterworth SW, Prochaska JO. Motivational interviewing-based health coaching as a chronic care intervention. J Eval Clin Pract. 2010;16(1):166–174.
53. Liddy C, Johnston S, Nash K, Ward N, Irving H. Health coaching in primary care: A feasibility model for diabetes care. BMC Fam Pract. 2014;15(1):1–14.
54. Bodenheimer T, Laing BY. The teamlet model of primary care. Ann Fam Med. 2007;5(5):457–461.
55. Webb TL, Joseph J, Yardley L, Michie S. Using the Internet to promote health behavior change: A systematic review and meta-analysis of the impact of theoretical basis, use of behavior change techniques, and mode of delivery on efficacy. J Med Internet. 2010;12(1):e4. doi:10.2196/jmir.1376.
56. Prochaska JO, Norcross JC. Systems of Psychotherapy. A Transtheoretical Analysis. 8th ed. Stamford, CT: Cengage Learning; 2014.
57. Mitchell SA, Black M. Freud and Beyond: A History of Modern Psychoanalytic Thought. New York: Basic Books; 2016.
58. Jung CG. The Archetypes and the Collective Unconscious. 2nd ed. Princeton, NJ: Princeton University Press; 1969.
59. Jung CG, Von Franz ML. Man and His Symbols. New York: Dell Publisher Laurel; 1964.
60. Adler A. The Individual Psychology of Alfred Adler. Ansbacher HL, Ansbacher RR. eds. New York: Harper Torchbooks; 1964.
61. Shulman BH, Dreikurs SD. The contributions of Rudolf Dreikurs to the theory and practice of individual psychology. J Individ Psychol. 1974;34(2):153–169.
62. Knowles MS. The Modern Practice of Adult Education: From Pedagogy to Andragogy. Rev. and updated ed. Wilton, CT: Chicago Follet Pub. Co.; 1980.
63. Knowles M. The Adult Learner: A Neglected Species. 3rd ed. Houston, TX: Gulf Publishing; 1984.
64. Knowles MS, Holton EF, Swanson RA. The Adult Learner: The Definitive Classic in Adult Education and Human Resource Development. 7th Ed. New York: Routledge; 2012.
65. Rogers C. Client-Centered Therapy: Its Current Practice, Implications and Theory. London, England: Constable; 1951.
66. O'Hanlon B. Taproots: Underlying Principles of Milton Erickson's Therapy and Hypnosis. New York: WW Norton & Company; 1981.
67. Berg IK, Dolan Y. Tale of Solution. New York: WW Norton; 2002.
68. Beck AT. Cognitive Therapy and the Emotional Disorders. New York: Plenum Press; 1976.
69. Seligman MEP. Learned Optimism. 2nd ed. New York: Pocket Books; 1998.
70. Csikszentmihalyi M. Flow: The Psychology of Optimal Experience. 1st ed. New York: Harper & Row; 1990.
71. Cooperrider DL, Whitney D. Appreciative Inquiry: A Positive Revolution in Change. San Francisco, CA: Berrett-Koehler Publishing Inc.; 2005.
72. Bandura A. Social Learning Theory. Englewood Cliffs, NJ: Prentice Hall; 1977.
73. Prochaska JO, Norcross JC, DiClemente CC. Changing for Good: The Revolutionary Program That Explains the Six Stages of Change and Teaches You How to Free Yourself From Bad Habits. New York: W Morrow; 1994.
74. Miller WR, Rollnick S. Motivational Interviewing: Preparing People for Change. New York: Guilford Press; 2002.
75. Rollnick S, Miller WR, Butler CC. Motivational Interviewing in Health Care; Helping Patients Change Behaviors. New York: Guilford Press; 2008.
76. Miller WR, Rollnick S. Motivational Interviewing: Helping People Change. 3rd ed. New York: Guilford Press; 2013.
77. Maslow AH. A theory of human motivation. Psychol Rev. 1943;50(4):370–396.
78. Max-Neef M. Development and human needs. Real-life economics: Understanding wealth creation. In: Ekins P, Max-Neef M, eds. Real-Life Economics. London, UK: Rutledge; 1992:197–214.
79. Deci EL, Ryan RM. The support of autonomy and the control of behavior. J Pers Soc Psychol. 1987;53(6):1024–1037.
80. Deci EL, Ryan RM. The "what" and "why" of goal pursuits: Human needs and the self-determination of behavior. Psychol Inq. 2000;11(4):227–268.
81. Deci EL. Intrinsic Motivation. New York: Plenum Press; 1975.
82. Robins JL, Kiken L, Holt M, McCain NL. Mindfulness: An effective coaching tool for improving physical and mental health. J Am Assoc Nurse Pract. 2014;26(9):511–518.
83. Silbee D. The Mindful Coach. Seven Roles for Facilitating Leader Development. San Francisco, CA: Jossey-Bass; 2010.
84. Stober DR. Coaching from the humanistic perspective. In: Evidence-Based Coaching Handbook: Putting Best Practices to Work For Your Patients. Hoboken, NJ: John Wiley and Sons; 2006:17–50.
85. Moore M, Jackson E, Tschannen-Moran B. Coaching Psychology Manual. 2nd ed. Philadelphia; Wolters Kluwer; 2016.
86. Seligman MEP, Csikszentmihalyi M. Positive psychology: an introduction. Am Psychol. 2000:55(1);5–14. doi:10.1037/0003-066X.55.1.5.
87. Peterson C, Seligman MEP. Character Strengths and Virtues: A Handbook and Classification. Oxford, England: Oxford University Press; 2004.
88. Seligman M. Flourish. New York: Free Press; 2011:16–20.

89. Compton WC, Hoffman E. An Introduction to Positive Psychology. Belmont, CA: Wadsworth Publishing, Cengage Learning; 2013.
90. Rock D, Page LJ. Coaching with the Brain in Mind. Foundation for Practice. Hoboken, NJ: John Wiley & Sons Inc.; 2009.
91. Goleman D. Working with Emotional Intelligence. New York: Bantam Books; 1998.
92. Ryan RM, Deci E. An overview of self-determination theory. In: Deci E, Ryan RM, eds. Handbook of Self-Determination Research. Rochester, NY: University of Rochester Press; 2002:3–33.
93. Markland D, Ryan RM, Tobin,VJ, Rollnick, S. Motivational interviewing and self-determination theory. J Soc Clin Psychol. 2005;24(6):811–831.
94. Williams GC, Grow VM, Freedman ZR, Ryan RM, Deci EL. Motivational predictors of weight loss and weight-loss maintenance. J Pers Soc Psychol. 1996;70(1):115–126.
95. Williams GC, Rodin GC, Ryan RM, Grolnick WS, Deci EL. Autonomous regulation and adherence to long-term medical regimens in adult outpatients. Health Psychol. 1998;17(3):269–276.
96. Bandura A. Self-efficacy: Toward a unifying theory of behavioral change. Psychol Rev. 1977;84(2):191–215. doi:10.1037/0033-295x.84.2.191.
97. Bandura A. Social Foundations of Thought And Action: A Social Cognitive Theory. Upper Saddle River, NJ: Prentice Hall; 1986.
98. Bandura A. Organizational application of social cognitive theory. Aust J Manag. 1988; 13(2):275–302.
99. Luszczynska A, Schwarzer R. Social cognitive theory. In: Conner M, Norman P, eds. Predicting Health Behaviour. 2nd ed. Buckingham, England: Open University Press; 2005:127–169.
100. Tough A. The Adult's Learning Projects: A Fresh Approach to Theory and Practice in Adult Learning. Toronto, Canada: OISE; 1971.
101. Tough A. Intentional Changes: A Fresh Approach to Helping People Change. Chicago, IL: Follett; 1982.
102. Walter JL, Peller JE. Becoming Solution-Focused in Brief Therapy. New York: Routledge; 1992.
103. Cox E, Bachkirova T, Clutterbuck D, eds. The Complete Handbook of Coaching. 2nd ed. London, England: Sage Publications; 2014.
104. Auerbach J. Cognitive coaching. In: Stober DR, Grant AM, eds. Evidence-Based Coaching Handbook: Putting Best Practices to Work for Your Clients. Hoboken, NJ: John Wiley & Sons; 2010:103–128.
105. Duke Integrative Medicine Wheel of Health. https://www.dukeintegrativemedicine.org/patient-care/wheel-of-health/. Accessed June 16, 2016.
106. Wolever RQ, Caldwell KL, Wakefield JP, et al. Integrative health coaching: An organizational case study. Explore. 2011;7(1):30–36.
107. Feinstein RE. Prevention-oriented primary care: A collaborative model for office-based cardiovascular risk reduction. Heart Dis. 1998;5:264–271.
108. Feinstein RE, Brewer AA, eds. Primary Care Psychiatry and Behavioral Medicine: Brief Office Treatment and Management Pathways. New York: Springer; 1999:332–335.
109. Drucker P. The Practice of Management. New York: Harper Collins; 1986.
110. Schwartz JM, Begley S. The Mind and the Brain: Neuroplasticity and the Power of Mental Force. New York: Harper Collins Publishers; 2002.
111. Grossman P, Niemann L, Schmidt S, Walach H. Mindfulness-based stress reduction and health benefits: A meta-analysis. J Psychosom Res. 2004;57(1):35–43.
112. Beck AT, Emery G, Greenberg RL. Anxiety Disorders and Phobias. New York: Basic Books; 1976.
113. Eshelman D, McKay M. Refuting irrational ideas. In: Davis M, Eshelman D, McKay M, eds. The Relaxation and Stress Reduction Workbook. 6th ed. Oakland, CA: New Harbinger Publications; 2008.
114. Greenberger D, Padesky CA. Mind Over Mood. 2nd ed. Change How You Feel by Changing the Way You Think. New York: Guilford Press; 2016.
115. Feinstein RE, Brewer AA, eds. Primary Care Psychiatry and Behavioral Medicine: Brief Office Treatment and Management Pathways. New York: Springer; 1999:480–481.
116. Kabat-Zinn J, Hanh TN. Full Catastrophe Living: Using The Wisdom of Your Body and Mind to Face Stress, Pain, and Illness. 2nd ed. New York: Bantam Books; 2013.
117. Tang YY, Posner MI. The neuroscience of mindfulness. NeuroLeadership J. 2008;1(1):33–37.
118. Robins JL, Kiken L, Holt M, McCain NL. Mindfulness: An effective coaching tool for improving physical and mental health. J Am Assoc Nurse Pract. 2014;26(9):511–518.
119. Greeson JM. Mindfulness Research Update: 2008. Complement Health Pract Rev. 2009;14(1):10–18.
120. Hobson JA, Pace-Schott EF. The cognitive neuroscience of sleep: Neuronal systems, consciousness and learning. Nat Rev Neurosci. 2002;3(9):679–693.
121. Davis JM, Fleming MF, Bonus KA, Baker TB. A pilot study on mindfulness-based stress reduction for smokers. BMC Complement Altern Med. 2007;25(7):1–7.
122. Kristeller JL, Wolever RQ. Mindfulness-based eating awareness training for treating binge eating disorder: The conceptual foundation. Eat Disord. 2010;19(1):49–61.
123. Bowen S, Chawla N, Collins SE, et al. Mindfulness-based relapse prevention for substance use disorders: A pilot efficacy trial. Subst Abus. 2009;30(4):295–305.

124. Winbush NY, Gross CR, Kreitzer MJ. The effects of mindfulness-based stress reduction on sleep disturbance: A systematic review. Explore. 2007;3(6):585–591.
125. Hofmann SG, Sawyer AT, Witt AA, Oh D. The effect of mindfulness-based therapy on anxiety and depression: A meta-analytic review. J Consult Clin Psychol. 2010:8(2):169–183.
126. Follette V, Palm KM, Pearson AN. Mindfulness and trauma: Implications for treatment. J Ration Emot Cogn Behav Ther. 2006;24(1):45–61.
127. Brown KW, Ryan RM, Creswell JD. Mindfulness: Theoretical foundations and evidence for its salutary effects. Psychol Inq. 2007;18(4):211–237.

26

Crisis Intervention in Integrated Care

SCOTT A. SIMPSON AND ROBERT E. FEINSTEIN

BOX 26.1

KEY POINTS

- **A crisis occurs when a person feels overwhelmed, becomes dysfunctional, and is unable to adequately manage or resolve life stressors.**
- **A stressor may be a new life event, an interpersonal problem, an internal conflict, or a developmental problem.**
- **Crises are self-limited and result in three possible outcomes: (1) improved functioning, (2) recovery to the previous level of functioning, or (3) stabilization at a lower level of functioning.**
- **All members of the integrated health team play a role in recognizing the patient in crisis.**
- **Primary care providers begin the evaluation and treatment of the patient in crisis and refer the patient to an appropriate team member and for the appropriate level of care.**
- **Patients in an integrated health system are monitored for crises in the tracking registry.**
- **The behavioral health specialist provides time-limited, targeted crisis intervention treatment. All members of the integrated health team support the therapist and patient throughout the course of treatment.**
- **A timeline, social network map, and wheel-and-spoke diagram are tools for evaluation and treatment planning for the patient in crisis.**
- **Crisis intervention treatment may help a patient realize personal growth and improved functioning.**

INTRODUCTION

This chapter describes how to identify persons in crisis, determine an initial level of psychiatric care, and deliver crisis intervention treatment within an integrated primary care and behavioral health practice. See Box 26.1 for an overview of key points in understanding the crisis intervention approach.

A crisis occurs when a person feels overwhelmed, becomes dysfunctional, and is unable to adequately cope, manage, or resolve a life situation. People in crisis experience overwhelming, paralyzing anxiety that leaves them feeling powerless to use their usual social supports, personal strengths, and coping skills to solve a problem at hand. Crises are universal phenomena: Everyone is vulnerable.[1]

ORIGINS OF A CRISIS

A crisis may be precipitated by any stressful life event, including interpersonal problems, medical illness, internal conflicts and psychological events, or a developmental issue. The stress cause by a life event reflects the nature of the event as well as the patient's reaction.

Stressful Life Events

A crisis may be precipitated by the intrinsic distress of a traumatic life event, such as a fire or an assault.

BOX 26.2
STRESS RANKING OF SELECTED LIFE EVENTS

1. Death of spouse/mate.
2. Death of close family member.
3. Major injury/illness to self.
4. Detention in jail or other institution.
5. Major injury/illness to close family member.
6. Foreclosure.
7. Divorce.
10. Infidelity.
16. Surviving a disaster.
18. Assuming responsibility for sick or elderly loved one.
24. Dealing with unwanted pregnancy.
32. Getting married/remarried.
38. Spouse/mate begins/ceases work outside the home.
40. Change in residence.
49. Retirement.

Adapted with permission from Hobson's (1998) list of 51 events on the Social Readjustment Rating Scale–Revised.

The onset of a crisis after an event is often immediate but may be delayed up to six weeks. The Social Readjustment Rating Scale–Revised ranks a range of external stressful life events reflecting the course of human life, for example the death of a spouse, medical illness, or retirement, as detailed in Box 26.2.[2] Similarly, trauma survivors experience predictable stages of grief, functional impairment, and crisis.[3]

Interpersonal Crisis

Crises in this domain are usually precipitated by conflicts between two people. These conflicts may arise in a marriage (e.g., affair, sickness, role reversal) or at work (e.g., between a boss and an employee). When these conflicts arise, the ability of both parties to actively communicate their feelings and behave civilly is impaired; the resulting dysfunctional dyad cannot resolve disputes or solve problems.

Internal Conflict or Psychological Event

Sometimes the precipitating event of a crisis can be obscured because the event is an internal experience that needs to be described by the patient. Psychological events, such as a disturbing thought, an impulse to hurt oneself or another, or a disturbing dream as reported by patients who have posttraumatic stress disorder, can precipitate a crisis. Internal crises can precipitate symptoms of anxiety or depression or more dramatic symptoms such as non-epileptic seizures (see Chapter 29: Integrative Care Model for Neurology and Psychiatry: Non-Epileptic Seizures Project) and conversion disorders. Psychological events may also relate to internal reactions and meaning attributed to a stressful life event or interpersonal crisis.

Developmental Crises

Erik Erikson observed that people routinely experience developmental crises as they advance through life's developmental stages and the age-related tasks that accompany those stages, from childhood to retirement.[4] Failure to master the tasks of an earlier developmental stage is a potential source of crisis that may interrupt future development in the next stage; for example, a failure to negotiate the role and identity confusion of adolescence may prevent successful transition into adulthood. In young adulthood, persons need to cope with either intimacy or isolation. Later they may face a crisis of stagnation if they fail to realize the generativity of middle adulthood.

The responses to stressful events, trauma, and developmental issues are considered "generic," since they are experienced similarly and ubiquitously in Western cultures.[5]

Personalized Meaning of the Stressor

Events affect individuals differently. Patients often ascribe personal meaning to events, and may magnify or deny the impact of a current problem or situation. Perhaps a crisis evokes a patient's prior memory or emotionally traumatizing life experience.[6] Perhaps a patient's inability to manage a present crisis reinforces a preexisting maladaptive belief that the crisis and resulting dysfunction are beyond control. These associations add significant meaning to a situation even though they are often unconscious or unappreciated by the patient. By looking for past patterns that are similar to the current crisis, primary care providers can help the patient recognize a crisis and the context through which a current situation is being experienced. From this position, the provider can help the patient develop more adaptive responses.

A "crisis" is often not centered around diagnoses codified in the American Psychiatric Association's *Diagnostic and Statistical Manual of Mental Disorders*, fifth edition (DSM-5).[7] Indeed, patients in crisis only sometimes fit the DSM-5's recognized diagnoses. Many patients in crisis may not have a history of mental illness or substance abuse. The closest DSM-5 diagnoses to a crisis are either trauma-related diagnoses or an adjustment disorder, whose relationship to the older concept of crisis is debated.[8] However, sometimes a DSM-5 diagnosis, like major depression or an anxiety disorder, may precipitate the crisis or be discovered in the course of a crisis. Patients with personality disorders struggle with poor problem solving and experience recurrent crises (See Chapter 17: Working with Personality Disorders in an Integrated Care Setting). When a DSM-5 diagnosis is present, the clinician can apply crisis treatment principles to the treatment of the disorder or can treat according to the best practices described elsewhere in this book.

COURSE OF A CRISIS

People employ coping skills, defense mechanisms, interpersonal relationships, and environmental supports to manage life's inherent stress; choices of coping skills reflect upbringing, temperament, innate strengths, and the cultural influences. Certain personal characteristics (e.g., resilience, optimism, and self-efficacy) further enable effective management of a stressful situation.[9] Optimal anxiety management can enhance performance and productivity, as when studying for an exam or completing a project on deadline. The successful maintenance of a stressor-coping equilibrium enables patients to complete and enjoy the activities of life (e.g., working, building relationships, starting families). Culture often provides individuals with traditions designed to manage crises, such as the cultural rituals around death, sickness, or divorce.[10] Figure 26.1 illustrates the development, process, and potential outcomes of a crisis.

A crisis begins with a stressor that disrupts a stable equilibrium. A patient's failure to manage a stressor precipitates a state of crisis and a feeling of being overwhelmed, which may manifest as anxiety, depression, or a sense of panic or incompetence.[1] Other environmental factors may compound this

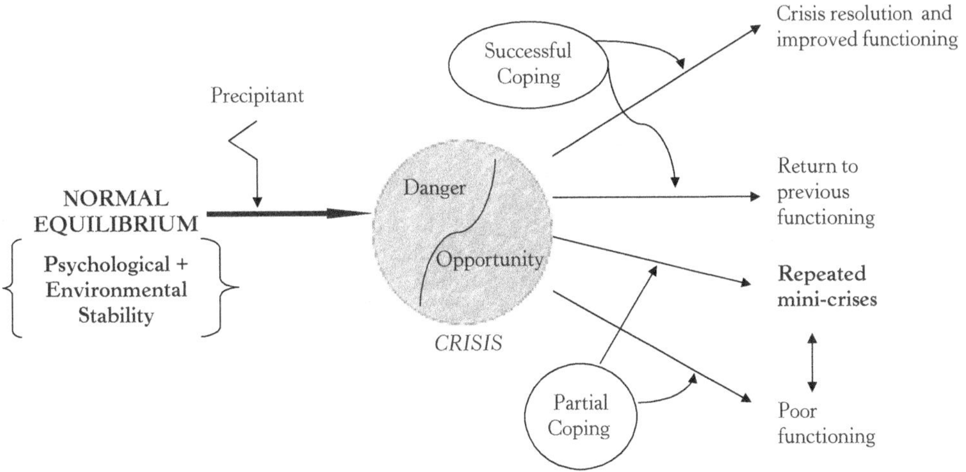

FIGURE 26.1 Crisis: development, process, and outcomes

stress. For example, the death of a spouse may rob the survivor of both an income and the emotional support of a close confidant.

The most intense anxiety may not be experienced immediately after the precipitant. Many persons initially deny, avoid, or "recoil" from dealing with an acute stressor. Only about 25% of patients can identify a crisis on the day of the stressor; 25% will realize the severity of the problem, usually with symptoms, after a week. The remaining 50% may take up to six weeks to recognize the precipitants of a crisis and related symptoms.

Most crises resolve over six weeks as the intensity of the precipitants diminishes or the patient copes independently. But while a new equilibrium will be found, there is no guarantee that functioning will improve. There are three typical outcomes for crisis:[11]

1. Ideally, someone will navigate the crisis and emerge with novel coping skills and an enhanced sense of mastery; thus a crisis becomes an opportunity for personal growth.
2. More commonly, the crisis will be managed and the pre-crisis level of functioning returns.
3. Some crises are incompletely or maladaptively resolved. The patient only partially copes and stabilizes at a lower level of functioning; some patients struggle with ongoing anxiety or other symptoms. Other patients accept a resolution of the crisis that is only a compromise. For instance, a patient may remain in a dysfunctional relationship to avoid the pain of separation. This type of patient remains vulnerable to the recurrence of future crises and may fail to return to his or her previous functioning.[12]

INTEGRATED CARE AND CRISIS INTERVENTION TREATMENT

Integrated behavioral health draws on the unique skills and positions of every primary care team member. Table 26.1 reviews potential roles of each integrated team member in crisis intervention treatment.

Each of these clinicians maintains a distinct relationship with the patient, in which different opportunities exist to recognize and treat a patient in crisis. The success of any one team member improves the capabilities of the others; for example, a care manager following up with patients within one week of an emergency department visit, improves rates of access to primary care, insurance coverage, and patient functioning.[13] Outreach by behavioral health specialists increases appointment attendance and patients' satisfaction.[14]

Patients in an integrated health system should be monitored in a registry, which is typically managed by a health coach, behavioral health specialist (BHS), or other trained personnel and actively monitored by the BHS, consulting psychiatrist, or other members of the health care team. A registry can be used to track crises, problems, symptoms (e.g., depression and anxiety rating scales), functional measures (e.g., Clinical Global Impression Scale or World Health Organization Disability Assessment Schedule), medication doses, information on the last visit, and details on the frequency of a patient's contact with specialists or use of community resources.[15–17] A well-designed registry allows the integrated team members to quickly identify patients who are not improving and intervene.[18,19] Epidemiologic merits of a registry include monitoring population health across a practice, identifying populations at high risk of psychiatric and medical comorbidity, and evaluating the effectiveness of practice innovations.

An integrated behavioral health team should maintain regular communication about the patient's care and progress. Ideally, the team should have a standing meeting as a group to review cases at a frequency determined by the practice. Ad hoc communication about particular patients is common and useful. Each team member should share his or her preferred method of communication (e.g., e-mail, pager, cellphone) and develop a standardized process to ensure that referrals to BHSs are tracked, that cases are entered into the population registry, and that primary providers receive updates on the patient's treatment. A registry accessible by all members of the integrated health team facilitates regular communication.

OVERVIEW OF CRISIS INTERVENTION TREATMENT

Crisis intervention is a therapeutic approach to help patients resolve a crisis. In contrast to other psychotherapy models, crisis intervention is designed to be time-limited and to be focused on resolution

TABLE 26.1 ROLES OF INTEGRATED HEALTH TEAM MEMBERS IN CRISIS INTERVENTION TREATMENT

	Initial Visit	Weeks 1 and 2	Weeks 3 and 4	Weeks 5 and 6	Weeks 7 and 8	Termination and Follow-up
Primary Care Provider/ Advanced Practice Nurse	1. Identify crisis. 2. Begin formulation. 3. Assess for safety. 4. Screen for mental health and substance abuse. 5. Encourage follow-up with integrated care team. 6. Recommend crisis intervention treatment. 7. Advise BHS or consulting psychiatrist.	1. Schedule brief follow-up appointment. 2. Reinforce positive changes. 3. Solicit feedback on initial therapy referral. 4. Review mental health screens. 5. Anticipate medical complications from crisis (e.g., medication nonadherence). 6. Assess safety.	As needed	1. Follow active medical issues, as necessary. 2. Reinforce positive change and use of social supports. 3. Review recommendations from therapist or psychiatrist. 4. Provide feedback to therapist.	As needed	1. Review therapist's formulation of crisis. 2. Chart "red flags" of crisis for future reference. 3. Administer periodic screens. 4. Validate patient's progress. 5. Reinforce positive work.
Medical Assistant, Nurse, and Staff	1. Help identify the crisis. 2. Administer mental health screens before the appointment. 3. Alert primary care provider to core issues. 4. Enhance motivation to engage in therapy.	1. Validate patient's engagement in therapy. 2. Assist with outreach after missed appointments. 3. Offer feedback on patient's progress.	As needed	As needed	As needed	1. Validate patient's success and positive change. 2. Be alert for "red flags" of new crisis. 3. Advise about administration of screens, periodically.
BHS/Therapist	1. Receive referral from primary provider. 2. Contact patient, introduce therapy, and schedule first appointment. 3. Advise primary care provider of safety issues. 4. Enter patient into registry.	1. Develop rapport. 2. Complete formulation. 3. Assess safety and mitigate risks. 4. Develop a timeline. 5. Assess social network. 6. Frame goals for treatment. 7. Provide feedback to primary care provider. 8. Review formulation and plan with consulting psychiatrist. 9. Update registry.	1. Reinforce positive work. 2. Teach anxiety coping skills, if necessary. 3. Connect patient with social supports. 4. Generate wheel-and-spoke treatment plan. 5. Assess safety. 6. Update registry.	1. Review progress. 2. Reinforce positive changes. 3. Reinforce nonpharmacologic anxiety management. 4. Pursue and find solutions to problems. 5. Administer screens. 6. Conduct midpoint review with psychiatrist. 7. Assess safety. 8. Update registry.	1. Review progress. 2. Review solutions and successes. 3. Reflect on challenges of therapy. 4. Reflect on crisis and precipitants. 5. Anticipate future challenges. 6. Assess safety. 7. Update registry.	1. Share formulation with primary provider and staff. 2. Share "red flags" with other providers. 3. Summarize case with consulting psychiatrist and remove from caseload. 4. Update registry.

(continued)

TABLE 26.1 CONTINUED

	Initial Visit	Weeks 1 and 2	Weeks 3 and 4	Weeks 5 and 6	Weeks 7 and 8	Termination and Follow-up
Health Coach, if available	1. Review wellness needs as recommended by primary care provider. 2. Input information into registry.	1. Assess needs related to nutrition, weight, exercise, sleep, harm reduction of substance use, and stress. 2. Implement wellness plan with goals and outcome measures.	1. Follows progress in registry. 2. Update wellness plan, as needed. 3. Provide feedback to BHS.	1. Follow progress in registry. 2. Update wellness plan, as needed. 3. Provide feedback to BHS.	1. Follow progress in registry. 2. Update wellness plan, as needed. 3. Provide feedback to BHS.	1. Assess goals and outcomes. 2. Provide feedback to BHS. 3. Advise patient of aftercare wellness plan.
Care Coordinator/ Case Manager	Meet patient and determine needs for care coordination.	1. Coordinate referrals to other physicians with primary care provider. 2. Refer to community resources as needed.	Outreach the patient (as necessary) to aid in follow-up	As needed	As needed	Refer to community resources for ongoing care, if indicated.
Consulting Psychiatrist	1. Aid in triage to appropriate level of care. 2. Assess for dangerousness, if needed. 3. Develop population-based standards of care.	1. Consult on initial formulation. 2. Consider pharmacotherapy. 3. Advise additional medical workup, if necessary. 4. Assess safety.	1. Support therapist and see patient, if necessary. 2. Monitor progress in the registry and standards of behavioral health care.	1. Review progress of treatment with therapist. 2. Consider role for pharmacotherapy. 3. Assess safety. 4. Monitor progress in the registry.	As needed	1. Provide feedback to BHS/therapist. 2. Finalize formulation with therapist and primary care provider. 3. Anticipate future crises.

BOX 26.3

STEPS OF CRISIS INTERVENTION

1. **Identify the stressor or precipitant (e.g., external event, interpersonal problem, medical illness, psychological event, or developmental issue).**
2. **Characterize the patient's reactions to the crisis.**
3. **Understand the personal meanings of the event for the patient.**
4. **Develop a timeline of the crisis to understand the "Why now?"**
5. **Collect a social history including occupational, interpersonal, developmental, and psychiatric and substance use history to understand events influencing the current crisis.**
6. **Screen for other life problems that may exacerbate the crisis (e.g., medical conditions, legal issues, or substance abuse).**
7. **Build a social network map that includes the patient's family members and other sources of support.**
8. **Identify and prioritize problems contributing to the crisis.**
9. **Integrate biological, psychiatric, social, and cultural elements into a case formulation.**
10. **List potential solutions with the patient.**
11. **Assess less adaptive coping styles and teach more adaptive coping styles.**
12. **Support the patient in using the team and proposed solutions to resolve the crisis.**
13. **As the crisis resolves, provide anticipatory guidance.**

of the acute crisis. In most cases, crisis intervention therapy is delivered over one to eight individual sessions with a BHS.[1,5,20] Crisis intervention treatment proceeds through the stages described in Box 26.3.

We present a model of crisis intervention adapted to the integrated care setting. A medical assistant may conduct primary screening for a crisis; the primary provider conducts an initial assessment and subsequently uses the integrated care team, including a health coach, BHS, consulting psychiatrist, and care manager, to facilitate treatment. Telehealth consultation may be used if a psychiatrist or other members of the team are not readily available.

Recognition of the Crisis

Identifying the presence of a crisis and determining the precipitating stressor are the first steps of crisis intervention. Patients in crisis often feel confused and disorganized; they may be unable to recognize their own crisis state. In a collaborative care environment, every team member must be attuned to the signs of a patient in crisis. Many warning signs might suggest a patient is in crisis: He or she may unexpectedly miss appointments, feel easily frustrated upon checking in or when interacting with the medical assistant or nurses, or a patient may confide distress to a favorite staff member. Some patients may not renew or fill prescriptions while accumulating several emergency department visits. Patients may also share new, medically unexplained somatic symptoms[21] or screen positive on mood and anxiety screeners.

The opportunity for crisis intervention and treatment may be lost if clinicians fail to recognize and investigate changes in symptoms and functioning. When a patient appears distressed, being open about the patient's behavior and affect will invite a conversation. There are multiple moments during an office visit when a patient can be approached about stressful life events. Every integrated care team member should feel empowered to open a conversation with the patient. For example:

> *SCHEDULER:* "It has been a long time since you missed an appointment without calling. I hope nothing serious is happening?" *(Next step: Alert care manager or nurse that patient may need additional outreach.)*
>
> *NURSE:* "You seem upset today; I don't usually see you like this. How are you feeling lately?" *(Next step: Provide a self-report screening instruments and alert the provider.)*

> *PRIMARY CARE PROVIDER:* "It is unlike you to not take your medication regularly. What might be going on?" *(Next step: Assess for the presence of crisis.)*

Formulation of the Crisis

Identifying the stressor precipitating the crisis can be challenging for people whose intense distress leaves them unable to navigate the events driving their crisis. Moreover, the stressor is also likely to have occurred in the six weeks before the person presents for care. Some information may be available to the primary care provider from previous records or collateral informants. However, most likely, it will be the primary care provider who will obtain the initial history of the crisis. The provider's inquiries may be prompted by the concerns of other staff members or by the patient's family members. Family members can participate in the crisis intervention interview and treatment (see Chapter 27: Best Practice for Family-Centered Health Care: A Three-Step Model).

The interview can start by asking, "Why now?" What was happening on the day the patient reached out for help? The interview should then focus on the immediate precipitants of a crisis. Developing a six-week timeline of recent events, related to the crisis, focuses the interview and explores for sources of distress, as Figure 26.2 illustrates. The interview can progress to open-ended questions, exploring other stressors, the nature and duration of symptoms, changes in functioning or daily routines, and how the patient is doing generally.

Consider external events, interpersonal conflicts, internal conflicts, and developmental issues as common sources of a crisis. Discussing changes in these domains may also provide clues to the timing and nature of the stressor. "When was the last time things were going well?" is a helpful question that may further elucidate the onset of the crisis state.

Clinicians must also consider the presence of new medical conditions, primary mental illness, or substance abuse among patients in crisis. The relationship between crisis and psychiatric/medical disorder is bidirectional. By their nature, some medical, mood, anxiety, psychotic, and substance use disorders can occur without a life stressor. These illnesses can result in substantial functional impairment that drives ancillary stressors, hinders patients' use of effective coping strategies, and results in a crisis. In the other direction, stressful life events are often significant risk factors or precipitants for depression and substance use.[22–24] Screening instruments such as the Patient Health Questionnare-9 (PHQ-9),[25,26] Generalized Anxiety Disorder-7 (GAD-7),[27] and Alcohol Use Disorders Identification Test (AUDIT)[28] or the QPD (see chapter 10 Automated Mental Health Assessment for Integrated Care: The Quick PsychoDiagnostics Panel (QPD) Meets Real-World Clinical Needs) can be administered to patients by staff before appointments and aid the clinician's evaluation of the crisis and its resolution.

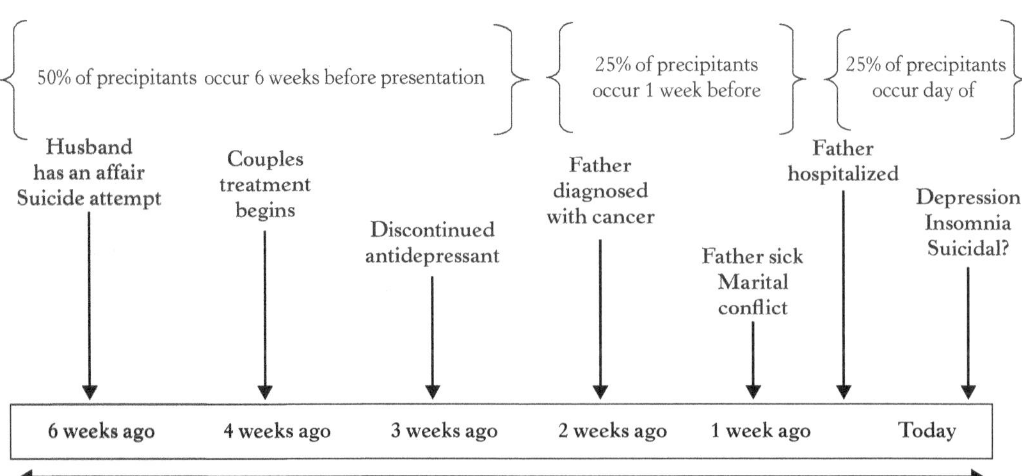

FIGURE 26.2 Six-week timeline

The primary care provider may use the triage assessment system (TAS) to identify maladaptive psychological reactions to crisis.[29] The TAS is a framework that briefly formulates the patient's reaction to a stressor and identifies maladaptive coping. In the TAS, the crisis state is described as an interaction among emotional, behavioral, and cognitive reactions. The primary emotional reaction is often clear and described by the patient: sadness, anger, guilt, or loneliness. These emotions often relate to the patient's crisis behaviors. These behaviors are most often (1) immobility or inability to solve the crisis, (2) avoidance of the relevant stressors, or (3) an adaptive "approach" reaction by which the patient works to resolve the crisis. Finally, cognitive reactions characterize the perception of the crisis. The crisis event can be perceived as an (1) irrevocable loss, (2) a transgression, or an offense against the patient, or (3) a threat that will bring future catastrophe. The synthesis of these emotional, behavioral, and cognitive reactions describes the patient's impairment and the effect of the crisis on social relationships, work, well-being, and self-perception. The presence of maladaptive behavioral and cognitive responses suggests the need for more intensive treatment by the integrated team or referral.

Although an adept primary care provider may be able to identify the stressor, complete the formulation, and deliver some brief suggestions within a medical appointment, the primary care provider is more likely to refer the patient for brief treatment with a "warm handoff" to the BHS. The BHS can spend more time exploring the crisis, its meanings, and the process by which the patient's individual strengths may allow crisis resolution. The process of building and working in a therapeutic relationship can reinvigorate the patient's commitment to his or her social network, an important step in resolving the crisis state.

Determination of the Level of Care

Not all patients can be safely managed in the office. Figure 26.3 demonstrates levels of care that may be available to a practice.

Patients may need to transition to other levels of care over time. Some patients may "step down" their care, as when graduating from intensive outpatient substance treatment to weekly therapy sessions or to community resources (e.g., Alcoholics Anonymous). Other patients may need a "step up" in care, as when hospitalization is required for acute suicidality.

All initial assessments of crisis states must address whether the patient is a danger to himself or herself, a danger to other persons, or so impaired as to be unable to maintain his or her essential activities of daily living (often called grave disability). Frank

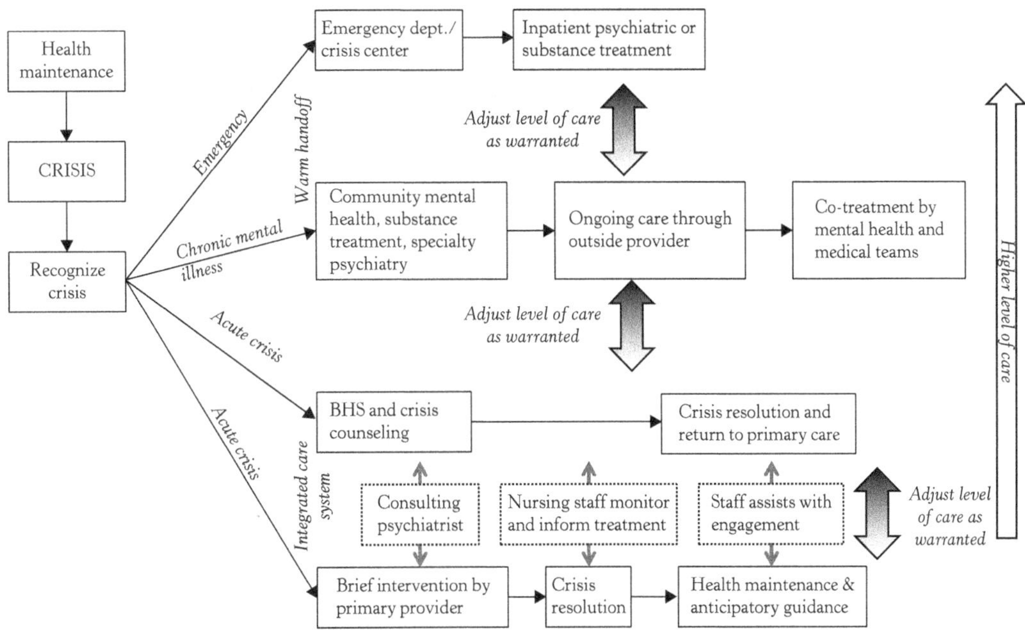

FIGURE 26.3 Levels of behavioral health care

suicidal or homicidal ideation is always of concern; it should be evaluated with input from a BHS and/or a psychiatrist and may result in the patient's need for inpatient care. Risk assessment is discussed in detail in Chapter 18: Violence and Suicide. Other less dangerous considerations include concurrent psychiatric illness, the presence of psychosis or substance use, and past behaviors.[30]

For the patient requiring immediate transfer to a higher level of care, established protocols should exist for monitoring the patient while in the office and completing a warm handoff to the BHS or a care coordinator who might facilitate referral to a crisis center or emergency department. A phone call and sharing of records from the primary care office is vital so that emergency providers understand the patient's full presentation as well as resources available to build a potential discharge plan. Some patients referred to a crisis center or emergency department will be admitted to inpatient treatment; others may be referred from the emergency department to an outpatient community mental health or substance treatment setting. In an integrated care environment, a care manager or other team member should follow up with the patient within one week after an emergency department visit to encourage re-engagement with the practice or connection to other recommended services.[31,32]

Referral to Specialty Care

An initial formulation of the crisis may suggest that the precipitant is an exacerbation of a chronic or severe mental illness or relapse of a substance use disorder. In these cases, specialty treatment outside the integrated care office may be indicated.

Patients with serious chronic mental illness and substantial social work needs may benefit from specialized care from a community mental health center, assertive community treatment team, or mobile crisis team, if available. These services offer intensive psychiatric case management, crisis resources, medications, and peer support. For these patients, primary care offices can provide ongoing medical care and health maintenance in coordination with a patient's primary mental health provider or a case manager.

Patients with moderate to severe substance use disorders may require intensive outpatient, residential, or inpatient detoxification services. Indications for these services include failure to achieve abstinence with less intensive treatment, high risk of complicated withdrawal, and significant social impairment (e.g., homelessness) that complicates efforts to achieve sobriety.[33] Patients who need substance use treatment in the community should also be followed by the integrated care team within a medical home. The team should continue to review the patient's progress in treatment, monitor medical complications of substance use and treatment, and reinforce adherence to his or her treatment plan.

Treatment Within the Integrated Care Medical Home

The medical appointment itself should not be forgotten as an opportunity for the primary care provider to deliver brief counseling.[34] Compassionate listening and empathizing are powerful acts of healing. Crises evolve in a setting of poor social connectedness; clinicians provide a positive relationship in which to validate the patient's distress, the complexity of a situation, and remind the patient of personal strengths. Providers can also make use of this healing relationship to deliver brief therapeutic techniques; for example, patients with significant anxiety may benefit from brief teaching of mindfulness meditation.[35] Some patients with medical illness experience demoralization, a sense of subjective incompetence and hopelessness. Engaging these patients in a short discussion of the meaning of their illness, hopes for the future, sources of support, and likely treatment options may ameliorate demoralization.[36]

Motivational interviewing is another useful technique that can be applied during a medical appointment by a primary care provider (with ability, interest, and time) or a BHS. Motivational interviewing is a therapeutic method in which the clinician and patient explore the positive and negative aspects to behavioral change in a collaborative fashion (See Chapter 25: Health Coaching in Integrated Care). This method is particularly useful for patients who are ambivalent about reducing their problematic substance use or making healthy behavioral choices.[37] Patients who are already actively working toward sobriety may benefit from a reminder of strategies for managing cravings, advice on avoiding triggers for use, and reinforcement of healthy decisions.

Integrated BHSs will be able to briefly treat many crises in the primary care setting, particularly for patients whose crisis results from a clear external stressor, who have mild or moderate substance use disorders, or who cannot access specialty care. The severity of illness that can be handled in a primary care setting depends on the comfort, skills, and capacity of the practitioners and the team within the care system. For instance, models exist for managing actively suicidal patients, borderline personality disorder, and serious chronic mental illness in outpatient therapy, but delivering these treatments may not be feasible for most primary care practices.[38–41]

Crisis Intervention Therapy

After deciding that crisis therapy is indicated, the primary care provider may encourage and arrange for crisis intervention treatment. Many patients in crisis are seeking help and are hopeful that treatment will be beneficial. Yet some patients may be reluctant to pursue therapy, feeling it is unnecessary or unlikely to be helpful. The crisis state perturbs a person's sense of self-worth and self-efficacy so that the idea of relying on others, or even admitting there is a problem, may be challenging. Patients may minimize their struggles or avoid stressors despite evidence of profound functional impairment. Other patients express an interest in therapy but feel overwhelmed at the idea of pursuing more care and more appointments.

There are several strategies for the primary care provider and BHS to help the patient begin treatment. Motivational interviewing by the primary care provider can help guide the patient's decision to participate in therapy.[42] Another helpful strategy is to facilitate a warm handoff to the BHS while in the office.[18] An in-person introduction "breaks the ice," humanizes the experience of therapy, and conveys the provider's trust in the BHS. The BHS, in the presence of the primary care provider, also has an opportunity to solicit a personal commitment from the patient to begin crisis treatment. If a face-to-face introduction is not possible, the primary care provider can provide an overview of the therapeutic process and have the care coordinator schedule the first therapy appointment. If an appointment cannot be scheduled before the patient leaves, the care coordinator or the BHS should actively contact the patient to schedule treatment. Thus the collaboration among the integrated care team begins at the first visit and continues throughout crisis treatment.

After referral to the therapist, the primary care provider should also schedule a follow-up medical appointment in several weeks to ensure that the patient has begun therapy. A subsequent visit provides an opportunity for feedback from the patient on his or her initial therapy visits. This feedback may help anticipate hurdles to the patient's therapy, including difficulties with adherence and motivation. Table 26.1 outlines the tasks that care team members perform throughout the process of crisis therapy; team members' specific work will vary somewhat based on the provider's expertise and among different care systems.

Having begun the crisis assessment during the first medical appointment, the primary care provider should share with the BHS an initial formulation of the crisis, including an understanding of the precipitant and its personal meaning to the patient. The provider shares a safety assessment and the status of medical issues and prognoses pertinent to the patient's ongoing crisis. An objective understanding of the patient's medical illness helps the therapist recognize a patient's tendencies toward catastrophic thinking; for example, the therapist could help a patient who ruminates on "worst case" scenarios of an upcoming surgery. Also, nurses and other staff can offer encouragement and validate the patient's decision to pursue therapy.

Therapy with a BHS

Therapy with a BHS begins with the therapist eliciting both the "Why now?" and a detailed developmental and social history relevant to the acute crisis. The history of prior crises and the resolution of those crises offer the therapist clues as to how the patient will successfully navigate the present episode. The process of gathering this history helps the patient and therapist build rapport that is essential for productive therapy.

Therapist's Assessment of the Social System

As therapy begins, the therapist should evaluate the patient's social support system. The BHS may use a social system map to visualize important relationships and sources of support in the patient's life (Fig. 26.4).

A social system map identifies all the patient's significant relationships, including family, friends, coworkers, medical providers, cultural and community supports. Patients' appreciation of these relationships alleviates the sense of loneliness imposed by the crisis state while beginning to remove the self-imposed pressure of solving the problem on their own. For patients who have lost a key member of their support system, a therapist might consider how other persons in the social system can

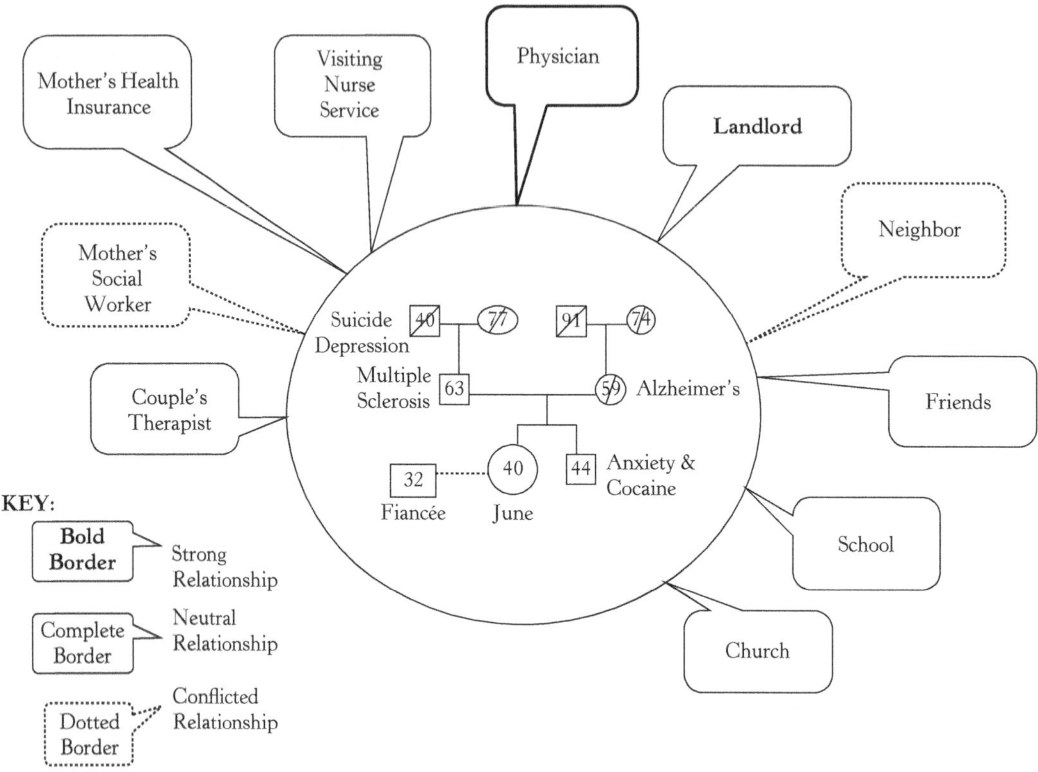

FIGURE 26.4 Social network map

fill the support needs left by a loss. The evaluation of the patient's support network may reveal that the patient's experience is inducing similar anxiety and tension among their supportive relationships. Perhaps in the past, the patient's anxiety served to solicit help from their social environment.[43,44]

Consultation with Psychiatry

The BHS or primary care provider can consult with a psychiatrist either live or via telehealth (see Chapter 9: Telehealth in an Integrated Care Environment). Psychiatric consultation can be used for therapeutic advice, new recommendations for refractory patients, indications for additional medical workup, psychopharmacotherapy, or for a focused brief psychotherapy targeting symptoms or the crisis. Patients should be followed in a tracking registry. The consulting psychiatrist is positioned as a supportive and helpful team player, not exclusively as a supervisory figure.[44]

A psychiatrist may contribute to the initial formulation and safety assessment. For high-risk or particularly difficult cases, the psychiatrist may treat the patient directly or via telehealth. After several weeks, the psychiatrist should review the tracking registry of patients in crisis with members of the integrated team in order to assess their progress. A failure to make progress as anticipated or the discovery of new information may require reassessment of the diagnosis, case formulation, treatment offered, or a change in the level of care. Challenging cases may be highlighted in the registry for consultation. A population-based review may suggest the use of algorithms or standards of care for subpopulations of patients in crisis.

Development of Solutions by Patient and Therapist

Identifying the stressor, understanding the crisis, and assessing the patient's social network allow the patient and therapist to define the problem and begin to seek solutions. Within the context of the patient's life, the therapist can help the patient understand maladaptive coping, sources of impairment, and possible solutions to the crisis. Organizing this active behavioral approach can be done with a "wheel-and-spoke" treatment plan, shown in Figure 26.5.

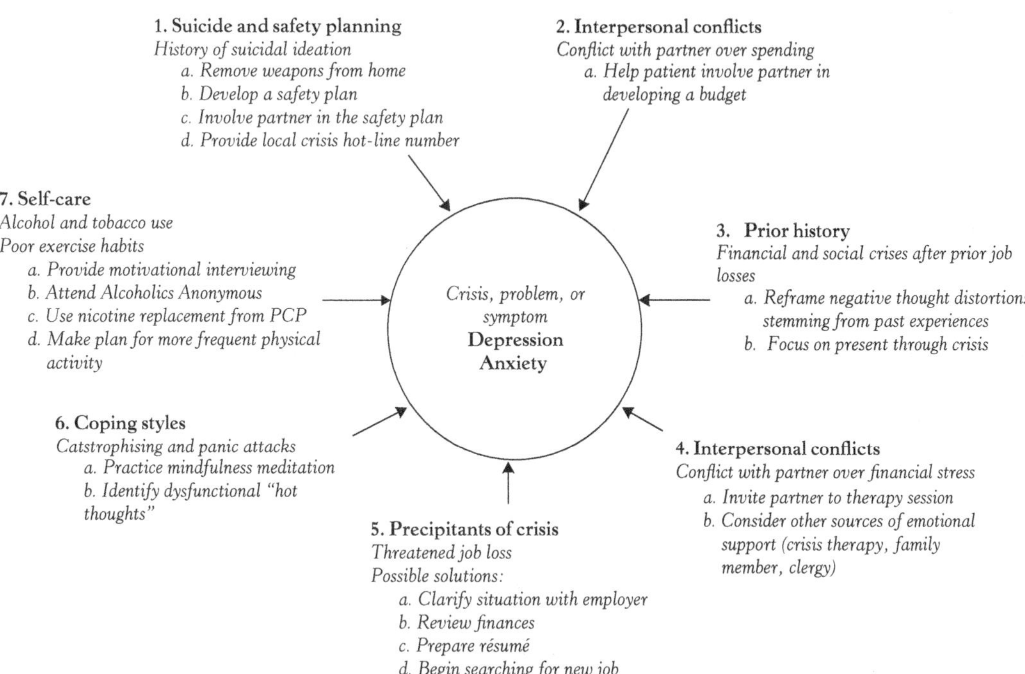
1. Suicide and safety planning
History of suicidal ideation
a. Remove weapons from home
b. Develop a safety plan
c. Involve partner in the safety plan
d. Provide local crisis hot-line number
2. Interpersonal conflicts
Conflict with partner over spending
a. Help patient involve partner in developing a budget
7. Self-care
Alcohol and tobacco use
Poor exercise habits
a. Provide motivational interviewing
b. Attend Alcoholics Anonymous
c. Use nicotine replacement from PCP
d. Make plan for more frequent physical activity
Crisis, problem, or symptom
Depression
Anxiety
3. Prior history
Financial and social crises after prior job losses
a. Reframe negative thought distortions stemming from past experiences
b. Focus on present through crisis
6. Coping styles
Catstrophising and panic attacks
a. Practice mindfulness meditation
b. Identify dysfunctional "hot thoughts"
4. Interpersonal conflicts
Conflict with partner over financial stress
a. Invite partner to therapy session
b. Consider other sources of emotional support (crisis therapy, family member, clergy)
5. Precipitants of crisis
Threatened job loss
Possible solutions:
a. Clarify situation with employer
b. Review finances
c. Prepare résumé
d. Begin searching for new job

FIGURE 26.5 List the core problem in the wheel center, prioritize contributing problems by numbering them, and list possible solutions.

In the center of the wheel, the crisis, problem, or diagnosis is defined. If the crisis involves suicide or violence risk, then this issue becomes the center of the wheel and the focus of crisis treatment (see Chapter 18: Violence and Suicide). Otherwise, the focus of crisis treatment is typically a problem or diagnosis mutually decided between the patient and provider. The "spokes" describe problems contributing to the crisis, and these problems are prioritized by numbers. Under each problem are potential solutions.

The patient and BHS brainstorm solutions to contributing problems. Ideas for solutions often come from the patient's past experiences in resolving difficult situations. The BHS can review the patient's maladaptive coping styles and suggest the more adaptive approaches described in Box 26.4.

The BHS provides feedback and steers the patient toward solutions that reflect the patient's positive psychological traits and values, reaction style, new coping strategies, use of the social network, and environmental supports.[9] In constructing solutions, the therapist must be entirely focused on resolution of the acute crisis.

This process of defining the crisis as induced by a stressor, describing available social supports, and listing a menu of solutions pulls from many theories of psychotherapy. The act of empathizing and active listening are core tenets of all types of psychotherapy, while formulation of the personal meaning of a stressor based on a patient's prior experiences evokes a more psychodynamic approach.[6] Primary care providers and office staff may use motivational interviewing to help reluctant patients engage in treatment.[45] Family therapy is often used to resolve interpersonal or familial conflicts in the social network or develop systemic interventions. Crisis intervention's persistent emphasis on trying possible solutions employs solution-focused problem-solving therapy.[10] Reminding patients of mindfulness and anxiolytic techniques like deep breathing are classic cognitive-behavioral interventions. Therapeutic strategies typically reflect the patient's needs and capabilities and the therapist's predilections, training, and assessments of the patient's responses.

Implementation of Solutions

With a formulation, new coping styles, and possible solutions in hand, the patient and therapist implement the different proposed solutions and proceed through crisis intervention treatment as described

BOX 26.4
COPING STYLES

MALADAPTIVE COPING STYLES

Deceptive/Antisocial: using dishonesty, lying, cheating, or stealing to solve a crisis
Suicidal: using the threat of suicide, or suicide attempts, to coerce someone or to solve a problem
Violent: using violence (threatened or actual) to establish control and solve problems
Impulsive: unpredictable or impulsive responses without anticipating possible outcomes
Random/Chaotic: an unproductive and extreme form of trial and error, an impulsive style often seen in prolonged psychotic states

ADAPTIVE COPING STYLES

Intuitive: using imagination, feelings, and perceptions to solve a problem
Logical/Rational: carefully reasoned, logical, deductive style
Trial and Error: trying a random solution, modifying it if it fails, and trying again
Help seeking: asking others for help
Informational: gathering information before deciding
Wait and See: allowing time or circumstance to determine the outcome
Action oriented: taking an action to immediately rectify the problem
Contemplative: quietly thinking over the problem before taking action
Spiritual: asking for God's direction
Emotional: using emotion such as tears, anger, or fear to help solve problems
Controlling: controlling people or oneself to gain the power to solve the problem
Manipulative: using a variety of manipulative styles to solve the problem

in Box 26.3. This working stage is the most challenging part of crisis intervention therapy. Flexibility is important for the BHS as well as for the patient. Many patients in crisis have come to rely on a single coping strategy, which may be ineffective or maladaptive. The process of pursuing different coping strategies (Box 26.4) and solutions to the crisis embodies the self-efficacy that the patient has lost through the intense anxiety of a crisis. The therapist helps the patient understand why certain solutions are unsuccessful, celebrates with the patient the success of other solutions, and realistically appraises the patient's progress toward crisis resolution. Any regression to maladaptive coping styles—for example, avoidance of a stressor or recurrent substance use—is interpreted as a contributor to the crisis. Adaptive, positive work is reinforced with praise and the experience of successful problem solving.

As therapy proceeds, the therapist may leverage the resources of the integrated care team to monitor and engage the patient (see Table 26.1). Nurses, office staff, and the care coordinator help track missed appointments and reach out to the patient to aid a return to treatment. These providers may also readminister anxiety, depression, or the QPD screeners and offer feedback on the patient's progress to the BHS. For instance, the patient may seem less irritable in interactions with scheduling staff or make a small joke walking from the waiting room. The BHS should communicate an enhanced formulation to the primary care provider to ensure that the level of care is safe and appropriate and that all team members are aware of updated treatment plans. The psychiatrist may monitor therapeutic progress through the registry and is available for consultation.

Resolution of the Crisis and Anticipatory Guidance

In the final stages of crisis intervention therapy, the patient reflects on his or her positive choices, new coping styles, and functional improvement. The therapist helps the patient recognize how particular

BOX 26.5

RELEVANT EVIDENCE

Strength of recommendation taxonomy (SOR A, B, or C)

- **Motivational interviewing should be used to encourage healthy behavioral choices, including reducing substance misuse. (SOR A)[37]**
- **A member of the integrated health team should follow up with patients after an emergency department visit. (SOR B)[13,31,32]**
- **Mindfulness meditation improves patient anxiety. (SOR B)[46]**
- **Standard depression and substance use screeners should be administered in primary care. (SOR B)[47,48]**
- **Crisis intervention therapy facilitates crisis resolution and improves patient functioning. (SOR C)[1,5,11,40,44]**
- **A social network map and wheel-and-spoke diagram assist in evaluation and treatment of the patient in crisis. (SOR C)[20]**
- **A "warm handoff" should be made by the primary provider to the behavioral health specialist. (SOR C)[18]**
- **Integrated health systems should use patient registries to track patients' treatment and improvement. (SOR C)[15,18]**
- **Intensive outpatient or residential substance abuse treatment is indicated for patients with a high risk of complicated withdrawal, significant social impairment, or failure to achieve abstinence with less intensive treatment. (SOR C)[33]**

solutions have improved the crisis. Improvement may also be reflected in reduced anxiety and depression as measured by outcome scales. The consulting psychiatrist and primary provider advise as to the continuation of psychiatric medications that may have been initiated.

Before the termination of therapy, the BHS, reinforced by the primary care provider, offers anticipatory guidance regarding future crises. "Red flags" that herald a relapse into crisis should be explicitly identified and shared with the primary care provider and integrated care team, who will continue to follow the patient after therapy ends. A plan should be made for routine monitoring of crisis symptoms in the future. Monitoring may be as straightforward as a routine inquiry about a troubled relationship or more frequent administration of a PHQ-9 depression screener. Keeping the patient's social system map and wheel-and-spoke solutions diagram in the medical record provides a lasting reminder of the supports and solutions available to the patient.

CONCLUSION

Crisis therapists are fond of the Chinese character for crisis, which combines the symbols for "danger" and "opportunity." Integrated behavioral health teams offering crisis intervention treatment help many patients grow and optimize their potential. Close communication among primary care providers, BHSs, care coordinators, staff, and the consulting psychiatrist is essential to ensure that the patient receives a thorough assessment at the appropriate level of care, aid necessary to resolve the acute crisis, and support in preventing future crises. See Box 26.5 for a summary of some of the evidence- based approaches that are used as part of the crisis intervention approach.

REFERENCES

1. France K. Crisis Intervention: A Handbook of Immediate Person-to-Person Help. 6th ed. Springfield, IL: Charles C Thomas; 2014.
2. Hobson CJ, Kamen J, Szostek J, Netercut CM, Tiedmann JW, Wojnarowicz S. Stressful life events: A revision and update of the social readjustment rating scale. Int J Stress Manag. 1998;5(1):1–23.
3. Lindemann E. Symptomatology and management of acute grief. Am J Psychiatry. 1944;101(2):141–148.
4. Erikson EH. Identity and the Life Cycle; Selected Papers. New York: International Universities Press; 1959.

5. Aguilera DC. Crisis intervention: Theory and Methodology. 8th ed. St. Louis, MO: Mosby; 1998.
6. Jerry PA. Dynamic change in crisis intervention. Am J Psychother. 1998;52(4):437–449.
7. American Psychiatric Association, DSM-5 Task Force. Diagnostic and Statistical Manual of Mental Disorders: DSM-5. 5th ed. Arlington, VA: American Psychiatric Association; 2013.
8. Gil T. From crisis to adjustment disorder: A medicalization of a concept? Turk Psikiyatri Derg. 2013;24(1):58–62.
9. Jeste DV, Palmer BW, Rettew DC, Boardman S. Positive psychiatry: Its time has come. J Clin Psychiatry. 2015;76(6):675–683.
10. Haley J. Problem-Solving Therapy. 2nd ed. San Francisco: Jossey-Bass; 1987.
11. Hobbs M. Crisis intervention in theory and practice: A selective review. Br J Med Psychol. 1984;57 (Pt 1):23–34.
12. Gilliland BE, James RK. Crisis Intervention Strategies. Pacific Grove, CA: Brooks/Cole; 1988.
13. Griswold KS, Homish GG, Pastore PA, Leonard KE. A randomized trial: Are care navigators effective in connecting patients to primary care after psychiatric crisis? Community Ment Health J. 2010;46(4):398–402.
14. Pastore P, Griswold KS, Homish GG, Watkins R. Family practice enhancements for patients with severe mental illness. Community Ment Health J. 2013;49(2):172–177.
15. Patient Population Tracking. University of Washington AIMS Center. https://aims.uw.edu/sites/default/files/Patient_Tracking_FAQ.pdf. Published 2013. Accessed December 23, 2015.
16. Busner J, Targum SD. The Clinical Global Impressions Scale: Applying a research tool in clinical practice. Psychiatry (Edgmont). 2007;4(7):28–37.
17. WHO Disability Assessment Schedule 2.0. World Health Organization. http://www.who.int/classifications/icf/whodasii/en/. Updated November 6, 2014. Accessed December 21, 2015.
18. Raney LE. Integrating primary care and behavioral health: The role of the psychiatrist in the collaborative care model. Am J Psychiatry. 2015;172(8):721–728.
19. Unutzer J, Chan YF, Hafer E, et al. Quality improvement with pay-for-performance incentives in integrated behavioral health care. Am J Public Health. 2012;102(6):e41–e45.
20. Feinstein RE, Carey L. Crisis intervention in office practice. In: Feinstein RE, Brewer AA, eds. Primary Care Psychiatry and Behavioral Medicine: Brief Office Treatment and Management Pathways. New York: Springer; 1999:430–447.
21. Katon WJ, Walker EA. Medically unexplained symptoms in primary care. J Clin Psychiatry. 1998;59(Suppl 20):15–21.
22. Kendler KS, Karkowski LM, Prescott CA. Causal relationship between stressful life events and the onset of major depression. Am J Psychiatry. 1999;156(6):837–841.
23. Sinha R. The role of stress in addiction relapse. Curr Psychiatry Rep. 2007;9(5):388–395.
24. Rahe RH, Meyer M, Smith M, Kjaer G, Holmes TH. Social stress and illness onset. J Psychosom Res. 1964;8(1):35–44.
25. Kroenke K, Spitzer RL, Williams JB. The PHQ-9: Validity of a brief depression severity measure. J Gen Intern Med. 2001;16(9): 606–613.
26. Kroenke K, Spitzer RL, Williams JB, Lowe B. The Patient Health Questionnaire somatic, anxiety, and depressive symptom scales: A systematic review. Gen Hosp Psychiatry. 2010;32(4):345–359.
27. Spitzer RL, Kroenke K, Williams JB, Lowe B. A brief measure for assessing generalized anxiety disorder: The GAD-7. Arch Intern Med. 2006;166(10):1092–1097.
28. Saunders JB, Aasland OG, Babor TF, de la Fuente JR, Grant M. Development of the Alcohol Use Disorders Identification Test (AUDIT): WHO collaborative project on early detection of persons with harmful alcohol consumption—II. Addiction. 1993;88(6):791–804.
29. Myer RA, Conte C. Assessment for crisis intervention. J Clin Psychol. 2006;62(8):959–970.
30. McDowell AK, Lineberry TW, Bostwick JM. Practical suicide risk management for the busy primary care physician. Mayo Clin Proc. 2011;86(8):792–800.
31. Griswold KS, Zayas LE, Pastore PA, Smith SJ, Wagner CM, Servoss TJ. Primary care after psychiatric crisis: A qualitative analysis. Ann Fam Med. 2008;6(1):38–43.
32. Stanley B, Brown GK, Currier GW, Lyons C, Chesin M, Knox KL. Brief intervention and follow-up for suicidal patients with repeat emergency department visits enhances treatment engagement. Am J Public Health. 2015;105(8):1570–1572.
33. Center for Substance Abuse Treatment. Substance Abuse: Clinical Issues in Intensive Outpatient Treatment. Treatment Improvement Protocol (TIP) Series 47. Rockville, MD: Substance Abuse and Mental Health Services Administration; 2006.
34. Prusnofsky L, Feinstein RE. Consulting and counseling in primary care. In: Feinstein RE, Brewer AA, eds. Primary Care Psychiatry and Behavioral Medicine: Brief Office Treatment and Management Pathways. New York: Springer; 1999:405–429.

35. Khoury B, Lecomte T, Fortin G, et al. Mindfulness-based therapy: A comprehensive meta-analysis. Clin Psychol Rev. 2013; 33(6):763–771.
36. Griffith JL, Gaby L. Brief psychotherapy at the bedside: Countering demoralization from medical illness. Psychosomatics. 2005;46(2):109–116.
37. Rubak S, Sandbaek A, Lauritzen T, Christensen B. Motivational interviewing: A systematic review and meta-analysis. Br J Gen Pract. 2005;55 (513):305–312.
38. Jobes DA. Managing Suicidal Risk: A Collaborative Approach. New York: Guilford Press; 2006.
39. Comtois KA, Jobes DA, O'Connor S, et al. Collaborative Assessment and Management of Suicidality (CAMS): Feasibility trial for next-day appointment services. Depress Anxiety. 2011;28(11):963–972.
40. Laddis A. Outcome of crisis intervention for borderline personality disorder and posttraumatic stress disorder: A model for modification of the mechanism of disorder in complex posttraumatic syndromes. Ann Gen Psychiatry. 2010;9:(19):1–12.
41. Brennaman L. Crisis emergencies for individuals with severe, persistent mental illnesses: A situation-specific theory. Arch Psychiatr Nurs. 2012;26(4):251–260.
42. Miller WR, Rollnick S. Motivational Interviewing: Preparing People for Change. 2nd ed. New York: Guilford Press; 2002.
43. Yerushalmi H. Whose crisis is it? A relational psychoanalytic perspective. Am J Psychother. 2010;64(3):283–305.
44. Caplan G. Principles of Preventive Psychiatry. New York: Basic Books; 1964.
45. Miller WR, Rollnick S. Motivational Interviewing: Helping People Change. 3rd ed. New York: Guilford Press; 2013.
46. Chiesa A, Serretti A. Mindfulness-based stress reduction for stress management in healthy people: A review and meta-analysis. J Altern Complement Med. 2009;15(5):593–600.
47. U.S. Preventative Services Task Force. Screening for depression in adults: recommendation statement. Am Fam Physician. 2010;82(8):976–979.
48. U. S. Preventive Services Task Force. Screening and behavioral counseling interventions in primary care to reduce alcohol misuse: Recommendation statement. Ann Intern Med. 2004;140(7):554–556.

27

Best Practice for Family-Centered Health Care

A Three-Step Model

JOANNA STURHAHN STRATTON, KATHERINE BUCK, AND ALISON M. HERU

BOX 27.1

KEY POINTS

- **Our three-step model organizes evidence-based family treatment for medical and mental health diagnoses.**
- **Medical teams, patients, and families are more satisfied when the whole family is involved in medical care.**
- **Everyone on the medical team has a role in family inclusion, from the front desk staff to the medical provider.**
- **Benefits to the patient include adherence to the treatment plan and medication.**
- **Benefits to the family include higher family cohesion and more positive health behaviors.**
- **Our model consists of three distinct levels of family-centered care and intervention: family inclusion, family education and support, and family systems therapy.**

INTRODUCTION

Although patients usually enter the exam room alone, their ability to maintain good health is significantly impacted by their family, friends, community, and culture. Due to time constraints, many medical practices treat the individual without involving or consulting with the patient's family, missing an opportunity to include important and influential family members in a patient's care. The good news is that the Patient Protection and Affordable Care Act has created an opportunity for health care practitioners to redesign current practice and develop new models of care to keep patients with chronic conditions healthy and out of the hospital.[1] Sadly, despite spending more money per capita, Americans are becoming less healthy.[2] Patients in family-centered care can reverse this trend.

Medical and mental health outcomes are improved when an integrated medical team involves family members in a patient's care.[3] Working with an individual, without his or her family, and treating physical and mental health care separately produces high systemic costs, poorer outcomes, and lower patient satisfaction.[4] Integration of systemic, familial, and relational factors into health care improves the overall health and well-being of the patient and the family.[5] In this chapter, we explain the benefits of an integrated health care model that incorporates family into behavioral and physical health treatment. Our model consists of three distinct levels of family-centered care and intervention: family inclusion, family education and support, and family systems therapy. We illustrate, through a disguised case example, the transformative impact on the lives of patients when important family members are included in their medical care. In the case example, we demonstrate how our three-step model operates in practice, and we describe strategies such as the pre-visit "huddle," joint visit or co-consultation, and treatment plans. Our case example acknowledges that families are complex and that medical providers are frequently expected to serve many roles within a short amount of time. An overview of the key elements of involving family in health care for the treatment of physical and mental health problems is described in Box 27.1.

DEFINITION OF FAMILY

The term *family* may have different meanings to different people. In this chapter, we define family as kinship that is secured in social and cultural values and understandings, rather than being produced solely by nature and biology.[6] Families are at the center of our this model of integrated care. This view recognizes that there can be different configurations of family that may change over time. For example, patients may define family more broadly as members of their community who support and love them. For patients, families are a point of reference for the definition of health and health care access, and for information about the significance and impact of illness and sickness. Treatment adherence is 1.74 times higher in patients from cohesive families and 1.53 times lower in patients from families in conflict.[7] We should include families in patient care because chronic health conditions affect the entire family.[8]

PRIMARY CARE SETTING

Integrated primary care settings represent the ideal location for family intervention. Primary care offices are the frontlines, not only for the nation's presenting medical complaints, but also for the majority of mental health complaints.[9] In fact, the majority of psychiatric prescriptions are written by nonpsychiatric physicians.[10] As many as 70% of appointments with primary care providers (PCPs) can be tied to a psychosocial concern.[11] A PCP may, in just a few hours, see patients with presenting problems such as obesity, substance abuse, diabetes, heart disease, and depression. All of these illness have clear evidence for family intervention.[12–16] Indeed, much of a PCP's work is linked to behavioral change, such as improving exercise, sleep patterns, diet and reducing smoking.[17] Behavioral health providers are increasingly shifting from mental illness consultation to team collaboration.[18] Our three-step family model describes the many opportunities for family intervention in primary care and specialty clinics.

Every team member has skills to bring the family into the treatment of the patient. The front desk staff, the medical assistant, the nurse practitioner, the care coordinator, the clinical pharmacist, the behavioral health specialist (BHS), and the PCP all have different and important skills. For example, the members of the front desk staff include the family in scheduling and remembering appointments and educate the family members about the cancellation and rescheduling policy. The medical provider educates family members to assist in the patient's care. The BHS uses techniques such as motivational interviewing and family therapy techniques to increase understanding of and adherence to treatment plans. The care coordinator participates in the team-based care and coordinates referrals for the family.

FAMILY-CENTERED CARE

There is general agreement that families should be included in situations such as medical emergencies, advance directives, and terminal illness, and the scope of family involvement is widening. Physicians should watch for signs of distress in caregivers.[19] Caregiver burden, which carries its own morbidity and mortality, is increasingly recognized in caregivers who assist family members with chronic illness.[20] Several specialties, such as family medicine, palliative care, and clinics that manage chronic illness, use specific protocols for working with caregivers.[21] Health care professionals should be aware that caregivers of a terminally ill patient can require as much support as the patient. Unfortunately, we have not focused as much on the health of family members when their loved one has been diagnosed with a broader range of medical and mental health disorders.

How health care professionals provide family intervention depends on their level of expertise. Family support enhances care, regardless of the patient's diagnosis or point of entry into the health care system. Families should be included from the moment a patient enters the medical system, when the patient makes his or her first appointment on the telephone, and in the waiting room.

Our three-step model provides a clear, easy-to-follow structure that includes the whole medical team. Specifically, it helps all members of the medical team assess and care for individuals and families using evidence-based family treatment approaches. Similar to working with chest pain or elevated lipids, a robust research base supports best practices for including families in patient care. In each step

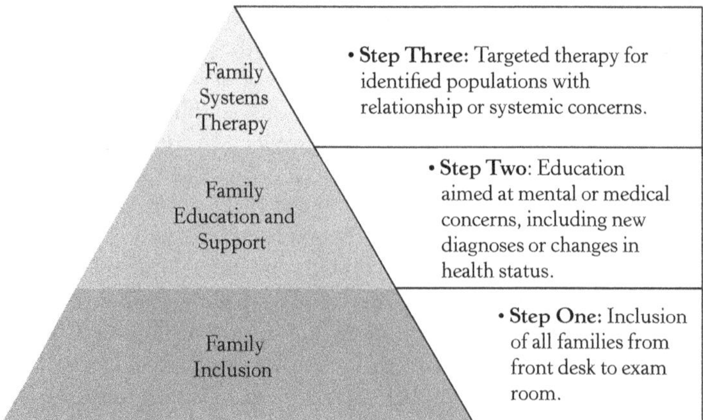

FIGURE 27.1 Key recommendations for family intervention

of our model, we highlight the evidence for the proposed treatment. Our three-step model, shown in Figure 27.1, can be used in any clinic setting.

FAMILY-CENTERED CARE: THREE-STEP MODEL

Step 1. Family Inclusion

Definition

The family inclusion step describes the treatment of a patient either when the family members are in the examining room or when the provider is conceptualizing the patient in relationship to the family. This family-oriented thinking guides patient conversation, promotes asking questions that value the perspective of each family member, and informs diagnosis and treatment. Family inclusion requires no formal assessment and minimal training to implement.[22] It occurs when members of the medical team welcome the family by encouraging them to attend visits, participate over the phone, and ask questions. All members of the health care team can "think family." For example, when a mother attends an appointment with a child, the medical assistant can engage her in conversation while obtaining the child's vital signs. Moreover, by including family, we reinforce the value of the family member's contribution to health of his or her loved one.

Assessment

Concise but thorough biopsychosocial-cultural questioning can enhance patients' experience of care and increase provider awareness of factors that impact health.[23] Family inclusion uses general screening questions that ask the patient about his or her family, pertinent medical history, where the patient lives, which family members are most involved in the patient's medical care, who is most supportive of the patient's health care, and what goals and values the family shares. Obtaining consent at the initial visit to include a significant family member can be followed by general psychosocial screening at a later visit. Some clinics use tools that include questions about family functioning. In 2014 the National Comprehensive Cancer Network (NCCN) established clinical practice guidelines recommending assessment of distress in all cancer patients using the Distress Thermometer for Patients.[24] The NCCN Distress Thermometer is a self-report instrument that has a visual analog scale and a problem list that includes three "family" questions about the patient's relationship with a partner, with children, and about coping with elderly relatives or dependents.[24]

Screening tools can also be used to identify families with psychosocial risk. The Psychosocial Assessment Tool (PAT) is one validated measure of psychosocial risk.[25] It was developed for use with families with children with cancer, but its use has expanded to families coping with other chronic medical illnesses such as obesity, chronic pain, transplantation, congenital heart disease, sickle cell disease, and irritable bowel syndrome. Results from multiple clinical sites and disease conditions show that generally one-half to two-thirds of all families have a low level of psychosocial risk. In low-risk families, family education and support are appropriate. For the medium and high-risk families, more focused family interventions are needed, as shown in detail in Table 27.1.

TABLE 27.1 FAMILY-CENTERED HEALTH CARE: THREE-STEP MODEL

Steps	Who Gets It?	Who Does It?	When?	Key Components
Step 1: Family Inclusion	All patients	All staff and providers at every level	New patient visits, well-child checks (anticipatory guidance), practice-wide interventions (quality improvement, etc.)	"Think family," family-friendly policies, universal screening, screening follow-up, "meet-and-greets"
Step 2: Family Intervention, Education, and Support	Patients experiencing a health event, trying to make a health change, or with mild "phase of life" concerns	Medical provider, behavioral health specialist, psychiatrist, nurse, medical assistant, health coach, care coordinator, staff	Well-child checks (when health need or psychosocial risk is identified), discussion of medical adherence, new diagnoses, health and behavior change	Family-centered screening, family inclusion in health and behavior interventions, family education and support, groups
Step 3: Family systems therapy	Patients with family communication or mental health concerns	Behavioral health specialist, psychiatrist (clinicians with family systems training)	Communication problems, couples concerns, sexual problems, substance abuse, child behavior concerns, abuse, family support for connection to mental health services	Couples intervention skills (brief), family and parent intervention skills (brief), family assessment skills, facilitation of referral to specialty mental health, consultation skills

A case study (Box 27.2) will illustrate the model and remind health care practitioners about the value of family inclusion. While we describe an example of one patient who presents for care, the health of the whole family is considered and treated. The family members display complex physical and mental health issues. However, when the integrated care team facilitates family interventions, the outcomes are positive and the patient, the family, and the providers are satisfied.

Treatment Plan
Patient (Serena's) Concern #1: Pain Management

Dr. Carey, the patient's PCP, collaborated with Serena to set long-term goals to help her learn new pain management skills and return to normal activities. One significant strength was that Serena was encouraged by her daughter, who also wanted to learn these same self-management skills. One anticipated obstacle was that Serena has had more than 20 years of struggling with pain management and as a result has physical and psychological dependence on pain medication. The immediate short-term plan was to have a family meeting with Dr. Francis (BHS) and Dr. Carey (PCP) to determine next steps.

What Happened Here with the Jay Family?

The whole family was included and considered during this encounter. Dr. Carey noticed that there was a familial aspect to the presenting concern as both Serena and Deidra struggled with pain and took pain medications. Dr. Carey hypothesized that Serena may have had undiagnosed and untreated depression as well as significant relational conflict that lowered her stress tolerance. Dr. Carey felt

> **BOX 27.2**
>
> THE JAY FAMILY, STEP 1: FAMILY INCLUSION
>
> **Three generations of women were introduced to Dr. Carey, the PCP: Serena, age 42, the patient with the appointment; Deidra, her daughter; age 23, and Haven, Deidra's daughter and Serena's granddaughter, age 3. During this medical visit, Dr. Carey discussed Serena's pain and request to obtain a medication refill. Dr. Carey engaged in conversation with all three family members. During the exam, the provider learned that Serena (the grandmother) had been diagnosed with arthritis and fibromyalgia in her 20s. Deidra (the daughter) mentioned that she, herself, was in a car accident in her teens and still experiences chronic low back, neck, and shoulder pain. Both women take oxycodone and acetaminophen with pregabalin for their pain.**
>
> **During this first visit, Dr. Carey asked Serena questions regarding her pain, administered the Psychosocial Assessment Tool (PAT), and determined that the family is at a clinical level of psychosocial distress. After this 30-minute encounter, Dr. Carey noticed a complex interaction between the women. Dr. Carey scored the PAT and wondered if the endorsed stress, relationship conflict, and other family issues may have exacerbated the patient's experience of pain. Since Dr. Carey felt as if she had "just scratched the surface," she recommended that Serena return with Deidra for a longer co-visit that would include the BHS, Dr. Francis.**

confusion about whom to "treat" during the visit and may have been inclined to treat Deidra's pain as well. Often, competing dynamics in the room can derail the original intent of the visit.[26] In 30 minutes, Dr. Carey made a global assessment of the problems and clearly defined next steps. Where does a family-oriented medical provider go from here?

Step 2. Family Education and Support

Family education and support provides patient and family with biopsychosocial-cultural information about the medical or mental health diagnosis in order to explore the implications of the diagnosis, to teach and assist the family in developing new healthy routines and behaviors, and to help establish healthy family norms. Most PCPs, advanced practice nurses, and BHSs are comfortable with educating and supporting families. Nurses, health coaches, care coordinators, and other less well-trained members of the integrated care team may need about four to six hours of training in working with families but do not need to have specific family therapy training.

Family education and support (Step 2) is appropriate for patients who are experiencing a new health diagnosis or a change in their health status, are having difficulty adjusting to a medical regimen, are trying to make a health or lifestyle change, are having adjustment concerns, or need help developing their advance directives or health care proxies. These concerns can be identified by the patient or the medical provider or through a screening process. Step 2 focuses on family-centered screening, family inclusion in health and behavioral interventions, and family education and support.

Family-Centered Screening

As part of this step, reviewing family screening and assessment tools can help the integrated team in their preliminary plan for the family. Since the early 1980s family screening tools have been found to be effective in identifying and quantifying family functioning. These tools include the Family Apgar[27] and the McMaster Family Assessment Device (FAD).[28] The Family Apgar is a 5-item measure of perceived family support in the domains of adaptation, partnership, growth, affection, and resolve. The FAD assesses six domains of family functioning[29] (problem solving, communication, roles, affective responsiveness, affective involvement, and behavior control). The original 60-item self-report measure that operationalized the McMaster Model of Family Functioning now has a validated 12-item form that measures general functioning and is easier to administer in a busy clinical setting.[30]

Family Education and Support Session

This second visit with the Jay family was longer and focused on behavioral health interventions that impacted every member of the family. Ideally, the second visit is a joint visit, or co-consultation, "teamlet" which, includes both the medical provider and the BHS.

Team Huddle

The medical provider and the BHS should have a short huddle before they enter the room with the family. In the huddle, the providers have five goals:

1. To establish the purpose of the family education and needed supports, and to consider possible interventions. In the case of the Jay family, the integrated team prepared to explore all systemic, biopsychosocial-cultural variables that contribute to pain.
2. To define each provider's role. The PCP and BHS would share responsibility for obtaining any information that each may need to make a family assessment and alliance and form a treatment plan.
3. To identify in the patient and family Prochaska's stage of change[31] or Rollnick's[32] assessment of the patient's interest or motivation to change.
4. To create and define treatment goals and engage in patient-led discussion to identify treatment goals and next steps.
5. To guide "teach-back" by encouraging the patient to discuss his or her understanding of the plan.

Family Interventions: Education and Support

Member of an integrated care team can receive four-to six hours of family therapy in-service training (as needed) provided by a trained family therapist. Family education and support principles outlined by William McFarlane, MD,[33] include providing illness education and a supportive environment that allows family members to express their feelings, frustrations, and difficulties when their family member has a mental illness.

Two examples of effective family education and support programs for pain are as follows:

1. A three-week *spouse-assisted coping skills training program* for management of cancer pain.[34] Patients who received this intervention had significant improvements in pain coping and self-efficacy compared with controls.
2. An *osteoarthritis couple-oriented education/ support intervention.*[35] In this five-session intervention, the spouse practices cognitive or behavioral pain-management strategies (e.g., managing fatigue, effective strategies for requesting spousal assistance, and providing spousal assistance). Patients in this family education and support program experienced more support and less punishing responses from spouses compared with the controls. Patients also had reduced pain severity and depressive symptomatology and enhanced self-efficacy in managing pain.

Short-term family education and support interventions are effective for many chronic illnesses (e.g., diabetes,[36,37] multiple sclerosis[38]).

Research demonstrates that family members' beliefs about pain are related to pain adjustment and treatment outcomes of the patient. Spousal pain beliefs about disability, emotion, control, and medication are significantly correlated with partners' pain severity and other indicators of pain adjustment.[39] Parental management of a child with functional abdominal pain, for example, can be taught with an intervention of three sessions of family education and support and brief cognitive-behavioral therapy.[40]

Box 27.3 gives an example of family education and support (Step 2) for the Jay family.

Treatment Plan

Patient (Serena's) Concern #1: Pain Management

Serena stated that she believes that having satisfying work would serve as a positive distraction from her pain. She has enjoyed work in the past and believes that it provided her with purpose and reduced her financial stress. She asserted that her marijuana use had become a problem since she couldn't abstain for any significant period of time without feeling more pain or excessive irritability. Her goals included using medical marijuana when pain flares to 9 or above on a pain scale. She planned to discontinue daily use of marijuana. Serena believed that chronic marijuana use was making her depression worse. An obstacle preventing abstinence was that her family members used marijuana daily. Serena planned to learn how to modulate and monitor her pain accurately using

BOX 27.3

THE JAY FAMILY, STEP 2: FAMILY EDUCATION AND SUPPORT

Dr. Francis, the BHS, asked the family to complete two screening tools prior to their appointment: the Family Assessment Device (FAD), which assesses general family functioning, and the Patient Health Questionaire-9 (PHQ-9),[41] which screens for depression. The Jay family's scores can be seen in Table 27.2.

Dr. Carey and Dr. Francis took turns asking questions. Dr. Carey asked questions about the medication and side effects. She also noticed tension and disagreement between mother and daughter. The patient and her daughter agreed that they struggle in their relationship with one another and admitted that they fought often, felt depressed, used marijuana daily, and battled constant pain. Dr. Carey asked about prior success with antidepressant medications and pain management. Dr. Francis asked the family about the connection between stress and pain.

They came to the consensus that the primary goal for both Serena and Deidra was to better manage their pain. They offered four to six family education and support sessions, delivered by Dr. Francis, the BHS, to manage their experience of pain and to focus on learning to communicate calmly and respectfully.

Serena and Deidra agreed to meet with Dr. Carey regularly to monitor their pain and the impact of the new exercise regimen and physical therapy. The family barriers to change were a long history of dependence on opioid medication and economic stressors. Their strengths included a family belief that engaging in this plan together would be more effective than doing this alone.

The medical team believed that the patients' understanding of the visit and the treatment plan was the most important element to assess and discuss during the final few minutes of the visit. Therefore, they engaged in a teach-back portion of the visit so providers could check for possible misunderstandings and miscommunications. Both women clearly expressed their understanding of the plan.

Dr. Carey refilled the pain medication with the plan to reduce the dosage in four weeks. At that time, the PCP and BHS conferred with one another about the family's progress toward their identified goals.

body-centered exercises and learning mindfulness-based techniques. These two skills would help her to increase distress tolerance and decrease catastrophic thinking. Additionally, she would meet with the BHS for four to six family education and support sessions. Finally, she would engage with physical therapy to practice strengthening exercises and learn to move in ways that protected her lower back.

What Happened Here with the Jay Family?

In this visit, both providers were using their different skills and training to ask questions and gather data. As a result, they generated two different diagnostic hypotheses: One is medical and the other is a diagnosis of the family dynamics. The pre-visit huddle set the agenda and enabled collaboratively developed treatment recommendations for the patient and family, using the skillsets of both providers and the family. Providers are more satisfied when health professionals are working together towards patient goals and when patients routinely have access to comprehensive services.[42] Patients are grateful that their families are involved.

In this encounter, the assessment measures provided concrete, quantitative data regarding family functioning, as detailed in Table 27.2.

The FAD provided information that the communication style and roles within the Jay family were not satisfying or functional for either woman. Serena scored a 2.1 and Deidra scored a 2.2 on the general functioning subscale, which indicated that they were both in the family dysfunctional range. The PHQ-9, offered to both patients, indicated that they both struggled with moderate to severe levels of depression: Serena scored a 20 while Deidra scored a 14. While this visit had tremendous value

TABLE 27.2 JAY FAMILY SCORES

Measure	Ranges	Serena	Deidra
Patient Health Questionnaire (PHQ-9): brief self-report depression screening: nine-question form[41]	Minimal depression 0–4 Mild depression 5–9 Moderate depression 10–14 Moderately severe depression 15–19 Severe depression 20–27	20	14
Family Assessment Device (FAD)[28]: The short FAD assesses general family functioning.	General Functioning scale over 2 = dysfunction	2.1	2.2

and encouraged further clarity, there was undoubtedly more focused work that could be done with this family. In fact, the family asked to continue in treatment and was eager to begin.

Step 3. Family Systems Therapy

Family systems therapy (FST) is used to identify family structure and dynamics with the goal of modifying family dysfunction and reinforcing adaptive functioning. Some BHSs will come to an integrated care environment with sufficient family therapy training. If no one in the practice has FST capability, the BHS can obtain training from a family therapist, which typically takes 1 to 2 years. If having someone in the practice with FST is not possible, then families in need of FST should be referred out.

FST highlights family patterns of behavior and generational themes and provides options for solving problems and changing family dynamics. Family well-being and couple well-being are linked to adults' mental and physical health.[43] Improving the quality of the family relationships has large health benefits. FST helps families identify aspects of the illness they can control, find a sense of communion, adapt, and overtly recognize that an illness can act as a new and unwanted family member.[44] For instance, illness may act as a "new family member" as it asserts influence over the family, may direct family activities (e.g., how often the family can leave the house), and may be the target of family emotion and hostility.

FST Is Effective

FST is effective for a broad range of medical illnesses. In a meta-analysis,[45] an FST was defined as

> any couple, family, group, multifamily group, or individual focused therapeutic intervention that refers to any one of the following systems-oriented authors (Anderson, Boszormeny-Nagy, de Shazer, Haley, Minuchin, Satir, Selvini-Palazzoli, Stierlin, Watzlawick, White, Zuk) or specified the intervention by use of at least one of the following terms: systemic, structural, strategic, tri-generational, triadic, paradoxical/Milan, functional, solution-focused, narrative, resource/ strength oriented, McMaster model.

Using this definition, 38 randomized controlled trials were included in a meta-analysis, which revealed the efficacy of FST.[45] Three other studies showed that patients benefitted from receiving FST: (1) FST reduced chronic pain patient and psychological distress,[46] (2) after orthopedic surgery, patients receiving FST improved adaptation and returned to work sooner,[47] and (3) breast cancer patients receiving FST showed less acute postoperative anxiety and depression.[48] A meta-analysis of 52 randomized controlled trials[49] found higher effect sizes for FST/relationship-focused interventions compared to educational interventions. An earlier 2004 meta-analysis[50] also found that FST reduced family members' burden of depression and anxiety but only marginally improved patient outcomes. This meta-analysis was not limited to FST and included family education and support interventions.

The same authors examined couples interventions in 2010, again including family education and support interventions.[14] They found benefits to patients and partners in one-third of the studies. FST is also effective for improving health behaviors such as smoking cessation and is helpful for couples with chronic health difficulties.[51]

Jay Family, Step 3

Of relevance to the Jay family are the FST studies on chronic pain and distress. In a controlled, prospective study of couples therapy for patients with chronic low back pain, Saarijärvi[46] found that marital communication improved in 56 patients in couples therapy but worsened in the control group. Couples therapy consisted of five sessions over 5 months. Outcome measures were self-reported psychological distress, marital satisfaction, health locus of control, pain and disability, as well as clinical examinations. At five-year follow-up, psychological distress was found to be decreased in the treatment group and increased in controls. The difference between the groups was significant ($p = .005$). A significant difference between the treatment group and controls was observed in measures of depression, anxiety, hostility, and obsessive-compulsive scores. Emotional distress is a major obstacle to rehabilitation in patients with chronic pain. FST facilitates care by improving family well-being.

The BHS asked the Jay family to commit to four to six sessions with the purpose of reducing family conflict at home and increasing positive communication. Box 27.4 describes the FST the Jay family received. FST occurred in conjunction with occasional co-visits with the PCP. Serena and Deidra believed that a better relationship would reduce anxiety and pain flares.

Treatment Plan

Patient (Serena's) Concern #1: Pain Management

Serena stated that she would like to learn to communicate more effectively in order to reduce the arguments that precede pain flares. Her motivation to learn these skills included her connection to three-year-old Haven and her deep desire to be an excellent grandparent. She was worried about her ability to communicate differently because she became so emotionally overwhelmed when she felt disrespected by her daughter. She agreed to learn and implement breathing and relaxation exercises, use a time-out technique, and establish family ground rules.

Patient (Serena's) Concern #2: Sleep

Serena stated that poor sleep quality had contributed to her pain for many years. Her goal was to sleep eight hours a night and wake up feeling rested. To accomplish this goal, she decided not to drink coffee or watch television in bed. Sleep was also

BOX 27.4

THE JAY FAMILY, STEP 3: FAMILY SYSTEM THERAPY

During the first FST session with the family therapist, they all agreed to focus on increasing positive and effective communication. They practiced a structured communication skill-building technique, alternately listening to each other and then paraphrasing what they heard the other person say. They also talked about their emotional involvement and their roles in the family system. Serena believed that she was the caretaker but that she often felt overwhelmed and taken for granted. Deidra believed that she was the peacekeeper because her sisters "used" their mother and they all fought about money and equity in the family. Given the roles that each of the women played, they brainstormed ideas that would help create peace at home. They made ground rules for facilitating effective communication and listed them on a piece of paper that they attached to the refrigerator. The other family members, who were not present, were allowed to add to the ground rules or negotiate changes.

The therapy also focused on the sleep patterns of both women. Serena and Deidra had a hard time falling asleep and staying asleep, and experienced early waking. At this session, the BHS used a sleep-action plan, a one-page guide that helped the family identify concrete goals, to help them modify their sleep patterns.

Serena and Deidra endorsed significant symptoms of depression. They believed that unemployment and financial stress made these symptoms worse. They also acknowledged a biological propensity to depression and anxiety since it runs in their family.

difficult because her family members worked different shifts and were awake at night. To be successful, Serena also agreed to use pre-bed rituals and a white noise machine.

Patient (Serena's) Concern #3: Depression

Serena stated that she would like to feel calmer and happier. Haven and the family dog provided relaxation and joy. There is a strong family history of biologically based depression and anxiety that makes her need for treatment important. She decided that her family will walk the dog once a day and she will personally engage in a special activity (with Haven) once a week. Serena agreed to attend a pain management support group at a local church. She found this church tremendously uplifting and encouraging.

What Happened Here with the Jay Family?

During FST (Step 3) both women struggled with how change would impact them personally and their relationship. The Jay family had barriers to the family changing and becoming healthier. Serena had decided that her pain medication use was the biggest obstacle to being happy. She wanted to reduce her dependence on narcotic medication. Deidra had not accepted that her medications were a "habit" and believed they were medically necessary. She felt annoyed at times that her mother expected her to behave exactly as she did. She thought that her injury from the car accident was much different from her mother's fibromyalgia diagnosis. In family therapy, their medical diagnoses became differentiators rather than unifiers. This is important because even though they shared similar physical experiences, they judged each other harshly for the way they responded to pain. Each of the women was given an opportunity to describe her triggers, her needs, and how she received respite. With an increased understanding, each of the women identified that she could allow the other person to develop healthier behaviors without feeling betrayed.

OUR MODEL: IMPLEMENTATION AND CHALLENGES

Implementing the three-step model requires effort and commitment from the entire medical team. As a start, an educational retreat may orient the integrated team to the benefits of family inclusion and the evidence-based research that supports the three-step model. Family-centered care can be normalized by displaying posters in the clinic portraying families in exam rooms and by providing family materials after the visit that highlight how to best support the patient's health goals. In the waiting room, patients and family members can watch educational videos on health and wellness. A clinic "Family Day" can communicate that families are welcome by inviting families into the practice for educational programming and social events.

Significant challenges remain to implementing family-centered care. Families have innate powers to produce change but can often be the largest and most impactful barrier to health.[52] For example, while the doctor can recommend a diet that is lower in carbohydrates and sodium for a diabetic patient, and the patient agrees, the spouse may continue to prepare traditional foods that are not ideal for diabetics. Competing family obligations can result in patients and family members "forgetting" appointments. Family members may also inadvertently contribute to misinformation about the patient's health when they use web-based resources that contradict the family member's diagnosis or recommendation for treatment.

Perhaps most importantly, family-centered care advances the Institute of Healthcare Improvement's Triple Aim:[53] improving the patient experience of care, improving the health of populations, and reducing the per capita cost of health care. Our three-step model supports the Triple Aim by improving the patient experience and the range of health services in an integrated health care system.[54] More specifically, family-centered care facilitates more effective teamwork in the diagnostic and treatment process among health care professionals, patients, and their families. The Institute of Medicine's recent report "Improving Diagnosis"[55] calls patients' families "critical partners in the diagnostic process." Integrated care hinges on successful collaboration among health care professionals, patients, and their families.

CONCLUSION

Our three-step model guides any primary care or specialty clinic on best practice for the inclusion of the patient's family in medical and behavioral health care. Although this chapter addresses the use of the three-step model in a primary care setting, the basic principles also apply to specialty settings. Family inclusion and family support and education (Steps 1 and 2) can be applied easily in any integrated care environment. Implementing FST (Step 3) may require a clinician specifically trained in FST, or these families may need to be referred out of the practice.

BOX 27.5
SUMMARY OF RECOMMENDED TREATMENT APPROACHES AND RELEVANT EVIDENCE

Strength of recommendation taxonomy (SOR A, B, or C)

- **"Thinking family" during routine appointments and routine screening, from the front desk to the exam room, improves adherence to the medical plan. (SOR A)[7]**
- **Family education and support should be provided for families experiencing health concerns, mental health concerns, or family transitions. This may take the form of brief psychoeducation or family education about health conditions. (SOR A)[13,14,32,33,36,46]**
- **Family systems therapy is effective for treating relational concerns and family conflict, such as marital distress. (SOR A)[14,41,45,46]**
- **Family systems therapy is effective in improving patient outcomes such as substance use, obesity, depression, and diabetes. (SOR B)[14,45,46]**

The full vision of including the family as a basic unit of care in our current health system is still ahead of us. However, the inclusion of the family in the patient-centered medical home can provide the impetus for bringing families into primary care.[56] The three-step model is compatible with other family-centered integrated care models. There are reasons for optimism as we reflect on the benefits for patients, families, and care teams. These include greater health outcomes, greater satisfaction, and increases in positive communication. Family members routinely express interest in talking with providers about how to help their relatives change unhealthy behaviors and support health but also mention that they do not attend medical visits.[57] When they do attend, the visit includes a significant increase in patient questions and discussion about preventive services.[58] Further, there is the belief that integrated health care facilitates the delivery of the "right care, at the right time, in the right place" and avoids more costly care, to the patients and families, later on.[59] We hope that these changes in primary care show the way for family involvement for all medical specialties. A summary of evidence-based treatment approaches for family inclusion in medical and behavioral health care is found in Box 27.5.

REFERENCES

1. Kocher R, Emanuel E, DeParle N. The Affordable Care Act and the future of clinical medicine: The opportunities and challenges. Ann Intern Med. 2010;153(8):536–539.
2. Bradley EH, Taylor LA. The American Health Care Paradox: Why Spending More Is Getting Us Less. Philadelphia: Public Affairs; 2013.
3. Kwan BM, Nease D. The state of the evidence for integrated behavioral health. In: Talen MR, Valeras AB, eds. Essentials of Integrated Care: Connecting Systems of Care, Clinical Practice and Evidence-Based Approaches. New York: Springer Science Business Media; 2013:65–98.
4. Lurie IZ, Manheim LM, Dunlop DD. Differences in medical care expenditures for adults with depression compared to adults with major chronic conditions. J Ment Health Policy. 2009;12(2): 87–95.
5. Fox M, Hodgson JL, Lamson AL. Integration: Opportunities and challenges for family therapists in primary care. Contemp Fam Ther. 2012;34(2):228–243.
6. Carsten J. Cultures of Relatedness. New York: Cambridge University Press; 2000.
7. DiMatteo M. Social support and patient adherence to medical treatment: A meta-analysis. Health Psychol. 2004;23(2):207–218.
8. Taylor-Brown S, Rosenberg T, McDaniel S. Chronic illness and primary care: Integrating mental health and primary care. In: Talley RC, Fricchione GL, Druss BG. Eds. The Challenges of Mental Health Caregiving. New York, NY: Springer; 2014;55–79.
9. Bray J, Frank R, McDaniel S, Heldring M. Education, practice, and research opportunities for psychologists in primary care. In: Frank R, McDaniel S, Bray J, Heldring M, eds. Primary Care Psychology. Washington, DC: American Psychological Association; 2004:3–21.
10. deGruy F. Mental health care in the primary care setting. In: Donaldson MS, Yordy KD, Lohr KN, Vaneslow NA, eds. Primary Care: America's Health in a New Era. Washington, DC: National Academy Press; 1996:285–311.

11. Gatchel RJ, Oordt M. Clinical Health Psychology and Primary Care: Practical Advice and Clinical Guidance for Successful Collaboration. Washington, DC: American Psychological Association; 2003.
12. Ebbeling C, Antonelli R. Primary care interventions for pediatric obesity: Need for an integrated approach. Pediatrics. 2015;135(4):757–758
13. Fals-Stewart W, Lam W. Brief behavioral couples therapy for drug abuse: A randomized clinical trial examining clinical efficacy and cost-effectiveness. Fam Syst Health. 2008;26(4):377–392.
14. Martire L, Schultz R, Helgeson V, Small B, Saghafi E. Review and meta-analysis of couple-oriented interventions for chronic illness. Ann Behav Med. 2010;40(3):325–340.
15. Shields N, Finley M, Chawla N, Meadors M. Couple and family interventions in health problems. J Marital Fam Ther. 2012;38(1):265–280.
16. Wood N, Crane D, Schaalje G, Law D. What works for whom: A meta-analytic review of marital and couples therapy in reference to marital distress. Am J Fam Ther. 2005;33(4):273–287.
17. Robinson P, Reiter J. Behavioral Consultation and Primary Care: A Guide to Integrating Services. New York: Springer; 2007.
18. Marlowe D, Hodgson J, Lamson A. White M, Irons T. Medical Family Therapy in Integrated Primary Care: An Interactional Framework. In Hodgson J, Lamson A, Mendenhall T, Crane DR. eds. Medical Family Therapy. New York: Springer International Publishing; 2014.
19. Mitnick S, Leffler C, Hood VL. American College of Physicians. Ethics, Professionalism and Human Rights Committee. Family caregivers, patients and physicians: Ethical guidance to optimize relationships. J Gen Intern Med. 2010;25(3):255–260.
20. Schulz R, Beach SR. Caregiving as a risk factor for mortality: The caregiver health effects study. JAMA. 1999; 282(23):2215–2219.
21. Heru AM. Working with Families in Medical Settings. New York: Routledge; 2013:109–129.
22. Heru AM. Family-centered care in the outpatient general psychiatry clinic. J Psychiatr Pract. 2015;21(5):381–388.
23. Woods SB, Priest JB, Denton W. Tell me where it hurts: Assessing mental and relational health in primary care using a biopsychosocial assessment intervention. Fam J Alex Va. 2015;23(2):109–119.
24. National Cancer Care Network. Distress Thermometer. http://www.nccn.org/patients/resources/life_with_cancer/pdf/nccn_distress_thermometer.pdf.
25. Kazak AE, Schneider S, Didonato S, Pai AL. Family psychosocial risk screening guided by the Pediatric Psychosocial Preventative Health Model (PPPHM) using the Psychosocial Assessment Tool (PAT). Acta Oncol. 2015;54(5):574–580.
26. McDaniel SH, Campbell TL, Hepworth J, Lorenz A. Family-Oriented Primary Care. 2nd ed. New York: Springer; 2005.
27. Mengel M. The use of the family APGAR in screening for family dysfunction in a family practice center. Am J Manag Care. 2011;17(2):105–113.
28. Mansfield AK, Keitner GI, Dealy J. The family assessment device: An update. Fam Process. 2015;54(1):82–93.
29. Epstein NB, Baldwin LM, Bishop DS. J Marital Fam Ther. 1983;9(2):171–180.
30. Boterhoven de Haan KL, Hafekost J, Lawrence D, Sawyer MG, Zubrick SR. Reliability and validity of a short version of the General Functioning Subscale of the McMaster Family Assessment Device. Fam Process. 2015;54(1):116–123. doi:10.1111/famp.12113.
31. Prochaska JO, Redding CA, Evers KE. The transtheoretical model and stages of change. In: Glanz K, Lewis FM, Rimer BK, eds. Health Behavior and Health Education: Theory Research and Practice. 2nd ed. San Francisco: Jossey Bass; 1997.
32. Rollnick S, Miller WR. What is motivational interviewing? Behav Cogn Psychother. 1995;23(4):325–334.
33. Macfarlane W. Family education and support workbook. http://www.nebhands.nebraska.edu/files/FamPsy_Workbook.pdf. Accessed September 29, 2015.
34. Keefe FJ, Ahles TA, Sutton L, et al. Partner-guided cancer pain management at the end of life: A preliminary study. J Pain Symptom Manage. 2005;29(3):263–272.
35. Keefe FJ, Caldwell DS, Baucom D, et al. Spouse-assisted coping skills training in the management of knee pain in osteoarthritis: Long-term follow-up results. Arthritis Care Res. 1999;12(2):101–111.
36. Keogh KM, Smith SM, White P, et al. Psychological family intervention for poorly controlled type 2 diabetes. Fam Pract. 1987;24(4):394–398.
37. Katz ML, Volkening LK, Butler DA, Anderson BJ, Laffel LM. Family-based family education and support and care ambassador intervention to improve glycemic control in youth with type 1 diabetes: A randomized trial. Pediatr Diabetes. 2013;15(2):142–150.
38. Schwartz CE. Teaching coping skills enhances quality of life more than peer support: Results of a randomized trial with multiple sclerosis patients. Health Psychol. 1999;18(3):211–220.
39. Cano A, Miller LR, Loree A. Spousal beliefs about partner chronic pain. J Pain. 2009;10(5):486–492.
40. Levy RL, Langer SL, Walker LS, et al. Cognitive behavioral therapy for children with functional abdominal pain and their parents decreases pain and other symptoms. Am J Gastroenterol. 2010;105(4):946–956.

41. Kroenke K, Spitzer RL, Williams JB. The PHQ-9: Validity of a brief depression severity measure. Gen Intern Med. 2001;16(9):606–613.
42. Vickers KS, Ridgeway JL, Hathaway JC, Egginton JS, Kaderlik AB, Katzelnick DJ. Integration of mental health resources in a primary care setting leads to increased provider satisfaction and patient access. Gen Hosp Psychiat. 2013;35(5):461–467.
43. Woods SB, Denton W. The biobehavioral family model as a framework for examining the connections between family relationships, mental, and physical health for adult primary care patients. Fam Syst Health. 2014;32(2):235–240.
44. Ruddy NB, McDaniel S. Medical family therapy in the age of health care reform. Couple Family Psychol. 2013;2(3):179–191.
45. Von Sydow K, Beher S, Schweitzer J, Retzlaff R. The efficacy of systemic therapy: A meta-analysis of 38 randomized controlled trials. Fam Process. 2010;49(4):457–485.
46. Saarijärvi S, Alanen E, Rytokoski U, Hyyppa MT. Couple therapy improves mental well-being in chronic low back pain patients. A controlled, five-year follow-up study. J Psychosom Res. 1992;36(7):651–656.
47. Cockburn JT, Thomas FN, Cockburn OJ. Solution-focused therapy and psychosocial adjustment to orthopedic rehabilitation in a work hardening program. J Occ Rehabil.1977;7(2):97–106.
48. Hu D, Wu H, Dong Y, Chen D, Li Y, Hu L. Study on the effect of family therapy on social support and mental status in peri-operative patients with breast cancer. J Nurs Admin. 2007;7(9): 9–11.
49. Hartmann M, Bäzner E, Wild B, Eisler I, Herzog W. Effects of interventions involving the family in the treatment of adult patients with chronic physical diseases: A meta-analysis. Psychother Psychosom. 2010;79(3):136–148. doi:10.1159/000286958.
50. Martire LM, Lustig AP, Schulz R, Miller GE, Helgeson VS. Is it beneficial to involve a family member? A meta-analysis of psychosocial interventions for chronic illness. Health Psychol. 2004;23(6):599–611.
51. Rohrbaugh MJ, Shoham V, Skoyen JA, Jensen M, Mehl MR. We-Talk, communal coping, and cessation success in a couple-focused intervention for health-compromised smokers. Fam Process. 2012;51(1):107–121.
52. Cherrington A. Developing a family-based diabetes program for Latino immigrants: Do men and women face the same barriers? Fam Community Health. 2011;34(4):280–290.
53. Triple aim. http://www.ihi.org/engage/initiatives/TripleAim/Pages/default.aspx.
54. Miller B, Brown-Levey S, Payne-Murphy J, Kwan BM. Outlining the scope of behavioral health practice in integrated primary care: Dispelling the myth of the one-trick mental health pony. Fam Syst Health. 2014;32(3):338–343.
55. Institute of Medicine. Improving Diagnosis. http://iom.nationalacademies.org/~/media/Files/Report%20Files/2015/Improving-Diagnosis/DiagnosticError_ReportBrief.pdf. Accessed October 1, 2015.
56. Blount A. Donald Bloch's vision, CFHA history, and the future. Fam Syst Health. 2015;33(2): 102–110.
57. Hirsch JK, Walker KL, Wilkinson RB, Lyness JM. Family criticism and depressive symptoms in older adult primary care patients: Optimism and pessimism as moderators. Am J Geriat Psychiat. 2014;22(6):632–635.
58. Katerndahl D, Parchman M. Effects of family presence on the content and dynamics of the clinical encounter among diabetic patients. J Eval Clin Pract. 2013;19(6):1067–1072.
59. Bazemore A, Petterson S, Peterson L, Phillips RL. More comprehensive care among family physicians is associated with lower costs and few hospitalizations. Ann Fam Med. 2015;13(3):206–213.

28

Group Interventions in Integrated Care Settings

BRIAN ROTHBERG AND HILLARY D. LUM

BOX 28.1
KEY POINTS

- **Group interventions in medical settings can provide patient education and support, resulting in improved patient outcomes.**
- **Group interventions can treat diverse patient populations in integrated care settings or specialty practices and in community-based settings.**
- **Group interventions can focus on education and treatments for a variety of acute or chronic illnesses and life stages, or in support of surgical/medical procedures.**
- **Training of group facilitators is a critical component of implementing group interventions; all team members should demonstrate basic competency in running groups.**
- **Both clinicians and patients benefit from the longer group formats that are typical for group interventions.**

INTRODUCTION

Thomas Mann's novel *The Magic Mountain*[1] begins in the early 1900s at a tuberculosis (TB) sanatorium in an idyllic mountain valley in the Swiss Alps. The patients, from very wealthy families from around the world, are receiving state-of-the-art forms of treatment for TB at that time: a significant amount of rest, fresh air, sleeping outdoors, and nutritional support. Although the ingredients for the treatment were straightforward, the fees at the sanatoriums were high and the residential stays could last several months to years.

Around the same time, Dr. Joseph Hersey Pratt was working with real TB patients in an ambulatory setting in Boston, MA. His patients, from poorer backgrounds, could not pay for extravagant sanatorium care. They were often family breadwinners who chose to forgo treatment in order to continue working. Also, many patients were too sick to be admitted to the sanatoriums. To offer these patients another way to access treatment, Dr. Pratt formed the Emmanuel Church Tuberculosis Class, which taught practical underpinnings of TB treatment that could be used in the person's home. He found that the class format saved time and later noted that the "membership is of widely different races and different sects, they have a common bond in a common disease. A fine spirit of camaraderie has been developed."[2]

Group psychotherapy slowly evolved as a therapeutic modality, predominantly within behavioral health clinical settings, and came to the forefront of treatment during World War II. Treatment groups were developed for the large influx of soldiers presenting with emotional injuries from the war. The success of these treatments showed promise that group interventions might serve as efficacious and efficient mainstream behavioral health treatments. Despite their successes in TB treatment, for many decades group interventions within general medicine and other nonpsychiatric medical specialties were rarely included in treatment protocols.

The tide began to shift in the early 1990s when John Scott, MD, initiated the first group medical visit model, called the Cooperative Health Care Clinic (CHCC), within Kaiser Permanente.[3] This model of care adopted many lessons learned from the group psychotherapy literature, adapted to meet the needs of patients in primary care settings. In prototypical group interventions 10 to 15 patients with a common medical condition, such as diabetes mellitus, meet and discuss ways to improve disease management and quality of life. Since the early 1990s, diverse primary and specialty medical settings have incorporated many novel and creative group interventions. The American Academy of Family Physicians recognizes group interventions as an important model of care within the patient-centered medical home.[4]

The use of group interventions in medical care appears to be increasing in small group practices, large academic medical centers, and especially integrated health care systems. The evidence base for their utility is expanding rapidly. Groups help patients achieve patient- and disease-centered outcomes through peer-to-peer support, increasing time with providers, and increasing self-efficacy through education. Patients can be educated on a variety of subjects efficiently and effectively in groups through the cross-pollination of ideas and emotional support. These group experiences provide mutual enrichment for patients and health care team members. Box 28.1 reviews some of the key points for utilizing group in medical settings.

GROUP THEORY

The clinician's role in applying group theory to clinical settings has been explored extensively in the group psychotherapy literature. One important milestone involved understanding groups as functioning units beyond the individual members, often referred to as group dynamics or group-as-a-whole. For example, groups demonstrate common stages of development (e.g., dependence, counter-dependence, interdependence)[5] in relation to power and authority figures, and groups have specific tasks or goals.[6] Groups can become derailed by different processes, such as overdependence upon or rebellion against the leader. These observations have helped clinicians design interventions to impact the group-as-a-whole, in addition to interventions aimed at individual members. These techniques can address the unique culture of each group and its predictable developmental stages, or the leader's emotional reactions to group processes. One particularly helpful concept for groups is the phenomenon of scapegoating.[7] Instead of focusing the leader's attention solely on a "problematic" patient in the group, scapegoating refocuses attention to the potential role the patient is serving for others in the group. For example, an overly talkative member may serve a "role" to help quieter members not have to talk. The general tendency of group facilitators is to try to quiet the talkative member, but the scapegoating concept redirects the facilitator to encourage quieter members to participate themselves *and* also to have the more talkative member elicit participation of the quieter members.

Clinicians should apply a few basic ingredients to all group interventions to create a supportive, educational, and ultimately therapeutic environment as shown in Table 28.1. These ingredients are necessary to develop a sense of safety in the group, which is vital for healing to take place. The work of groups, such as imparting information,[7] is more efficient and effective when the group members experience emotional safety, share commonalities with other members, and participate voluntarily. A clear group contract is critical for the group to function at its highest level. The group contract will contain many of the "basic ingredients" described in Table 28.1, including commitments to confidentiality and visit frequency. The contract sets the boundaries of the group, such as start and end times. The leader must adhere to the negotiated parameters to provide the safest environment. Confidentiality is usually set prior to the start of the group or at the first session so that group members do not share protected health information outside of the group meeting.

Clinicians benefit from the longer amounts of time spent with patients. Group discussions promote time for building rapport and understanding unique patient experiences beyond disease processes. Clinicians are able to actively promote peer-to-peer learning among group members, including sharing of challenges and successes from group members' personal experiences that may serve to motivate and support other members. In the group intervention setting, clinicians are not the only "experts" but instead can encourage patients to share and build on their own successes.

THERAPEUTIC FACTORS OF GROUPS

The experience of illness and infirmity is often an isolating process that can lead to intense feelings of vulnerability, anxiety, loneliness, and demoralization.[8]

TABLE 28.1 BASIC COMPONENTS AND STRUCTURE OF GROUP INTERVENTIONS

	Overview	Example
Purpose	Improve patient, disease, or health care utilization outcomes through education and/or support	• Improved quality of life and greater self-efficacy in the elderly
Number of members	Based on purpose and physical space	• 8–12 patients
Confidentiality	Open sharing dependent upon feelings of safety	• Confidentiality agreements signed at the start
Patient population	Individuals voluntarily participate in group setting around common medical issues	• Older adults • Diabetes or other chronic conditions • Pregnancy or other women's health issues
Setting	Receptive health care system	• Accountable care organizations • Health maintenance organizations • Patient-centered medical home • Sponsored by community organizations
Visit interval and content	Based on purpose. Topics may be determined by group facilitators with input from patients.	• Weekly • Monthly • Quarterly
Time and format	Based on purpose. May include individual clinical visits to address specific needs.	• 60–180 minutes
Staffing	Team members from multiple disciplines	• Physician • Advanced practice nurse • Physician assistant • Psychologist • Nurse • Social workers • Health coaches • Medical assistants • Educators (diabetes, nutrition) • Pharmacists • Volunteers

Physical and behavioral health illnesses, especially the more severe forms, are often marked by estrangements from family members and friends, loss of the ability to work, and overall loss of functionality. Patients may begin to lose hope and become demoralized in the face of increased morbidity. As patients become more isolated and demoralized, they become increasingly unable to comply with treatment recommendations and may have difficulty participating in rehabilitation programs[2] due to perceived futility of such interventions. The opportunity to participate in a group intervention can directly combat isolation and demoralization while simultaneously providing treatment aimed at specific health-related issues. Group therapy involves 11 unique therapeutic factors[7] (Table 28.2) that improve patients' experiences and well-being compared to one-on-one patient–clinician interactions.

One of the most important therapeutic factors is group *cohesion*. Group cohesion was first measured in the late 1940s[9] and was later described as an analog of the patient–provider working alliance described in individual therapy.[7] Cohesive groups give people a sense of belonging, acceptance, and validation, which can help to restore meaning in patients' lives. Other therapeutic factors are *universality*, which reduces the patients' feelings of isolation by showing how their struggles are similar to

TABLE 28.2 THERAPEUTIC FACTORS OF GROUP

Therapeutic Group Factors	Description
Provides hope	Increases patients' belief and confidence in their ability to heal by raising positive expectations and by exposing patients to the improvement of others
Experience shared difficulties (universality)	Reduces patients' feelings of isolation by showing how their struggles are similar to those of other group members. It is a disconfirmation of a patient's feelings of uniqueness.
Imparts information	Offers instruction, advice, suggestions, and direct guidance about diseases and health management principles from clinicians and other group members
Fosters altruism	Enhances well-being through the act of helping others
Corrects bad experiences related to old family conflicts	Offers opportunities to relive and replay early family patterns and traumas with opportunities to enact healthier outcomes
Develops social skills	Enhances basic communications and socializing skills through role playing and direct feedback from others
Fosters healthy imitative behavior	Offers opportunities to learn new healthy behaviors from other members by observation
Promotes interpersonal learning	Improves abilities to express needs, listen to others, tolerate disagreements, and learn other aspects of interpersonal communication and behavior in relationships
Provides positive effects of group membership (group cohesion)	Allows for a group to develop a working alliance that fosters the sense of belonging to, and acceptance and validation by, the group
Offers a safe place for ventilating and emotional release (catharsis)	Encourages the ability to express intense feelings in a supportive environment
Attends to existential factors	Offers supports when considering the meanings of life, morbidity, mortality, suffering, and meaning of attachment. These factors can be especially important to patients with severe medical or psychiatric illnesses and in geriatric populations.

Yalom ID, Leszcz W. The Theory and Practice of Group Psychotherapy. 5th ed. New York: Basic Books; 2005.

those of other group members, and *instillation of hope*. The two concepts were beautifully captured by a group member in a 12-week group for patients with non-epileptic seizures. The member, in reflecting on her experience in the group, stated, "I learned two things that I will take away from this group. The first is that I am not alone [universality]; the second is there is a way out [hope]."

Group medical interventions promote patient education in several ways. Patients learn from the clinician facilitators and also from other patients in the group. This process of learning from other patients is described as *imparting information*. Imparting information is "didactic instruction" about general health principles and "advice, suggestions, or direct guidance from either the clinician or the group members."[7] Table 28.2 lists the other group therapeutic factors.

GROUP INTERVENTIONS IN INTEGRATED CARE SETTINGS

A key feature of group interventions is the amount of time patients spend with clinicians. The typically hurried pace of one-to-one appointments in primary care and specialty settings may constrain meaningful contact with clinicians to very short periods of time, often 15 minutes or less. Group interventions traditionally are scheduled for 90 minutes to two hours, and the clinicians and staff interacting with the group are present for most of the appointment time. Patients can more thoroughly discuss and process information with their clinicians about the interplay of complex medical conditions, current behavioral health concerns, and the impact of medical illness on day-to-day living and overall well-being.

Effective group treatments in primary care or medical-surgical specialty settings can focus on types of illnesses (e.g., diabetes, hypertension), stages of life (e.g., pregnancy, adolescence, geriatrics), preparation for or recovery from surgical procedures (e.g., preoperative assessments, postoperative follow-ups), self-management skills (e.g., dialysis management, medical devices), and behavior change (e.g., smoking cessation, weight loss). Four overarching purposes for group interventions are to provide patient education, provide patient support, foster behavioral change, and teach skills.

Groups that focus on education maximize the extended time with health care providers and employ discussions that include ample time for questions. Topics that are relevant to the group members may include the disease, prognosis, possible illness trajectories, symptoms or side-effect management, and self-management skills, as well as learning how to work with the health care team. For example, a diabetes self-management group intervention may deliver diabetes education in the context of patient goal setting and troubleshooting.[10]

Groups that focus on patient support draw upon each patient's ability to share personal challenges and successes. For example, a geriatric-focused group intervention entitled "Mind, Body, Soul: A Shared Medical Appointment Series in Successful Aging"[11] facilitated patient engagement through a supportive environment where experiences, questions, answers, and solutions were shared.

In addition to emotional support, healthy behaviors can be learned and facilitated through group participation. Group interventions help patients focus on a medical condition, such as diabetes or cardiovascular disease, while they also stimulate discussions about emotional challenges, stressors, coping mechanisms, and practical problem solving related to dealing with acute illness and chronic disease. Clinician facilitators help patients acknowledge, express, and reflect on their emotions and receive acknowledgment and understanding of these struggles. As patients share or hear stories from others in the group, they gain a better understanding of their own illnesses, the realistic aspects of their treatment options, or the potential seriousness of their prognosis. Patients can feel empowered to start or maintain treatment plans in a safe and supportive environment of their peers and group facilitators. Unhealthy behaviors can be reduced or extinguished through education, modeling, and concern from clinicians and peers. Patients may quit smoking tobacco or abstain from drinking alcohol and substitute healthier behaviors to cope with chronic illness.

Groups may teach patients how to set up successful exercise regimens, make important dietary changes, or practice proper sleep hygiene. Also, patients learn new skills, such as using mindfulness exercises to reduce stress or managing medications with a pill box. Disease-specific skills can be taught, such as monitoring blood pressure at home, keeping a food diary, and using insulin.

RECENT AND EMERGING MODELS OF GROUP MEDICAL VISITS

The early modern group medical visit model was developed in 1991 to address the complex needs of older adults.[12] In the initial CHCC, a physician and nurse conducted monthly meetings of 15 to 20 older individuals with multiple medical problems and polypharmacy to address concerns that could not be adequately addressed within the time constraints of conventional office visits. Group interventions were staffed by a medical provider, a behavioral health specialist (e.g., psychologist, licensed clinical social worker), a health coach, an educator such as a nurse, a dietitian, and/or a scribe such as a medical assistant or care coordinator.[13,14] These groups attempted to bring patients together to better engage with challenges related to living with multiple chronic conditions.

Subsequently, group interventions have been developed for multiple populations and types of care, including chronic disease management, subspecialty care, "drop-in" groups for same-day access, and annual physical examinations (e.g., annual Medicare wellness visits). Chronic disease management group interventions are employed for patients with diabetes, hypertension, obesity, and heart failure. Specialty group visits exist related to bariatric surgery, nephrolithiasis, dermatologic issues, and others. The Veterans Health Administration embraces group medical visits as part of several outpatient care teams, with special attention to implementation of group interventions among elderly veterans. Group interventions for veterans related to weight loss, tobacco cessation, and mental health issues (e.g., posttraumatic stress disorders) are well received.[15]

In addition to group interventions in ambulatory settings, a growing number of group interventions occur in community-based settings, sponsored or hosted by community health organizations. Peer-led, community-based groups, in conjunction with traditional medical care, can empower patients to adopt healthy behaviors. Alcoholics Anonymous (AA) and Recovery International are strong models of peer-led groups. Groups such as AA provide supportive environments, but other groups may use confrontational techniques to challenge members to stop abusing substances. Community-based groups often focus on providing support and education around behavioral and social needs related to specific diseases. Examples of these types of groups are listed in Table 28.3. These groups are not specifically facilitated by health care providers who bill insurance, and as such these groups are not reimbursable. The groups may be led by a behavioral health provider or a trained layperson as a peer facilitator. Group interventions may be one-time meetings or serve a group of committed participants over time.

TABLE 28.3 COMMUNITY-BASED GROUP INTERVENTIONS

Type of Group	Example
Behavioral health conditions	Alcoholics Anonymous Posttraumatic stress disorder
Situation-specific	Suicide survivors Spousal loss Bereavement and grief
Role-specific	Caregiver support
Disease-specific	Alzheimer disease Huntington disease Parkinson disease Cancer Cancer survivors

FINANCING GROUP INTERVENTIONS

At present, group interventions that are reimbursable must be conducted by a health care provider. Physicians (except psychiatrists) and advanced practice clinicians can bill through a patient's physical health benefits and must meet evaluation/management (E/M) criteria for the services rendered. The activities and documentation related to the medical services provided in group intervention settings must meet the same criteria as for medical services provided in non-group settings. The service is billed under a diagnosis within the scope of practice for the physician (e.g., an internist or family physician diagnosing diabetes or an oncologist treating breast cancer). Psychiatrists and advanced practice psychiatric nurses can bill E/M services and psychotherapy codes but should submit charges under behavioral health diagnoses (e.g., major depression or generalized anxiety disorder) to the behavioral health carve-out companies. Mental health insurers are typically distinct subcompanies with billing rules that differ from those of insurers of physical health benefits. Psychologists, social workers, and master's-level therapists may bill mental health insurers using psychotherapy codes for behavioral health conditions or can use health and behavioral (H&B) codes that are billed to the insurers of physical health. H&B codes reflect treatment of psychological conditions directly related to chronic health conditions. In practice, H&B codes are less routinely used and may provide low reimbursement.

With changes related to the Affordable Care Act, value-based billing, and increasing emphasis on new payment models (e.g., pay-for-performance, capitation, shared saving and global budgets), group interventions should become more valuable and more easily reimbursable. (See Chapter 6: Financing Integrated Care Models.) These changes in our health care reimbursement systems should make it easier to incorporate groups into routine clinical care in the future.

OUTCOMES OF GROUP INTERVENTIONS

Group interventions can improve patient-oriented, disease-oriented, and health care utilization outcomes, including improving patient and physician satisfaction, quality of care, and quality of life.

Several high-quality randomized controlled trials (RCTs) of group interventions, primarily focusing on geriatric patients with multiple medical conditions or patients with diabetes, have shown improved self-efficacy and self-care practices and increased satisfaction with medical care.[16,17] Additional clinical experience and evidence for group medical visits is based on practice-based interventions, quality-improvement programs, and feasibility studies. The outcomes measured in group interventions vary widely. Taken together, the evidence for group interventions in integrated settings represents a B-level recommendation. B-level recommendations are based on studies of limited-quality patient-oriented evidence, as further described in Box 28.2.[18]

Patient-Oriented Outcomes

Patient-oriented outcomes are those that matter to patients and help them live longer or better lives. Examples include reduced morbidity or mortality, improved symptoms, improved functioning, and improved quality of life. Early RCTs of group interventions involving elderly patients showed better quality of life, greater self-efficacy, and higher overall quality of care.[3,16] These group interventions involved a series of monthly meetings that consisted of a warmup period using reminiscence therapy techniques such as recalling past life events or memories to build rapport and an educational component on a geriatric health-related topic. Next, the health care team reviewed vital signs, recent tests, and need for future medical appointments. Each meeting ended with a question-and-answer period followed by plans for the next meeting. These studies[3,16] reported positive effects on patient experience with group interventions compared with usual care. Both trials reported improvements on overall health status and functional status, but there was no difference compared with usual care for either of these measures. Group interventions for older adults have been expanded to include annual Medicare wellness visits and specific topics of high relevance to older adults, including group interventions to prevent falls, for advance care planning, and for treatment of late-life depression.

In a separate RCT,[17] groups of seven or eight patients with diabetes met every other month with a primary care provider, a pharmacist, and a nurse or certified diabetes educator. Patients had their blood pressures checked and home blood-glucose values reviewed and then attended an educational session delivered by the nurse or educator. The

BOX 28.2
SUMMARY OF RECOMMENDED TREATMENT APPROACHES AND RELEVANT EVIDENCE

Strength of recommendation taxonomy[18] (SOR A, B, or C)

- **Group medical visits for patients with poorly controlled diabetes and hypertension (run by a primary care provider, pharmacist, nurse, or other certified diabetes educator) showed improved blood pressure and no change in hemoglobin A1c at 1 year. (SOR A)[17]**
- **Pharmacist-led group medical visits (offered quarterly at a cardiovascular risk-reduction clinic) for patients with a goal of maintaining guideline-based control of cardiovascular risk factors were successful. Both individual and group interventions maintained glycemic and blood pressure control for patients with diabetes compared to no maintenance intervention at 1 year. (SOR A)[32,33]**
- **An integrative medical group-visit care model for chronic pain combined patient-centered, nonpharmacologic strategies and principles of mindfulness-based stress reduction to reduce pain and associated symptoms. Improved pain, depression score, sleep quality, and perceived stress were reported after eight weeks. (SOR B)[20]**
- **A neurologist- and nurse practitioner-led educational session, as part of a headache management program, followed by a comprehensive individual treatment plan improved migraine-specific symptoms, overall health status, patient satisfaction, and health care utilization at 8 weeks and 6 months. (SOR B)[34]**

patient, pharmacist, and physician then reviewed the patient's diabetes control and developed an individualized plan for medication and/or lifestyle management directed toward improving blood pressure and hemoglobin A1c level (HbA1c). In this trial, patients who participated in the group intervention showed improved self-efficacy, self-care practices, and satisfaction with medical care.[17] Among patients with hypertension and diabetes in this study, higher self-efficacy was one proposed mechanism for improvement in blood pressure control.[17]

A focus group of veterans who attended group interventions was studied to more broadly understand patient-oriented outcomes. They reported that the group dynamics gave them confidence and knowledge to help them achieve their health management goals.[19]

In addition to higher satisfaction with care and improved self-management skills, some group interventions also specifically improve behavioral health outcomes among patients with multiple medical conditions and high symptom burden. For example, Boston Medical Center developed an integrative medical group visit that merges principles of group interventions, evidence-based complementary medicine, and mindfulness-based stress reduction for patients with chronic pain and chronic conditions.[20] Patients who participated in these group interventions experienced decreased pain and depressive symptoms, improvements in sleep quality, and decreased perceived stress. Similarly, Latino adults with diabetes and heart disease risk factors who frequently attended a twice-weekly group had lower levels of depression and loneliness and improved quality-of-life indicators compared to participants with low attendance.[21]

Group interventions have been shown to qualitatively improve patient-centered psychosocial outcomes. A group intervention to support women with a history of breast cancer, as they transitioned to breast cancer survivorship, found that the group intervention enabled participants to share experiences, focus on emotional needs, and have open discussions about cancer recurrence, while increasing confidence in being discharged back to primary care from the oncology clinic and using alternative support services.[22]

Disease-Oriented Outcomes

Disease-oriented outcomes include intermediate, histopathologic, physiologic, or surrogate results (e.g., blood sugar, blood pressure, coronary plaque thickness) that may or may not reflect improvements in patient outcomes. Patients with diabetes have been a frequent target population for group medical visits. A recent systematic review of RCTs and observational studies for group medical visits for patients with diabetes reviewed 13 trials.[23] This meta-analysis found that group medical visits had a positive effect on disease-oriented outcomes, with significant reductions in glycated hemoglobin (HbA1c reduction: 0.46% with a 95% confidence interval [CI] of 0.80% to −0.31%).[23] A similar systematic review of diabetes group medical visits found five studies with improvements in systolic blood pressure (mean difference = −5.2; CI: −7.40 to −3.05) and five studies reporting large improvements in health-related quality of life (standardized mean difference = −0.84; CI: −1.64 to −0.03).[24]

Group interventions are being piloted to improve the care of patients who have serious illnesses and face challenges related to adhering to medical treatment protocols. As an example, a group intervention for patients with hepatitis C infection was developed because these individuals often experience a high burden of psychiatric disease, substance abuse, and/or housing instability. The significant psychosocial challenges often make it difficult for these patients to achieve high levels of medication adherence. A group intervention pilot program for individuals with hepatitis C infection found that group attendance supported antiviral medication adherence and virologic response rates.[25]

Health Care Utilization Outcomes

Group interventions have also been shown to be effective in improving health care utilization outcomes. The RCTs of group interventions for older adults, introduced above, also evaluated the effects of group interventions on health care utilization.[3,16] In a two-year RCT of the CHCC model that aimed to improve the health of elderly patients, attendees of the group intervention had significantly fewer hospital admissions, emergency department visits, and medical specialist visits.[16] The overall cost of care within the health maintenance organization was $41.80 per member per month lower for group intervention participants compared to control group patients. In addition to these utilization outcomes, patients reported higher satisfaction with their primary care physician, felt the physician was less hurried, and reported greater time spent with the physician. An RCT of group visits for patients with diabetes and hypertension showed fewer emergency department and primary care clinic visits compared to patients who were not involved in group visits.[17]

Given the evidence that group interventions can improve patient, disease, and health care utilization outcomes, many integrated care settings may desire to leverage group interventions to improve outcomes for a population of patients through disease-based patient registries. For example, a patient-centered medical home may maintain a diabetes patient registry. The registry could be designed to track disease-oriented factors such as blood pressure, weight, and laboratory tests, as well as symptom or functional impairment such as pain, depression, falls, and self-management ability. Group interventions may be able to target and improve some of these outcomes. By tracking patient outcomes in the patient registry, the practice might find evidence that registry patients who participate in a group intervention have improved outcomes compared to registry patients who are not in a group. Because the use of a patient registry can systematically track patient outcomes over time, these integrated care settings may find new opportunities to integrate group interventions into the care of more of their patient populations through quality-improvement projects.

MAXIMIZING THE POTENTIAL OF MULTIDISCIPLINARY TEAMS

A core requirement for a successful and sustainable group intervention is a high-functioning multidisciplinary team. Each team member has a specific role, and each role is designed to be consistent with the individual's scope of practice. Ongoing team meetings and coordination are important to sustain the effectiveness of group interventions, to foster group dynamics, and to facilitate patient interactions with their various interdisciplinary providers. Group interventions can be staffed by a combination of primary care providers or other medical specialists, psychologists and other behavioral health providers, nurses, care coordinators, medical assistants, pharmacists, social workers, nutritionists, and/or health coaches, whose roles are described in Table 28.4. Several key roles include group facilitation, providing medical care, documenting medical care, and scheduling patient visits. Many groups rely on co-facilitation by trained facilitators who have different backgrounds. The use of facilitators from different disciplines enhances group experience because of the varied perspectives and expertise brought to the group. For example, a diabetes group may be co-facilitated by a physician, pharmacist, nurse, health coach, or diabetes educator. Also, cross-training in groups can allow them to run continuously even when individual clinicians are unavailable for occasional sessions. Groups may improve team members' work satisfaction by adding flexibility in day-to-day clinic operations.

Key characteristics of staff members who successfully conduct group interventions include high levels of interest, availability, and willingness to be trained in group interventions as models of care. Potential facilitators should be familiar with group facilitation skills and should understand the relevant medical, behavioral health, and social needs of the patient population. All team members should demonstrate basic competencies in running groups, such as understanding the different levels of group functioning (intrapersonal, interpersonal, subgroup, and group-as-a-whole) and should possess several verbal interventions for each of the levels. Additional skills include establishing rapport between patients, asking open-ended questions to encourage group sharing of challenges and successes, providing and modeling empathy, and helping patients share group time, with redirection and inclusion of all participants' experiences.

Certain team members may have an interest in more advanced group facilitation training and will find resources through the American Group Psychotherapy Association,[26] the American Psychological Association Division 49,[27] and others.[28–30] Clinicians attending intensive group-training workshops will experience a combination of didactic lectures and experiential exercises. During these trainings, master group clinicians lead experiential exercises giving clinicians the opportunity to become members of a group and to see group facilitation modeled by an expert.

A clinic-based champion is critical for initiating and developing new group interventions. This onsite champion, often a behavioral health specialist, staff supervisor, or clinical team leader, serves as a resource in helping form the new group intervention team and in program development, and should understand local concerns and potential obstacles.[14] The champion plays a crucial role in explaining the benefits of the program to patients and staff and assists with training group facilitators and other clinical staff.

TABLE 28.4 DESCRIPTION OF GROUP INTERVENTION TEAM MEMBER ROLES

Team Member	Role*
Provider (physician, advanced practice nurse, physician assistant)	Takes medical histories, conducts brief examinations, performs assessments, provides group-based and individualized treatment plans
Psychologist or other behavioral health provider (e.g., social worker)	Facilitates discussion of self-care techniques, coping, problem solving, and decision making
Registered nurse, case manager, or care coordinator	Moderates session, facilitates discussions, assists with assessments related to patient- or disease-specific goals
Medical assistant	Registers participants, measures vital signs, assists with visit documentation as a scribe, initiates orders and referrals.
Psychiatrist	Consults with health care team, facilitates groups, educates group members about psychotropic medication and interplay of physical and behavioral health disorders
Health coach	Focuses on lifestyle change, facilitates and supports patient-centered autonomy, supports decisions based on patient values
Patient navigator	Helps patient access and use the health care systems. Could be a peer or a trained volunteer.

*Specific roles will be based on local/institutional policies related to each discipline's scope of practice.

APPROPRIATE PATIENT POPULATIONS AND REFERRAL PROCESS

Establishing a Group

Group interventions in medical settings require dedicated clinic-based resources such as trained staff and workflows, clinic meeting space, and patient educational resources that can serve multiple patients at one time. Creating a clinic infrastructure for a group intervention may involve adapting existing clinic workflows or developing new ones. Broader education of the clinical and administrative staff will usually be needed to increase buy-in and the likelihood of success. Staff and clinicians will need to clearly understand why the groups are being started, when they will start, and how referrals will be placed. In addition, groups will require brief written explanations to assist with patient recruitment. The clinic-based champion might monitor referrals through a new system or designate another individual to oversee the process. Routinely, the responsibility for new workflows will be assigned to a nurse navigator or case manager in the clinic because the skills and system understanding needed for the tasks closely aligns with their existing responsibilities.

Physical space needed typically consists of a conference room that can comfortably accommodate multiple patients. If the main purpose of the group is patient education, teaching tools such as large whiteboards, projectors for slides and videos, or patient handouts can be helpful. The clinic should also have private exam space available for obtaining vital signs and for conducting optional brief individual patient–provider visits. Depending on the group intervention format, the team can decide whether individual visits are possible before, during, or after group sessions.

Selecting Appropriate Patient Population

The patient recruitment and referral process should include team- and provider-focused education to identify appropriate patients for group interventions. Within integrated care settings, new or existing patient registries, based on patient diseases, could be a source of recruitment and referrals. Appropriate patient characteristics for group interventions include (1) willingness to participate in a group setting and (2) having the medical condition that the group intervention targets. Several group intervention feasibility pilots have demonstrated that a wide range of patients can participate in appropriately designed group interventions. For instance, racially diverse populations, non-English-speaking populations, individuals with low health literacy, and older adults with some functional limitation have been able to participate in various group interventions. At the same time, some patients may not be appropriate and should not be referred to groups. Patients with dementia or other significant cognitive impairment, patients with severe or uncontrolled mental illness, and those with mobility, sensory, or transportation limitations may not be good candidates. However, a patient who might not be a good fit for a specific group in one clinical setting might be a perfect fit for a group in another setting. For example, someone with uncontrolled diabetes who might not be a good fit for a group in a primary care clinic might fit better in an endocrine clinic that is better suited to run a group and provide care for more severe illness.

Educating Patients About Groups

Educational outreach, marketing, and recruitment programs should be rolled out to patients. John Scott, MD, the founder of the CHCC model, noted in a conversation (February 2015) that one of the most important components of a successful group intervention is: "You gotta have the trout stream stocked." For group visits to be sustainable, the clinic must be able to consistently recruit and retain patients. Due to inherent anxieties related to joining a new group of people, some patients will hesitate when group intervention models are recommended. Clinicians should expect these common reactions and can discuss such initial fears with patients. First, normalizing the reaction can help patients understand that joining a group of strangers to share intimate information can be very anxiety provoking. Mentioning group interventions on par with or in combination with individual interventions can be effective. The recommendation to participate should be framed like any other clinical recommendation, such as for a medication or a procedure, and must connect the patient's concerns to the intended benefits. Also, patients may be unaware of the similar efficacy of individual and group interventions and the benefits that groups offer that individual treatments do not; brief discussions of recent research findings on groups can have some impact. While patients may defer participating in a group intervention to a later time, it remains important to lay the groundwork for future discussions, invitations, and referrals.

Referrals will originate from both existing patients and new patients. Front desk staff members who have the first interactions with patients can tremendously influence a patient's willingness to join a group. Any team member can begin the conversation about joining a group and any other team member can complete the conversation. New patients can learn about groups during their basic orientation to clinic flow and protocols. It is better to introduce the group interventions early on in the treatment process, when patient expectations are more malleable. Existing patients who have strong bonds with their current provider might be concerned that a group referral could sever that bond. In our experience, face-to-face contact with an individual clinician, who is also one of the leaders of the group, allows the patient a smoother transition from the individual's current clinician to the group intervention clinicians. Group interventions used in conjunction with individual-care opportunities can complement each other. For example, a group for patients with non-epileptic seizures was developed to complement ongoing treatment, not supplant it. See Chapter 19: Integrative Care Model for Neurology and Psychiatry: Non-Epileptic Seizures Project for more discussion of this specialty group.

Since patient no-shows or dropouts frequently occur as a new group is starting, clinicians may have to recruit twice the number of patients expected to ensure adequate attendance. Reasons why patients might not be able to participate include acute health concerns, transportation problems, work responsibilities, or financial constraints.

FUTURE DIRECTIONS

In the future, fully realized integrated care models in primary and specialty care settings will likely offer group interventions as part of a panoply of services. Patients may enter a clinical setting through an individual and/or group intake or as triggered by a disease-specific registry within the clinic. As part of routine care, group interventions can help with setting goals for preventive health/self-management, developing healthy behaviors, managing symptoms of illness, coping with life stressors and chronic illness, and successfully navigating various stages of life. Clinics will have robust choices of treatment interventions using clinic-based in-person groups, community-based groups, and telehealth groups.

Telehealth groups using videoconferencing technology can be especially helpful to reach patients who have limited transportation or live in rural settings. For example, the Veterans Health Administration has pioneered telemedicine groups using video conferencing for weight loss (the 12-week MOVE! program) and pain management using an interdisciplinary, integrated cognitive-behavioral and physical therapy group-based approach.[31,32] Telemedicine advances can be integrated into the design of group interventions, can provide convenient access for participants, and eliminate the need for meeting space.

In a future reimbursement system that emphasizes improving patient outcomes and providing high-value care, well-developed, tested, and properly implemented group interventions can be important models of care within health care systems. Group interventions can have a dramatic impact on various levels of the health care system as medicine moves more in alignment with the Institute for Healthcare Improvement's "triple aim." Patients will experience a greater level of satisfaction with the availability of different services and support from health care workers and peers. Health care workers can experience a greater level of satisfaction and job fulfillment by spending more time with patients, working within multidisciplinary teams, and realizing improved patient outcomes.

Future development of group interventions could even further expand health care access by integrating nontraditional infrastructure and resources, such as the use of trained peer facilitators/navigators or technology. The combination of clinician-led groups alongside peer-led groups could allow easier access and more varied and perhaps more robust care options. The diverse group interventions could build a continuum of support for patients and caregivers with different levels of need. For example, a patient newly diagnosed with diabetes could be offered an educational group and a peer support group during early phases of the illness. Later he could transition into a diabetes group intervention and individual services for long-term chronic disease management and support. Peer-support groups allow patients to become mentors to one another, in addition to already established relationships with medical providers and existing support networks of family and friends. Combining face-to-face groups with social media groups, such as Facebook, allows resources to be available anytime and anywhere for patients to access support when traditional resources (e.g., an outpatient clinic) may not be accessible.

The sustainability and the expansion of effective group interventions into integrated care settings would benefit from new policies to create specific reimbursement mechanisms for group intervention visits. Many valuable components of group interventions, including peer-based learning and the support that occurs as a result of the group interaction, are difficult or time-consuming to document under current documentation and reimbursement requirements. The ability to specifically bill for medical care delivered through group interventions through a dedicated group intervention billing code would likely promote the sustainability of group interventions in integrated care settings.

REFERENCES

1. Mann T. The Magic Mountain. Woods JE, trans. New York: Alfred A. Knopf; 1995.
2. Pratt J. The class method of treating consumption in the homes of the poor. JAMA. 1907;49(9):755–759.
3. Beck A, Scott J, Williams P, et al. A randomized trial of group outpatient visits for chronically ill older HMO members: The Cooperative Health Care Clinic. J Am Geriatr Soc. 1997;45(5):543–549.
4. American Academy of Family Physicians. Shared medical appointments/group visits. AAFP Policies. http://www.aafp.org/about/policies/all/shared-medical.html Accessed April 17, 2015.
5. Bennis W. Patterns and vicissitudes in T-Group development. In: Bradford LP, Gibb JR, Benne KD, eds. T-Group Theory and Laboratory Method. New York: John Wiley and Sons; 1964:248–278.
6. Bion WR. Experiences in Groups, and Other Papers. New York: Basic Books; 1961.
7. Yalom ID, Leszcz W. The Theory and Practice of Group Psychotherapy. 5th ed. New York: Basic Books; 2005.
8. Frank JD, Frank J. Persuasion and Healing: A Comparative Study of Psychotherapy. 3rd ed. Baltimore, MD: Johns Hopkins University Press; 1991.
9. Festinger L. Social Pressures in Informal Groups: A Study of Human Factors in Housing. 1st ed. New York: Harper; 1950.
10. Naik AD, Palmer N, Peterson NJ, et al. Comparative effectiveness of goal setting in diabetes mellitus group clinics: Randomized clinical trial. Arch Intern Med. 2011;121(5):453–459.
11. May SG, Cheng PH, Tietbohl CK, et al. Shared medical appointments to screen for geriatric syndromes: Preliminary data from a quality improvement initiative. J Am Geriatr Soc. 2014;62(12):2415–2419.

12. Carlson B. Shared appointments improve efficiency in the clinic. Managed Care. 2003;12(5):46–48. http://www.managedcaremag.com/archives/0305/0305.sharedappointments.html. Accessed September 26, 2015.
13. Bronson DL, Maxwell RA. Shared medical appointments: Increasing patient access without increasing physician hours. Cleve Clin J Med. 2004;71(5):369–370, 372, 374.
14. Berger-Fiffy J. The "nuts and bolts" of implementing shared medical appointments: The Harvard Vanguard Medical Associates experience. J Ambul Care Manage. 2012;35(3):247–256.
15. Cherniack PE. The use of shared medical appointments in the care of the elderly. J Ambul Care Manage. 2014;37(1):32–37.
16. Scott JC, Conner DA, Venohr I, et al. Effectiveness of a group outpatient visit model for chronically ill older health maintenance organization members: A 2-year trial of the cooperative health care clinic. J Am Geriatr Soc. 2004;52(9):1463–1470.
17. Edelman D, Fredrickson SK, Melnyk SD, et al. Medical clinics versus usual care for patients with both diabetes and hypertension: A randomized trial. Ann Intern Med. 2010;152(11):689–696.
18. Ebell MH, Siwek J, Weiss BD, et al. Simplifying the language of evidence to improve patient care: Strength of recommendation taxonomy (SORT): A patient-centered approach to grading evidence in medical literature. J Fam Pract. 2004;53(2):111–120.
19. Cohen S, Hartley S, Mavi J, et al. Veteran experiences related to participation in shared medical appointments. Milit Med. 2012;177(11):1287–1292.
20. Gardiner P, Dresner D, Barnett KG, et al. Medical group visits: a feasibility study to manage patients with chronic pain in an underserved urban clinic. Glob Adv Health Med. 2014;3(4):20–26.
21. Geller JS, Orkaby A, Cleghorn GD. Impact of a group medical visit program on Latino health-related quality of life. Explore (NY). 2011;7(2):94–99.
22. Thompson J, Coleman R, Colwell B, et al. Preparing breast cancer patients for survivorship (PREP)—a pilot study of a patient-centred supportive group visit intervention. Eur J Oncol Nurs. 2014;18(1):10–16.
23. Housden L, Wong ST, Dawes M. Effectiveness of group medical visits for improving diabetes care: A systematic review and meta-analysis. Can Med Assoc J. 2013;185(13):E635–E644.
24. Edelman D, Gierisch JM, McDuffie JR, et al. Shared medical appointments for patients with diabetes mellitus: A systematic review. J Gen Intern Med. 2015;30(1):99–106.
25. Ho CJ, Preston C, Fredericks K, et al. A unique model for treating chronic hepatitis C in patients with psychiatric disorders, substance abuse, and/or housing instability. J Addict Med. 2013;7(5):320–324.
26. American Group Psychotherapy Association. www.agpa.org. Accessed January 19, 2016.
27. American Psychological Association Division 49. http://www.apadivisions.org/division-49/. Accessed January 19, 2016.
28. Centering Healthcare Institute. http://centering-healthcare.org/. Accessed January 19, 2016.
29. Stanford Small Group Self-Management Programs. http://patienteducation.stanford.edu/programs/. Accessed January 19, 2016.
30. Improving Chronic Illness Care. http://improvingchroniccare.org/index.php?p=Critical_Tools&s=162. Accessed January 16, 2016.
31. Ahrendt A, Kattelmann K, Rector T, et al. The effectiveness of telemedicine for weight management in the MOVE! Program. J Rural Health. 2014;30(1):113–119.
32. Palyo S, Schopmeyer K, McQuaid J. Tele-pain management: Use of videoconferencing technology in the delivery of an integrated cognitive-behavioral and physical therapy group intervention. Psychol Serv. 2012;9(2):200–202.
33. Taveira TH, Wu WC. Interventions to maintain cardiac risk control after discharge from a cardiovascular risk reduction clinic: A randomized controlled trial. Diabetes Res Clin Pract. 2014;105(3):327–335.
34. Blumenfeld A1, Tischio M. Center of excellence for headache care: Group model at Kaiser Permanente. Headache. 2003;43(5):431–440.

INDEX

Page references for figures are indicated by *f*, for tables by *t*, and for boxes by *b*.

Acamprosate, for alcohol use disorders, 234, 318*t*
Acceptance, 449
Accountable care organization (ACO), 83
Action stage, 473–474
Acupuncture, for chronic pain, 438
Addiction. *See also* Substance use disorders; *specific addictions*
  as brain disease, 224–225
Adler, Alfred, 466*t*, 469
Administrator, 49, 52*t*
Adult education, 466*t*, 472
Advance care planning, 444–446, 446*b*
Advance directives, 446, 446*b*, 451
Advanced practice nurse, 49, 51*t*
Affordable Care Act (ACA)
  financing integrated care models, 76, 86
  group interventions, 532
  integrated care support, 122
  mental health policy, 92
  population health, 47
  prevention, 460
  substance use disorders, 224
Agenda mapping, 475
Aging Brain Care (ABC), 107–119
  Aging Brain Center Medical Home, 110–119 (*See also* Aging Brain Center Medical Home)
  background, 108
  Center for Brain Care Innovation, 117–119
  fragmented *vs.* integrated care, 107–108
  Healthy Aging Brain Center, 108–110, 109*b*
  strength of recommendation (SOR) taxonomy, 119*b*
Aging Brain Center Medical Home (ABC Med Home), 110–119
  expansion, 110–117
    acute care transition, 115
    assessment, initial, 114–115
    awards and funding, 110–111
    care delivery, 113–114
    enrollment, 112–113
    follow-up, 115
    population health management, 111
    population health management, eMR-ABC software, 115–116
    staffing, 112, 113*f*, 114*f*
    success stories and lessons learned, 116–117
    team meetings, 115
    workforce development, 111–112
  future plans, 117–119
  pilot program, 110
  replication, 117, 118*b*
  strength of recommendation (SOR) taxonomy, 119*b*
Alcoholics Anonymous (AA), 233, 532, 532*t*
Alcohol use and alcohol use disorders, 228–235
  complications, medical, 229, 230*t*
  epidemiology, 228
  erectile dysfunction in, 397, 402*t*
  interventions, 231–235
    brief, 231–232, 232*t*
    detoxification, 232–233
    follow-up, 234–235
    medication-assisted, 233–234
    mutual support groups, 233
    psychotherapeutic, 233
  laboratory tests, 229–231
  psychiatric screening, 229
  screening and assessment, 228–231, 229*b*
  suicide risk, 328
  urine toxicology, 241*t*
Alcohol Use Disorders Identification Test (AUDIT), 228
Alprazolam
  for anxiety disorders, 156, 157*t*
  in pregnancy, 375*t*
Alprostadil, for erectile dysfunction, 402*t*
Amitriptyline. *See also* Tricyclic antidepressants (TCAs)
  for borderline personality disorder, 317*t*
  for depression, 182*t*
  for insomnia, 422, 423*t*
  for somatic symptoms, 296
Amoxapine, for borderline personality disorder, 317*t*
Amphetamine, urine toxicology, 241*t*
Anger
  coping stages, 449
  management, 342

Anorexia nervosa (AN), 262–266
in adults, 265–266
in children and adolescents, 265
diagnosis and clinical presentation, 262, 265
epidemiology, 262, 265
guiding principles, 262
team member activities, 266–272
assessment, 266
basic clinical management, 270–271
education, 266, 269
level of care guidelines, 267*t*–269*t*
medical assistants and front desk personnel, 266
primary care clinicians, 266–271, 267*t*–269*t*
referral, 271
resources lacking, local, 271
screening, initial, 266
urgent and emergency situations, 271–272
in young adults, 265
Anorgasmia, female, 404
Anticonvulsants. *See also specific types*
in pregnancy, 374, 376*t*, 381
for suicidal ideation, 341
for violence, 341
Antidepressants. *See also specific types*
for binge eating disorder, 259
for depression, in bipolar disorder, 186*b*, 194
in pregnancy, 374, 375*t*
for suicidal ideation, 341
for violence, 341
Antihypertensives, on sexual function, 397, 397, 401*t*
Antioxidants, dietary, 415, 416*t*
Antipsychotics. *See also specific types*
in pregnancy, 374, 376*t*, 381
for schizophrenia and psychotic disorders, 207–215
changing, 214–215
discontinuing, 215
initial choice, 207, 211, 211*t*
initiating, 207
maintenance, 214, 214*t*
monitoring, 207, 214*t*
side effects, 207, 212*t*–213*t*
stabilization, 211, 214
for violence, 341
Antisocial personality disorders (ASPD). *See also* Personality disorders
biological basis and psychosocial formulation, 304–305
description, 304*b*–305*b*
prevalence and co-occurring disorders, 304
schema, 308–312, 309*t*–310*t*
treatment, 318*t*, 320–321
Anxiety disorders, 149–165. *See also specific types*
chronic pain with, 420, 431
clinical pathways, 161*t*–162*t*
differential diagnosis, 151*f* (*See also specific disorders*)
etiology, drugs of abuse, medications, and toxins, 153*t*
generalized anxiety disorder, 151–153
integrated care, 160–165
follow-up, 165
initial team member roles, 160–163, 161*t*–162*t*
initial treatment planning, 163
research, 160
team-based, 160
team monitoring and treatment, 163–165
key elements, 149, 149*b*
medical conditions, associated, 152*t*
mixed anxiety depressive disorder, 156
obsessive compulsive disorder, 154–155
panic disorder, 150–151
post-traumatic stress disorder, 155
prevalence, 149–150, 367
screening, 156
self-awareness, 150
social phobia, 153–154
strength of recommendation (SOR) taxonomy, 164*b*
treatment, 156–160
behavioral activation, 158
choosing modality, 159–160
cognitive-behavioral therapy, 159
exercise, 158
eye movement desensitization and reprocessing, 159
mindfulness meditation, 158
pharmacologic, 156–157, 157*t*
prolonged exposure therapy, 159
psychoeducation, 158
relaxation response training, 158
women
peripartum, 370
postpartum, 370–371
Appreciative inquiry, 469, 476
Aripiprazole
for bipolar disorder
depression, 190*t*, 194–195
maintenance, 191*t*
mania, 187, 190*t*
dosing, 211*t*
for schizophrenia, 207
side effects, 207, 212*t*–213*t*
Arousal (sexual), 388, 389*t*–390*t*, 397
Art Rx, 438–439
Asenapine
dosing, 211*t*
for mania, in bipolar disorder, 187, 190*t*
side effects, 207, 212*t*–213*t*
Assertive Community Treatment (ACT), 217
Assessment. *See also specific disorders and integrated care models*
in care coordination, 126–127
Assessment, mental health, 134–143
automated, 134–143 (*See also* Quick PsychoDiagnostics Panel (QPD Panel))
challenges, 135–136
comprehensive, 137
medical providers on tools for, 136
provider wish list, 136–137
Asynchronous telepsychiatry (ATP), 129–130
Attention density, 478
Attitudes, 9
Atypical antipsychotics. *See also specific agents*
for anxiety disorders, 157, 157*t*
for bipolar disorder
depression, 187, 190*t*, 191*t*, 194–195
maintenance, 191*t*
mania, 187, 190*t*

AUDIT-Consumption (AUDIT-C), 228
Auerbach, Jeff, 478
Autistic spectrum disorder, 206*t*
Automated mental health assessment, 134–143. *See also* Quick PsychoDiagnostics Panel (QPD Panel)

Bandura, Albert, 467*t*, 472
Barbiturates, urine toxicology, 241*t*
Bargaining, 449
Bariatric surgery, 420
Beck, Aaron, 467*t*, 478
Beginner's mind, 477
Behavioral activation, 158
Behavioral health care, 4–6, 5*f*, 7*t*, 12
Behavioral health consultants (BHC), 22, 25*b*
Behavioral Health Laboratory model, 97
Behavioral health specialist (BHS). *See also specific disorders*
  anxiety disorder care, 160, 161*t*–162*t*, 163–164
  bipolar disorder care, 188*t*
  depression care, 177–180, 179*f*, 180*b*
Behavioral therapy
  for chronic pain, 439–440
  for suicidal ideation, 342–343
  for violence, 342–343
Behavior health clinicians, 29
Beliefs, 9
Benzodiazepines
  for anxiety disorders, 156, 157*t*, 159–160
  in pregnancy, 374, 375*t*, 381–382
  prescription cautions, 248–249
  for sexual disorders, 401*t*
  for suicidal ideation, 342
  urine toxicology, 241*t*
  use and abuse disorders, 244–245
  for violence, 341, 342
Benzphetamine, for weight loss, 418, 419*t*
Bereavement, 452–453. *See also* Death and dying
Berg, Insoo Kim, 467*t*
Best practice, family-centered health care, 514–526. *See also* Family-centered health care
Beta-blockers, for anxiety disorders, 157, 157*t*
Binge eating disorder (BED), 256–273
  clinical presentation, 257–258
  critical pathway, 267*t*–269*t*
  diagnosis, 257
  epidemiology, 257
  integrated care, 257–258
  team member activities, 258–262
    assessment, initial, 258
    behavioral health specialist, 261
    care coordinator, 260–261
    education, 258–259
    follow-up, 259–260
    health coach, 261–262
    medical assistants and front desk personnel, 258
    medication decisions, 259–260
    primary care clinicians, 258–260, 267*t*–269*t*
    psychiatrist, consulting, 262
    referral, 260
    registry enrollment, 260
    resources and referrals, 260–261, 261*b*
    resources lacking, local, 262
    screening, 258
    treatment plan formulation, 259
    urgent and emergent situations, 262
Biofeedback, 438
Biomedical communication, 460–461
Biopsychosocial awareness, somatic symptom disorder and illness anxiety, 280–281, 282*f*, 283*t*
  Columbia Stages of Biopsychosocial Awareness (CS-BPSA) model use, 283*t*, 284–286
  levels, 281, 282*f*
  stages, 281–284, 282*f*, 283*t*
Biopsychosocial model, 4
Bipolar disorder, 169–178, 186–195
  assessment, 176
  on comorbid medical disorder outcomes, 169–170
  costs, 174
  course, 174
  diagnosis, 170, 171*t*–172*t*
  differential diagnosis, 170, 172*t*–173*t*
  epidemiology, 169, 170, 174
  medical illness interactions, 174–175
  postpartum, 371–372, 371*t*
  in pregnancy, medications, 374–377, 375*t*–376*t*
  screening, 175–176
  strength of recommendation (SOR) taxonomy, 195*b*
  treatment, primary care, 186–195
    critical pathway, depression, 192*t*–193*t*
    critical pathway, mania, 188*t*–189*t*
    goals, 186
    risks and hospitalization, 186
  treatment, primary care, pharmacotherapy (*See also under* Depression; *specific agents*)
    depression, 187, 190*t*–193*t*
    depression, antidepressants, 186*b*, 194
    depression, first-line, 187, 194
    depression, maintenance, 194–195
    depression, second-line, 194
    discontinuation, 195
    mania, 187, 188*t*–191*t*
Borderline personality disorder (BPD). *See also* Personality disorders
  biological basis and psychosocial formulation, 304
  description, 304*b*
  differential diagnosis, 206*t*
  non-epileptic seizures with, 353
  prevalence and co-occurring disorders, 304
  schema, 308–312, 309*t*–310*t*
  suicide risk, 328
  treatment, 317*t*, 319–320
Brain care, aging, 107–119. *See also* Aging Brain Care (ABC)
Brief interventions. *See also specific types*
  for alcohol use disorders, 226, 231–232, 232*t*
  for sedative use and abuse disorders, 245
  for tobacco use disorders, 236
Brief psychotic disorder, 206*t*. *See also* Psychotic disorders
Bronx Behavioral Health Integration Project (Bronx- BHIP), 85

Bulimia nervosa (BN), 262–266
in adults, 265–266
in children and adolescents, 265
diagnosis and clinical presentation, 265
epidemiology, 265
guiding principles, 262
team member activities, 266–272 (*See also under* Eating disorders)
in young adults, 265
Bundled payment plans, 83
Buprenorphine, for opioid use disorders, 243, 318*t*
Bupropion. *See also* Norepinephrine-dopamine reuptake inhibitors
for depression, 183*t*, 184
in pregnancy, 374, 375*t*
for sexual desire and arousal, 400*t*
for tobacco use disorders, 236
for weight loss, with naltrexone, 417, 419*t*
Buspirone
for anxiety disorders, 157, 157*t*
for sexual desire and arousal, 400*t*

Calendar of Premenstrual Experiences (COPE) diary, 372
Canada, collaborative care, 31–44
benefits, 37
collaboration improvement activities and strategies
communication between providers, 34
coordination of care, 34–35, 35*t*
inpatient discharge plan, 34–35, 35*t*
mental health consultation with primary care, 34
definition, 33
framework, 33*t*
future steps, 43–44
guiding principles, 33
Hamilton Family Health Team (HFHT) Mental Health Program, 38–43, 40*t*–41*t*
history and overview, 31–32
integrating mental health services within primary care, 36–37
integrating primary care providers within mental health services, 37–38
key components, 37, 38*t*
Practice Support Program: Adult Mental Health Module, 35–36
primary care and mental health systems roles, shared vision, 33–34
primary care provider mental health care capacity and capability, 35
strength of recommendation (SOR) taxonomy, 43*b*
Canada Health Act, 31
Canadian Collaborative Mental Health Initiative (CCMHI), 32
Cannabis use and cannabis use disorders, 245–247
edibles, 246
epidemiology, 245
interventions, 246–247
medical uses, 245–246
potency, 246
screening and assessment, 246
urine toxicology, 241*t*
Capitation plans, 83
Carbamazepine
for mania, in bipolar disorder, 187, 190*t*
for obsessive compulsive personality disorder, 318*t*
in pregnancy, 376*t*
Care coordination. *See* Coordinated care
Care coordinator assistants (CCAs), ABC Med Home, 111–117
acute care transition, 115
assessment, initial, 114–115
care delivery, 113
development, 111–112, 116
eMR-ABC, 115–116
follow-up, 115
staffing, 112, 113*f*, 114*f*
success stories and lessons learned, 116–117
Care managers. *See also specific types*
depression care, 177
interprofessional role, 49, 52–53, 52*t*
CAT (Commitment, Activation, Taking Action Steps), 476
Center for Brain Care Innovation (CBCI), 117–119
Change talk, 476
Change tolerance, 11
Cherokee Health Systems, 17–30
financing, 29–30
history, 17–18
implementation challenges, 25–27
innovations, breakthrough, 29, 29*f*
mission and strategic priorities, 18–20, 20*t*
psychiatric treatment pathways, 24–25, 25*b*
structure, 18, 18*t*, 19*f*
success, keys, 27–29
team-based care, 21–24
clinical encounter, 23
clinical model structure, 23
guiding principles, 21–22
psychiatric care structure, 24
team members and functions, 22–23
values and critical success factors, 20–21, 21*t*
Child, death of, 453–454
Child and Youth Mental Health (CYMH) module, 36
Chlorpromazine, for borderline personality disorder, 317*t*
Chronic disease, 460. *See also specific types*
Chronic pain, 430–440. *See also* Pain, chronic
Citalopram. *See also* Selective Serotonin Reuptake Inhibitors (SSRIs)
for anxiety disorders, 156, 157*t*
for binge eating disorder, 260
for depression, 181, 182*t*
for obsessive compulsive personality disorder, with depression, 318*t*
in pregnancy, 375*t*
Clerical personnel, 50, 51*t*–52*t*, 60. *See also specific types and disorders*
Client, 463
Client-centered therapy, 466*t*
Clinical Institute Withdrawal Assessment for Alcohol, Revised (CIWA-Ar), 232–233
Clinical support personnel, 49, 51*t*–52*t*
Clonazepam
for anxiety disorders, 156, 157*t*
for insomnia, 422, 423*t*

in pregnancy, 375*t*
Clozapine
for borderline personality disorder, 317*t*
dosing, 211*t*
for schizophrenia, 207
side effects, 207, 212*t*–213*t*
for suicidal ideation, 341
for violence, 341
Coach, health, 459–492. *See also* Health coach(ing)
Cocaine, urine toxicology, 241*t*
Cognitive approaches, health coaching, 477–481
cognitive-behavioral coaching, 478, 479*t*–480*t*
mindfulness-based stress reduction, 478–481
self-directed neuroplasticity, 477–478
Cognitive behavioral coaching, 478, 479*t*–480*t*
Cognitive Behavioral Interpersonal Skills (CBIS) manual, 35–36
Cognitive Behavioral Therapy (CBT), 467*t*
for alcohol use disorders, 233
for anxiety disorders, 159, 160
for binge eating disorder, 259
for chronic pain, 437–438
behavioral weight and sleep management with, 439–440
for illness anxiety, 297
for schizophrenia spectrum and psychotic disorders, 217
for somatic symptoms, 297
for suicidal ideation, 342
for violence, 342
Collaborative care, 5*f*, 79, 128
collaboration, improving, 34–35, 35*t*
mental health, 32, 33
Collaborative habit, 46
Co-located care
definition, 5*f*
telehealth, 127–129
University of Rochester, 61
White River Junction, 97
Columbia Stages of Biopsychosocial Awareness (CS-BPSA) model, 281–286, 282*f*, 283*t*
Columbia-Suicide Severity Rating Scales (C-SSRS), 334
Commitment, 11
suicidal ideation, 343
violence, 343
Communication
of bad news, 446–448 (*See also* Death and dying)
biomedical (paternalistic), 460–461
physician-directed, 460–461
positional dialog, 460
between providers, 34
shared care models, 60
transactional dialog, 460
Community-based group interventions, 532, 532*t*
Community health coordinators, 22–23
Complementary health. *See also specific types*
for chronic pain, 430–431
Comprehensive multi-disciplinary evaluation (CMDE), 288, 290*t*–291*t*, 294–296, 295*b*–296*b*
Comprehensive Symptoms and Experiences Timeline (CSET), 288, 290*t*–291*t*, 294–296, 295*b*–296*b*
Computerized patient record system (CPRS), 96
Conception, female, 368
Conceptual framework, 3–14
applying, 13–14
behavioral health, 4–6, 7*t*
biopsychosocial model, 4
core elements, integrated care models, 9–13 (*See also* Core elements, integrated care models)
integration, 3–4
levels and categories, 8–9, 10*t*
outcomes measurement, 13–14
stepped integration, 8–9, 10*t*
strength of recommendation (SOR) taxonomy, 13*b*
Triple Aim, IHI, 6–8, 461
variety of styles, 4
Confidence ruler, 476
Confidentiality
suicidal ideation, 343
violence, 343
Conjugated equine estrogen, for vaginal dryness/atrophy/dyspareunia, 399*t*
Consultation
mental health, with primary care, 34
psychiatric, 57–60 (*See also* Psychiatric consultation)
Consultation-liaison psychiatry, 76–78
Contemplation stage, 473
Conversion disorders, non-epileptic seizures with, 352, 354
Cooperrider, David, 467*t*
Coordinated care, 34–35, 35*t*
for anxiety disorders, 163
for bipolar disorder, 189*t*
Canada model, 34–35, 35*t*
definition, 5*f*
telehealth, 126–127
Coping
crisis intervention, 509, 510*b*
death and dying, 448–449
Core elements, integrated care models, 9–13
adapting behavioral health services, tools, and personnel, 12
attitudes, beliefs, and culture change, 9
commitment, flexibility, and change tolerance, 11
organizational support, 11
outcomes measurement, 12–13
patient-centered care, 11
population-based approach, 12
stepped care, 12
stigma, counteracting, 9–11
team-based care, 11
Cost-effectiveness, 8, 76
Crisis, 497, 499
Crisis intervention, 497–511
coping styles, 509, 510*b*
course, 499–500, 499*f*
crises, 497
definition and focus, 501, 503
origins, 497–499, 498*b*
steps, 503, 503*b*
strength of recommendation (SOR) taxonomy, 511*b*
stress ranking, life events, 498, 498*b*
for suicidal ideation, 342–343
treatment, integrated care, 500–511
behavioral health specialist, 501*t*, 507–510, 508*f*, 509*f*

Crisis intervention (*Cont.*)
crisis intervention therapy, 507
formulation of crisis, 504–505, 504*f*
fundamentals, 500, 501*t*–502*t*
within integrated care medical home, 506–507
level of care determination, 505–506, 505*f*
recognition of crisis, 503–504
referral, 506
resolution of crisis and anticipatory guidance, 510–511
for violence, 342–343
Critical pathways/algorithms
anxiety disorders, 161*t*–162*t*
binge eating disorder, 263*t*–264*t*
bipolar disorder, depression, 192*t*–193*t*
bipolar disorder, mania, 188*t*–189*t*
crisis intervention, 501*t*–502*t*
death and dying, 445*t*
integrated behavioral pain medicine, 433*f*
intimate partner violence, violence, suicide, 337*t*–338*t*
lifestyle and wellness, 411*t*–412*t*
non-epileptic seizures, 361*f*
personality disorders, 314*t*–315*t*
psychosis, 208*t*–210*t*
sex
men, desire, arousal pain, 401*t*–402*t*
women, desire, arousal, pain, 399*t*–400*t*
somatic symptom disorder and illness anxiety, 289*f*, 292*t*–293*t*
Csikszentmihali, Mihalyi, 467*t*
Culture change, 9
Cyclobenzaprine, for somatic symptoms, 296

DARN (Desire, Ability, Reason, or Need), 467*t*, 476
DARN CATS (Desire, Ability, Reason, Need, Commitment, Activation, Taking Action Steps), 476
Davidson Trauma Scale (DTS), 160
Death and dying, 443–455
advance care planning for, 444–446, 446*b*
advance directives, 446, 446*b*, 451
bereavement, 452–453
child, death of, 453–454
communicating bad news, 446–448
coping stages, 448–450
end-of-life care, 451–452
hospice care, 452
integrated care, 444, 445*t*
palliative care, 449–450
primary care providers in, 443
reaction to, 455
spiritual care, 451–452
spiritual life, reconnecting, 451, 452*b*
unnatural death, 454–455
Deci, E.L., 469, 471*t*
De facto mental health care providers, 78–79
Dehydroepiandrosterone (DHEA), for sexual desire and arousal, 400*t*
Delirium, 206*t*
Delusional disorder, 206*t*. *See also* Psychotic disorders
Dementia, in elderly, 107–119. *See also* Aging Brain Care (ABC)
Denial, 448–449
Depression, 169–186
assessment, 176
collaborative care model, 176–178
comorbid medical disorder outcomes, 169–170
coping stages, 449
costs, 174
diagnosis, 170, 171*t*–172*t*
differential diagnosis, 170, 172*t*–173*t*
disease course, 174
in elderly, 107–119 (*See also* Aging Brain Care)
epidemiology, 169, 170, 174, 367
IMPACT Study (Improving Mood Promoting Access to Collaborative Treatment) for, 9, 12, 37, 79, 81, 86*b*, 108
medical illness interactions, 174–175
non-epileptic seizures with, 352, 354
screening tools, 175–176
treatment, primary care, 177–180
behavioral health specialist, 177–180, 179*f*, 180*b*
patient handouts, 179*f*
psychotherapy, 178, 180
treatment, primary care, pharmacotherapy, 178, 181–186
augmentation strategies, 185–186
continuation and discontinuation, 185
failure, 185
initiation, 184–185
medication selection, 181
norepinephrine-dopamine reuptake inhibitors, 183*t*, 184
norepinephrine-serotonin modulators, 181, 183*t*, 184
selective serotonin reuptake inhibitors, 181, 182*t*
serotonin-norepinephrine reuptake inhibitors, 181, 182*t*
tricyclic antidepressants, 182*t*–183*t*, 184
in women
perimenopausal, 370
peripartum, 369–370
postpartum, 370, 380
premenstrual dysphoric disorder, 369
prevalence, 367
Depression care managers (DCMs), 49, 52–53, 52*t*
Depression Improvement Across Minnesota, Offering a New Direction (DIAMOND), 37, 83, 86*b*
de Shaser, Steve, 467*t*
Desipramine. *See also* Tricyclic antidepressants (TCAs)
for depression, 183*t*
Desire (sexual), 388, 389*t*–390*t*, 397
from acquired sexual neutrality to, 395
innate, 395
receptive, 395
Desvenlafaxine. *See also* Serotonin-Norepinephrine Reuptake Inhibitors (SNRIs)
for depression, 181, 182*t*
Detoxification, medical
for alcohol, 232–233
for opioids, 242
for sedatives, 245
Developmental crisis, 498
Dialectical behavioral therapy, 342
DIAMOND (Depression Improvement Across Minnesota, Offering a New Direction), 37, 83, 86*b*
Diathesis-stress model, 432
Diazepam, in pregnancy, 375*t*

DiClimente, Carlo, 467*t*
Dietary Intervention in Primary Care (DINE) questionnaire, 415
Diethylpropion, for weight loss, 418, 419*t*
Diphenhydramine, for insomnia, 422, 423*t*
Directed repetitive sex, 404
Discharge plan, inpatient, 34–35, 35*t*
Dissociative symptoms, non-epileptic seizures with, 353, 354
Disulfiram, for alcohol use disorders, 234, 318*t*
Divalproex
  for borderline personality disorder, 317*t*
  for mania, in bipolar disorder, 187, 190*t*
Doherty, McDaniel, and Baird's taxonomy, 53–57, 54*b*–57*b*
  level1: minimally collaborative, 53–54, 54*b*
  level2: basic collaboration, primary and behavioral health care, parallel, 54, 54*b*
  level3: basic collaboration, co-located services, 54–55, 55*b*
  level4: close collaboration, partially integrated system, 55, 56*b*
  level5: close collaboration, fully integrated system, 55, 56*b*
  level6: full collaboration, transformed/merged practice, 55–57, 56*b*
  SAMHSA health care integration levels, 124–126, 125*t*
Do-not-resuscitate (DNR) orders, 451
Doxepin, for insomnia, 422, 423*t*
Dreikurs, Rudolf, 466*t*
Drug use disorders. *See* Substance use disorders; *specific drugs*
Duloxetine. *See also* Serotonin-Norepinephrine Reuptake Inhibitors (SNRIs)
  for anxiety disorders, 156, 157*t*
  for depression, 181, 182*t*
  for illness anxiety, 297
  in pregnancy, 375*t*
  for somatic symptoms, 296
Duty-to-protect statutes, 343
Duty to warn, 343
Dyspareunia, 388, 389*t*–390*t*, 391, 398*t*–399*t*

Eating, healthy, 414
Eating disorders, 256–273. *See also specific types*
  anorexia nervosa and bulimia nervosa, 262–266
  behavioral health specialists, 257
  binge eating disorder, 257–262
  other, 272–273
  prevalence, 256
  primary care provider, 256–257
  strength of recommendation (SOR) taxonomy, 272*b*
  team member activities, 266–272
    assessment, 266
    basic clinical management, 270–271
    education, 266, 269
    level of care guidelines, 267*t*–269*t*
    medical assistants and front desk personnel, 266
    primary care clinicians, 266, 267*t*–269*t*
    referral, 271
    resources lacking, local, 271
    screening, initial, 266
    urgent and emergency situations, 271–272
ECHO (Extension for Community Healthcare Outcomes), 126
e-cigarettes, 237
Edinburgh Postnatal Depression Scale (EPDS), 372
Education, 466*t*. *See also specific disorders and models*
  adult, 466*t*, 472
  patient-centered medical home, 73
  patient-specific primary care clinician, 59
Electroconvulsive therapy
  for psychosis, 342
  for violence, 342
Electronic health record (EHR), 29
Electronic record consultation (e-consults), 58–59
Ellison, Jeff, 475
Emotional intelligence, 469
eMR-ABC population health management software, 115–116
End-of-life care, 451–452
Erectile dysfunction (ED), 389*t*
  in alcohol use disorders, 397, 402*t*
  assessment and diagnosis, 391–393
  detection and screening, 391, 392*b*
  interactions between causes, 391
  management, 93, 401*t*–402*t*, 403
  treatment algorithm, 394*f*
Erikson, Erik, 498
Erikson, Milton, 466*t*
Escitalopram. *See also* Selective Serotonin Reuptake Inhibitors (SSRIs)
  for anxiety disorders, 156, 157*t*
  for binge eating disorder, 260
  for depression, 181, 182*t*
  in pregnancy, 375*t*
Estradiol, for sexual function (female), 388, 399*t*, 399*t*
Estrogen, for sexual function (female), 397, 398*t*, 405
Eszopiclone, for insomnia, 422, 423*t*
Evoking, 475
Exercise
  for anxiety disorders, 158
  for wellness, 412–414
Exercise-based sex therapy, 396
Extrinsic motivation, 469
Eye movement desensitization and reprocessing (EMDR)
  for anxiety disorders, 159
  for chronic pain, 438

Family, 514–515
Family Assessment Device (FAD), 518
Family-based treatment (FBT), for anorexia nervosa and bulimia nervosa, 270
Family-centered health care, 514–526
  family, 514–515
  implementation and changes, 523
  overview and recommendations, 515–516, 516*f*
  primary care setting, 515
  strength of recommendation (SOR) taxonomy, 524*b*
  three-step model, 516–523, 517*t*
    family education and support, 517*t*, 518–521, 520*b*, 521*t*
    family inclusion, 516–518, 517*t*, 518*b*
    family systems therapy, 517*t*, 521–523, 522*b*
Family-centered screening, 518
Family education and support, 517*t*, 518–521
  definition and fundamentals, 518
  family-centered screening, 518
  interventions, 519, 520*b*

Family education and support (*Cont.*)
session, 518–519
team huddle, 519
treatment plan, 519–521, 521*t*
Family inclusion, 516–518, 517*t*
assessment, 516–517, 517*t*
case study, 517, 518*b*
definition, 516
treatment plan, 517–518
Family systems therapy (FST), 517*t*, 521–523
case study, 522, 522*b*
definition and fundamentals, 521
effectiveness, 521
treatment plan, 522–523
Family therapy
for non-epileptic seizures, 356
for suicidal ideation, 342
for violence, 342
Federally Qualified Health Center (FQHC), 20
Fee-for-service models, 80–81
Financing integrated care, 76–87
Affordable Care Act, 76
bundled payment and capitation plans, 83
Cherokee Health Systems, 29–30
consultation-liaison psychiatry, 76–78
cost-effectiveness, 76
de facto mental health care providers, 78–79
fee-for-service models, 80–81
high-cost patients, 81–82
history, 76
integrated care models, overview, 79–80
managed behavioral health organizations, 78
medical cost offset, 81
Mental Health Parity and Addiction Equity Act model, 76, 78
models, 82
Montefiore Medical Center, 84–85
pay-for-performance, 82
shared savings model, 83–84
strength of recommendation (SOR) taxonomy, 86–87, 86*b*–87*b*
5 A's of behavioral counseling, 231–232, 232*t*
Flexibility, 11
Flibanserin, for sexual desire and arousal, 400*t*
Fluoxetine. *See also* Selective Serotonin Reuptake Inhibitors (SSRIs)
for anxiety disorders, 156, 157*t*
for borderline personality disorder, 317*t*
for bulimia nervosa, 271
for depression, 181, 182*t*
for illness anxiety, 297
in pregnancy, 375*t*
for premature ejaculation, 401*t*
Fluvoxamine, for obsessive compulsive personality disorder, 318*t*
Focal psychodynamic psychotherapy, 342
Focusing, 475
Force multiplication, 126
FRAMES (Feedback, Responsibility, Advice, Menu, Empathic, Self-efficacy), 231
Frequency, intensity, type, and time for exercise (FITT prescription), 413
Freud, Sigmund, 466*t*

Gabapentin
for alcohol use disorders, 234
for anxiety disorders, 157, 157*t*
for somatic symptoms, 296
Gallwey, Timothy, 462–463
Generalized anxiety disorder, 151–153, 151*f*, 152*t*. *See also* Anxiety disorders
Generalized Anxiety Disorder-2 (GAD-2), 156
Generalized Anxiety Disorder-7 (GAD-7), 156
Global budgets, 83–84
Gluten, 414, 416*t*
Glycerol, for vaginal dryness/dyspareunia, 399*t*
Grief, 452–453
Group interventions, 527–538
community-based, 532, 532*t*
financing, 532
future directions, 537–538
group theory, 528, 529*t*
history, 527–528
key features, 530–531
for non-epileptic seizures, 355–356
outcomes, 532–535
disease-oriented, 534
health care utilization, 534–535
patient-oriented, 533–534
patient populations and referrals, 536–537
recent and emerging models, 531–532
strength of recommendation (SOR) taxonomy, 533, 533*b*
teams, maximizing, 535, 536*t*
therapeutic factors, 528–530, 530*t*
Group theory, 528, 529*t*

Haloperidol
for borderline personality disorder, 317*t*
dosing, 211*t*
for mania, in bipolar disorder, 187
in pregnancy, 376*t*
side effects, 207, 212*t*–213*t*
Hamilton Family Health Team (HFHT) Mental Health Program, 38–43, 40*t*–*41*t
advice to others, 42–43
challenges, 41–42
competencies, mental health providers working in primary care, 39
evaluation data, 38–39
history and overview, 38
implementation, collaborative, 42
successes, 39–41
team members and roles, 38, 40*t*–41*t*
Health coach(ing), 459–492
for anxiety disorders, 164
for binge eating disorder, 261–262
for bipolar disorder, 188*t*
at Cherokee Health Systems, 22–23
chronic diseases, 460
cognitive approaches, 477–481
cognitive-behavioral coaching, 478, 479*t*–480*t*

mindfulness-based stress reduction, 478–481
self-directed neuroplasty, 477–478
definition, 463
development, 462–463
developments, health care, 460–462
as discipline, 463–464
efficacy, 464–465
health/wellness and integrative medicine, 462
interprofessional role, 49, 51*t*
motivational interviewing, 467*t*, 474–477
for personality disorders, 315*t*, 319
vs. psychotherapy, 465–468, 466*t*–467*t*
roles, 464
six stages, 481–492, 481*f*
ending engagement, 491–492
establishing agreement, 481–482, 482*b*
introductory session, 482–484
ongoing conversations, 484–491
action planning, 486–490
checking in with patient, 484
helping patient become aware of need to change, 485–486
helping patient identify agenda, 485
wrap-up, 490
pre-engagement discovery, 481
process checks, 491
recontracting for new health goals, 491
solution-focused health coaching, 477
strength of recommendation (SOR) taxonomy, 491*b*
team-based integrated primary care, 49, 51*t*
theories and methodology, 468–472
humanism, 468–469
human needs fulfillment and lifestyle change, 468, 470*t*–471*t*
positive psychology, 469
self-determination theory and self-efficacy, 469–472, 471*t*
as thinking partner, 463, 464, 472
transtheoretical model of change (Stages of Change Model), 473–474
for women's mental health, reproductive lifespan, 382
Health Resource and Services Administration (HRSA), 6*t*
Healthy Aging Brain Care Monitor (HABC Monitor), 114
Healthy Aging Brain Center (HABC), 108–110, 109*b*
Hierarchy of needs, 470*t*
High-cost patients, 81
Historical Clinical Risk-20 (HCR-20), 334
Hormonal fluctuations, women, 368
Hospice care, 449–452. *See also* Palliative care
Humanism, 468–469
Human needs fulfillment, 468, 470*t*–471*t*
Human scale development, 470*t*–471*t*
Hydroxyzine, for insomnia, 422, 423*t*
Hypothyroidism, menstrual changes and, 377

Illness anxiety (IA), 276–299
care pathways, 288–299
comprehensive multi-disciplinary evaluation, 288, 290*t*–291*t*, 294*b*
evaluation, assessment instruments, 288, 290*t*–291*t*
evaluation, critical care pathways, 288, 292*t*–293*t*, 294*b*
overview, 288, 289*f*
psychoeducation, 297–298
treatment, 297–299
challenges, 276–277
clinical presentation, 277–278
comorbidity and differential diagnosis, 278
diagnostic labels, 277
DSM-5 criteria, 277
etiology, 278
fundamentals, 276
identification, 280–288
biopsychosocial awareness, 280–281, 282*f*, 282*t*
biopsychosocial awareness, Columbia Stages of Biopsychosocial Awareness (CS-BPSA) model, 283*t*, 284–286
biopsychosocial awareness, levels, 281, 282*f*
biopsychosocial awareness, stages, 281–284, 282*f*, 283*t*
culture change, 284–285
emotions and stress, somatic, 280
mind–body dualism, abandonment, 280
organization of care, 286
patient–clinician relationship, 285
systems approach, 286–288
team approach, 284
translational research, patient education, 285–286
somatic symptoms *vs.*, 279–280
strength of recommendation (SOR) taxonomy, 298*b*
Imipramine. *See also* Tricyclic antidepressants (TCAs)
for depression, 183*t*
IMPACT Study (Improving Mood Promoting Access to Collaborative Treatment), 9, 12, 37, 57, 79, 81, 86*b*, 108. *See also* Aging Brain Care (ABC)
Importance ruler, 476
Indiana University Center for Aging Research (IUCAR), 108. *See also* Aging Brain Care (ABC)
Inhibited/delayed ejaculation, 389*t*, 404, 401–402, 401*t*
Inner game, 462–463
Inpatient discharge plan, 34–35, 35*t*
Insomnia, 420–422, 423*t*
Institute for Healthcare Improvement (IHI), 461
Triple Aim, 6–8, 461
Integrated Behavioral Pain Medicine (IBPM), 432–437
goals, 432
Integrated Behavioral Pain Medicine (IBPM) treatment, 433*f*, 437
primary care case manager, 433*f*, 434–435, 434*t*–435*t*
primary care provider, 433*f*, 434
psychiatric screening and referral, 433*f*, 435–437, 436*t*
triage, 432–434, 433*f*
Integrated care
definition, 3–4, 5*f*
lexicon, 5*f*
telehealth, 129–130, 130*f*
web resources, 6*t*
Integrated care models, 79–80. *See also specific types*
Integrated primary care, 5*f*
Integration
of care into existing care systems, 8
definitions, 3–4
Integrative medicine, 462
Interdisciplinary care, 124

Internal conflict, 498
International Coaching Federation (ICF), 463
  on coaching *vs.* psychotherapy, 465–468
Interpersonal crisis, 498
Intimate partner violence (IPV), 327–345. *See also* Violence
  clinical approach, 328–334
  clinical presentation, 327
  definition, 327
  epidemiology, 328, 329*b*
  etiology, 328
  interventions, physician/behavioral health specialist, 344–345
  management and treatment, 334–343, 335*f*, 337*t*–340*t*
  patient risk registry, 334
  phases, 344
  safety checklist, 335*b*
  screening, 344
  self-help, support, and web information, 345
  team, 334
Intrinsic motivation, 469

Jung, Carl, 466*t*

Kabat-Zinn, Jon, 478–481
Knowles, Malcolm, 466*t*, 472
Kübler-Ross, Elisabeth, 448–449
K-Y, for vaginal dryness/dyspareunia, 399*t*

Lamotrigine
  for bipolar disorder
    depression, 191*t*, 194–195
    maintenance, 191*t*
  in pregnancy, 376*t*
Learned optimism, 469
Learning, adult, 466*t*, 472
Levomilnacipran. *See also* Serotonin-Norepinephrine Reuptake Inhibitors (SNRIs)
  for depression, 181, 182*t*
Lidocaine, for premature ejaculation, 401*t*, 404
Liebowitz Social Anxiety Scale (LSAS), 160
Lifestyle
  changes, 468, 470*t*–471*t*
  wellness factors, 410
Liraglutide, for weight loss, 418, 419*t*
Lisdexamfetamine, for binge eating disorder, 260
Lithium
  for antisocial personality disorder, 318*t*
  for bipolar disorder
    depression, 190*t*, 191*t*, 194–195
    maintenance, 191*t*
    mania, 187, 190*t*
  for borderline personality disorder, 317*t*
  in pregnancy, 374, 375*t*, 381
  for suicidal ideation, 341
Lorazepam
  for anxiety disorders, 156, 157*t*
  for insomnia, 422, 423*t*
  in pregnancy, 375*t*, 381
Lorcaserin, for weight loss, 418, 42019*t*
Loxapine, for borderline personality disorder, 317*t*
Lurasidone
  for depression, in bipolar disorder, 191*t*, 194
  dosing, 211*t*
  in pregnancy, 376*t*
  side effects, 207, 212*t*–213*t*

Maintenance stage, 474
Managed Addiction Treatment Services (MATS), 84
Managed behavioral health organizations (MBHOs), 78
Managed care, 461
Mania, in bipolar disorder. *See* Bipolar disorder
Maslow, Abraham, 470*t*
Max-Neef, 470*t*–471*t*
McMaster Family Assessment Device (FAD), 518
Medicaid Delivery System Reform Incentive Payment (DSRIP) program, 85
Medical assistant
  anxiety disorder care, 160, 161*t*–162*t*
  bipolar disorder care, 188*t*
  depression care, 177
  interprofessional role, 49, 51*t*
Medical cost offset, 81
Medical neighborhood, 70–71, 70*b*
Meditation. *See* Mindfulness-based interventions
Melatonin, for insomnia, 421, 423*t*
Menopause, 369
Menstrual cycle, 368
Mental health care, 5*f*
Mental health care practitioner. *See also specific types*
  de facto, 78–79
  interprofessional role, 49, 52*t*
  primary care *vs.* traditional mental health, 47–49
Mental Health Parity Act of 1996, 78, 92, 461
Mental Health Parity and Addiction Equity Act (MHPAEA) model, 76, 78
Mental Health Parity and Addiction Equity Act of 2008, 76, 92, 461
Methadone, for opioid use disorders, 242–243, 318*t*
Methamphetamine, urine toxicology, 241*t*
Miansarin, for borderline personality disorder, 317*t*
Micro Symptoms and Experiences Timeline (MSET), 294, 295*b*–296*b*
Miller, William, 467*t*, 474–475
Milna, for somatic symptoms, 296
Mind–body dualism, abandonment, 280
Mindfulness-based interventions
  for anxiety disorders, 158
  for chronic pain, 438
  for illness anxiety, 297
  for somatic symptoms, 297
Mindfulness-based stress reduction (MBSR), 478–481
Miracle question, 477
Mirtazapine
  for depression, 181, 183*t*, 341
  for insomnia, 422, 423*t*
Mixed anxiety depressive disorder, 156, 157*t*
Models, integrated care, 79–80. *See also specific types*
Monoamine oxidase inhibitors (MAOI), for borderline personality disorder, 317*t*
Montefiore Medical Center, 84–85
Mood Disorder Questionnaire (MDQ), 176

Mood disorders, 169–196. *See also* Bipolar disorder; Depression
- assessment, primary care, 176
- comorbid medical disorder outcomes, 169–170
- costs, 174
- diagnosis, 170, 171*t*–172*t*
- differential diagnosis, 170, 172*t*–173*t*
- disease course, 174
- epidemiology, 169, 170, 174
- medical illness interactions, 174–175
- with psychotic features, 206*t*
- screening tools, 175–176
- treatment
  - collaborative care, depression, 176–178
  - primary care, 178–186
    - bipolar disorder, 186–195
    - major depression, 178–186
  - setting, 169

Mother-child dyadic therapy, 378–379
Motivation, 469
Motivational enhancement therapy, 233
Motivational interviewing
- for crisis intervention, 506
- in health coaching, 467*t*, 474–477

Multiple Mini Interview (MMI), ABC Med Home, 111, 119*b*
Mutual support groups, for alcohol use disorders, 233

Naltrexone
- for alcohol use disorders, 233–234, 318*t*
- for opioid overdoses, 244
- for opioid use disorders, 243–244
- for weight loss, with bupropion, 418, 419*t*

Narcissistic personality disorder (NPD). *See also* Personality disorders
- biological basis and psychosocial formulation, 307
- description, 305*b*
- prevalence and co-occurring disorders, 304
- schema, 308–312, 309*t*–310*t*
- treatment, 318*t*, 321–322

Narcotics Anonymous (NA), 242
National Comprehensive Cancer Network (NCCN), 516
National Consortium for Credentialing Health and Wellness Coaches (NCCHWC), 463
National Institute on Alcohol Abuse and Alcoholism (NIAAA) screen, 228
National Wellness Institute, 462
Neighborhood, medical, 70–71, 70*b*
Neurocognitive disorder with behavioral disturbance, 206*t*
Nicotine replacement, 236
Non-epileptic seizures (NES), 351–364
- classification, 353
- clinical presentation, 352
- comorbidities, psychiatric, 352–353
- definition and prevalence, 351
- diagnosis, 354
- differential diagnosis, 353
- epidemiology and course, 353–354
- etiology, 354
- health care costs and patient harm, 352
- history and terminology, 351
- integrated treatment, 357–364
  - care location, 360
  - care pathways, 360, 361*f*
  - consultants, 359
  - financial viability, 363–364
  - group therapy, 360–362
  - multidisciplinary project team, 359
  - observations, 363
  - outcome measures, 363
  - quality and safety experience, 359–360
  - recommendations overview, 357, 358*b*
  - referrals, 362
  - stakeholders, convening, 357–358
  - strength of recommendation (SOR) taxonomy, 364*b*
  - sustainability, long-term, 364
  - target population, 358–359
- subgroups, 353
- treatment, 354–357
  - diagnosis delivery, 354–355
  - for neurology, ongoing, 355
  - psychiatric evaluation, 355
  - psychotherapeutic, 355–357
  - self-help and support, 357, 357*b*

Norepinephrine-dopamine reuptake inhibitors. *See also specific agents*
- for depression, 183*t*, 184

Norepinephrine-serotonin modulators. *See also specific agents*
- for depression, 181, 183*t*, 184

Nortriptyline. *See also* Tricyclic antidepressants (TCAs)
- for depression, 183*t*
- in pregnancy, 375*t*

Nurse
- anxiety disorder care, 160, 161*t*–162*t*
- bipolar disorder care, 188*t*
- Cherokee Health Systems roles, 22
- depression care, 177
- interprofessional roles, 49, 50*t*, 51*t*

Nutrition, 414–417, 415*t*
- for chronic pain, 439

Nutritional status assessment, 414–415

OARS (Open-ended questions; Affirmations; Reflective listening; Summarize), 467*t*, 475
Obesity
- prevalence, 417
- weight management for, 417–420, 419*t*

Obsessive compulsive disorder (OCD), 151*f*, 152*t*, 154–155. *See also* Anxiety disorders
- postpartum, 370–371

Obsessive-compulsive personality disorder (OCPD). *See also* Personality disorders
- biological basis and psychosocial formulation, 307–308
- description, 305*b*
- prevalence and co-occurring disorders, 304
- schema, 308–312, 309*t*, 311*t*
- treatment, 318*t*, 322–324

Olanzapine
- for bipolar disorder
  - depression, 190*t*, 194–195
  - depression, with fluoxetine, 191*t*, 194
  - maintenance, 191*t*
  - mania, 187, 190*t*

Olanzapine (*Cont.*)
for borderline personality disorder, 317*t*
dosing, 211*t*
for insomnia, 422, 423*t*
in pregnancy, 376*t*
for schizophrenia, 207
side effects, 207, 212*t*–213*t*
Omega-3 fatty acids
for borderline personality disorder, 317*t*
in nutrition, 415, 415*t*
Opioid therapy, CDC guidelines, 239*b*, 240, 248
Opioid use and opioid use disorders, 237–244
approaches, iatrogenic opioids, 238–242
aberrant opioid medication behavior, 240
detoxification, 242
prescription drug monitoring programs, 238
urine toxicology, 238–240, 241*t*
approaches, non-iatrogenic opioids, 242–244
fundamentals, 242
medication-assisted, 242–244
mutual support groups, 242
epidemiology, 237
interventions, 238
overdose education and naltrexone distribution, 244
in pregnancy, 244, 248
screening and assessment, 238
Organizational support, 11
Orgasm, 388, 389*t*–390*t*
Orlistat, for weight loss, 418, 419*t*
Ospemifene, for dyspareunia with vaginal atrophy, 388, 398*t*
Outcomes measurement, 12–13
Overall Anxiety Severity and Impairment Scale (OASIS), 156

Pain, chronic, 430–440
biopsychosocial dimensions, 430–431
definition, 430
diathesis-stress model, 432
epidemiology, 430
psychiatric comorbidity, 431*t*, 431–432
strength of recommendation (SOR) taxonomy, 439*b*
treatment, 437–440
acupuncture, 438
Art Rx, 438–439
behavioral, weight, and sleep management, 439–440
cognitive-behavioral therapy, 437–438
complementary health, 430–431
drug abuse and dependence, 430–431
mindfulness-based therapies, 438
nutrition/dietitian intervention, 439
pharmacologic consultation, 437
psychophysiologic and biofeedback, 438
safety and effectiveness, 430–431
trauma-focused therapies, 438
treatment model, Integrated Behavioral Pain Medicine (IBPM), 432–437
goals, 432
Integrated Behavioral Pain Medicine (IBPM) treatment, 433*f*, 437
primary care case manager, 433*f*, 434–435, 434*t*–435*t*
primary care provider, 433*f*, 434
psychiatric screening and referral, 433*f*, 435–437, 436*t*
triage, 432–434, 433*f*
Pain, sexual (dyspareunia), 388, 389*t*–390*t*, 390, 405
Paliperidone
dosing, 211*t*
side effects, 207, 212*t*–213*t*
Palliative care, 449–451
Panic disorder, 150–151, 151*f*, 152*t*. *See also* Anxiety disorders
Panic Disorder Severity Scale (PDSS), 160
Paroxetine. *See also* Selective Serotonin Reuptake Inhibitors (SSRIs)
for anxiety disorders, 156, 157*t*
for depression, 181, 182*t*
for illness anxiety, 297
in pregnancy, 375*t*
Paternalistic communication, 460–461
Patient Aligned Care Teams (PACT), 91, 99–101, 463
Patient care technician, 49, 51*t*
Patient-centered care, 5*f*, 11
Patient-centered medical home (PCMH), 5*f*, 65–73, 461
accreditation, 68–69
building blocks, 66, 66*f*
definition, concept, and principles, 65–66
education, 73
framework and success factors, 66–67, 67*f*
functions and attributes, 66
future, 73
medical neighborhood, 70–71, 70*b*
payment, 71–73
physical space, 69–70
practice transformation, 67–68, 68*b*
research, 71, 72*b*
strength of recommendation (SOR) taxonomy, 72*b*
team-based care, 69
Patient-centeredness, 7
Patient-Centered Primary Care Collaborative (PCPCC), 66–67, 67*f*. *See also* Patient-centered medical home (PCMH)
Patient engagement, 6
Patient experience of care, 6–7
Patient Health Questionnaire-2 (PHQ-2)
depression screen, 135
Veterans Administration, 95
violence screening, 328
Patient Health Questionnaire-9 (PHQ-9)
ABC Med Home, 112, 114, 115
depression screen, 135, 136
for mood disorders, 175
team-based integrated primary care, 49, 52, 57, 59, 62
violence screening, 328, 334
Patient services representatives, 22
Pay-for-performance (P4P), 82
Payment reform, 66
Pediatric autoimmune neuropsychiatric disorders (PANDAS), 154
Perimenopausal depression, 370
Perimenopause, 369
Peripartum anxiety, 370
Peripartum depressive symptoms and depression, 369–370
PERMA (Positive emotions, Engagement, Relationships, Meaning, Achievement), 469

Perphenazine
  for borderline personality disorder, 317*t*
  dosing, 211*t*
  for schizophrenia, 207
  side effects, 207, 212*t*–213*t*
Personality disorders, 303–324. *See also specific disorders*
  antisocial personality disorders
    biological basis and psychosocial formulation, 304–305
    description, 304*b*–305*b*
    prevalence and co-occurring disorders, 304
    schema, 308–312, 309*t*–310*t*
    treatment, 318*t*, 320–321
  borderline personality disorder
    biological basis and psychosocial formulation, 304
    description, 304*b*
    prevalence and co-occurring disorders, 304
    schema, 308–312, 309*t*–310*t*
    treatment, 317*t*, 319–320
  chronic medical illnesses with, 304
  chronic pain with, 431*t*, 432
  clinical presentation, 303–304
  integrated care team, 313–319, 314*t*–315*t*
    behavioral health specialist, 314*t*, 315–316
    care coordinator, 315*t*, 316
    front desk staff and medical assistants, 313, 314*t*
    health coach, 315*t*, 319
    meetings, 313
    nurse, 313, 314*t*
    primary care provider, 313–315, 314*t*
    psychiatrist, 315*t*, 316, 317*t*–318*t*
  interventions and general principles, 312, 313*b*
  narcissistic personality disorder
    biological basis and psychosocial formulation, 307
    description, 305*b*
    prevalence and co-occurring disorders, 304
    schema, 308–312, 309*t*–310*t*
    treatment, 318*t*, 321–322
  non-epileptic seizures with, 353
  obsessive-compulsive personality disorder
    biological basis and psychosocial formulation, 307–308
    description, 305*b*
    prevalence and co-occurring disorders, 304
    schema, 308–312, 309*t*, 311*t*
    treatment, 318*t*, 322–324
  risks, 304
  schema, 308–312, 309*t*–311*t*
  strength of recommendation (SOR) taxonomy, 323*b*
  substance use illnesses with, 304
  treatment
    long-term, 316, 317*t*–318*t*
    short-term, 315–316
Personal physician, 65
Peyronie disease, 389*t*
Pharmacists, clinical, 22–23
Phendimetrazine, for weight loss, 418, 419*t*
Phentermine and topiramate, for weight loss, 418, 419*t*
Phenytoin, for antisocial personality disorder, 318*t*
Phosphodiesterase inhibitors (PDE-5 & PDE-11)
  for erectile dysfunction, 393, 401, 402*t*
  for sexual desire and arousal (women), 400*t*, 403
Physical space
  Cherokee Health Systems, 29, 29*f*
  patient-centered medical home, 69–70
Physician assistant, 49, 51*t*
Physician-directed communication, 460–461
Physician-directed medical practice, 65
Pit stops, 482
Population-based approach, 12
Population health, 7, 47
Population health management
  Aging Brain Center Medical Home, 111
  eMR-ABC software, 115–116
  Preferred Population Health Management, 117
  team-based integrated primary care, 47
Positional dialog, 460
Positive functioning, 6
Positive psychology, 467*t*, 469
Postpartum anxiety, 370–371
Postpartum bipolar disorder, 371–372, 371*t*
Postpartum depression, 370, 380
Postpartum period, 368–369
Postpartum psychosis, 372
Postpartum thyroiditis, 377
Posttraumatic stress disorder (PTSD), 155. *See also* Anxiety disorders
  differential diagnosis, 151*f*, 206*t*
  integrated care for, 92–104 (*See also* Primary Care-Mental Health Integration (PC-MHI); Veterans Health Administration)
  medical conditions, associated, 152*t*
Practice-based collaborative care (PBCC), 128
Practice Support Program (PSP)
  Adult Mental Health Module, 35–36
  learning modules, 36
Practice transformation, 67–68, 68*b*
Prazosin, for anxiety disorders, 157
Pre-contemplation stage, 473
Preferred Population Health Management (PPHM), 117
Pregabalin
  for anxiety disorders, 156–157, 157*t*
  for somatic symptoms, 296
Pregnancy, 368. *See also* Women's mental health, reproductive lifespan
  drugs in
    anticonvulsants, 374, 376*t*, 381
    antidepressants, 374, 375*t*
    antipsychotics, 374, 376*t*, 381
    benzodiazepines, 374, 375*t*, 381–382
    for bipolar disorder, 374–377, 375*t*–376*t*
    lithium, 374, 375*t*, 381
    lorazepam, 381
    SNRIs, 374
    SSRIs, 374, 381
    trazodone, 381
    zolpidem, 382
  emotionality in, 378
  loss of, emotionality, 378
  substance use disorders in, 244, 248
Premature ejaculation, 389*t*
  clinical presentation, 404
  interactions between causes, 390

Premature ejaculation (*Cont.*)
management, 401*t*, 404
psychosocial, 396
psychosocial plus medical, 403
types, 404
Premenstrual dysphoric disorder, 369
Preparation stage, 473
Prescription drug monitoring program (PDMP), 238–239
PREVENT (Providing Resources Early to Vulnerable Adults Needing Treatment for Memory Loss), 108
Primary care, 5*f*, 36–37. *See also specific models and topics*
Primary care behavioral health, 5*f*
Primary care clinicians (PCCs)
Cherokee Health Systems, 22
interprofessional role, 49, 50*t*
primary care *vs.* traditional mental health environment, 47–49
Primary Care-Mental Health Integration (PC-MHI), 97, 99–104. *See also* Veterans Health Administration
achieving, 99, 100*b*
education, 104
evaluation, 101
future research, 104
key elements and activities, 102*b*
mission and vision, 99, 99*b*
organizing, within care systems, 101–104, 102*b*
origins and history, 97–99
strength of recommendation (SOR) taxonomy, 101–104, 103*b*
target conditions, 99–101
Primary care physician (PCP). *See also specific models and disorders*
anxiety disorder care, 160, 161*t*–162*t*, 164–165
bipolar disorder care, 188*t*–189*t*
building mental health care capacity and capability, 35
depression care, 177, 180
interprofessional role, 49, 50*t*
Problem-solving treatment
for suicidal ideation, 342
for violence, 342
Prochaska, James, 467*t*, 473–474
Professionalism, transdisciplinary, 47, 48*b*
Project for the Extension for Community Healthcare Outcomes (Project ECHO), 126
Prolonged exposure therapy, for anxiety disorders, 159
Pseudo-seizure. *See* Non-epileptic seizures (NES)
Psychiatric consultation
Cherokee Health Systems, 22, 24, 25*b*
communication in shared care models, 60
levels of integration, 57–60
collaboration and connection, 59
electronic record, 58–59
formal direct, 58
formal indirect, 57–58
informal, 57
patient-specific education, 59
in primary care, behavior health clinicians development, 29
team-member efficiency, 60
Psychiatric nurse, 50*t*
Psychiatrist
anxiety disorder care, 160–163, 161*t*–162*t*
bipolar disorder care, 188*t*–189*t*
Cherokee Health Systems, 22
depression care, 178
interprofessional role, 50*t*, 53
Psychiatry, 466*t*
Psychoanalysis, 466*t*
Psychodynamic/interpersonal psychotherapy, for somatic symptoms, 297
Psychodynamic psychotherapy, 466*t*
Psychoeducation, for anxiety disorders, 158
Psychogenic seizure. *See* Non-epileptic seizures (NES)
Psychological event, 498
Psychologist, 49, 50*t*
Psychophysiologic interventions, for chronic pain, 438
Psychosis. *See* Psychotic disorders
Psychosocial Assessment Tool (PAT), 516, 518*b*
Psychosocial-cultural context, 461
Psychosocial factors, 4
Psychotherapy. *See also specific types*
for non-epileptic seizures, 355–356
for suicidal ideation, 342
for violence, 342
Psychotic disorders, 199–216
assessment, 202
biopsychosocial-cultural evaluation, 205
clinical presentation, 200
Denver Health Medical Center, 218–220
differential diagnosis
medical, 203–205, 204*b*
psychiatric, 205, 206*t*
emergencies, 203
in geriatric patients, 217–218
postpartum psychosis, 372
primary care treatment, 200–201
psychosis
assessment, 202
positive screens, 202–203
screening, 201
specialty psychiatric care
Assertive Community Treatment (ACT), 217
cognitive-behavioral therapy, 217
social skills training, 216
vocational rehabilitation and supportive employment, 216–217
strength of recommendation (SOR) taxonomy, 221*b*
women with psychoses, 217
Psychotic disorders, integrated care, 207–216
family and community involvement, 216
health and wellness, 215–216
psychopharmacology, psychosis, 207–215
antipsychotics, initial choice, 207, 211, 211*t*
antipsychotics, monitoring, 207, 214*t*
antipsychotics, side effects, 207, 212*t*–213*t*
changing, 214–215
critical pathway, 208*t*–210*t*
discontinuing, 215
initiating, 207
maintenance, 214, 214*t*
stabilization, 211, 214
referral, 216

substance use treatment, 215
symptom management, 215
PVCSMART (Positive statements, Values, Control, Specific, Measurable, Attainable, Realistic, Time sensitive), 476–477, 483

Quetiapine
for bipolar disorder
depression, 187, 190*t*, 191*t*, 194
mania, 187, 190*t*
dosing, 211*t*
for insomnia, 422, 423*t*
in pregnancy, 376*t*
for schizophrenia, 207
side effects, 207, 212*t*–213*t*
for suicidal ideation, 341
for violence, 341
Quick PsychoDiagnostics Panel (QPD Panel), 134–143, 138
assessment
challenges, 135–136
comprehensive, 137
tools, medical providers on, 136
assessment report, 138–141, 139*f*
diagnostic notes, 138–140
outcome assessment, 140
patient review, 140–141
symptom list, 140
symptom scores, 138
base version, 137*b*, 138
disorders screened, 137, 137*b*
institutional benefits, 142
outcomes, 142, 142*f*
overview, 137–138
as panel, 138
patient satisfaction, 141–142
physician acceptance, 141, 141*t*
prevalence, mental health conditions, 134
provider wish list, 136–137
software, 138
summary and relevant facts, 142–143, 143*b*

Ramelteon, for insomnia, 422, 423*t*
Reasonable care, 343
Receptionist, 49, 52*t*
Recovery International, 532
Refocus, 478
Reframe, 478, 479*t*
Relationship problem, 388
Relaxation response training (RRT), 158
Reproductive life cycle, 368–369
Respecting Choices Program, 444–445
Reverse integrated care, 80
Righting reflex, 461, 475
Risperidone
for borderline personality disorder, 317*t*
dosing, 211*t*
for mania, in bipolar disorder, 187, 190*t*
in pregnancy, 376*t*
for schizophrenia, 207
side effects, 207, 212*t*–213*t*
Robbins, J.M., 471*t*
Rochester integrated care, 60–63
Rogers, Carl, 466*t*
Rollnick, Stephen, 467*t*, 474–475
Ryan, R.M., 469, 471*t*

SAFE questions (Safe/Stressed, Afraid/Abused, Friends/ Family, Emergency Plan), 328–330
Salas, Eduardo, 46
Schizoaffective disorder, 206*t*. *See also* Psychotic disorders
Schizophrenia spectrum disorders, 199–221
assessment and differential diagnosis
medical, 203–205, 204*b*
psychiatric, 205, 206*t*
psychosis, 202
biopsychosocial-cultural evaluation, 205
clinical presentation, 200
Denver Health Medical Center, 218–220
emergencies, medical and psychiatric, 203
geriatric patients with psychoses, 217–218
positive screens, psychosis, 202–203
primary care treatment, 200–201
screening, 201
specialty psychiatric care
Assertive Community Treatment, 217
cognitive-behavioral therapy, 217
social skills training, 216
vocational rehabilitation and supportive employment, 216–217
strength of recommendation (SOR) taxonomy, 221*b*
suicide risk, 327–328
women with psychoses, 217
Schizophrenia spectrum disorders, integrated care, 207–216
family and community involvement, 216
health and wellness, 215–216
psychopharmacology, psychosis, 207–215
antipsychotics, initial choice, 207, 211, 211*t*
antipsychotics, monitoring, 207, 214*t*
antipsychotics, side effects, 207, 212*t*–213*t*
changing, 214–215
critical pathway, 208*t*–210*t*
discontinuing, 215
initiating, 207
maintenance, 214, 214*t*
stabilization, 211, 214
referral, 216
Schizophreniform disorder, 206*t*. *See also* Psychotic disorders
Schizotypal personality disorder, 206*t*
Schwartz, Jeffrey, 477–478
SCOFF eating disorder questionnaire, 266
Screening. *See also specific disorders*
care coordination, 126–127
family-centered, 518
Screening, brief intervention, and referral to treatment (SBIRT)
for alcohol use disorders, 226, 231–232
for drug use disorders, 227, 247
Sedative-hypnotic medications, 244. *See also specific types*
use and abuse disorders, 244–245
Sedative use and sedative use disorders, 244–245
Seizures
non-epileptic, 351–364
pseudo-seizure (*See* Non-epileptic seizures (NES))

Selective Estrogen Reuptake Modulators (SERMs), for dyspareunia with vaginal atrophy, 388, 399*t*
Selective Serotonin Reuptake Inhibitors (SSRIs). *See also specific agents*
for anxiety disorders, 156, 157*t*, 159
for binge eating disorder, 259–260
for borderline personality disorder, 317*t*
for bulimia nervosa, 271
for depression, 181, 182*t*
for illness anxiety, 297
in pregnancy, 374, 381
for premature ejaculation, 401*t*, 403
on sexual function (men), 397, 403, 404*t*
for suicidal ideation, 341
for violence, 341
Self-determination theory (SDT), 469–472, 471*t*
adult learning, 472
autonomy, 469, 471*t*
competence, 469–472, 471*t*
relatedness, 471*t*, 472
Self-directed learning, 472
Self-directed neuroplasticity, 477–478
Self-efficacy, 469–472
Seligman, Martin, 467*t*, 469
Sensate focus exercises, 397, 403, 403–404, 405
Serotonin-Norepinephrine Reuptake Inhibitors (SNRIs). *See also specific agents*
for anxiety disorders, 156, 157*t*
for depression, 181, 182*t*
for illness anxiety, 297
in pregnancy, 374
for premature ejaculation, 401*t*
on sexual function (men), 401*t*
for somatic symptoms, 296
Sertraline. *See also* Selective Serotonin Reuptake Inhibitors (SSRIs)
for anxiety disorders, 156, 157*t*
for binge eating disorder, 260
for borderline personality disorder, 317*t*
for bulimia nervosa, 271
for depression, 181, 182*t*
for illness anxiety, 297
in pregnancy, 375*t*
for premature ejaculation, 401*t*
Severe and enduring anorexia nervosa (SEAN), 262. *See also* Anorexia nervosa (AN)
Sex and sexual functioning, 386
Sexual problems, 386–407
arousal, 388, 389*t*–390*t*
assessment, diagnosis, and treatment planning, 388–394
assessment and diagnosis, 391–394
detection and screening, 391, 391*b*
interactions between causes, 390
overview, 388, 389*t*–390*t*
assessment to treatment gap, bridging, 394–396
from acquired sexual neutrality to desire, 395
from biology and culture to relationships, 394
sexual problem–inducing phenomena, 395–396
treatment success, 394
desire, 388, 389*t*–390*t*
major sexual problems, 388, 389*t*
orgasm, 388, 389*t*–390*t*
pain, 388, 389*t*–390*t*, 390
patient discussion, 387
patients on, 388
primary care physician role, 386–387
relationship problems and, 388
strength of recommendation (SOR) taxonomy, 406*b*
treatment, 396–406
arousal (men), 403–404, 401*t*–402*t*
arousal (men, women, and couples), 397, 403
arousal (women), 403
desire (men), 397
desire, arousal, organism and pain (women), 397, 399*t*–400*t*
hormone, 405
orgasm (men), 404, 401*t*–402*t*
orgasm (women), 399*t*, 404–405
psychosocial, 396
sexual pain (women), 388, 389*t*–390*t*, 390, 405
Shared care, 5*f*, 60
Shared savings model, 83–84
Short-term therapy, 466*t*
Sildenafil, for erectile dysfunction, 400*t*, 402*t*
Single-Item Alcohol Screener, 228, 229*b*
Single-Item Drug Use Screener, 228, 229*b*
Sleep and sleep disorders, 420–422, 423*t*
with chronic pain, 439–440
SMART Goals (Specific, Measurable, Attainable, Realistic, Time sensitive), 476
Social network map, crisis intervention, 507–508, 508*f*
Social phobia, 151*f*, 152*t*, 153–154
Social skills training, for schizophrenia and psychotic disorders, 216
Social worker, 49, 52*t*
Solution-focused health coaching (SFHC), 467*t*, 477
Somatic symptom disorder (SSD), 276–299
care pathways, 288–299
comprehensive multi-disciplinary evaluation, 288, 290*t*–291*t*, 294*b*
evaluation, assessment instruments, 288, 290*t*–291*t*
evaluation, critical care pathways, 288, 292*t*–293*t*, 294*b*
overview, 288, 289*f*
psychoeducation, 297–298
treatment, organization, 297–299
treatment, somatic symptoms, 296–297
challenges, 276–277
chronic pain with, 431*t*, 431–432
clinical presentation, 277–278
comorbidity and differential diagnosis, 278
diagnostic labels, 277
DSM-5 criteria, 277
etiology, 278
fundamentals, 276
identification, 280–288
biopsychosocial awareness, 280–281, 282*f*, 282*t*
biopsychosocial awareness, Columbia Stages of Biopsychosocial Awareness (CS-BPSA) model use, 283*t*, 284–286
biopsychosocial awareness, levels, 281, 282*f*
biopsychosocial awareness, stages, 281–284, 282*f*, 283*t*
culture change, 284–285

emotions and stress, somatic, 280
mind–body dualism, abandonment, 280
organization of care, 286
patient–clinician relationship, 285
systems approach, 286–288
team approach, multidisciplinary, 284
translational research, patient education, 285–286
illness anxiety *vs.*, 279–280
non-epileptic seizures with, 353
strength of recommendation (SOR) taxonomy, 298*b*
Space, physical
Cherokee Health Systems, 29, 29*f*
patient-centered medical home, 69–70
Specialty medical providers, 22. *See also specific types*
Stages of coping, 448–449
Stepped care, 12
Stigma, counteracting, 9–11
Stimulants. *See also specific types*
prescription cautions, 248
urine toxicology, 241*t*
Stop, Start, Squeeze (SSS), for premature ejaculation, 404
Stress
assessment and management, 422–424
diathesis-stress model, 432
life events
ranking, 498, 498*b*
stressful, 497–498, 498*b* (*See also* Crisis intervention)
stressor personalized meaning, 499
Substance Abuse and Mental Health Services Administration (SAMHSA), 6*t*
integrated care levels, 10*t*, 124–126, 125*t*
Substance-induced psychosis, 206*t*
Substance use disorders, 5*f*, 223–250. *See also specific types*
addiction as brain disease, 224–225
alcohol, 228–235
cannabis, 245–247
chronic pain and, 431*t*, 430–431
diagnosis, 225–226
integrated care overview, 226
opioids, 237–244
other drugs, 247
prevalence and morbidity, 223
primary care provider
diagnosis, 224
prescription cautions, 239*b*, 240, 248–249
skills and training, 224
recovery support, 247–249
relapse and relapse monitoring, 247–248
sedatives, 244–245
sequelae, 223
societal problems, 223
stigma, 224
strength of recommendation (SOR) taxonomy, 249*b*
suicidal ideation, 328, 333
system barriers, 224
team
functioning, 227–228
members and roles, 226–227
tobacco, 235–237
undertreatment, 223–224
violence and, 327, 333
in women, 248
Sudden infant death syndrome (SIDS), 454
Sugar, 414, 416*t*
Suicidal ideation, 326–346
borderline personality disorder, 328
challenge, 326
chronic pain and psychiatric comorbidity, 432
chronic patterns, 343
clinical approach, 328–334
assessment, clinical, 332
behavioral phases, 331*t*
clinical interview, 330–332
clinical reactions, 333
current, 332
neurologic and medical, 333, 334
past history, 333
recent behavior, 332–333
risk assessment tools, 334
screening, 328–330
substance abuse and, 333
support system, 333
treatment cooperation, 333
clinical presentation, 327
definition, 327
differential diagnosis, 327–328
epidemiology, 328, 330*b*
etiology, 328
integrated care team, 334
legal issues, 343–345
management and treatment, 334–343
critical pathway, 336, 337*t*–340*t*
decision algorithm, level of care, 334, 335*f*
motivation, 336
pharmacotherapy, 341–342
safety checklist, 335*b*
settings, 336, 341
patient risk registry, 334
prevention, 345
schizophrenia, 327–328
strength of recommendation (SOR) taxonomy, 346*b*
substance abuse, 328
Supportive employment, for schizophrenia and psychotic disorders, 216–217
Sustain talk, 475, 476
Suvorexant, for insomnia, 422, 4232*t*
Sweeteners, 415, 416*t*

Tadalafil, for erectile dysfunction, 403, 402*t*
Tarasoff-limiting statutes, 343
Team-based care, 11, 79. *See also specific types*
Canada, Hamilton Family Health Team Mental Health Program, 38–43, 40*t*–41*t* (*See also* Hamilton Family Health Team (HFHT) Mental Health Program)
Cherokee Health Systems, 21–24
patient-centered medical home, 69
Team-based integrated primary care, 46–64, 49, 51*t*
Affordable Care Act and, 47
clinical-administrative team support, 60
collaborative habit in, 46
future evolution, 63

Team-based integrated primary care (*Cont.*)
- interprofessional roles, 49–53
  - administrator, 49, 52*t*
  - advanced practice nurse, 49, 51*t*
  - care managers, 49, 52–53, 52*t*
  - clinicians, clinical support personnel, and clerical personnel, 49, 51*t*–52*t*, 53
  - health coach, 49, 51*t*
  - mental health clinicians, 49, 52*t*
  - nurse LPN/LVN, 49, 50*t*
  - nurse RN, 49, 51*t*
  - patient care technician/medical assistant, 49, 51*t*
  - physician assistant, 49, 51*t*
  - primary care clinicians, 49, 50*t*
  - psychiatrist and psychiatric nurse, 50*t*, 53
  - psychologist, 49, 50*t*
  - receptionist, 49, 52*t*
  - social worker, 49, 52*t*
- population health, 47
- primary care and behavioral health integration, 53–60 (*See also specific types*)
  - communication, shared care, 60
  - Doherty, McDaniel, and Baird's taxonomy, 53–57, 54*b*–57*b*
  - psychiatric consultation, levels of integration, 57–60
  - team-member efficiency, 60
- primary *vs.* traditional mental health care environment, 47–49
- Rochester integrated care, 60–63
- strength of recommendation (SOR) taxonomy, 63*b*
- team focus, 46
- transdisciplinary professionalism, 47, 48*b*

TEAMcare, 79

Telehealth, 121–132
- advantages, 124
- applied, virtual integrated specialist clinical workflow, 130, 130*f*
- care integration support, 124–130
  - co-located care: primary care, collaborative care, 128–129
  - co-located care: primary care, consultation, 127–128
  - coordinated care: basic collaboration from a distance, 127
  - coordinated care: screening and assessment, 126–127
  - integrated care, 124
  - integrated care: asynchronous telepsychiatry, 129–130
  - integrated care: clinical models, 130, 130*f*
  - integration continuum, 124–126, 125*t*
  - separate health care systems, 126
- Cherokee Health Systems, 29
- definitions and purpose, 122
- health care environment, current, 122
- history, 123
- implementation, web-based resources, 122, 123*t*
- participation, patient, 124
- reimbursement, state, 123–124
- strength of recommendation (SOR) taxonomy, 131*b*
- summary and conclusions, 130–131
- Veterans Administration leadership, 123

Temazepam, for insomnia, 422, 423*t*

Termination stage, 474

Testosterone
- for sexual desire (men), 401*t*, 405
- for sexual desire and arousal (women), 397, 400*t*, 406

Testosterone/estrogen cream, for dyspareunia, 399*t*, 406

Thinking partner, 463, 464, 472, 477

Thiothixene, for borderline personality disorder, 317*t*

Thyroid disorders, pregnancy and, 377

Thyroiditis, postpartum, 377

Tobacco use and tobacco use disorders, 235–237

Topiramate
- for alcohol use disorders, 234
- for binge eating disorder, 259, 260
- for weight loss, with phentermine, 418, 419*t*

Transactional dialog, 460

Transdisciplinary professionalism, 47, 48*b*

Transformation, practice, 67–68, 68*b*

Translating Initiatives in Depression into Effective Solutions (TIDES), 97

Transtheoretical model of change, 281, 467*t*, 473–474

Tranylcypromine, for borderline personality disorder, 317*t*

Trauma-focused therapies, for chronic pain, 438

Trauma Screening Questionnaire (TSQ), 156

Trazodone
- for depression, 184
- in pregnancy, 381

Triage assessment system (TAS), 505

Triazolam, for insomnia, 422, 423*t*

Tricyclic antidepressants (TCAs). *See also specific types*
- for depression, 182*t*–183*t*, 184
- in pregnancy, 374, 375*t*
- for somatic symptoms, 296

Trifluoperazine, for borderline personality disorder, 317*t*

Triple Aim (IHI), 6–8, 461

12-step facilitation, for alcohol use disorders, 233

Universal needs, 471*t*

University of Colorado School of Medicine, non-epileptic seizures integrated approach, 357–364. *See also under* Non-epileptic seizures (NES)

University of Rochester integrated care, 60–63
- co-located, integrated clinics, 61
- electronic records and team-based care, 61–63
- origins, 60–61

University of Washington Advancing Integrated Mental Health Solutions (UW AIMS Center), 6*t*, 128

Unnatural death, 454–455

Urine drug toxicology, 238–240, 241*t*

U.S. Department of Health Human Services Health Services Administration, 6*t*

Vacuum erection device, 402*t*

Vaginal atrophy, 399*t*–400*t*, 403

Vaginal dryness, 399*t*

Vaginismus, 405

Valproic acid (valproate), pregnancy and, 376*t*, 381

Vaping, 237

Vardenafil, for erectile dysfunction, 400, 402*t*

Varenicline, for tobacco use disorders, 236

Vasomotor symptoms, 399*t*–400*t*

Venlafaxine. *See also* Serotonin-Norepinephrine Reuptake Inhibitors (SNRIs)

for anxiety disorders, 156, 157*t*
for borderline personality disorder, 317*t*
for depression, 181, 182*t*, 341
in pregnancy, 375*t*
for somatic symptoms, 296
Veterans Health Administration, 90–105
barriers and resources, 95–97
electronic health records, 96
new care model adoption and testing capabilities, 95–96
research and education, 96–97
drivers, 91–95
crossover conditions and engagement behaviors, 94
health outcomes and costs, 93
mental health access preservation, 94
mental health comorbidities, 93
mental health policy, 92–93
performance measurement, 95, 95*t*
prevention, 94
primary care context, 91–92
early programs, 123
implementation, 97–98
mental health care, 91
Patient Aligned Care Teams, 91, 99
telehealth, 123 (*See also* Telehealth)
vision of future (Primary Care-Mental Health Integration), 98–104 (*See also* Primary Care-Mental Health Integration (PC-MHI))
Video-electroencephalography (VEEG), for non-epileptic seizures, 352
Vilazodone. *See also* Selective Serotonin Reuptake Inhibitors (SSRIs)
for depression, 181, 182*t*
Violation, unnatural death, 454–455
Violence, 326–346
challenge, 326
chronic patterns, 343
clinical approach, 328–334
assessment, clinical, 332
behavioral phases, 331*t*
clinical interview, 330–332
clinical reactions, 333
current ideation, 332
neurologic and medical exam, 334
neurologic and medical issues, 333
past history, 333
recent behavior, 332–333
risk assessment tools, 334
screening, 328–330
substance abuse and, 333
support system, 333
treatment cooperation, 333
clinical presentation, 327
definition, 327
differential diagnosis, 327
epidemiology, 328, 329*b*
etiology, 328
integrated care team, 334
legal issues, 343–345
management and treatment, 334–343
critical pathway, 336, 337*t*–340*t*
decision algorithm, level of care, 334, 335*f*
motivation, 336
pharmacotherapy, 341–342
safety checklist, 335*b*
treatment settings, 336, 341
patient risk registry, 334
prevention, 345
self-help, support, and web information, 345
strength of recommendation (SOR) taxonomy, 346*b*
unnatural death, 454–455
Violence and Suicide Risk Assessment Scale (VASA), 334
Vitamin D, 415, 415*t*
Vitamin E, for dyspareunia, 399*t*
Vocational rehabilitation, for schizophrenia and psychotic disorders, 216–217
Volition, unnatural death, 454–455
Vortioxetine, for depression, 183*t*, 184

Weight management, 417–420, 419*t*
behavioral, with chronic pain, 439–440
Well-being, 469
Wellness, 409–425, 462. *See also specific disorders*
5 A's, 411
critical care pathway, 411*t*–412*t*
exercise, 412–414
health coaching for, 462
lifestyle factors, 410
nutrition, 414–417, 415*t*
plan design, 410–412
sleep, 420–422, 423*t*
strength of recommendation (SOR) taxonomy, 425*b*
stress reduction, 422–424
weight, 417–420, 419*t*
"Wheel-and-spoke" treatment plan, crisis intervention, 508–509, 509*f*
Wheel of health self-assessment, 475
White River Junction co-located mental health care model, 97
Whole-health continuum, 7
Whole-person approach, 7, 65
Women's mental health, reproductive lifespan, 367–383
anxiety spectrum disorders
peripartum, 370
postpartum, 370–371
bipolar disorder, 371–372, 371*t*
depression
perimenopausal, 370
peripartum, 369–370
postpartum, 370, 380
premenstrual dysphoric disorder, 369
hormonal fluctuations, 368
integrated care team, functions and roles, 372
integrated care team, member roles, 372–382
behavioral health specialist, 377–379
case manager, 382
health coaches, 382
nurses and medical assistants, 372–373
obstetrician/gynecologist, 377
primary care providers
other medications, 377
psychotropic medications, 373–377, 375*t*–376*t*
thyroid disorders, 377

Women's mental health, reproductive lifespan (*Cont.*)
psychiatrists and pharmacotherapy, 380–382
resources, community and internet, 379, 379*t*
postpartum psychosis, 372
prevalence, 367
reproductive life cycle, 368–369
screening tools, 368
socially constructed differences, 368
strength of recommendation (SOR)
taxonomy, 383*b*

Yale-Brown Obsessive Compulsive Scale (Y-BOCS), 160

Zaleplon, for insomnia, 422, 423*t*
Ziprasidone
dosing, 211*t*
for mania, in bipolar disorder, 187, 190*t*
side effects, 207, 212*t*–213*t*
Zolpidem
for insomnia, 422, 423*t*
in pregnancy, 375*t*, 382